Acoustical Imaging
Volume 15

Acoustical Imaging

A Continuation Order Plan is available for this series. A continuation order will bring
delivery of each new volume immediately upon publication. Volumes are billed only upon
actual shipment. For further information please contact the publisher.

International Symposium on Acoustical Imaging

Imaging

Acoustical Imaging
Volume 15

Edited by

Hugh W. Jones
Technical University of Nova Scotia
Halifax, Nova Scotia, Canada

QC244.5
I5
v.15
1987

PLENUM PRESS · NEW YORK AND LONDON

The Library of Congress cataloged the first volume of this series as follows:

International Symposium on Acoustical Holography.

   Acoustical holography; proceedings. v. 1–
New York, Plenum Press, 1967–

   v. illus. (part col.), ports. 24 cm.

   Editors: 1967–   . A. F. Metherell and L. Larmore (1967 with H. M. A. el-Sum)
   Symposium for 1967–   held at the Douglas Advanced Research Laboratories, Hun-
tington Beach, Calif.

   1. Acoustic holography—Congresses—Collected works. I. Metherell. Alexander A., ed.
II. Larmore, Lewis, ed. III. el-Sum, Hussein Mohammed Amin, ed. IV. Douglas Advanced
Research Laboratories, v. Title.
QC244.5.I.5   69-12533

ISBN 0-306-42565-3

Proceedings of the 15th International Symposium on Acoustical Imaging,
held July 14–16, 1986, in Halifax, Nova Scotia, Canada

©1987 Plenum Press, New York
A Division of Plenum Publishing Corporation
233 Spring Street, New York, N.Y. 10013

All rights reserved

No part of this book may be reproduced, stored in a retrieval system, or transmitted
in any form or by any means, electronic, mechanical, photocopying, microfilming,
recording, or otherwise, without written permission from the Publisher

Printed in the United States of America

PREFACE

Volume 15 follows the format of earlier volumes in the series. The contents give the next installment in the varied aspects of acoustical imaging research. On this occasion, some emphasis was placed on the relationship of underwater acoustics to acoustical imaging and a volume of papers under the title "Underwater Acoustics Proceedings from the 12th ICA Symposium held in Halifax," will appear at roughly the same time as this volume. There is no duplication in these volumes but they are interlinked, at least to the extent that papers from common conference sessions appear in one or another volume.

An innovation is the review paper presented at the beginning of the volume "A History of Acoustical Imaging," by G Wade. This fairly detailed review comes at a point in time when so much has been achieved and in some cases passed by, that a record of some of the earlier work might help to keep a balance with the large collections of research papers which have appeared in the many volumes.

The assistance of the international advisory commitee, whose membership included, apart from myself, Dr. A Berkhout, Dr. J. Greenleaf, and Dr. G. Wade, is gratefully acknowledged. Their support in referencing papers and developing interest in some of the topics, chosen for the programme, was an important factor in the success of the Halifax meeting. The work of the members of the local organizing committee, whose names are listed below, was responsible for the smooth and efficient conference arrangements and the excellent entertainment of the delegates.

As earlier editors have noted, these volumes entail much preparation and detailed work. The assistance of Hwa Wan Kwan and Damion Loomes is particularly appreciated as is the assistance of Mrs. Carol Kwan and Mrs. Lisa Berry. Their enthusiastic support, given in difficult circumstances has been a major factor in completing the work relatively quickly.

H. W. Jones

ORGANIZING COMMITTEE

Dr. H. W. Jones (Chairman)   Mr. D. M. F. Chapman
Dr. H. M. Merklinger (Vice Chairman)   Dr. D. D. Ellis
Mr. H. W. Kwan (Secretary)   Dr. N. A. Cochrane
Dr. L. J. Leggat (Treasurer)   Ms. S. Robertson (Co-ordinator)

ACKNOWLEDGEMENTS

We thank the Nova Scotia Department of Development for funding, in part, the publication of this volume.

Our thanks are due to the Natural Science and Engineering Research Council of Canada, the protocol office of the Government of Nova Scotia and the following for their financial assistance:

> Arctec Canada Limited
> Orion Electronics Limited
> Hermes Electronics Limited
> Focal Marine Limited
> E. Y. E. Marine Consultants
> Nova Scotia Research Foundation Corporation
> Seastar Instruments Limited

CONTENTS

TRANSDUCERS AND ARRAYS

IMAGE AND SIGNAL PROCESSING

DIRECT IMAGING

POSTER SESSION

A HISTORY OF ACOUSTIC IMAGING

Glen Wade

Electrical & Computer Engineering Department
University of California, Santa Barbara
Santa Barbara, CA 93106

ABSTRACT

The technology for "seeing" with sound has an important and interesting history. Certain of nature's creatures have been good at acoustic
imaging for many millenia. Bats and dolphins are prodigies in using sound
waves for probing their universe. The human species, lacking sophisticated natural ability, has overcome this deficiency by developing appropriate technology. Rudimentary cross-sectional acoustic images have been
available since prior to World War I, stemming from the development of
pulse-echo techniques. More recently intensity-mapping and phase-amplitude systems have become the bases for acoustic imaging. This talk presents some historical highlights of the fascinating progress in this work.

"THE" VERSUS "A"

When Hugh Jones asked me to give this talk, his assigned title was
"The History of Acoustic Imaging." I probably would not have accepted the
assignment had I noticed the word "The." I am sure that I am not quali-
fied to tell you about "The History of Acoustic Imaging." I simply do not
know the history. I do, however, know some history.

Hugh's sense of kindness is unbounded. When he realized my problem,
Hugh readily agreed that I could change the subject to a history. Perhaps, a still better title for what I will say would be "A Partial History
of Selected Topics Concerning Acoustic Imaging."

Several years ago, I heard a talk on this same subject. The speaker
treated a number of aspects of acoustic imaging of which I was mostly
unaware. Although my knowledge of certain historical facts is fairly
good, my knowledge of the facts concerning that speaker's selected topics
was poor. Perhaps some of you will have a similar experience today, as
you listen to my talk. For many of you, I will probably leave out the
most important aspects of acoustical imaging history (that is, those with
which you are familiar) and cover less important (that is, less familiar)
topics. Perhaps you will wonder why Hugh chose me to give this talk. I
have been wondering that myself.

1

WHAT IS AN IMAGE?

All of this illustrates the extraordinary breadth and scope that the history of acoustical imaging has. The breadth is due, at least partially, to the fact that the concept "image" itself is broad. Simply put, an image is a reproduction of the appearance of an object or region. Images are generally of either two or three dimensions, but one-dimensional images are no rarity and are highly useful.

An example of a one-dimensional image is the A-scan of elementary pulse-echo sonar. A simple A-scan, by itself, is not usually thought of as being an image, at least in the non-technical sense of the word, but it does reproduce, or map, a one-dimensional region and, hence, qualifies as an image. A sonar transducer emits a pulse of energy which travels along a straight-line path and insonifies an object. Echoes are returned from reflecting elements in the object. These echoes, traveling back along the same path, are sensed by a receiver and recorded as blips, spaced horizontally on a cathode-ray tube screen. The position of any blip yields the range of the reflecting elements; the brightness yields the echo amplitude and therefore the reflecting effectiveness of the element. By putting together, side by side, a number of such A-scan traces, each corresponding to a different travel path for the irradiated and reflected energy, we obtain a B-scan pattern which maps in two dimensions the position and amplitude of the reflectors. This obviously is a two-dimensional image.

NEW VERSUS OLD

A-scan and B-scan patterns are relatively modern. But there are other acoustic imaging systems that are extremely old. Much of the purpose of acoustic imaging is to see in places where light cannot penetrate or does not exist. For this purpose, we can employ X rays, gamma rays, electron beams, microwaves, acoustic waves and other forms of propagating energy. Of these, acoustic waves are the most natural. For untold millenia, various members of the animal kingdom have used these waves in imaging otherwise unobservable objects and inhomogeneities. These are the systems that I refer to as having great antiquity. Figure 1 shows a picture of an animal, the fennec, with impressive-looking data-acquisition apparatus.

BATS AND ROBOTS

Echo-locating bats (see Figure 2) are among the most remarkable of nature's prodigies in acoustic imaging. They are good at both data acquisition and processing. Because of their keen ability to generate, hear and interpret sound, they can catch their prey on the wing in complete darkness. They utter twittering noises, too high-pitched for human ears to detect. They process the echoes of this sound from nearby objects to avoid hitting obstructions or each other and to intercept insects in midflight. Sound gives the bat a mental image of its surroundings. By using a specialized larynx, unusually sensitive ears and a highly-developed audio cortex, bats can quickly and safely find their way through the furniture in a dark room and even through ropes, cords and threads strung across it.

Bats are so good at acquiring and processing the acoustic data that they can detect the flutter of an insect's wing even when the total amplitude of the flutter is as small as about 100 microns[S79].

A more modern object that can make use of acoustic imaging is a robot. To build a robot that can steer itself through a room full of chairs, tables, lamps and other obstacles, is an extremely difficult task.

2

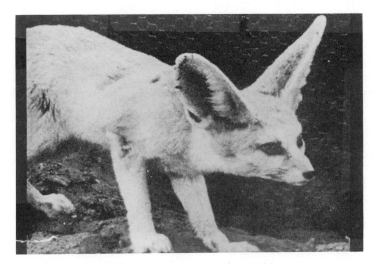

Fig. 1 The Fennec

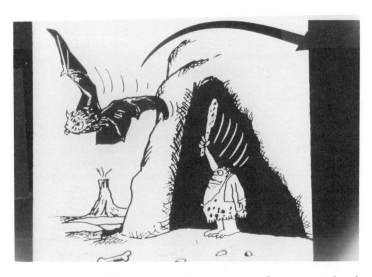

Fig. 2. A highly effective ancient system for acoustic imaging.

The world's fastest such robot takes a little more than an hour to cross a 35-foot laboratory. With its acoustic apparatus, a bat can do it in a second or two. What bats accomplish in the dark area of a cave is matched by what porpoises, dolphins and whales can accomplish in the murky waters of the ocean. Table 1 shows Carl F. Schueler's comparison of a figure of merit for the bat with that of modern equipment for medical diagnosis.

HUMANS

The above animals perform with ease what is well outside the natural abilities of humans; we cannot shout into a dark room and by listening to echoes tell very much about the nature of the objects in it. About the most we can do is to determine whether or not we are in a room and, if so, something about its size. However, with light we are well equipped to explore. We can light a candle and, by means of its flickering flame, quickly determine the room size and shape and the location and character of its furnishings. Man is equipped by nature to more rapidly process optical data than acoustical data.

The 525 x 525 picture elements of a television frame with 256 recog-nizeable variations in color and intensity changing at a rate of 30 times per second can be at least partially perceived by the human visual system. The corresponding data rate is

$$(525 \times 525) \times (\log_2 256) \times 30 = 66 \times 10^6 \text{ bits/sec.} \tag{1}$$

In watching a television program, we do not detect everything that is going on. We see the details in only the portion of the screen which is focused onto the fovia. If the data rate is compressed by a factor of 5, a typical viewer will scarcely notice a difference in picture quality. This suggests a realistic data rate of human visual perception of less than 15 megabits/sec. Although the human eye contains more than a hundred million sensors, there are fewer than a million nerve fibers carrying signals from these sensors to the visual cortex of the brain.

A normal human ear can hear sound up to a frequency of about 15 kHz. This corresponds to a maximum of 30,000 samples/sec. Approximately 325 differences in volume are detectable by the ear. The data rate is there-fore approximately

$$2 \times (\log_2 325) \times 30,000 = 0.5 \times 10^6 \text{ bits/sec} \tag{2}$$

If we assume roughly the same compression factor for the ear as we have already assumed for the eye, we get about 0.1 megabits/sec. Thus human eyes appear to be more than a couple of orders of magnitude faster in processing data than human ears. We rely upon our eyes almost exclusively for producing mental images of the outside world.

Almost, but not quite. Sometimes sound does provide data for human image processing, assuming a broad definition of the term. Who has not seen on a cloudy night, a sky suddenly becoming bright because of an otherwise unobserved flash of lightening? The corresponding clap of thunder comes along a few seconds later. The number of seconds divided by 3 gives the distance in kilometers to where the flash occured. Our ears tell us the direction and our imagination may fill in with enough details to provide a rudimentary mental "image" of the event. A sort of mental A-scan, if you will.

This can be called "passive imaging." An equivalent active technique for a dark or foggy night would be to clap hands or shout sharply and count the seconds before an echo returns from a nearby cliff. The number

4

Table 1.   Figures of Merit for Ancient Bats and Modern B-Scanners.

TYPICAL B-SCANNER SPECIFICATIONS		BAT EPTESICUS SONAR SPECIFICATIONS	
PARAMETER	CAPABILITY	PARAMETER	CAPABILITY
RANGE (R)	$<$ 1 METER	RANGE (R)	$>$1 METER
MASS (M)	10 KILOGRAMS	MASS (M)	10^{-2} KILOGRAM
POWER (P)	100 WATTS	POWER (P)	10^{-5} WATT
MINIMUM TARGET (T)	10^{-4} METER	MINIMUM TARGET (T)	10^{-2} METER
FIGURE OF MERIT	10	FIGURE OF MERIT $\dfrac{R}{MPT} = 10^{9}$	

of seconds divided by 6 (because of the round-trip), gives the number of kilometers to the cliff and our ears tell the direction. Such an approach to data acquisition and processing is a simple version of the elaborate natural technology possessed by bats and porpoises. A practical implementation of the approach has been useful to sailors since the days of the Phoenicians. Under conditions of fog or darkness, when the shore or rocks are suspected to be nearby, it has long been the practice for men in boats

to make sharp sounds of short duration and listen for echoes. Experienced fishermen are said to be able to detect a buoy in this way at several hundred meters.

SONAR FOR LARGE-SCALE IMAGING

These and similar kinds of experiences may have suggested to early pioneers in sonar the possibility of developing a pulse-echo technology for underwater viewing in the ocean. The importance of being able to "see" beneath the water's surface was illustrated by the sinking of the Titanic on April 15, 1912 and later by the German U-boat menace to French shipping in World War I.

Sailing at high speed about 1600 miles northeast of New York City, the Titanic, the world's largest ship, on its maiden voyage struck an unseen iceberg and sank with 1517 passengers and crew losing their lives.

Both Lord Rayleigh and O. P. Richardson had previously thought of using ultrasonic waves for oceanic search, but this tragic shipwreck stimulated much new thought on how to prevent future occurences of this kind. In a 1912 interview published in Scientific America, Sir Hiram S. Maxim, an American-born engineer and inventor, again proposed sound as a way of preventing this type of catastrophy. Inspired by what he supposed to be techniques employed by bats, Sir Maxim stated that ships could be protected from collisions with icebergs and other ships by generating sound pulses under water and detecting their echoes. Shortly afterwards, two inventors filed patents on devices to produce sound waves in either air or water and to detect echoes from distant objects. In 1912 L. F. Richardson submitted a British patent application to do this and Canada's Reginald A. Fessenden filed a similar U.S. application early in 1913. A year later, an iceberg was successfully detected at two kilometers in a field test of Fessenden's underwater apparatus.

An additional impetus for the development of more sophisticated underwater detection equipment arose during World War I because of the awsome destructive power of German submarines. Paul Langevin, a major French physicist, was asked by his government to provide an effective way for detecting submerged vessels. An engineer, M. C. Chilowski, had developed an ultrasonic device for the French Navy, but its acoustic intensity was too weak to be practical. Heading a joint U.S., British and French venture, Langevin looked into the question of how to increase the acoustic power in the water. In less than three years, he succeeded in obtaining high ultrasonic intensity by means of piezoelectric transducers operating at resonance[L16]. By 1918, active systems for producing and analyzing returned acoustic echoes were functioning and proving to be useful in neutralizing the U-boat threat.

We frequently think of sonar as being simply an acoustic form of radar. However, as we have seen its development actually preceeded that of radar, and was employed by the French Navy in an extremely important defensive application in World War I. Nevertheless, the many useful applications of radar, in both military and civil sectors, caused its development to proceed very rapidly, so that today the sonar field often benefits from progress in the more recently developed technologies of radar. Because of such contributions from radar, sonar systems have become highly sophisticated in recent years.

The term "radar" was derived from the phrase "radio detection and ranging." Following extensive use of the word radar, the term "sonar" was coined as a companion to radar being derived from the phrase "sound navigation and ranging."

Actually, the study of passive sonar goes back at least to Leonardo da Vinci, whose writings state that sound can propagate over huge distances in the water[U83]. Leonardo could hear the movement of ships by using a listening tube passing from his ear through the air and down into the water. He noticed that this type of passive sonar would be more effective if the ship carrying the listener was stationary (quiet) rather than in motion (and therefore generating noise).

The listening tube was later improved upon by Colladen and Sturm[L77]. These two experimenters employed a tube with a trumpet-like opening at its lower end as an underwater sound receiver. Their transmitter was a submerged bell whose ringing could be detected miles away by an observer using the tube.

One version of their system had the essential elements of active sonar. In describing an experiment on Lake Geneva in 1827, Colladen and Sturn used sketches showing how their system could detect a hypothetical submerged object. By means of such equipment in two boats ten miles apart, using a light source and stop-watch to perform the time of propagation measurement, they were able to measure the speed of sound to an accuracy of about two-tenths of one percent. Colladen was surprised that such a small amount of energy at the source could be transmitted such a great distance through the water and still be detected by the trumpet receiver.

So far, I have succeeded in mentioning a few odds and ends concerning the historical perspectives associated with acoustic imaging. I would like now to go back and add to this information, systematize various ideas and examine some aspects of acoustic imaging in detail.

SMALL-SCALE IMAGING

The sonar systems were applied to large-scale imaging of huge structures within vast regions of the ocean. Much innovative work was required of other researchers before other acoustic systems could be applied to the small-scale imaging of tiny structures within the more limited region of objects of interest in factories, hospitals and laboratories. One of the most gifted of these latter researchers was the Russian scientist S. J. Sokolov, whose productive work extended over three decades beginning in the 1920's. Sokolov was one of the first to recognize and systematically explore the usefulness of ultrasound for imaging the internal structure of optically opaque objects. Some of his schemes were designed to detect inhomogeneities, such as flaws and voids, within manufactured parts.

In one of his systems, the inhomogeneities were made "visible" by reflecting collimated light from a liquid surface in a fashion similar to that of liquid-surface holography. The system provided a way to encode image information so that the image could be read in real time by light diffracted from the sound. As we will see in detail shortly, the method was an authentic precursor of acoustic holography and predated Dennis Gabor's invention of hologrophy by more than ten years!

In Langevin's system, the transmitter emitted a pulse and the amplitude of the reflected pulse was used in producing an image. In Sokolov's, the transmitter emitted continuous waves and both the amplitude and the phase of the transmitted waves were used in producing the image. Over the years, since the days of Langevin and Sokolov, other systems, based on other principles, have been investigated with varying degrees of success. At present, a wide variety of systems exists including some that are conceptually similar to standard X-ray machines. In these systems, the sound, cw or pulsed, is transmitted through the object and the amplitude of the sound on the other side is measured as a function of lateral position. The resulting amplitude map is the image.

THREE FUNDAMENTAL APPROACHES

As indicated in Table 2, pulse-echo, phase-amplitude, and amplitude-mapping approaches constitute the conceptual bases for three fundamental types of acoustic imaging systems. These approaches can therefore be used as a method for categorizing systems. By now, however, systems exist that combine these approaches in such ways as to make an unambiguous categorization difficult or impossible.

The pulse-echo systems include not only sonar for oceanic search, but also linear arrays of dynamite and geophones for reflection seismology, and B-scan equipment for clinical diagnosis. The phase - amplitude systems include holographic instruments for flaw detection and weld inspection. The amplitude-mapping systems include acoustic microscopes for materials inspection and biomedical analysis.

PROTO-HOLOGRAPHY

Sokolov's liquid-surface system for detecting flaws in metal test pieces is illustrated in Figure 3. The scheme was first proposed in 1929. Later, Sokolov patented the system and published a paper concerning its operation[S35a]. This system is remarkably like the modern liquid-surface

Table 2.   Conceptual Bases for Three Fundamental Types of
Acoustic Imaging Systems.

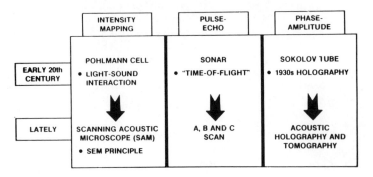

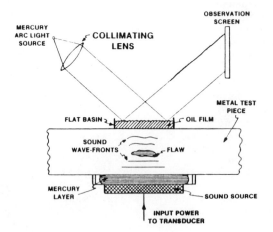

Fig. 3.   Sokolov's liquid-surface system for detecting flaws in
metal test pieces.

holographic systems. However, two major differences exist. Modern systems have a second sound source which produces a reference beam. They also use lasers to read out the image information. Lasers, of course, were not available to Sokolov, and his light source was not as coherent as it should have been for high-quality imagery. However, the absence of a second sound source does not change the character of the operation of the system in any fundamental way. Even without the second sound source, the formation of static ripples could be expected to take place on the oil surface of the system in such a way as to form a hologram. Flaws of sufficiently small dimensions would obviously permit the passage of a substantial portion of undisturbed sound through the metal piece. This sound can be regarded as constituting a reference beam. The object beam is then that part of the incoming sound scattered from the flaws. Thus, we have the acoustic equivalent of the "Gabor-type" hologram of optical holography.

Conceivably, therefore, Sokolov can be regarded as having produced the first hologram, however crude, and doing so a number of years before Gabor's invention of holography. It is therefore possible to argue that, from a chronological standpoint, rudimentary acoustic holography preceded optical holography. Of course, Sokolov had no way of understanding holographic principles as we understand them currently. His images were not of high quality. Not only did he operate without the use of a laser, but also he provided no spatial filtering to eliminate unwanted beam components in the reconstruction process.

PROTO-ACOUSTO-OPTIC DIFFRACTION IMAGING

In another of Sokolov's early attempts to detect flaws with ultrasound, he used a bulk system strikingly similar in overall appearance to that of the present Bragg-diffraction systems[S35b]. A diagram of Sokolov's system is shown in Figure 4. Again, Sokolov was interested in detecting inhomogeneities, such as cracks and casting errors, in manufactured metallic parts, rather than in forming images per se. He apparently intended the direction of propagation for the light through the sound cell to be perpendicular to that of the acoustic propagation. Thus it appears that he used the arrangements of Debye and Sears and of Lucas and Biquard to display the diffraction spectra of the light as produced by interaction with the sound. Strictly speaking therefore, Debye-Sears diffraction rather than Bragg diffraction was probably involved. The intensity and the number of orders of the diffraction spectra displayed would, of course depend upon the strength and the wavefront configuration of the sound in the metal.

PROTO-ACOUSTIC MICROSCOPY

Although I have emphasized Sokolov's ideas on the use of phase information for imaging, he also contributed to the development of systems which measured intensity only. He originally proposed using sound at 3 GHz where the wavelength of the sound in water is very short (half a micrometer) and capable of resolving truly minute objects. The name he gave to the corresponding device was the "ultrasonic microscope[S49]." Technological impracticalities prevented Sokolov from operating at sufficiently high frequencies (such as 3 GHz) for the purposes of microscopy. However, the principle he put forth (that of reading out localized electronic charge developed on a piezoelectric crystal in response to an acoustic input) has since become embodied in a well-known device called the Sokolov tube, which has had substantial use for low-frequency acoustic imaging[J74].

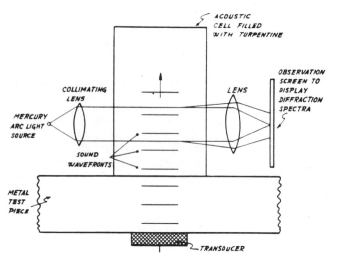

Fig. 4. Sokolov's bulk diffraction system for detecting flaws in metal.

INTENSITY MAPPING

Intensity-mapping systems represent perhaps the simplest conceptual approach to forming an image with acoustic energy. This approach takes advantage of the transparency of many objects to sound by mapping the intensity of the acoustic waves transmitted through the objects. Though elementary in concept and similar to the principle upon which the standard x-ray picture is made, intensity mapping was not the first method used to make acoustical images. Langevin's pulse-echo approach and Sokolov's phase-amplitude schemes were proposed and used several years before the first practical intensity-mapping technique was developed. However, imaging by mapping transmitted acoustic intensity forms the basis of the successful modern acoustic microscope developed by C. F. Quate and colleagues at Stanford University within the last 15 years. We shall refer to this instrument later but let us first look at another approach of this type which was developed more than 30 years earlier by Reimar Pohlman.

It was based on a special technique that Pohlman invented for making acoustic intensity visible with light. This device, called the Pohlman cell, was the first practical high-resolution acoustical imaging tool that employed intensity-mapping[P37]. The Pohlman cell acts as an acoustico-optic energy converter. I avoid the use of the word transducer because of the peculiar way in which the device operates. As shown in Figure 5, the cell consists of a sandwich-like structure containing a suspension of fine metallic flakes in a suitable liquid. One of the sides of the sandwich is a glass plate and the other is a thin membrane which is acoustically transparent. Because of thermal motion, the metallic flakes would normally be oriented randomly in the medium. If the suspension is illuminated by light projected through the glass plate, the light reflected from the metallic particles, as seen by an observer, will have a diffusely-scat-

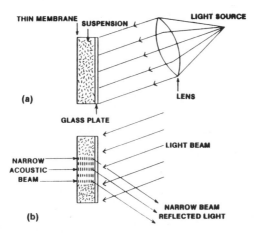

Fig. 5. Diagrams illustrating how the Pohlman cell works.
(a) cell with no insonification.
(b) cell with localized insonification.

tered, matte appearance. However, when sound, passing the stretched thin
membrane, is incident on the suspension, the metallic flakes will tend to
orient themselves locally with their broad surfaces parallel to each
other. Each flake will present the maximum area to the sound field.
Thus, in regions of high acoustic intensity, the planar surface of each
particle tends to become perpendicular to the direction of the acoustic
propagation. If the suspension is then irradiated by light, the reflected
light delineates the pattern of acoustic intensity impinging upon the cell
through the membrane on the other side. The regions of high acoustic
intensity, with their aligned metal flakes, will present a more reflective
surface to the incident light than other regions with their randomly-ori-
ented flakes. Under these conditions, an observer will see areas of varying brightness, corresponding to spatially-varying acoustic intensity,
superimposed on the gray matte-appearing background.

     The Pohlman cell has relatively high intrinsic resolution because of
the small size of the metallic particles used in the suspension. The
thickness of the membrane through which the sound passes can be very small
compared with a wavelength. A chief disadvantage of this imaging technique is that the response time for the particles to orient themselves
when insonification is present, or to become randomly oriented in the
absence of the insonification, is too long for real-time operation.
Nevertheless, the idea is intriguing and has attracted much attention over
the years since it was first proposed. The Pohlman cell continues to be
studied in various research laboratories for a variety of specialized
applications.

MICROSCOPY AGAIN

Perhaps the most spectacular of the acoustic images are those from ultrasonic microscopes. Owing to the long wavelength of ordinary sound, it may be difficult for the layman to imagine that sonic waves could possibly be useful to obtain highly resolved images of microscopic objects. It is easy for him to imagine this with ordinary light whose wavelengths are well known to be very short or with electrons whose size is regarded as negligibly small. Sound might at first glance appear to the layman to be entirely too cumbersome. This would be true if we were referring to sound in air where the frequency spectrum is severely limited. However, in water the acoustic spectrum is much larger. Because sound velocity is extremely slow compared to light, sound wavelengths are extremely short compared to those of electromagnetic waves for the same frequency. For example, at 1.5 MHz the electromagnetic vacuum wavelength is 200 m. The sound wavelength is 1 mm. At 3 GHz, a realizable acoustic frequency, the wavelength in water is down to that of visible light! Figure 6 illustrates the quality of images obtained several years ago for a frequency of 600 MHz where the sound wavelength is equivalent to that of short-wave infrared. The pictures were furnished by Professor C.F. Quate at Stanford and show various images of unstained human red blood cells.

Quate's system is of the lens type and reads image information with a piezoelectric transducer. A diagram of the system is shown in Figure 7. This system is generally referred to as the SAM (Scanning Acoustic Microscope)[L71]. It is the acoustical equivalent of the scanning electron-beam microscope (SEM).

MECHANICAL-SCANNING FOCUSED INSTRUMENTS

Also spectacular are the images produced by the mechanically-scanning, focused instruments of P. S. Green of Stanford Research Institute[G72], E. E. Aldridge of Harwell[A65], England, and others. These acoustic cameras generally have operated at lower frequencies, producing images of remarkably high quality, sometimes in near real-time (such as, 3 images per second). One of Aldridge's images is shown in Figure 8, and two images produced by Green, in Figures 9 and 10.

PULSE-ECHO APPROACHES

Modern ultrasonic systems for medical diagnosis are built upon Langevin's pulse-echo technique. Many of these instruments operate in real-time, producing so-called B-scan grey-scale images in the plane of the insonification by scanning a focused acoustic beam rapidly over azimuth and slowly over range to obtain a television display. Although the concept dates back to World War I, the technology necessary to steer and focus an acoustic beam and to reproduce a televised image was not readily available until about 25 years ago. In fact, the more sophisticated of these instruments has been in commercial use for only about 15 years. The first laboratory version of a digitally controlled B-scan system was reported by W. J. Fry and colleagues in 1968[F68]. By now, after many years of the success of ultra-sound use in clinical medicine, many persons have seen acoustically-produced images of the organs of their bodies and are accustomed to the concept. An example of such imaging is shown in Figure 11. It is not uncommon to determine the sex and other features of a fetus prior to the birth of the baby. Figure 12 depicts a typical situation.

Another very important application of the pulse-echo technique is for industrial non-destructive evaluation (NDE). The simplicity of the pulse-echo concept lends itself well to field instrumentation for detecting

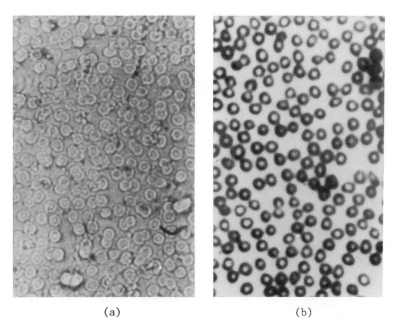

(a)   (b)

Fig. 6. Red blood cells by optical microscopy and scanning acoustic
microscopy at 600 MHz. (a) optical (b) acoustical.
(Images courtesy of C.F. Quate.)

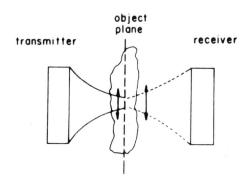

Fig. 7. Scanning focused beam system of SAM.

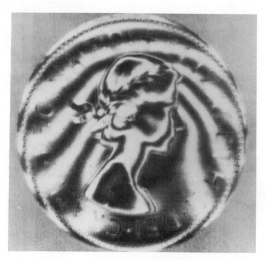

Fig. 8. Image of a British penny produced by the Aldridge system. The image is actually an image-plane Gabor hologram. The acoustic image of the penny was formed directly on the hologram plane and a fixed-phase electronic reference signal was mixed with the sound signal detected at the hologram plane.

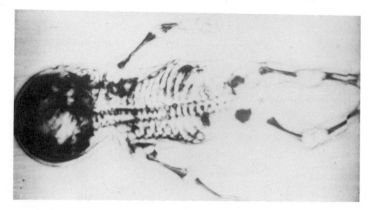

Fig. 9. Green's transmission image of an aborted human fetus. Green's system was very much like that of Aldridge's except that no reference signal was present in the system.

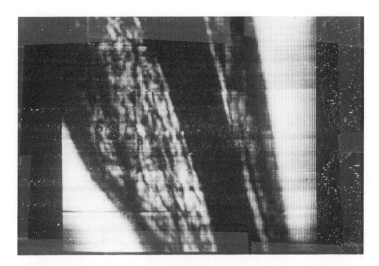

Fig. 10.   Intensity image of a human calf from a later, more
           sophisticated, focused system of P. S. Green.

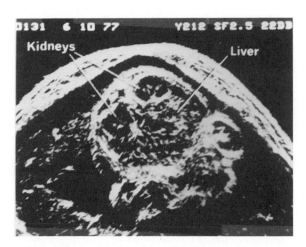

Fig. 11.   Cross-sectional, longitudinal-scan image from a Picker
           instrument showing the kidneys and liver of a human
           patient at the Seoul National University Hospital.

flaws in manufactured parts. Although for pedagogical reasons, we classify modern pulse-echo NDE equipment as descending from Langevin's original work, it was F. A. Firestone's Reflectoscope built at the University of Michigan that spurred the development of today's industrial pulse-echo systems. The Reflectoscope operated by generating a succession of ultrasonic pulses of short duration and detecting their echoes from sub-surface discontinuities within a solid. The Reflectoscope made it possible to examine an object from one surface only to determine, within limits, the size of any internal inhomogeneities and to measure the depth of the inhomogeneities below the surface.

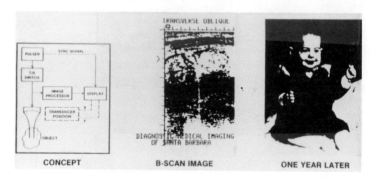

CONCEPT	B-SCAN IMAGE	ONE YEAR LATER

Fig. 12. The concept, the B-scan image and a photograph of the child one year later. (Courtesy of C. F. Schueler.)

Ever since Firestone's day, the pulse-echo approach has had substantial success in non-destructive evaluation. As with sonar and radar, the systems based on this approach provide a map of the region under investigation, producing cross-sectional images of the internal structure of the object similar to those of the B-scan medical instrument.

COMPUTER-AIDED TOMOGRAPHY

The latest stage in the application of pulse-echo techniques for acoustical imaging has followed the advent of X-ray computer-aided tomography. The measurement of acoustic echo intensity from one direction only produces a B-scan image that is somewhat similar to a tomogram in that it is a slice image in the plane of insonification. Thus, it was natural that computer-aided X-ray tomography developed in the early 1970's would stimulate research on computer-aided acoustic tomography[W80a].

Nevertheless, the result of this research so far had been disappointing. The key reason that acoustic tomographic systems have not replaced X-ray scanners in the hospital, in spite of advantages in terms of low patient radiation, is the lack of sufficient resolution of detail for the purposes to which these tomographic systems are applied. However, the research is continuing. Figures 13 and 14 show some early images obtained by means of computer-aided acoustic tomography.

Such workers as Greenleaf, Carson, Jakowatz and Kak were the first to produce tomograms mapping such parameters as attenuation and acoustic refractive index[G75],[G78],[C76a],[C76b],[J76]. Mappings of variations of either parameter require transmitting ultrasound through the object. But ultrasound can also be reflected from objects. Inhomogeneities within an object provide echoes, and research is going on to produce computer-reconstructed tomographic mapping of variations in ultrasonic reflectivity. In addition, tomographic extensions of Doppler processing are being pursued. Figures 15, 16, and 17 illustrate some of the first experiments performed in producing acoustic reflection tomograms[W80b].

Thus, starting with the simple seaman's concept of pulse-echo ranging, man has wrought evermore sophisticated acoustical imaging tools. Langevin's early work 75 years ago and Firestone's work three decades later have been combined with creative applications of television and digital electronics. These innovations have spawned a still-developing technology for "seeing" into optically opaque objects, including a mother's womb or a concrete structure, to produce slice images of complex structure.

But as we shall see, Sokolov's ideas on the use of acoustic phase information had their own interesting evolutionary consequences. Because of the phase-amplitude concepts, acoustic imaging appears to offer future performance which may be unrivaled by any other imaging modality for certain applications.

ACOUSTIC HOLOGRAPHY

Although Sokolov can be credited with being the first to produce holograms, he was probably unaware that he had done so, and the first worker to purposely set out to produce an acoustical hologram and publish on that effort was Pal Greguss in 1965[G65]. Greguss' method was fundamentally different from many of the approaches that have developed into useful concepts. However, his unique idea illustrates the kind of open-minded creative energy that contributes to progress in research.

To record the hologram, Greguss chose a "sonographic plate", whose exposure depended upon a "sonochemical" reaction rather than a photochemical one. If such a plate is developed in the presence of the sound fields, the pattern of the standing-wave components in the sound will be converted into a black-and-white image suitable for use in making a hologram. The drawback that limited this method to a laboratory curiosity is that the sound used for the recording process must be very intense.

The type of holographic system which, from publication dates in the research literature, has been investigated over the longest sustained period of time, is the kind that uses scanning receiving transducers moving through a raster pattern in a holographic plane. The procedure involved was first described in an elementary form by Thurstone in 1966 and is illustrated in Figure 18[T66]. Normally water is used as the medium for acoustic propagation in the embodiment shown. The sound source is placed on one side of the object and the scanning hydrophone on the other. The effective diameter of the hydrophone should be less than or at most equal to the fringe spacing to be recorded.

A second holographic approach was also the subject of much sustained research over a number of years. The principles of operation were enunci-

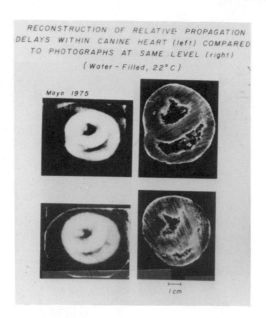

Fig. 13. Tomographic reconstructions of acoustic refractive index within
a canine heart (left) compared to photographs of cross-sections
through the corresponding levels (right). (Courtesy of J. F.
Greenleaf.)

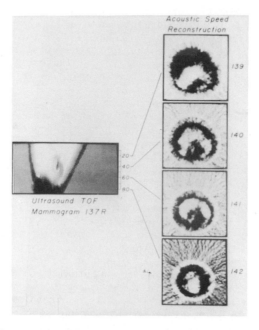

Fig. 14. An ultrasonic mammogram and four tomographic reconstructions of acoustic refraction index in a breast.
(Courtesy of J. F. Greenleaf.)

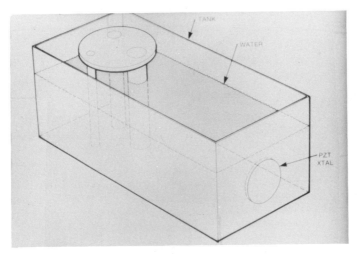

Fig. 15. Experimental arrangement to demonstrate reconstructive reflection tomography using pulses.

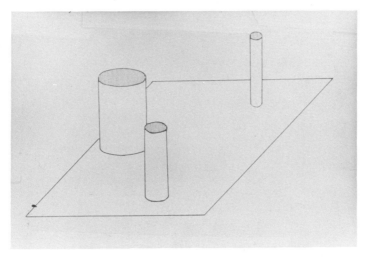

Fig. 16. Ideal perspective reconstruction of the reflection tomogram. The vertical coordinate represents the reflectivity distribution.

19

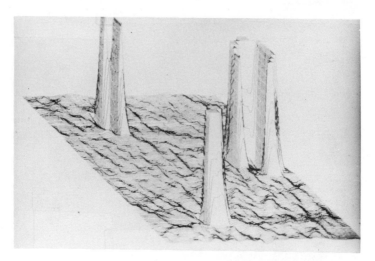

Fig. 17. Computer-calculated perspective reconstruction of an
experimental reflection tomogram after simple image
processing.

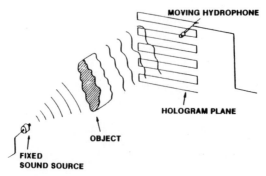

Fig. 18. Acoustical holography with a fixed transmitter and a
scanning receiver. An electronic reference is
provided to measure the phase of the received signal
with respect to the transmitted signal.

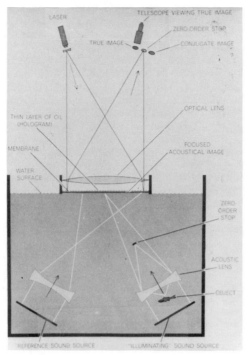

Fig. 19. Liquid-surface acoustical holography. Static ripples on the liquid-air interface constitute a record of the interference of the object and the reference beams and permit the rippled liquid surface to operate as a hologram in real time.

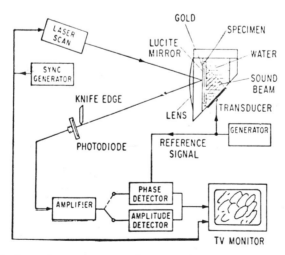

Fig. 20. Solid-surface system. Image information contained in the dynamic ripples on the surface of the lucite mirror is read out by a scanning laser beam.

21

ated by Mueller and Sheridon in their classic paper of 1966[M66]. The system uses a liquid-air surface as the recording medium and is similar to Sokolov's system of Figure 3. The modern arrangement is shown in Figure 19.

A third acoustic imaging system that employs laser-beam readout and operates in real-time, utilizes a solid surface from which to detect the sound field. The technique is sometimes referred to as "solid-surface" holography. The system is illustrated in Figure 20. Such a system has been profitably packaged by Sonoscan and is presently commercially available for acoustic microscopy[K72]. It is known as the scanning laser acoustic microscope (SLAM). The microscope was developed by Dr. Lawrence W. Kessler and colleagues while Dr. Kessler was still with the Zenith Radio Corporation. Figure 21 shows how the SLAM system can be adjusted to give simultaneously both an acoustic and an optical image of the same object. Figure 22 shows some of the images produced in this fashion.

TOMOGRAPHIC MICROSCOPY

As remarkable as the images from acoustic microscopes have been, there are still problems that make their use in non-destructive evaluation less than ideal. When an acoustic microscope operates in the transmission mode, the micrograph is simply a shadowgraph of all the structure encountered by the paths of the acoustic rays passing through the object. The resultant image is a two-dimensional mapping of three-dimensional internal structure and is particularly difficult to comprehend in the case of specimens of substantial thickness and structural complexity. We have seen in previous slides several two-dimensional images of three-dimensional objects. It is very difficult to ascertain the depth of the scattering center within a larva, for example. The third (out-of-the screen) dimension is completely unspecified.

The principles of computer-aided tomography can be applied to acoustical microscopy to solve this problem. Tomograms are unambiguous slice images. A tomographic microscope is one that produces slice images of the various layers of tiny three-dimensional objects. Research is presently underway on this type of microscope and one version of it has been given the acronym STAM for scanning tomographic acoustic microscope. In principle, STAM is capable of producing microscopic cross-sectional images to overcome the difficulties referred to in connection with microscopic shadow graphs[L85]. Figure 23 shows an early computer simulation performed to verify the concept.

BRAGG-DIFFRACTION IMAGING

A fourth acoustical imaging system using laser-beam readout makes use of the principle of Bragg-diffraction of coherent light from ultrasonic wavefronts in water. Although somewhat similar to the Sokolov system previously described, Bragg-diffraction imaging is different in important ways. The concepts were initially enunciated and experimentally studied by Korpel in 1966[K66]. The ideas were independently thought of by Hance, Parks and Tsai at Lockheed Research Laboratories[H67] and by myself at UCSB[W67]. Figure 24 shows the diagram of a Bragg-diffraction imaging system.

Phase information is retained by the Bragg-diffracted light that leaves the sound cell and this fact suggests a way of looking at Bragg-diffraction imaging that is reminiscent of holography where phase information is also retained. As described in the literature, the analogue between a Bragg-diffraction imaging system and a thick optical hologram is very close.

22

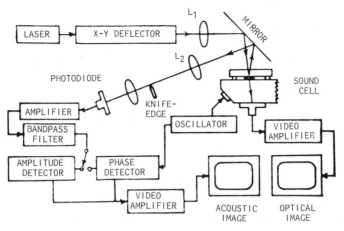

Fig. 21. Experimental arrangement for Kessler's acoustic microscope.
Note that both acoustic and optical transmission images are
formed simultaneously. (See Figure 27 of recent developments.)

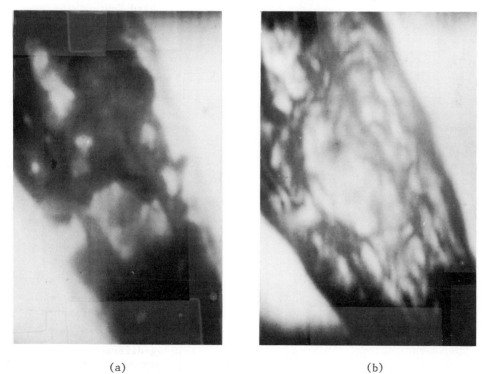

(a)   (b)

Fig. 22. Optical and acoustic images of a section of a fruit-fly
larva obtained by Kessler's microscope. (a) optical image.
(b) acoustic image.

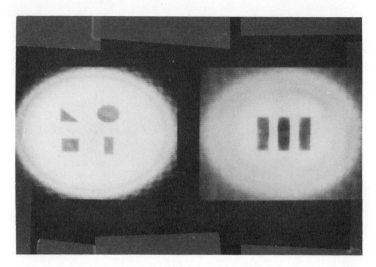

Fig. 23. Simulated two-layer object reconstructed from 18 projections using STAM's reconstruction algorithm. Top layer is on the left and bottom layer is on the right.

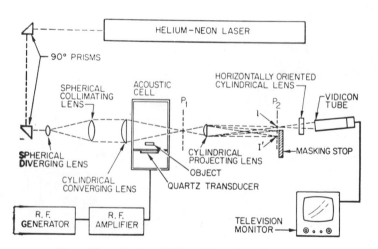

Fig. 24. Bragg-diffraction imaging system.

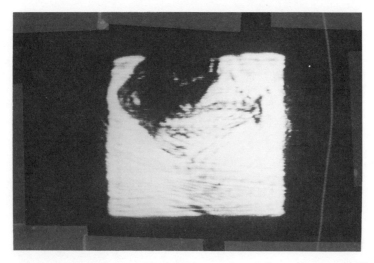

Fig. 25. Acoustic image of a fish produced by a Bragg-diffraction imaging system.

Bragg-diffraction imaging produces images in real-time. Figure 25 shows one such image of a swimming fish. The systems are easy to operate and inexpensive to construct. However, they have some severe drawbacks, including low sensitivity and limited field of view. In an era when patient radiation is a major concern, this lack of sensitivity produces a requirement for high insonifying power and makes Bragg-diffraction imaging unacceptable for clinical diagnostic purposes. However, this approach does have potential in the area of non-destructive evaluation and perhaps in microscopy for the in-vitro study of tissues where radiation hazard is not an important factor.

THE PROGRESS WILL CONTINUE

From this brief chronological review, we can see that acoustic imaging has previously attracted and is presently attracting the attention of a number of workers. The attempt to use sound for imaging possesses a history that goes back a number of decades. However, over the past 20 years there has been a spurt of new research activity in this field stemming primarily from the advent of the laser, strides in optical holography, and progress in digital computer technology. Much work has been done; much progress has been made; and much utility from acoustical imaging has been realized. But there remain many difficult questions to be resolved before the full capability of acoustical imaging can be applied to many of the practical problems. Much innovative work therefore remains to be done.

But this work is being done. From a historical review of what has already been accomplished, we can reasonably expect that modified versions of the old systems will be employed in the old ways and that some of the

25

new systems, still in the research stage, will find useful employment in entirely new ways.

The past history of acoustical imaging is extremely interesting. We can predict with confidence that the historical developments are not over, progress will continue and further important history will be made. Some of that history is being reported at this conference and recorded in the pages of this volume.

ACKNOWLEDGMENT

I would like to express great appreciation to Paul C.H. Chen and Charles Richman for their help in putting together this written version of what originally was a talk and to Eliane Yochum and Heather Simioni for their patience and skill in typing the several drafts that were necessary for producing the paper.

REFERENCES & BIBLIOGRAPHY

A65 E. E. Aldridge, A. B. Clare, and D. A. Shepherd, "Ultrasonic holography in non-destructive testing," in Acoustical Holography, Vol. 3, Chap. 7, A. F. Metherell, Ed., New York: Plenum Press, 1971.

C76a P. L. Carson, T. V. Oughton and W. R. Hendee, "Ultrasonic transaxial tomography by reconstruction," in Ultrasound in Medicine, Vol. 2, pp. 341-350, D. N. White and R. W. Barnes, Eds., New York: Plenum Press, 1976.

C76b P. L. Carson, T. V. Oughton and W. R. Hendee, "Ultrasonic transaxial tomography by reconstruction," in Ultrasound in Medicine, Vol. 2, pp. 391-400, D. N. White and R. W. Barnes, Eds., New York: Plenum Press, 1976.

F68 W. J. Fry, et al., "Ultrasonics visualizations systems employing new scanning and presentation methods," J. Acoust. Soc. Amer., Vol. 44, pp. 1324-1388, 1968.

G65 P. Greguss, "Ultrasonic holograms," Res. Film, Vol. 5:4, pp. 330-337, 1965.

G72 P. S. Green, L. F. Schaefer, and A. Makovski, "Considerations for diagnostic ultrasonic imaging," in Acoustical Holography, Vol. 4, pp. 97, G. Wade, Ed., New York: Plenum Press, 1972.

G74 P. S. Green, L. F. Schaefer, E. D. Jones and J. R. Suarez, "A new, high-performance ultrasonics camera," in Acoustical Holography, Vol. 5, pp. 493-503, P. S. Green, Ed., New York: Plenum Press, 1974.

G75 J. F. Greenleaf, S. A. Johnson, W. F. Samayoa and F. A. Duck, "Algebraic reconstruction of spatial distributions of acoustic velocities in tissue from their time-of-flight profiles," in Acoustical Holography, Vol. 6, pp. 71-90, N. Booth, Ed., New York: Plenum Press, 1975.

G78 D. E. Gustafson, M. J. Berggren, M. Singh, and M. K. Dewanjee, "Computed transaxial imaging using single gamma emitters," Radiology, Vol. 129, pp. 187-194, Oct. 1978.

H67 H. V. Hance, J. K. Parks, and C. S. Tsai, "Optical Imaging of A Complex Ultrasonic Field by Diffraction of a Laser Beam," J. Appl. Phys., Vol. 38, No. 4, pp. 1981, 1967.

J74 J. E. Jacobs and D. A. Peterson, "Advances in the Sokoloff Tube," in Acoustical Holography, Vol. 5, pp. 633-645, P. S. Green, Ed., New York: Plenum Press, 1974.

J76 C. V. Jakowatz, Jr. and A. C. Kak, "Computerized tomography using X-Rays and Ultrasound," School Elec. Eng., Purdue University, West LaFayette, IN, Res. Rep. TR-EE 76-25, 1976.

K66 A. Korpel, "Visualization of the Cross-Section of a Sound Beam by Bragg-Diffraction of Light," Appl. Phys. Lett., Vol. 9, p. 425, 1966.

K72 R. K. Kessler, P. R. Palermo and A. Korpel, "Practical High-Resolution Acoustic Microscopy," in Acoustical Holography, Vol. 4, pp. 51-71, G. Wade, Ed., New York: Plenum Press, 1972.

L16 P. Langevin and M. C. Chilowski, "Procédés et appareils pour la production de signaux sous-marins diregés et pour la localisation à distance d'obstacles sous-marins," French patent 502913, 1916.

L71 R. A. Lemons and C. F. Quate, "Acoustic Microscope-scanning Version," Appl. Phys. Lett., Vol. 24, No. 4, pp. 163-165, Feb. 1974.

L77 M. Lasky, "Review of Underwater Acoustics to 1950," J. Acoust. Soc. Am., Vol. 61, pp. 283-297, 1977.

L85 Z. Lin, H. Lee, and G. Wade, "Scanning Tomographic Acoustic Microscope: A Review," Vol. SU-32, pp. 168-188, March 1985.

M66 R. K. Mueller and N. K. Sheridon, "Sound Holograms and Optical Reconstruction," Appl. Phys. Lett., Vol. 9, pp. 328-329, November 1966.

M79 R. K. Mueller, M. Kaveh and G. Wade, "Reconstructive Tomography and Applications to Ultrasonics," Proc. IEEE, Vol. 67, No. 4, pp. 567-587, April 1979.

P37 R. Pohlman, "Über die richtende Wirkung des Schallfeldes auf Suspensionen nicht kugelformiger Teilchen," Zeitschrift für Physik, Vol. 107, pp. 497-507, 1937.

S35a S. J. Sokolov, "Ultrasonic Oscillations and Their Applications," Tech. Phys. USSR., Vol. 2, p. 522, 1935.

S35b S. J. Sokolov, "Über die praktische ausnutzung der beugnung des lichtes an ultraschällwellen," Phys. Z., Vol. 36, p. 142, 1935.

S49 S. J. Sokolov, "Ultrasonic Microscope," Akademia Nauk USSR., Doklady (Tekhnicheskaya Fizika), Vol. 64, p. 333-335, 1949.

S79 James A. Simmons, "Perception of Echo Plane Information in Bat Sonar," Science, Vol. 204, pp. 1336-1338, June 22, 1979.

T66 F. L. Thurstone, "Ultrasound Holography and Visual Reconstruction," Proc. Symp. Biomed. Eng., Vol. 1, pp. 12-15, 1966.

U83 Urick, R.J., Principles of Underwater Sound, 3rd Edition, p. 2, McGraw-Hill Book Company, New York, 1983.

W67 G. Wade, J. Landry and A. A. DeSouza, "Acoustical Transparencies for Optical Imaging Ultrasonic Diffraction," The First International Symposium on Acoustical Holography, December 1967.

W75 G. Wade, "Acoustical Imaging with Holography and Lenses," _IEEE Trans. on Sonics and Ultrasonics_," SU-22, Vol. 6, 1975.

W76a G. Wade, "Historical Perspective," in _Acoustical Imaging_, pp. 21-42, G. Wade, Ed., New York: Plenum Press, 1976.

W76b G. Wade, "Acoustical Imaging: Cameras, Microscopes, Phased Arrays and Holographic Systems," G. Wade, Ed., New York: Plenum Press, 1976.

W80a G. Wade, "Ultrasonic Imaging By Reconstructive Tomography in Acoustical Imaging," Vol. 9, pp. 379-431, K. Y. Wang, Ed., New York: Plenum Press, 1980.

W80b G. Wade, S. Elliott, I. Khogeer, G. Flesher, J. Eisler, D. Mensa, N. S. Ramesh, and G. Heidbreder, "Acoustic Echo Computer Tomography," in _Acoustical Holography_, Vol. 8, pp. 565-576, A. Metherell, Ed., New York: Plenum Press, 1980.

DIFFRACTION TOMOGRAPHY WITH MULTIPLE SCATTERING

S. Leeman, P.E. Chandler*, and L.A. Ferrari*

King's College School of Medicine and Dentistry, Dept. of
Med. Eng. and Phys., Dulwich Hospital, London SE22 8PT, U.K.
*University of California Irvine, Dept. of Elec. Eng.
Irvine, California 92717, U.S.A.

ABSTRACT

A method for reconstructing the image of an object from the
measurement of its scattering amplitude is developed for the case of
acoustic wave scattering from an inhomogeneous medium consisting of
velocity fluctuations. The inversion procedure is exact, and explicitly
takes into account *all* orders of multiple scattering. An interesting
feature is that progressively higher resolution of the recovered image is
obtained as higher order scattering is progressively incorporated into
the inversion procedure.

INTRODUCTION

Ultrasound inverse scatter imaging methods may be regarded as
consisting of three basic components[1] : (a) an underlying physical model
which specifies the propagation and scattering of the wave in the object;
(b) a data acquisition configuration, which may be chosen in order to
minimise eventual artefacts in the final image; and (c) a computational
model, which is essentially the algorithm whereby the desired mapping is
recovered from the measured data set.

The ultrasound methods may be further classified into three major
groupings, according to their data acquisition configurations[1]: (a)
computerised tomography, or transmission, methods, which may be regarded
as utilising the forward-scattered field; (b) reflectivity tomography
methods, which utilise the backscattered field; and (c) diffraction
tomography techniques, which measure the angle-scattered fields. Despite
the consistent designation of these methods as "tomographic", they are
all, potentially, three-dimensional imaging techniques, and each class
of methods spans a number of variations.

We limit ourselves, here, to diffraction tomography - i.e. angle
scattering methods. The computational models employed in this context
fall into essentially two main groups. (i) Inverse Fourier techniques
are analogues of the filtered-backprojection and Fourier-slice-theorem
reconstruction algorithms of conventional straight-line transmission CT
methods. The transposing of these "ray optics" methods to the

diffractive, scattering regime is possible only under the assumption that either the first Born, or the first Rytov, approximation holds for the scattered fields[2]. The precise validity ranges for these approximations are not known, but it is clear that methods dependent on them will have limited applicability in practice.   (ii) Successive approximation schemes, which are the analogue of the ART CT reconstruction algorithm, have also been proposed (see, for example, the paper by Berggren et. al. in this volume).   These are much more tolerant of multiple scattering effects,   and   overcome   the   restriction   to   the   Born   or   Rytov approximations, but they are computationally extremely demanding, and may well turn out to be prohibitively time consuming when applied to real data collected from three dimensional objects.

In this communication we describe a different reconstruction method – not based on any CT analogue – which is applicable to scattering from three dimensional objects, with multiple scattering allowed. There is no limitation on the strength of the interaction. The technique is based on earlier work, developed in a rather different context (full details and references are given in reference 3), but has not been previously applied for acoustical imaging. A rigorous development of the method would be beyond the scope of this presentation, and we choose to demonstrate the feasibility of the approach by analysing a particularly simple example.

THE PHYSICAL MODEL AND DATA ACQUISITION CONFIGURATION

Consider the case that the radiation propagating in the object may be described by the wave equation:

$$\nabla^2 \phi + k^2 \phi = \rho \phi$$

with $\phi(\underline{r})$ denoting the wave at location $\underline{r}$, $\rho(\underline{r})$ representing the scattering interaction density, and with $k=\omega/c$.   Here, ω is the (circular) frequency of the field, and c is a mean value for the wave velocity over the scattering region.   Clearly, this wave equation contains, as a special case, the Helmholtz equation, which is applicable to longitudinal ultrasound waves propagating in velocity-inhomogeneous media.

For simplicity in presentation, rotational symmetry is assumed

$$\rho(\underline{r}) = \rho(r)$$

More crucially, the interaction density is assumed to have the fairly general representation

$$r\rho(r) = \int_{\mu}^{\infty} d\alpha \; \sigma(\alpha). \exp\{-\alpha r\}$$

with

$$\int_{\mu}^{\infty} d\alpha \; |\sigma(\alpha)| \qquad \text{finite}$$

The inversion technique will attempt to construct $\sigma(\alpha)$ from the measured data, i.e. it will aim to essentially uncover the Laplace domain representation of the interaction.

The data acquisition configuration consists of a plane wave incident along the direction $\underline{n}_I$, with the scattering into all directions $\underline{n}_s$ being detected, the measured entity actually being the scattering amplitude, $T(\theta;k)$. This notation is intended to denote that T is measured at all scattering angles, θ, but at fixed incident k (≡ frequency) only. The assumed rotational symmetry of the scattering interaction has imposed the same symmetry on the scattering amplitude, which consequently depends on only one angular variable.

It is convenient to introduce the wave vectors

$$\mathbf{k_I} = k\mathbf{n_I} \quad \text{and} \quad \mathbf{k_s} = k\mathbf{n_s}$$

as well as the variable

$$\Delta \equiv -|\ \mathbf{k_s} - \mathbf{k_I}\ |^2$$

Also, we prefer to use the notation

$$f(\mathbf{k_s}, \mathbf{k_I}) \equiv T(\theta; k)$$

Note that the scattering amplitude may be regarded as a function of the two independent variables Δ and k (with the latter regarded as fixed in the data acquisition configuration under consideration), and may thus also be written as $f(k; \Delta)$. Physically, k may, in principle, take on any real positive value; on the other hand, physical values of Δ are real and negative, in the range $-4k^2 \leqslant \Delta \leqslant 0$. It is useful at this stage to point out that the computational model to be described below follows from a consideration of the analyticity properties of the scattering amplitude in the *complex* Δ domain.

SOME ELEMENTS OF SCATTERING THEORY

The scattering amplitude satisfies the well-known Lippmann-Schwinger equation:

$$f(\mathbf{k_s}, \mathbf{k_I}) = -\rho^+(\mathbf{k_s}-\mathbf{k_I})/4\pi - \int d\mathbf{k'} . \rho^+(\mathbf{k_s}-\mathbf{k'}) . G^+(\mathbf{k'}, k) . f(\mathbf{k'}, \mathbf{k_I})/2\pi^3$$

with $^+$ denoting the Fourier transform of the appropriate function, and where G is the free space Green's function.

Symbolically, the Lippmann-Schwinger equation may be written as

$$f = f_B + f_B G^+ f$$

and may be solved by iteration to give

$$f = f_B + f_B G^+ f_B + \ldots\ldots$$

The Nth term in this expansion is usually referred to as the Nth Born approximation to the scattering amplitude. It is a relatively simple exercise in Fourier transform evaluation to show that the first Born approximation ("1BA") may be written as

$$1BA \equiv f_B = \int_\mu^\infty d\alpha\ \sigma(\alpha) . [\alpha^2 - \Delta]^{-1}$$

The behaviour of the 1BA in the complex Δ domain is easy to establish from this integral representation: the 1BA is analytic everywhere in the finite complex Δ-plane, except for Δ real and $> \mu^2$. The existence of such a branch cut along the real axis of the Δ plane is associated with the circumstance that the denominator in the integrand of the integral defining the 1BA vanishes for these Δ values (leading to a singular integral).

The second Born term, f_{2B}, has a more complicated structure, but it is still possible to exploit the idea that its analyticity in the complex Δ domain breaks down when the integrand in its defining integral shows a non-removable singularity. Thus the powerful method devised by Landau[4] may be invoked to show that f_{2B} is analytic everywhere in the finite Δ plane, except for a branch cut along the real axis, for $\Delta > (2\mu)^2$. Indeed, it may be shown quite generally[3] that the Nth Born term has a similar behaviour, but with its branch cut extending over $\Delta > (N\mu)^2$. The analyticity properties of the scattering amplitude in the Δ plane, as well as the interesting structure of the cut along the real axis, are summarised in Fig.1. This statement, that the singularities of the scattering amplitude in the finite Δ plane are the same as those of the Born expansion, may be shown[3] to be independent of the convergence of the Born expansion.

THE BRANCH-CUT DISCONTINUITY

It is instructive to compute the discontinuity across the branch cut, viz.

$$D(\Delta) \equiv \{ \, f(k;\Delta+i\epsilon) - f(k;\Delta-i\epsilon) \, \}/\pi i$$

In the range $\mu^2 < \Delta < (2\mu)^2$, the branch cut arises only from f_B. Thus,

$$i\pi D_{12} = \int_{\mu}^{\infty} d\alpha \; \sigma(\alpha) \; \{ \, [\alpha^2 - (\Delta+i\epsilon)]^{-1} - [\alpha^2 - (\Delta-i\epsilon)]^{-1} \, \}$$

where we use the notation D_{MN} to denote the discontinuity for $(M\mu)^2 < \Delta < (N\mu)^2$, and where the usual "$i\epsilon$" convention is used to imply that the limit as $\epsilon \to 0$ is always intended. Invoking the identity

$$1/(x\pm i\epsilon) = P(1/x) + i\pi\delta(x)$$

where P denotes taking the principal-value integral, it readily follows that

$$\Delta^{\frac{1}{2}}.D(\Delta) = \sigma(\Delta^{\frac{1}{2}})$$

This fixes the function σ in the range $\mu < \alpha < 2\mu$, thus enabling the following low-resolution version of the object to be computed,

$$r\rho_{12}(r) = \int_{\mu}^{2\mu} d\alpha \; \sigma(\alpha).\exp\{-\alpha r\}$$

This remarkable finding may be extended further. We note that D_{23} arises from two contributions: (i) the 1BA of the density $\rho_{23}(r)$ – which is, as yet, not known (ii) the 2BA of the density $\rho_{12}(r)$ – which is known fron D_{12}. The contribution (ii) may be calculated from the known function ρ_{12}, and this may be subtracted from D_{23} to give a corrected discontinuity, D'. Then, it readily follows that

$$\sigma(\Delta^{\frac{1}{2}}) = \Delta^{\frac{1}{2}}D'(\Delta) \qquad \text{for } (2\mu)^2 < \Delta < (3\mu)^2$$

In this way, the function σ may be obtained over an even wider range, and an even higher resolution version of the object may be formed, viz. $\rho_{13}(r)$. The extension to higher orders is apparent.

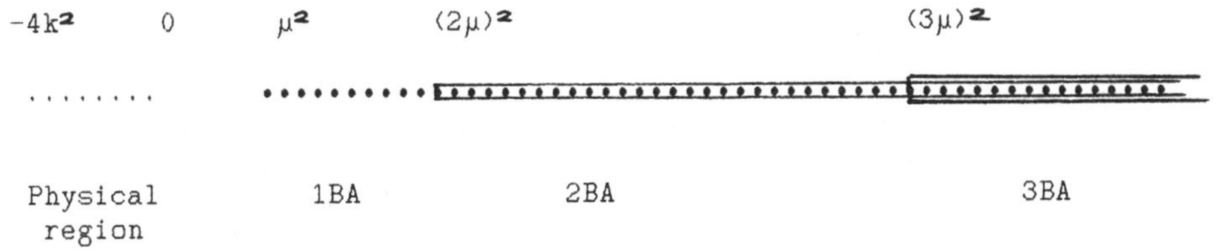

$$-4k^2 \qquad 0 \qquad \mu^2 \qquad (2\mu)^2 \qquad\qquad\qquad (3\mu)^2$$

| Physical region | 1BA | 2BA | 3BA |

Fig. 1. Analytic properties of the scattering amplitude in the complex Δ-plane.

THE INVERSION PROCEDURE

The method for recovering the interaction density $\rho(r)$ is summarised, for clarity.

(a) Measure the scattering amplitude at all angles, for a fixed frequency plane wave input.

(b) Calculate, by analytic continuation into the complex Δ-domain, the experimentally determined values, $D_{EXP}(\Delta)$, of the discontinuity across the branch-cut seen to lie on the real Δ-axis, for $\Delta > \mu^2$.

(c) Obtain a low resolution version of the object, $\rho_{12}(r)$, from D_{EXP} in the range $\mu^2 < \Delta < (2\mu)^2$. Use this to calculate a (subtracted) correction to the values of D_{EXP} in the range $(2\mu)^2 < \Delta < (3\mu)^2$.

(d) Obtain a higher resolution mapping, $\rho_{13}(r)$, by utilising the corrected values of D_{EXP} for $(2\mu)^2 < \Delta < (3\mu)^2$. Note that the mapping ρ_{13} is obtained by adding a correction term, ρ_{23}, to the previous estimate, ρ_{12}.

(e) The general structure for obtaining progressively higher resolution mappings is now apparent. Note, however, that the computational input rises rapidly as higher order corrections are incorporated.

CONCLUSIONS

We have demonstrated that inverse scatter imaging methods which are not analogues of conventional CT techniques may, in fact, be formulated. Notwithstanding many statements to the contrary, multiple scattering is *not* an obstacle that can be overcome only by ART-like successive approximation techniques (whose convergence has yet to be rigorously established by analytic argument).

Note that the method described here is essentially three-dimensional, and may accommodate more sophisticated physical models (particularly including loss effects), but at the cost of more elaborate data acquisition configurations and computing time.

The method suffers from the disadvantage that it is dependent on (probably) noise-sensitive analytic continuation procedures. The (truncated) Laplace domain representation for the interaction is a crucial assumption, and, although reasonably general, may not apply to all objects.

REFERENCES

1. S. Leeman and V.C. Roberts, "Inverse scatter imaging", in: Ultrasound in Medicine, F.A. Duck and H.Berktay, eds., Inst. of Acoustics, Edinburgh. (1986)
2. S. Leeman and M.A. Fiddy,"New representations for reconstruction techniques from projection data", in: Inverse Optics, Proc. SPIE, 413:20 (1983).
3. S. Leeman, "Non-local potentials and two-body scattering", Proc. Roy. Soc. Lond., A 315: 497 (1970).
4. L.D. Landau, Nucl. Phys., 13: 181 (1959).

ARC BACK PROJECTION WITH AN EFFICIENT COMPUTATION

FOR ULTRASOUND REFLECTION MODE TOMOGRAPHY

M.Ikegami, T.Yamamoto, and Y.Aoki

Faculty of Engineering, Hokkaido University

N-13, W-8, Sapporo, Japan 060

1. INTRODUCTION

Many types of imaging systems using ultrasound have been developed to visualize 2-dimensional cross-sections for medical diagnosis, nondestructive testing and other purposes. However, spatial resolution in such acoustical imaging systems is relatively poor, when compared with the CT systems using X-rays. The fundamental limitation is due to the long wavelength of ultrasound. Since the wavelength used in such applications is often very close to the required resolution limits, the diffraction effect may cause distortion. This problem may be solved by using ultrasonic diffraction tomography(UDT) [1,2]. Investigations of UDT which take the diffraction effect into account have been developed; In the investigations, a higher-order approximation of ultrasonic wave propagation is utilized. However, such methods require complicated calculations of wave propagation, resulting in great difficulty in computing.

Ultrasonic B-mode imaging systems have been utilized extensively in medical diagnosis. A disadvantage of conventional B-mode imaging systems, however, is that they poorly visualize objects lined up along the propagation direction of ultrasonic waves, because of the weak reflection from objects hidden by objects in front [3]. Furthermore, these systems suffer from limitations of lateral resolution due to beam-width.

There is another way to reconstruct images using B-mode imaging [4]. To reduce the shadow region, the images are obtained by scanning a transducer around the objects on a circular aperture in the cross-sectional plane. At each angular position, the transducer is also scanned in a lateral direction, using transducer array or some kind of mechanism. The scanning mechanism is relatively complex because the transducer must be scanned.

In this paper, we propose a method for reducing such shadow regions by using the circular scan of a single omnidirectional transducer, which may act as both a transmitter and a receiver. As a transmitter, the transducer emits circular waves within the plane of the objects. As a receiver, the transducer receives reflections which are proportional to the integral of the reflectivity which lies along a circular arc centered at the transducer. In the system proposed, ultrasound modulated by chirp

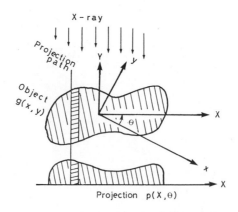

Fig. 1   Projection data and straight projection path
in transmission mode CT.

signals is used to illuminate objects. The received signals are
processed by the technique of digital signal processing to obtain the
projections.   To reconstruct 2D cross-sections of the objects, these
projections are processed using modified filtered back projection, taking
into account the integration path of the circular arc.

2.   PROJECTION OF REFLECTION MODE CT

Assume that $p(X, \theta)$ represents the projected data in tomographic
imaging. In transmission mode tomography(X-ray CT system), we can use the
projection-slice theorem: the Fourier transform of a projection is equal
to a slice of two-dimensional Fourier transform of the projected objects.
In reflection mode tomography, if the projection-slice theorem was applied
to reconstruction, errors would be produced in the reconstructed images.
This is due to the fact that there is a fundamental difference between
transmission mode tomography and reflection mode tomography.

Figure 1 shows the coordinate system of transmission mode tomography.
In X-ray CT system, the projected data $p(X, \theta)$ is the line integral of the
attenuation distribution $g(x, y)$. If we assume that reflection and
multipath effects can be neglected, the projection data $p(X, \theta)$ is defined
by

$$p(X, \theta) = \int g(X \cdot \cos\theta - Y \cdot \sin\theta , X \cdot \sin\theta + Y \cdot \cos\theta) dY \qquad (1)$$

where, (X, Y) denotes the rectangular cartesian coordinate system rotated
by the angle relative to the (x, y) axis. As the propagation path is a
straight line along the X-ray propagation direction, the projections are
obtained on the axis which is perpendicular to the X-ray.   Recently, fan-
beams are more used than parallel-beams in X-ray CT. The projection paths
are also straight lines in such a parallel-beam X-ray CT.

36

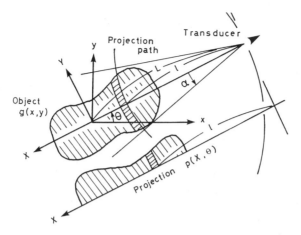

Fig. 2 Projection data and circular arc projection path
         in reflection mode CT.

Reflected A-mode images obtained by a pair of transducer and receiver
are regarded as reflection mode projections. If the beam-profile was wide
enough to illuminate the whole area of objects, the transmitting waves to
each direction would be reflected from the reflectivity of objects, and an
A-mode image would be measured by one receiver. The A-mode image is equal
to the sum of all A-mode images from each direction. We may consider the
reflected A-mode image as the projection of reflectivity along circular
arcs.

Since the projection path is a circular arc in reflection mode
tomography, the projected data $p(X, \theta)$ consist of the integration along a
circular arc, of which center is the position of an omnidirectional
transducer, and its radius is L+X, as shown in Fig. 2:

$$p(X, \theta) = \int g (L \cdot \cos\theta - (L+X) \cdot \sin(\theta + \alpha) $$
$$, L \cdot \sin\theta - (L+X) \cdot \cos(\theta + \alpha)) \, d\alpha \qquad (2)$$

where L is the radius of the circular scan and α is the direction of
transmitting wave. In this case, the projection path is not a straight
line but a circular arc. The projection direction is parallel to that of
ultrasound propagation.

If the distance between the objects area and the transducer is fairly
longer than the diameter of the objects area, the circular arc of the
projection path can be regarded as a straight line. Such a distant region
is called farfield. This farfield is defined by

$$\frac{a}{N} > \sqrt{L^2 + \left(\frac{a}{2}\right)^2} - L$$

$$L > \frac{a(N^2 - 4)}{8N} \qquad (3)$$

where, axa is the size of reconstructed image, and NxN is the number of pixel. Although we can define the field, the farfield is not exactly distinguishable from the nearfield.

Since the reflection mode projection data by A-mode image(on the farfield) is equal to the transmission mode projection data by X-ray, the Fourier Transform and Filtered Back Projection methods, which are popular with X-ray CT, can be applied to reconstruct a 2-D image from A-mode images. The following effects, however, must be carefully considered because ultrasound is used to illuminate objects, and projection data is a reflection mode of A-mode image.

(1) Refraction,
(2) Multiple scattering,
(3) attenuation distribution,
(4) Beam-profile of transducer,
(5) Error of projection data on the nearfield,

The effects in (1)-(3) are problems commonly occurring in the ultrasonic imaging technique. Since A-mode image is obtained on time axis, these effects cause errors in the projection data and degrade quality of reconstructed images. In X-ray CT system projection path is parallel to X-ray, the effect (4) can be compensated by multiplying some function with the projection data, whileas in the reflection mode, the effect can not be compensated. For this reason, a wide beam-profile must be used to illuminate the whole area of objects. The first three effects cause errors in projection data, and these errors often occur in the objects which have a complex distribution of propagation velocity and attenuation. In the reconstruction of cracks and defects in homogeneous media, these errors are not important.

In this paper a wide-band chirp compression technique that could be applied to reconstruct an A-mode image is described in section 3. In section 4, Fourier transform method on the farfield is described. We can compensate the fifth effect's error on the nearfield, as described in section 5.

3. WIDE BAND CHIRP COMPRESSION

In conventional B-mode scanning techniques, bursts of ultrasound are transmitted, and echo signals from the objects are collected by the transducer. Although several types of ultrasound can be utilized in such imaging systems, the impulse of ultrasound is most commonly used for the sake of simplicity. However, the use of encoded waves such as chirp signal waves improves the range resolution as well as the signal to noise ratio(SNR). In the system proposed here, we employ transmitting bursts modulated by chirp signals. The wave form can be written as follows,

$$
s(t) = \begin{cases} \exp(\ jw_0 t + \frac{1}{2}jkt^2) & : |t| <= T/2 \\ 0 & : |t| > T/2. \end{cases} \tag{4}
$$

where, w_0 denotes the angular frequency of the center of the chirp signal, k denotes the chirp rate, and T is the pulse(burst) duration time. In general, there are two methods of compressing chirp signal: a chirp compression filtering analogue signal, and a mutual correlation technique after the conversion of analogue signal to digital signal. The latter method requires one time of multiplication with the reference, two times of Fourier transform, and one time of the square root of squared complex number. In this method, we have reduced the Fourier transform from two times to one time.

The reflected signals r1(t) from the object g(x,y) can be written as:

$$r1(t) = \int \exp[\ jw_0\{\ t - \frac{2(X+L)}{v}\}]$$
$$\cdot \exp[\ \frac{1}{2}jk\{\ t - \frac{2(X+L)}{v}\}^2\ ] \cdot g(X)dX \tag{5}$$

where, X represents the distance between the transducer and the objects, and v represents the velocity of ultrasound. The received echo signals have an amplifier component and carrier component. Since the carrier component contains no information, it is eliminated by the coherent detection. Therefore, the detected signals(echogram) can be calculated as follows:

$$r2(t) = r1(t) \cdot \exp(\ -jw_0t)$$
$$= \int \exp\{\ -jw_0 \frac{2(X+L)}{v}\}$$
$$\cdot \exp[\ \frac{1}{2}jk\{\ t - \frac{2(X+L)}{v}\}^2] \cdot g(X)dX \tag{6}$$

After this detection and the collection using an A/D converter, all processes are conducted by a digital computer. The phase term proportional to time t^2 is eliminated by multiplying the complex function which equals to r2(t) in Eq.(6) [$X_0 = 0$] as follows:

$$r3(t) = r2(t) \cdot \exp\{\ -\frac{1}{2}jk(t - \frac{2L}{v})^2\}$$
$$= \int g(X) \cdot \exp\{k(X)\} \cdot \exp(\ -jk \frac{2X}{v} t\}dX$$

where
$$k(X) = -jw_0 \frac{2(X+L)}{v} + jk\frac{2X(X+2L)}{v^2} \tag{7}$$

Since Eq.(7) is regarded as Fourier transform of [g(X)exp{k(X)}], its inverse Fourier transform becomes [g(X)exp{k(X)}], and g(X) is calculated by the square root of [g(X)exp{k(X)}]^2. Consequently, g(X) is obtained by one time of multiplication with the reference, one time of Fourier transform, and one time of the square root of squared complex number. The spatial resolution of this system depends on the band width of the chirp signal as follows:

$$\delta X = v\pi/B \tag{8}$$

where, B is the band width of the chirp signal. If the interval and the number of sampling at an A/D converter are not properly measured, the spectrum can not be analyzed by Fourier transform, and the resolution is restricted by spectral analysis.

4. REFLECTION MODE CT ON THE FARFIELD

4.1 Reconstruction method

There are two methods of reconstructing two dimensional images using A-mode projections. One method is the conventional CT method on the farfield. The projections obtained on the farfield are regarded as equal to 90 degree rotated projections obtained by X-ray CT system. The reconstruction method of X-ray CT system can be applied to the reflection mode CT using A-mode projections on the farfield. This type of reconstruction is described in this section. The other method is the modified filtered back projection method on the nearfield. The same technique, as described above, can not be applied to the reconstruction on the nearfield. The modified filtered back projection method is

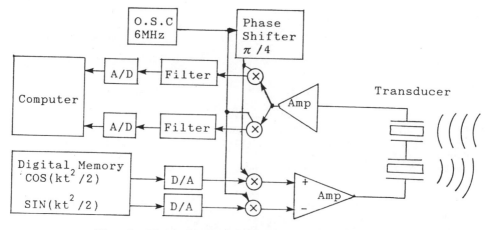

Fig. 3 Block diagram of data acquistion system.

theoretically analyzed in detail in section 5.

Since the projection path can be regarded as a straight line on the farfield defined by Eq.(3), the reconstruction method used in X-ray CT, which is based on Fourier slice theorem, can be applied to the reconstruction by A-mode projection data.

Though the distance between the area of objects and the transducer is longer than the diameter of objects area on the farfield, such a wide beam-profile of transducer is not necessary. As it is possible to assume that the homogeneous strength of ultrasound wave illuminates whole area of the objects,the compensation in section 2-(4) is, therefore, not necessary.

4.2 Experimental result

We conducted an experiment using 6 MHz ultrasound underwater with the following parameters.

carrier frequency	w_0	6.0MHz, 37.7E5rad/sec.
wave length	λ	0.25mm
chirp rate	k	1.10E10rad/sec.
pulse duration time	T	683E-6sec.
band width	B	1.2MHz, 7.54E6rad/sec.
sampling frequency	f	3.0MHz, 18.8E6rad/sec.
spatial resolution	ΔX	0.625mm

Figure 3 shows the block-diagram of experimental system. The chirp signals were memorized by digital memory, and the analogue chirp signals were generated using a D/A converter. Thus, the signal was the same at each time; it is possible to correlate the received signals and the reference signals with success.

In the experiment, the diameter of the circle, where 7 tin-plated wires with 2-mm. diameters were placed, was 5-cm. Figure 4(a) shows the projection data compressed by the chirp signal. 36 echograms were recorded, where the angle of circular-scan varied from 0° to 175° by 5°. Figure 4(b) shows reconstructed image. Five wires are clearly visible. This is probably because the scanning angle is not 360° but 180°, or because the lack of amplitude of the receiver section. A careful adjustment as well as a maximum number of projections are required for the reconstruction of good quality images.

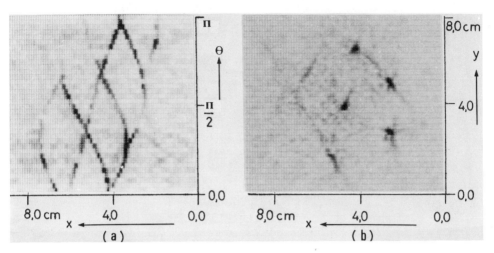

Fig. 4   Projection data and reconstructed image on farfield.
(a) Projection data after chirp compression of reflected signal.
Transducer is scanned from 0° to 175° by 5°.
(b) Reconstructed image: L = 1m.

5.   REFLECTION MODE CT ON THE NEARFIELD

5.1 Reconstruction method

        The method used in X-ray CT can be applied to reflection mode CT
by A-mode projection data on the farfield, but on the nearfield; this is
because the projection path is not a straight line but a circular arc with
center being at the transducer(Eq.(2)).

        There is a filtered back projection method consisting of two stages:
filtering the projections, and back-projecting the filtered projections
along straight lines. To reconstruct on the nearfield, the back projection
path is required to transform straight lines to circular arcs. After
filtering, the projection data is back-projected along the circular arc
path corresponding to the circular arc projection path instead of along
straight line on nearfield. The back projection is made by:

$$f(x,y) = \int p'(\ 1- L, \ \theta)d\theta$$

$$1 = sqr[(\ L \cdot cos \theta \ - \ x)^2 + (\ L \cdot sin \theta \ - \ y)^2] \qquad (9)$$

where, 1 denotes the distance between the transducer and the pixel on the
image, and L represents the radius of scanning circle. That is, the
reconstruction can be done using reflection mode projection data by A-mode
image.

5.2 Computation method

        Although the trigonometry function in Eq.(9) may be calculated as
many times as the number of projections, the square root of two squared
number must be calculated as many times as the projection number
multiplied by the pixels in the process of back-projection.   However, one
of the methods of reducing the steps is the use of a look-up table. This
method can not be applied to Eq.(9). By transforming the coordinates from
the rectangular system to the polar system, Eq.(9) can be rewritten as:

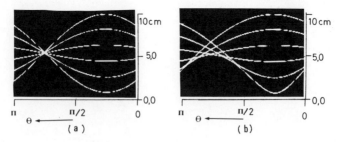

Fig. 5 Reflection mode projection data on farfield and nearfield.
(a) Projection data on farfield: L = 1m.
(b) Projection data on nearfield: L = 6cm.

$$x = r \cdot \cos \beta \quad , \quad y = r \cdot \sin \beta$$
$$r = n \cdot \varDelta r \quad : \quad n = 0, 1, 2, \cdots, N-1$$
$$\beta = m \cdot \varDelta \beta \quad : \quad m = 0, 1, 2, \cdots, N-1 \tag{10}$$

$$f(r,\beta) = \int p'(1 - L, \ \theta) d\theta$$
$$1 = sqr \{(L \cdot \cos \theta - r \cdot \cos \beta)^2 + (L \cdot \sin \theta - r \cdot \sin \beta)^2\} \tag{11}$$

If the relation between θ and β is as follow:

$$\varDelta \theta = i \cdot \varDelta \beta \quad i = 1,2,3, \cdots \cdot$$
or
$$\varDelta \beta = i \cdot \varDelta \theta \quad i = 1,2,3, \cdots \cdot \tag{12}$$

we can make a look-up table for 1. For example, assuming that i = 1, Eq.(11) can be written in the form

$$1 = sqr [\{L \cdot \cos(j \cdot \varDelta \theta)-n \cdot \varDelta r \cdot \cos(k \cdot \varDelta \theta)\}^2$$
$$+ \{L \cdot \sin(j \cdot \varDelta \theta)-n \cdot \varDelta r \cdot \sin(k \cdot \varDelta \theta)\}^2]$$

$$= sqr [\{L-n \cdot \varDelta r \cdot \cos(|j-k| \cdot \varDelta \theta)\}^2$$
$$+ \{n \cdot \varDelta r \cdot \sin(|j-k| \cdot \varDelta \theta)\}^2] \tag{13}$$

$N \times \pi / \varDelta \theta$ is the number of elements required for the look-up table. Once the look-up table has been prepared, the back projection is calculated only by addition and multiplication of integer numbers.

5.3 Computer simulation

To confirm the theory and the reconstruction algorithm, a computer simulation was conducted. The resulting projections from the transmission mode and the reflection mode are shown in Fig. 5(a) and 5(b), respectively. As shown in Fig 5(a), all 6 lines intersect at the same point where the transducer was placed on the line of the 6 objects. In the projections in Fig.5(b), the positions where two lines cross each other distribute. Therefore, it is not feasible to apply the projection-slice theorem to the reflection mode tomography.

The filter function of reflection mode tomography is different from that of transmission mode tomography. In the reflection mode radii of circular arcs of projection path vary in the area of objects, whereas in the transmission mode, the projection path are straight lines in the area. As a result, a space variant filter is required. Figure 6 shows the difference of point spread function between the center of the area and the center's surrounding.

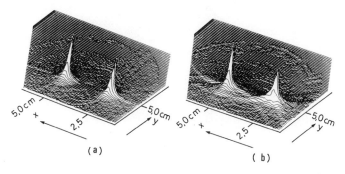

(a)   (b)

Fig. 6   Point spread function at center of image and at edge of image.
        (a) Point spread function on farfield: L = 1m.
        (b) Point spread function on nearfield: L = 6cm.

Figure 7 shows the computer simulation of reconstructed images with 10x10cm^2 and 128x128 pixels. Fig.7(a) is a properly reconstructed image on farfield (L = 1m), Fig.7(b) is a nearfield reconstruction back-projected along the circular arc path(L = 6(cm)). No difference can be observed between these two images. Fig.7(c) is a nearfield reconstruction using L = 6cm., and back-projected using L = 1m. Some points surrounding the center were not reconstructed correctly.

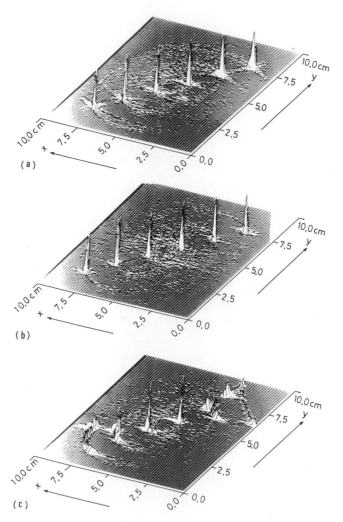

Fig. 7   Computer simulation of image reconstruction on some field.
(a)Reconstructed images on nearfield: L = 6cm.
(b)Reconstructed images on farfield: L = 1m.
(c)Reconstructed images on nearfield back-projected
      along straight line.

6. CONCLUSIONS

In this paper a new method of ultrasonic reflection mode tomography is proposed. This method combines pulse compression techniques with a modified filtered back projection technique. A good spatial resolution and images of high quality can be obtained using the method. And yet the problem in this type of imaging system is that the amount of calculation is relatively larger than that of other tomographic imaging systems. It is expected that a special hardware designed for look-up tables and high-speed summation of integer numbers may help to reduce the calculation time. The problem of constructing an imaging system of UCT with such a hardware is a subject of further investigation.

REFERENCE

(1) A.J.Devaney, "A Filtered Backpropagation Algorithm for Diffraction Tomography," Imaging, Vol.4, pp.336-350(1982)
(2) M.L.Oristaglio: "A Geometric Approach to The Filtered Backpropagation Algorithm," Ultrason. Imaging,Vol.5, pp.30-37(1983)
(3) T.yamamoto, Y.Aoki, "Holographic B-scope Imaging Using Wide-Band Chirped Ultrasound," IEEE Trans. Sonics & Ultrason., Vol. SU-31, No.4, pp.362-366, (July 1984).
(4) D.Hiller and H.Ermert, "System Analysis of Ultrasound Reflection Mode Computerized Tomography," IEEE Trans. Sonics & Ultrason., Vol.SU-31, No.4(July 1984).

PASSIVE IMAGING THROUGH MEDIA WITH DISTRIBUTED INHOMOGENEITIES USING AN

EXTENSION OF THE PHASE CLOSURE TECHNIQUE

K.A. Marsh and J.M. Richardson

Rockwell International Science Center
Thousand Oaks, CA 91360

ABSTRACT

We have investigated the application of the phase closure technique
to the problem of passive imaging of a spatially uncorrelated noise
source through an inhomogeneous medium whose properties are known only
statistically. The measurement system consists of an array of transducers whose signals are processed in a manner similar to that used in
radio interferometry of celestial sources. Although the standard phase
closure technique is not directly suited to a medium with distributed
inhomogeneities, a simple pre-processing step can be used to overcome
this limitation in many cases. This procedure, to which we refer as
"cross-correlated subarrays" involves processing the transducer signals
in groups, corresponding to operating the array as a series of smaller
subarrays. The beamwidth of a subarray is chosen to restrict the
response of the system to the angular field over which the assumptions of
phase closure are valid. If we let Δx_c be the coherence scale of the
field (a function of the parameters of the medium, together with range R
and wavelength λ) then for phase closure to be valid (with or without
cross-correlated subarrays) we require $\Delta x_c > (\lambda R)^{1/2}$. Cross-correlated
subarrays are required explicitly if the maximum source separation, s, is
such that $s > \Delta x_c$. These expectations have been tested by means of a
series of numerical experiments, and the results will be presented.

INTRODUCTION

The phase closure technique was developed originally for very long
baseline radio interferometry (VLBI) in astronomy in order to overcome
the phase distortion caused by the Earth's atmosphere (Readhead and
Wilkinson, 1978). We have investigated the possibility of applying it to
passive acoustic imaging in order to overcome the distorting effects
caused by both the propagation medium and phase errors in the instrument
itself (Marsh, Richardson and Martin, 1985). An important difference,
however is that for radio astronomy, the distorting medium represents a
thin sheet at one end of the propagation path, whereas for the acoustic
case, the inhomogeneities responsible for phase distortion are, in general, distributed throughout the region between the source and receiver.
In the present paper we address the problem of extending the validity of
the phase closure technique to the case of distributed inhomogeneities.

A closely related technique for overcoming phase distortion effects has recently been discussed by Paulraj and Kailath (1985). Their technique models the phase errors in exactly the same way as the phase closure technique, although the solution to the imaging problem is accomplished by eigenvector methods. Also closely related is the concept of phase recovery from bispectra (Bartelt, Lohmann, and Wirnitzer, 1984). As in the case of the conventional phase closure method, both of these methods would be applicable to instrumental phase errors, but would not be able to handle the case of distributed inhomogeneities without some modification.

THEORETICAL CONSIDERATIONS

As discussed by Marsh, Richardson and Martin (1985), the far-field intensity distribution $I(\underset{\sim}{e}_n)$ of a spatially incoherent sound source in the case of an inhomogeneous medium is related to the measured visibility V_{ij}^{meas} by:

$$V_{ij}^{meas} = \sum_n g_{in} \; g_{jn}^* \; I(\underset{\sim}{e}_n) \; e^{-2\pi i \underset{\sim}{u}_{ij} \cdot \underset{\sim}{e}_n} \; \Delta\Omega_n \tag{1}$$

where $\underset{\sim}{e}_n$ is a unit vector in the direction of the nth source component as viewed from the receiver, $\Delta\Omega_n$ is the solid angle subtended by the nth source, $\underset{\sim}{u}_{ij}$ is the baseline vector joining transducers i and j in units of wavelengths, and g_{in} and g_{jn} are complex gain factors representing the effect of propagation anomalies in the medium. The visibility itself is defined as

$$V_{ij}^{meas} = E \; S_i S_j^* \tag{2}$$

where S_i, S_j are the frequency-domain signals received by transducers i and j respectively, and E is the expectation operator.

The principal assumption underlying the standard phase closure technique is that we can factor g_{in} into a source-adjacent part and a receiver-adjacent part, i.e.,

$$g_{in} \simeq g_i g_n \tag{3}$$

If we further assume that the principal effect of the medium is a phase distortion then $|g_n| = 1$, and using (1) and (3) can express V_{ij}^{meas} in terms of the true visibility V_{ij}^{true} (corresponding to a uniform medium) as:

$$V_{ij}^{meas} = e^{i(\phi_i - \phi_j)} V_{ij}^{true} \tag{4}$$

where $\phi_i = \arg(g_i)$. The measured phase $\phi_{ij}^{meas} = \arg(V_{ij}^{meas})$ can therefore be expressed in terms of the true phase $\phi_{ij}^{true} = \arg(V_{ij}^{true})$ as:

$$\phi_{ij}^{meas} = \phi_{ij}^{true} + \phi_i - \phi_j \quad . \tag{5}$$

The standard phase closure technique attempts to obtain the phase errors ϕ_i using a measurement model of the form (5), and correct the data accordingly.

Physically, Eq. (3) implies that we are representing the medium as a pair of phase screens, one in front of the source and the other in front of the receiver. While such a model may not constitute a good description of the medium itself, it does provide a substantial number of degrees of freedom within which to represent the effects of the medium on acoustic signals. These degrees of freedom correspond to the number of source elements plus the number of receiving elements. If this model were exact, the phase errors introduced by the medium would be direction-independent, since phase shifts near the source do not affect the intensity distribution as seen at the receiver, while phase shifts in front of the receivers introduce errors which are the same for all source directions. On the other hand, inhomogeneities in the region between the source and receivers would result in direction-dependent phase errors, although it is always possible to define an angular field of view $\Delta\theta_{pc}$ over which the variation in phase error is sufficiently small according to some suitable criterion.

Provided all of the acoustic sources are located within the angular field $\Delta\theta_{pc}$, the standard phase closure technique is valid. Unfortunately, this is unlikely to be true in practice, since sources may occur over a wide range of azimuths. It is, however, possible to extend the phase closure technique to handle this situation. A conceptually simple way of accomplishing this is to divide the array up into a number of identical subarrays, and operate each as a small phased array, with the beams all pointed in the same direction. The beam pattern of each subarray will, of course, be much broader than the resolution of the full array. We will refer to the beam pattern of each subarray as the primary beam. We will treat each subarray as an individual element in a larger scale array, and cross-correlate the signals from each subarray as if we were dealing with an array of single transducers. The effect of this is that the angular response of the larger array will have been multiplied by the primary beam pattern corresponding to an individual subarray. By an appropriate choice of the number of elements in a subarray, we could, provided certain conditions are met, restrict the primary beamwidth $\Delta\theta_{pri}$ to the field $\Delta\theta_{pc}$ over which (3) is satisfied. In the case of a homogeneous medium, $\Delta\theta_{pri}$ can be obtained simply from the Fourier transform of the aperture distribution for a single subarray. In the case of an inhomogeneous medium, however, the phase distortions will broaden the response, ultimately setting a lower limit $\Delta\theta_b$ on the primary beamwidth obtainable.

Both $\Delta\theta_{pc}$ and $\Delta\theta_b$ can be related to the phase structure function $D(x - x')$, defined by Flatte et al. (1979) as:

$$D(x - x') = E[\phi(x) - \phi(x')]^2 \tag{6}$$

where x and x' represent the positions of two receivers located at a distance R from a point source and displaced perpendicular to the direction of propagation, and $\phi(x)$ represents the spatial variation of the phase of the received signal. We can then express $\Delta\theta_{pc}$ and $\Delta\theta_b$ in terms of some convenient criterion limiting the amount of permissible phase variation $\Delta\phi$ over the source and receiver, respectively. Provided the inhomogeneities have the same statistical character throughout the region between source and receiver, and taking $\Delta\phi$ to be 1 radian, we can then write

$$R \, \Delta\theta_{pc} = \frac{\lambda}{\Delta\theta_b} = \Delta x_c \tag{7}$$

where λ is the wavelength and Δx_c is defined by

$$D(\Delta x_c) = 1 \quad . \tag{8}$$

Provided $\Delta\theta_{pc} > \Delta\theta_b$, the primary beamwidth can be restricted to $\Delta\theta_{pc}$, enabling the phase closure technique to produce an image over the restricted field $\theta_r - \Delta\theta_{pc}/2$ to $\theta_r + \Delta\theta_{pc}/2$ where θ_r represents the center of the restricted field. A mosaic of subimages could then be produced, corresponding to various values of θ_r, and the final image produced by a combination of these subimages. In order to produce the rth subimage, the phase closure technique would be applied to the set of visibilities $V_{ij}^{(r)}$ defined by:

$$V_{ij}^{(r)} = \sum_{k=k_o(i)+1}^{k_o(i)+n_s} \sum_{\ell=\ell_o(j)+1}^{\ell_o(j)+n_s} a_k(i) \, a_\ell(j) \, E(S_k S_\ell^*) \, e^{-2\pi i u_{k\ell} \sin \theta_r} \tag{9}$$

where

$$k_o(i) = (i - 1)n_s$$

$$\ell_o(j) = (j - 1)n_s$$

and S_k, S_ℓ represent the signals received by the kth and ℓ^{th} transducers; $a_k(i)$, $a_\ell(j)$ are weights representing the apodizing function for each subarray, n_s is the number of elements in each subarray.

The procedure sketched above would enable phase-closure imaging over a wide field-of-view, and should provide a substantial improvement in imaging performance over that obtained by conventional beamforming. We will refer to it subsequently as "phase closure with cross-correlated subarrays." We now consider the question as to the physical regime over which this algorithm will be valid. A useful quantity to bear in mind in this regard is Δx_c defined by (8), which represents the coherence scale for the system at the particular range and frequency. The condition that $\Delta\theta_{pc} > \Delta\theta_b$ is equivalent to

$$\Delta x_c > (\lambda R)^{1/2} \quad . \tag{10}$$

Equation (10) thus represents a criterion by which one can determine whether or not phase closure (with cross-correlated subarrays) is capable of improving a distorted image. In order to relate it to more fundamental physical parameters, however, requires a knowledge of the form of the phase structure function D, which in turn is related to the spatial correlation function of the refractive index. If we assume that

$$E\phi(x) \, \phi(x') = \Phi^2 \exp\left(-(x-x')^2/L^2\right) \tag{11}$$

where Φ is the standard deviation of phase fluctuations at a single point, then provided $|x - x'| \ll L$,

$$D(x - x') \simeq 2\Phi^2(x - x')^2/L^2 \tag{12}$$

and hence

$$\Delta x_c \simeq \frac{L}{\sqrt{2} \, \Phi} \quad . \tag{13}$$

If the inhomogeneities are statistically uniform and isotropic, then from Flatte et al., (1979):

$$\Phi^2 \simeq 0.4 \left(\frac{2\pi}{\lambda}\right)^2 \langle\mu^2\rangle RL \tag{14}$$

where $\langle\mu^2\rangle$ represents the variance of the refractive index fluctuations. Equations (13) and (14) then give

$$\Delta x_c \simeq 0.2 \lambda \left(\frac{L}{\langle\mu^2\rangle R}\right)^{1/2} . \tag{15}$$

Thus from (10), we find that the maximum range over which the phase closure technique (with cross-correlated subarrays) can be applied to a distributed medium is

$$R_{max} = 0.2 \left(\frac{\lambda L}{\langle\mu^2\rangle}\right)^{1/2} . \tag{16}$$

In the case of horizontal imaging in the ocean at 500 Hz (assuming $L = 5$ km and $\langle\mu^2\rangle^{1/2} = 5 \times 10^{-4}$) we obtain $R_{max} = 49$ km, which suggests that substantial improvement in bearing estimation with horizontal arrays should be possible over ranges up to this value.

NUMERICAL EXPERIMENTS

In order to test the concepts discussed in the previous section, a series of numerical experiments was performed. In these experiments, an assumed source consisting of 4 pointlike components spread over a distance of 200 m was observed at a distance of 1 km and a frequency of 300 Hz, using a regularly spaced array of length 200 m containing 21 transducers. The sound velocity was assumed to be 1500 m/s. Inhomogeneities were simulated by placing four equally spaced phase screens between the source and receivers. Along each phase screen, the phase was made to vary randomly, with a correlation length L. The rms phase deviation through the entire system was chosen to be approximately 1 radian, so that L corresponds to Δx_c. Various values of L were assumed, in some cases chosen to purposely violate the assumptions for phase closure. The propagation was calculated according to the Fresnel approximation, as discussed by Marsh, Richardson and Martin (1985). In the case of the cross-correlated subarrays algorithm, each subarray had 5 elements, weighted with a rectangular function, i.e., no apodizing was used. A mosaic of 3 subimages was produced in each case, spaced by the half-power widths of the corresponding primary beams (sinc functions). Simple addition was used in order to construct the final image from the 3 subimages.

Since in these experiments $L \simeq \Delta x_c$, Eq. (10) implies that phase closure would be invalid if $L < (\lambda R)^{1/2}$. In the case of $L > (\lambda R)^{1/2}$, phase closure would be applicable, but cross-correlated subarrays would be required if the source components are separated by a distance s greater than L. These two criteria form a rather crucial test of the theoretical basis of our algorithm, and values of L were chosen to test them. In these experiments, $(\lambda R)^{1/2}$ corresponds to 71 m. We now discuss the results.

Case a: $L > (\lambda R)^{1/2}$, $s = L$.

The assumed value of L was 200 m. In this case we expect phase closure to be valid, and cross-correlated subarrays should not be necessary. The results are shown in Fig. 1, which fulfills our expectations. The use of phase closure has substantially improved the image over that obtained by conventional beamforming, but the use of cross-correlated subarrays has produced only a marginal improvement over standard phase closure.

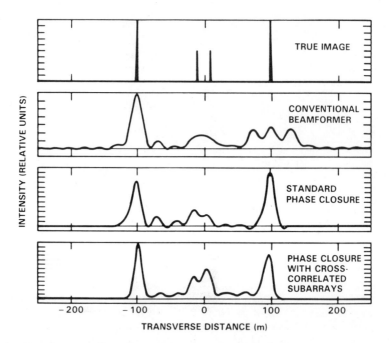

Fig. 1 Imaging results for the case of mild phase distortion. The length scale of the inhomogeneities, L, was chosen such that $L > (\lambda R)^{1/2}$ where λ is the wavelength and R is the range, thus phase closure was expected to be valid. In addition, the maximum source separation, s, did not exceed L, and hence, standard phase closure performs satisfactorily without the need for cross-correlated subarrays.

Case b: $L > (\lambda R)^{1/2}$, $s = 2L$.

The assumed value of L was 100 m. We expect phase closure to be valid, but the sources are now so widely spaced in comparison to the length scale of the inhomogeneities that cross-correlated subarrays should be required. The results, shown in Fig. 2 support these expectations. Standard phase closure gave a very poor result, whereas cross-correlated subarrays gave a reasonable reconstruction.

Case c: $L < (\lambda R)^{1/2}$.

The assumed value of L was 50 m. In this case we expect phase closure to be completely invalid, and the results in Fig. 3 show this to be true. It is interesting, however, that the cross-correlated subarrays image bears some resemblance to the assumed source, although the separation between components is incorrect.

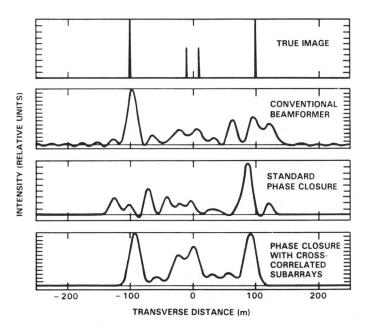

Fig. 2 Imaging results for the case of moderate phase distortion.
Parameters are the same as for Fig. 1, except that s = 2L,
i.e., the sources are now so widely spaced in comparison to the
length scale of the inhomogeneities that cross-correlated
subarrays are required.

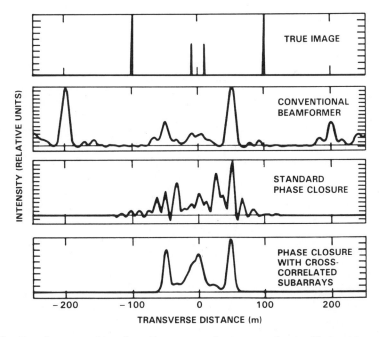

Fig. 3 Imaging results for the case of strong phase distortion. In
this case $L < (\lambda R)^{1/2}$, and hence, phase closure is not able to
restore the image.

CONCLUSIONS

The results of the numerical simulations were consistent with expectation, and indicate that the phase closure technique is applicable to the case of a medium with distributed inhomogeneities provided the angular response of the array approximately restricted, and that the coherence scale of the system is greater than or equal to $(\lambda R)^{1/2}$. We expect that the proper application of phase closure should result in improved bearing estimation with passive acoustic arrays.

ACKNOWLEDGMENT

This work was supported by DARPA Contract N00014-85-C-0182.

REFERENCES

Bartelt, H., Lohmann, A.W., and Wirnitzer, B. 1984, Applied Optics, 23:3121.

Flatte, S.M., Dashen, R., Munk, W.H., Watson, K.M., and Zachariasen, F. 1979, "Sound Transmission Through a Fluctuating Ocean," (New York, Cambridge Univ. Press).

Marsh, K.A., Richardson, J.M., and Martin, J.M. 1985, "Application of the Phase Closure Technique to Passive Acoustic Imaging Through Inhomogeneous Media," Acoustical Imaging, 14:133.

Paulraj, A. and Kailath, T. 1985, "Direction of Arrival Estimation by Eigenstructure Methods with Unknown Sensor Gain and Phase," to appear in IEEE ASSP.

Readhead, A.C.S. and Wilkinson, P. 1978, Astrophy. J., 223:25.

COMPUTATION SIMPLIFICATION

FOR HIGH-SPEED ACOUSTICAL IMAGE RECONSTRUCTION

Hua Lee and Jen-Hui Chuang

Department of Electrical and Computer Engineering
University of Illinois at Urbana-Champaign
Urbana, Illinois 61801

Abstract - In many conventional coherent acoustical image formation algorithms using weight, delay, and summation operators, the computation complexity is mainly governed by the associated exponential and trigonometric operations which are commonly computed by power series expansion in computers. The reconstructed source distribution can be regarded as a result of accumulation of relative co-linear or random vectors. In this paper, we present the computation simplification by analyzing the phase density distribution of these vectors during the image formation process. Then we are able to reduce the computation complexity by replacing the exponential and trigonometric operators by real and symmetric weighting functions. The computation reduction will not only significantly enhance the potential for high-speed acoustical image reconstruction, but also simplify the filter structure for VLSI hardware implementation. There is no significant resolution degradation due to the algorithm simplification. This technique can be also applied to inverse scattering, spectral estimation, nondestructive evaluation, and beam forming. In addition, it can be used to modify backward propagation method and phase-only reconstruction technique for holographic imaging.

Introduction

Traditionally, image resolution has been the main objective for imaging system optimization due to the emphasis of high-resolution imaging. High-resolution imaging involved many key optimization parameters such as frequency bandwidth, aperture size, signaling format, and analog-continuous conversion bit-rates. Various techniques such as least-square matched filtering, wave-field orthogonalization, and band-limited extrapolation have been developed to improved resolution with additional assumptions, constraints, and the support of extensive computation capability [1-10]. Relatively, very little effort has been devoted to computation simplification. More recently, due to the large array size, requirement for real-time processing, limitation of hardware complexity, computation reduction has become an important optimization objective and has significant impact to the development of imaging technology.

The techniques developed for computation reduction largely concentrated on optimization of wave-field detection. For example, optimal sampling is derived for maximum information content detection, hexagonal array is proposed for tomographic processing to eliminate the computation for data interpolation, and phase-only methods are for coding bit-rate reduction[11-14]. However, the mathematical operation structure in image formation remains and is often complicated for real-time hardware implementation.

Phase-only techniques are originated in holography [15-17]. Bit-rate and data size reductions are the main considerations when phase-only methods are recently applied to system simplification. However, when we use the phase-only techniques to perform image enhancement, we found that the phase density distribution has direct relation to the image formation [18]. In this paper, we consider the potential to use the phase density distribution weighting to replace the conventional image reconstruction procedure. We provide the basic guidelines for algorithm modification and an example of the design of the phase weighting. We also observe the degradation error due to the approximation. This technique is capable of high-quality image reconstruction for phase-only models especially for cases with large array the data size. In addition, the same concept can be extended to the amplitude-phase mode. It can be also applied to simplify the structure of spectral estimation algorithms.

Image Formation

For most acoustical imaging systems, the image reconstruction process is a linear spatial filtering operation which is often written as a linear convolution integral

$$p(x) = q(x) * h(x) \tag{1}$$

$$= \int q(x') \, h(x,x') \, dx'$$

where $p(x)$ is the resultant image, $q(x)$ is the received complex wave-field amplitude distribution, $h(x)$ is the impulse response of the image formation filter, and x is the space variable. Eq.(1) is the one-dimensional representation of the linear relationship, and it can be extended to multi-dimensional format with slight modification. To visualize the image formation in terms of phase correction, we first rewrite both the impulse response and received wave-field distributions in polar form

$$q(x) = A(x) \, \exp[j\theta(x)] \tag{2-a}$$

$$h(x) = B(x) \, \exp[j\phi(x)] \tag{2-b}$$

Then Eq. (1) becomes an integral over vectors with amplitude $[A(x')B(x-x')]$ and phase $[\theta + \phi]$

$$p(x) = \int [A(x')B(x,x')] \, \exp\{j[\theta(x') + \phi(x,x')]\} \, dx' \tag{3}$$

This suggests that the image $p(x)$ has greater resultant values when the vectors are in phase which leads to an accumulation effect, and will generate small values if the vectors spread in various directions and lead to vector cancellation. It can be seen that the resultant image distribution is effectively governed by the phase variation which explains the sensitivity of the phase correction process and the importance of the phase information.

It is also known that the amplitude variation of the impulse responses commonly used in image formation are very smooth and often approximated by a constant. Hence, the impulse response becomes

$$h(x) \tilde{} = C \exp[j\phi(x)] \qquad (4)$$

and it represents a phase correction filter.

Many research results in the signal and image processing areas pointed out that the phase variation of the wave-field distribution carries the most vital portion of the information content for high-resolution image reconstruction. Therefore, for imaging systems limited by detection, storage, transmission and coding bit-rate capacities, or processing hardware constraints, phase-only techniques have proven capable of high-quality imaging under these limitations and constraints. For phase-only processing, the amplitude variation of the resultant wave-field is assumed not available for image reconstruction, and Eq. (2-a) becomes

$$q(x) \tilde{} = \exp[j\theta(x)] \qquad (5)$$

As a result, Eq. (1) has now been simplified down to

$$p(x) \tilde{} = C \int \exp\{j[\theta(x') + \phi(x,x')]\}dx' \qquad (6)$$

And in the case of digital data acquisition and image formation, it becomes

$$p(x) \tilde{} = C \sum_{n=1}^{N} \exp\{j[\theta(n) + \phi(k,n)]\} \qquad (7)$$

$$= C \sum_{n=1}^{N} \exp\{j\psi(n,k)\}$$

Phase Density Distribution

Suppose that the total number of detected data samples is N, then for each k value, the image p(k) is now a summation over N unit vectors. Let $D(\Phi)$ be the distribution of the N phase terms $\Phi(n,k)$ which ranges over the interval $(-\pi, \pi)$ and can be regarded as the population density of these phase terms. The phase distribution $D(\Phi)$ has direct relation to image formation that larger values are due to clustered distribution and smaller values are due to the more uniform ones.

Conventionally, the execution of the vector accumulation or cancellation effects for the image formation largely depends upon the exponent operation. However, the operations such as EXP, SIN and COS are computed by power series expansion and become the main portion of the computation specially when N is large. Similar computations occur in the Fourier transformations and complex frequency weighting if frequency-domain techniques are used for reconstruction. These factors have even more significant impact to the implementation of the hardware for small-scale on-board computing systems.

In order to reduced the computational complexity, we should avoid the exponent operator and the associated operations by using alternative with simpler mathematical operations to replace the conventional techniques. There have been statistical methods to utilize the mean and variance of the phase density distribution $D(\Phi)$ to perform image formation and enhancement. Because the function $D(\Phi)$ is periodic with the period 2π, the computation for the mean becomes complicated due to the 2π ambiguity of the phase. The approach using the mean and variance has proven very effective for image enhancement, but not significant for computation simplification.

It is highly desirable to develop simple algorithms to perform image reconstruction. These algorithms should follow some basic guidelines:

(A) Complicated mathematical operations should be eliminated.

(B) The algorithms should produce small value for smooth phase density distribution. When the distribution is uniform, the resultant value should be zero.

(C) Greater values should be generated for clustered phase density distributions.

(D) Algorithm computations should be based on the phase density distribution $D(\Phi)$ and prevent high-order nonlinear operations.

(E) The algorithms should be stable and consistent in the presence of noise.

An Example

There will be many possible methods in terms of the constraints. They will all be considered feasible methods and their performance will be evaluated by the computation complexity, computation time, and degradation or error due to approximation. Here an example using first order weighting is provided to demonstrate computation simplification.

Consider a weighting function defined within the interval $(-\pi, \pi)$ and given by

$$W_r(\psi) = 1 - \frac{2}{\pi} \, |\psi_{\text{mod } 2\pi}| \qquad (8)$$

If we regard this function as a period of a periodic function, then the complete periodic function will have even symmetry at $\Phi = 0$, π or $-\pi$, and odd symmetry at $\Phi = \pi/2$ and $-\pi/2$. The weighting function is shown in Fig. (1). In addition, because of the property

$$W_r(\psi) = -W_r(\psi \pm \pi) \qquad (9)$$

this weighting operation will produce zero for any uniform phase density distribution. The even symmetry along the real axis and odd symmetry along the imaginary imply that this weighting emphasizes only the real component of the resultant image. Replacing the exponent operation with this weighting function, we can approximate Eq. (7) by

$$\text{Real } \{p(k)\} \tilde{=} C \sum_{n=1}^{N} W_r[\psi(n,k)] \qquad (10)$$

$$= C \sum_{n=1}^{N} 1 - \frac{2}{\pi} |\{\psi(n,k)\}_{\text{mod } 2\pi}|$$

$$= C \left\{ N - \frac{2}{\pi} \sum_{n=1}^{N} |\{\psi(n,k)\}_{\text{mod} 2\pi}| \right\}$$

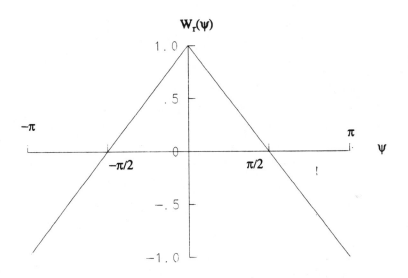

FIG. (1) PHASE WEIGHTING FOR REAL COMPONENT

59

It can be seen that only simple additions are involved in the image formation process except for two multiplications for scaling for each k. The "mod 2π" operation will be taken care of by the register overflow.

Similarly, the imaginary part of the source will be processed by using another weighting operation given by

$$W_i(\psi) = 1 - \frac{2}{\pi} | \{\psi - \frac{\pi}{2}\}_{mod2\pi} |$$

(11)

This weighting function is shown in Fig. (2). And the imaginary part of the image can be formulated as

$$Im\{p(k)\}\tilde{=}C \sum_{n=1}^{N} W_i[\psi(n,k)]$$

(12)

$$= C \sum_{n=1}^{N} 1 - \frac{2}{\pi} | \{\psi(n,k) - \frac{\pi}{2}\}_{mod\ 2\pi} |$$

$$= C \left\{ N - \frac{2}{\pi} \sum_{n=1}^{N} | \{\psi(n,k) - \frac{\pi}{2}\}_{mod\ 2\pi} | \right\}$$

If the amplitude of the resultant wave-field is also available for image reconstruction, Eq. (6) becomes

$$p(k)\tilde{=}C \sum_{n=1}^{N} A(n)\ exp[j\psi(n,k)]$$

(13)

To modify the algorithm, we can regard the amplitude distribution $A(n)$ as a discriminating factor which provides an additional weighting to the phase-only weighting scheme. Therefore, Eqs. (10) and (11) can be modified as

$$Real\{p(k)\}\tilde{=}C \sum_{n=1}^{N} A(n)\ W_r[\psi(n,k)]$$

(14)

$$= C \sum_{n=1}^{N} A(n) \left[1 - \frac{2}{\pi} | \{\psi(n,k)\}_{mod\ 2\pi} | \right]$$

$$= C \{ \sum_{n=1}^{N} A(n) - \frac{2}{\pi} \sum_{n=1}^{N} A(n) | \{\psi(n,k)\}_{mod\ 2\pi} |$$

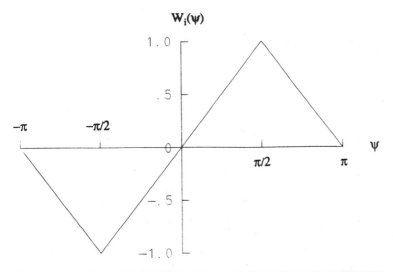

FIG. (2) PHASE WEIGHTING FOR IMAGINARY COMPONENT

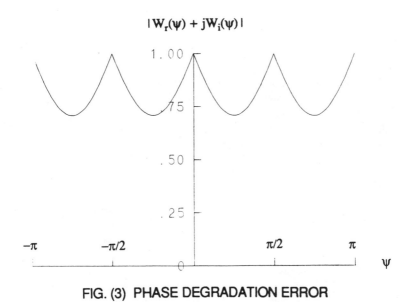

FIG. (3) PHASE DEGRADATION ERROR

and

$$\text{Im}\{p(k)\} \cong C \sum_{n=1}^{N} A(n) \ W_i[\psi(n,k)] \tag{15}$$

$$= C\left\{\sum_{n=1}^{N} A(n) - \frac{2}{\pi} \sum_{n=1}^{N} A(n) \mid \{\psi(n,k) - \frac{\pi}{2}\}_{\text{mod } 2\pi} \mid \right]$$

This technique is mainly designed for phase-only processing and the computational simplification is largely due to the elimination of the EXP operations and the reduction of the number of multiplications. If the amplitude is also included in the image formation, there is not significant reduction of the number of multiplications and the saving will be in terms of the replacement of the complicated EXP operations which remains effective for large multidimensional arrays.

Degradation Error

Computation is one of the key parameters in high-resolution imaging reconstruction. Because computation simplification is the main objective of the proposed technique, it is important to examine the trade-off in terms of image degradation.

The basic difference between the conventional phase-only technique and the proposed simplified version is the replacement of the exponent operations with phase weighting functions given by Eqs. (10) and (11). The amplitude of $\exp(j\Phi)$ is unity for all phase angles. This simple property is important to the consistency of the vector accumulation and cancellation effects. However, for the weighting function pair, the amplitude is a function of the phase and is not a constant. It can be calculated that the variation of the amplitude is a periodic function with period $\pi/2$ with the peak values are unity and are located at $\Phi = 0$ and $\pi/2$.

$$\mid \dot{W}_r(\psi) + jW_i(\psi) \mid = \left[1 - \frac{4}{\pi} \psi + \frac{8}{\pi^2} \psi^2\right]^{1/2} \tag{16}$$

The minimum value is 0.707 at $\Phi = \pi/4$. This implies that the norm of the weighting is not invariant to the mean of the phase clustering position and it gives a 3dB maximum error. This effect can be seen from Fig. (3). For complex source distribution, this may result in degradation to the images. However, it can be restored by a simple compensation factor. For real source distribution, the results have little degradation especially when N is large.

Spectral estimation using discrete Fourier transform (DFT) can be also described as a simple phase correction operation because the kernel of DFT is a phase-only variation. DFT is often applied to holographic image reconstruction, especially when the receiving apertures are in the Fresnel or Fraunhofer regions where the impulse response of the image formation filter can be approximated by the Fourier transform kernel [19,20]. Here we first use DFT as an example to demonstrate the approximation by using the weighting method. Suppose that only the phase of a finite (128-point) complex sequence is given and the amplitude is not available for processing. Fig. (4-a) is the phase-only estimate of the spectrum using direct DFT. The phase-only estimate of the spectrum using phase density distribution weighting is shown by Fig. (4-b).

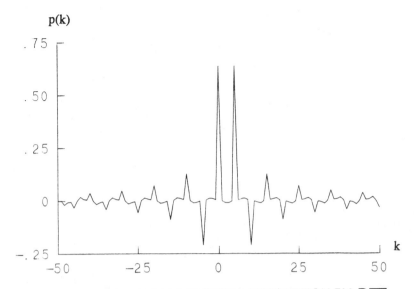

FIG. (4A) PHASE-ONLY SPECTRAL ESTIMATION BY DFT

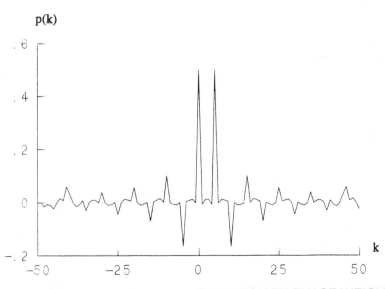

FIG. (4B) PHASE-ONLY SPECTRAL ESTIMATION BY PHASE WEIGHTING

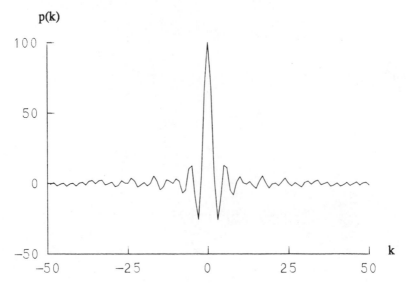

FIG. (5A) PHASE-ONLY RECONSTRUCTION BY PROPAGATION

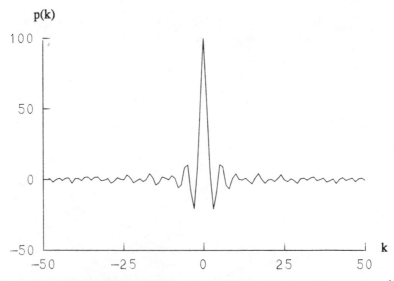

FIG. (5B) PHASE-ONLY RECONSTRUCTION BY PHASE WEIGHTING

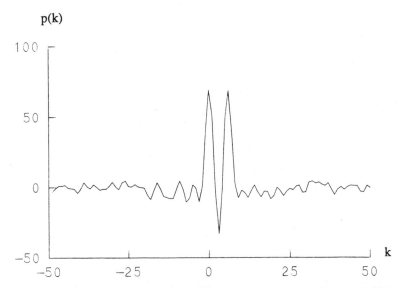

FIG. (6A) PHASE-ONLY RECONSTRUCTION BY PROPAGATION

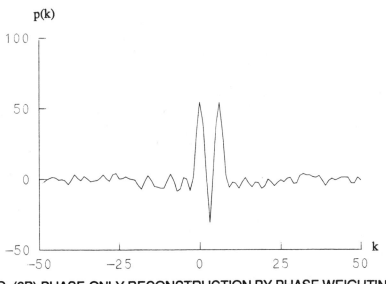

FIG. (6B) PHASE-ONLY RECONSTRUCTION BY PHASE WEIGHTING

Then we apply this technique to phase-only acoustical image reconstruction. Fig. (5-a) is the phase-only reconstruction of a centered target by using backward propagation, and Fig. (5-b) is the reconstruction using the weighting approach. Fig. (6-a) is the phase-only backward propagated image of two adjacent point sources, and Fig. (6-b) shows the reconstruction of the same source distribution by the weighting technique. These results indicate that the weighting method has compatible performance and sensitivity.

Conclusion

The key objective of computation simplification for phase-only acoustical holography considered in this paper is to replace the exponential and trigonometric operations in image formation by simpler low-order mathematical functions. This is because the exponential and trigonometric operations are routinely computed by using power series expansion and can be tedious when the processing array size and dimension becomes large.

Phase-only techniques are originally used in holography and have been applied to computation simplification in terms of coding bit-rate reduction. However, when we study the image formation process of phase-only reconstruction, we observe the direct relationship between the resultant image values and the vector accumulation and cancellation effects. Therefore, we propose to use the phase density distribution of the vectors as the indicator to predict the image formation. This allows us to bypass the mathematical operations used in conventional image reconstruction.

In this paper, we first introduce the basic concept of phase-only imaging based on the concept of phase density distribution. Then we provide the fundamental guidelines for the alternative mathematical operation for consistent image formation and present an approach using phase weighting as an example. The degradation due to this approximation is also briefly discussed. Phase-only reconstructions with backward propagation and Fourier transformation (Fresnel or Fraunhofer approximation of backward propagation) are used to demonstrate the performance and sensitivity of this approach.

Acknowledgment

This research is supported by the National Science Foundation under Grants IST-8409633 and ENG-8451484, Motorola Inc., and Hughes Aircraft Co.

References

1. A. J. Devaney, "A Filtered Backpropagation Algorithm for Diffraction Tomography," *Ultrasonic Imaging,* vol. 4, 1982, pp. 336-350.
2. A. J. Devaney, "Inverse Source and Scattering Problem in Ultrasonics," *IEEE Transactions on Sonics and Ultrasonics,* vol. SU-30, no. 6, November 1983, pp. 355-364.
3. Hua Lee, Carl Schueler, Glen Wade, and Jorge Fontana, "Digital Reconstruction of Acoustical Holograms in the Space Domain with a Vector Space Approximation," *Acoustical Imaging,* vol. 9, K. Wang, Ed., Plenum Press, New York, pp. 631-641, 1980.
4. Hua Lee and Glen Wade, "High-Resolution Imaging for Systems with Small Apertures," *Journals of Acoustical Society of America,* 72(6), pp. 2033-2035, December 1982. IEEE Computer Society Press, pp. 240-246, 1982.
5. Hua Lee and Glen Wade, "Constructing an Imaging Operator to Enhance Resolution," *Journals of Acoustical Society of America,* 75(2), pp. 499-504, February 1984.

6. Hua Lee, "Formulation of the Generalized Backward Projection Method for Acoustical Imaging," *IEEE Transactions on Sonics and Ultrasonics,* vol. SU-31, no. 3, pp. 157-161, May 1984.

7. Hua Lee, "Resolution Enhancement by Wavefield Extrapolation," *IEEE Transactions on Sonics and Ultrasonics,* vol. SU-31, no. 6, pp. 642-645, November 1984.

8. Hua Lee, "Resolution Enhancement of Backward Propagated Images by Wavefield Orthogonalization," *Journals of Acoustical Society of America,* 77(5), pp. 1845-1848, May 1985.

9. Hua Lee, "Inverse Filter Design for Holographic Imaging Systems with Small Apertures," *Acoustical Imaging,* vol. 14, A. J. Berkhout, J. Ridder, L. F. van der Wal Eds., Plenum Press, New York, pp. 715-718, 1985.

10. Hua Lee, "Optimal Reconstruction Algorithm for Holographic Imaging of Finite Size Objects," *Journals of Acoustical Society of America,* June 1986.

11. Hua Lee and Glen Wade, "Evaluating Quantization Error in Phase-Only Holograms," *IEEE Transactions on Sonics and Ultrasonics,* vol. SU-29, no. 5, pp. 251-254, September 1982.

12. Hua Lee and Glen Wade, "Analysis and Processing of Phase-Only Reconstruction in Acoustical Imaging," *Proceedings on Physics and Engineering in Medical Imaging,* IEEE Computer Society Press, pp. 240-246, 1982.

13. Hua Lee and Glen Wade, "Sampling in Digital Holographic Reconstruction," *Journals of Acoustical Society of America,* 75(4), pp. 1291-1293, April 1984.

14. Hua Lee, "Image Reconstruction for Planar Acoustic Tomography using Hexagonal Arrays," *Acoustical Imaging,* vol. 14, A, J. Berkhout, J. Ridder, and L. F. van der Wal Eds., Plenum Press, New York, pp. 319-328, 1985.

15. A. F. Metherell, "The Relative Importance of Phase and Amplitude in Acoustical Holography," *Acoustical Holography,* vol. 2, Metherell Ed., Plenum Press, Chapter 14, 1969.

16. John Power, John Landry, and Glen Wade, "Computed reconstructions from Phase-Only and Amplitude-Only Holograms," *Acoustical Holography,* vol 2, Metherell Ed., Plenum Press, Chapter 13, 1969.

17. A. V. Oppenheim and J. S. Lim, "The Importance of Phase in Signals," *IEEE Proceedings,* vol. 69, no. 5, pp.529-541, May 1981.

18. Hua Lee and Glen Wade, "Resolution Enhancement on Phase-Only Reconstructions," *IEEE Transactions on Sonics and Ultrasonics,* vol. SU-29, no. 5, pp. 248-250, September 1982.

19. Glen Wade, "Plane-Wave Approach to Fresnel and Fraunhofer Diffraction," *IEEE Transactions on Sonics and Ultrasonics,* vol. SU-15, no. 1, January 1968.

20. Hua Lee and Glen Wade, "Resolution for Images from Fresnel or Fraunhofer Diffraction using FFT," *IEEE Transactions on Sonics and Ultrasonics,* vol. SU-29, no. 2, p. 151, May 1982.

A FREQUENCY DIVERSITY METHOD OF REDUCING

SPECKLE IN WIDEBAND ULTRASOUND IMAGES

B.A. McDermott and F.L. Thurstone

Department of Biomedical Engineering
Duke University
Durham, NC   27705

ABSTRACT

A set of concurrent real-time B-mode image lines has been formed
using a parallel processing system. In this system, a wideband received
echo is partitioned by frequency diversity filtering and separate image
lines are formed. Due to their differing constituent frequencies, these
lines have decorrelated speckle patterns. The amount of speckle in the
displayed image is reduced upon averaging these image lines. The reduction
in image speckle and the accompanying improvement in perceived resolution
is accomplished with no sacrifice of temporal resolution or display
format. The effects of filter separation and amplitude apodization of the
received frequency spectrum are investigated through statistical analysis
of images containing speckle producing targets. A measurable increase in
image signal-to-noise ratio has been achieved.

INTRODUCTION

Medical ultrasound images are used in the diagnosis of numerous
health problems. Ultrasound brightness-mode (B-mode) images are produced
by transmitting insonifying pulses into the target in a line by line
format with the amplitude of the returned echo used to modulate the
intensity of a CRT display. A major advantage of this imaging format is
that it permits the real-time display necessary to view moving objects
such as a beating heart. The resulting images contain a granular structure
known as speckle. This speckle is the result of constructive and destructive interference of the ultrasound waves as they reflect off scattering
sites in the target. The presence of speckle, a phenomemon peculiar to
coherent imaging systems, has been shown by Kozma and Christensen [1] to
reduce perceived resolution in optical systems by up to a factor of seven.
In ultrasound images this speckle is viewed as an undesirable property of
the image, since the speckle masks small differences in the displayed grey
levels. Consequently, the reduction of image speckle has been a major area
of investigation in ultrasound imaging research.

Image integration or compounding has been studied as the primary
technique for reducing speckle. Images of the same object containing
different speckle patterns have been created by varying such imaging
parameters as transmit and receive frequency, transducer aperture, burst

length, and interrogation angle [2-12]. Unfortunately, the majority of these efforts have relied on the averaging of serially obtained images, making them incompatible with a real-time display format without a reduction in image size.

A new process has been implemented which produces simultaneous image lines with dissimilar speckle patterns. These image lines, which contain echo data about the same spatial line in the target, may then be averaged to accomplish speckle reduction, while still maintaining a real-time display format. This process, which we have called frequency diversity, is an extension of a signal processing technique first used to increase signal-to-noise ratios in radio communications. As applied to ultrasound imaging, it allows full-size, real-time images to be produced with a reduction in image speckle.

THEORETICAL BACKGROUND

The degree of success in reducing speckle with this frequency diversity process hangs on the rate of speckle decorrelation with frequency. There have been numerous investigations into methods of frequency compounding to reduce speckle. Since the transmit-reflection-receive process in ultrasound imaging is linear, it is possible to implement the frequency compounding in either the transmit or receive functions. Magnin [5] varied the transmit center frequency and burst length to produce images with decorrelated speckle patterns. The transmit center frequency was varied on a frame to frame basis and thus precluded any real-time imaging. He also showed that the use of longer burst lengths, which led to a more rapid decorrelation of images, had the adverse effect of decreasing range resolution. Trahey [6] performed experiments investigating the simultaneous use of spatial and frequency compounding. In these experiments, a variation in transmit center frequency was accompanied by a lateral translation of the transducer. Once again, a real-time display format was sacrificed in order to accomplish speckle reduction.

Entrekin and Melton [7] produced images with decorrelated speckle patterns by transmitting a wideband pulse and receiving on an annular array whose annuli had different center frequencies. This work was applicable to real-time imaging systems, however sector scanning with such a device would require mechanical manipulation of the transducer and it would not be compatible with phased array systems. Gelbach's [8,9] extensive computer simulations and experiments demonstrated mathematically that speckle patterns decorrelate rapidly with changing frequencies. He achieved large increases in image signal-to-noise ratio through digital filtering of the received echo information, although processing times were as large as one hour per frame. Yoshida [10] carried out computer simulations which partitioned the received frequency spectrum and compared an incoherent versus a coherent summation. These works all suggested that significant improvements in displayed images can be obtained, provided that the image degrading speckle can be adequately decorrelated through selective frequency filtering. In order to preserve the real-time display format, we have chosen to use narrowband filtering in the receive process to create parallel imaging channels with decorrelated speckle patterns.

PROCEDURE AND RESULTS

The Filters

The frequency diversity process uses bandpass filters to partition the received frequency spectrum into separate imaging channels. Figure 1

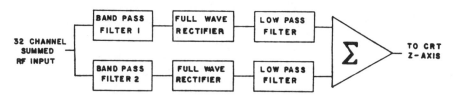

Fig. 1. Block diagram of a two channel frequency diversity process.

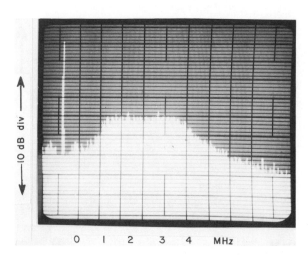

Fig. 2. Received frequency spectrum from a sponge at 7cm range in
a water tank.

shows a block diagram of a frequency diversity processing scheme as it is
applied to the 32 channel Duke phased array imaging system. This
simplified diagram shows a 2 channel processor, while the actual frequency
diversity hardware used is designed to allow for the addition of up to 10
narrowband image lines. The filters selected have a quality factor (Q =
center frequency/bandwidth) of approximately six. After the summed RF data
is partitioned by the bandpass filters, each frequency diversity channel
is passed through detection circuitry consisting of a full-wave rectifier
and a triple-pole lowpass filter. An analog summation of the individual
channels is then performed with the output going to the z-axis (brightness) control of the CRT display.

Each of the image lines produced by the method described above is
formed of dissimilar constituent frequencies due to the actions of the
bandpass filters. Consequently, the speckle patterns of each should be
different. Should the lines have completely decorrelated speckle patterns,
the summed line should demonstrate a $\sqrt{N}$ improvement in signal-to-noise
ratio; where N is the number of averaged lines.

Measurement Techniques

A sponge was selected for use as a speckle producing target in our
experiments. This selection was based on two important considerations.
First, the cell size of the sponge is sufficiently small (.2 mm) that it
is well below the resolution limits of the ultrasound machine used. This
results in an image which contains no resolvable targets and is completely

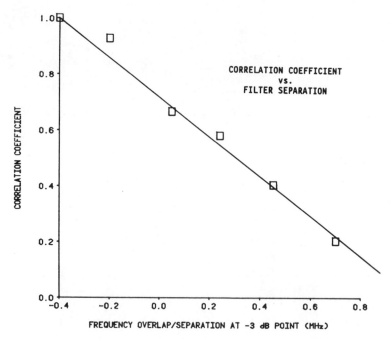

Fig. 3. Graph of correlation coefficient between images made with
varied center frequency of the narrowband filter.

filled with speckle. The second factor influencing our decision to use
this sponge was the broad, relatively flat frequency response it
produced. Figure 2 shows the received frequency spectrum from the sponge
at 7 cm in a water tank, when imaged by the Duke phased array machine. The
transducer used for the experiments was built with trapezoidal elements
which produces an extended bandwidth at the expense of decreased sensitivity.

To determine the relationship between filter separation and correlation coefficient [13], images of the same region of interest in the sponge
were produced using a single narrowband channel at various center frequencies. The desired images were digitized by a Vidco Graphic Memory and
read into a Digital VAX 11/780 for analysis. Since the filters used have a
constant Q, the bandwidth of the filters increases with increasing frequency. Consequently, center frequency separation alone is not an accurate
descriptor of the relationship between a given filter pair. This is
accommodated for by using the frequency overlap or separation at the -3 dB
point, as a measure of filter separation. As seen in the results in figure
3, negative values along the x-axis represent an overlap at the -3 dB
point while positive values represent a separation between the -3 dB
points of a filter pair.

The filter configuration we selected to investigate, consisted of four
narrowband filters evenly spaced across the received frequency spectrum of
the sponge. Figure 4 shows the frequency response of the sum of four
filters with a combined -3 dB bandwidth spanning from 1-3 MHz. The speckle
reduction in the frequency diversity images was computed using the method
proposed by Burckhardt [11]. He proposed that the reduction in speckle

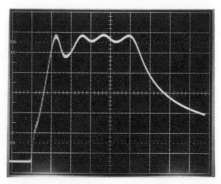

Fig. 4. Combined frequency response of four narrowband filters with
center frequencies of 1.25, 1.75, 2.25, and 2.75 MHz.

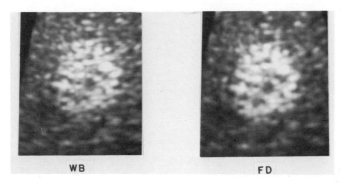

Fig. 5. Images of a positive contrast lesion made with wideband (WB)
processing and frequency diversity (FD) processing.

could be quantized in terms of increased signal-to-noise ratio in an area
with no resolvable targets. The signal-to-noise ratio of the region is
defined as follows:

$$SNR = \mu/\sigma \qquad (1)$$

where: μ = mean brightness of the speckle pattern
σ = standard deviation of the brightness levels in
the speckle pattern

The frequency diversity images displayed an average of a 17 percent
increase in signal-to-noise ratio over the conventional wideband images.
Again, this was computed using the sponge as a target, and the result of 25
comparisons between wideband and frequency diversity images of a given
region of interest with no resolvable targets. Figure 5 shows a comparison
between images of a low contrast lesion in a Lopez-Smith Contrast-Detail
Phantom. It can be seen that the frequency diversity process has increased
the contrast of this lesion.

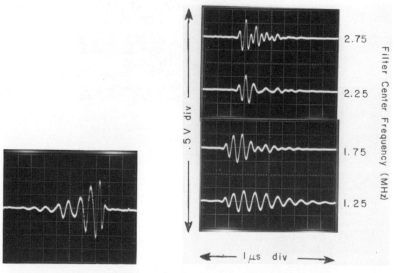

Fig. 6. Received RF sum from a wire target at 7 cm in a water tank. The horizontal scale is 1 us/div.

Fig. 7. Narrowband filtered pulses from a wire target.

Pulse Stretching

There was some concern that the narrowband filters would stretch the received pulse, and thus reduce speckle at the expense of a reduction in the range resolution of the system. The presence of any pulse stretching was investigated by looking at the received echo pulse from a wire target in a water tank. Figure 6 shows the received RF sum at the input to the bandpass filters. In Figure 7 the pulse has been passed through the four narrowband filters. The narrowband filters with the lower center frequencies do indeed elongate the pulse when compared to the wideband pulse. However the upper bandpass filters have a narrower pulse than the wideband and the effects of summing these four filters depend on the interactions of the four signals. The detected sum of these narrowband filters is compared to the detected wideband response in figure 8. When using the −6 dB pulse width as a measure of the range resolution, we found that the range resolution of the narrowband sum was equivalent to that of the wideband process. The pulse stretching in the frequency diversity processed pulse does not become apparent until the received pulse has decreased by −10 dB from its peak. At the −12 dB point, the frequency diversity pulse has stretched to 2.1 us, compared to a 1.6 us pulse width for the wideband pulse. This corresponds to a .75 mm reduction in range resolution of a low contrast target. It can be seen from figure 7 that the source of this stretching is predominantly the 1.2 MHz center frequency narrowband filter. The fact that filters with a constant Q were used implies that as the center frequency decreases, the bandwidth will also be reduced, thus increasing pulse stretching.

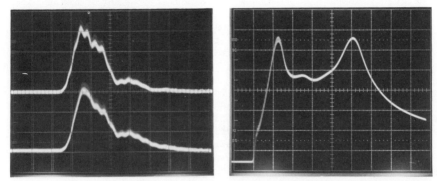

Fig. 8. Detected pulses from conventional wideband processor (top) and frequency diversity processor (bottom). The horizontal scale is 1 us/div.

Fig. 9. Frequency response of the sum of four narrowband filters with increased weighting on the outer filters.

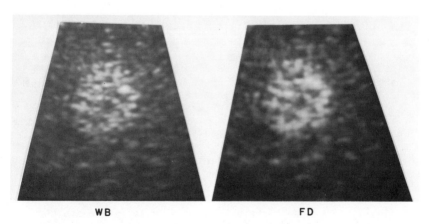

WB   FD

Fig. 10. Images of a positive contrast lesion made with wideband (WB) processing and a weighted sum in the frequency diversity (FD) process.

Amplitude Weighting

The flexibility of our filter hardware allows the weighting of the narrowband filters to be easily manipulated. By increasing the weighting of the outside two narrowband filters over the two center bands, we hoped to further increase the signal-to-noise ratio over the evenly weighted case. Figure 9 shows the linear sweep frequency response with the two center filters weighted -3 dB less than the peaks for the outer narrowband filters. Since the inner filters contain image data which is more highly correlated than that in the outer filters, reducing the contribution of the center filters should increase the effective number of independent images used to produce the displayed image.

A pair of images of a positive low contrast lesion in the Lopez-Smith phantom can be seen in figure 10. The frequency diversity image displays greater contrast than the conventional wideband image. The frequency diversity image also appears to be smoothed, partially a result of the increased contribution of the lower frequency narrowband filter. The measured increase in image signal-to-noise ratio for the sponge target was only 12 percent, less than that for the evenly weighted filters.

DISCUSSION

Our experiments demonstrated that the signal-to-noise ratio of a B-mode image can be increased by a frequency diversity process. An estimate of the increase in SNR for the frequency diversity images can be calculated using the graph of the relationship between correlation coefficient and filter separation, and Trahey's [13] equation for the variance of the sum of n partially correlated images:

$$\sigma^2 \frac{\sum\limits_{k=1}^{n} X_k}{n} = \frac{n+2 \sum\limits_{k=1}^{n} \sum\limits_{j=k+1}^{n} \rho(X_j, X_k)}{n^2} \sigma^2(X) \qquad (2)$$

Each X_i in equation 2 is an N by N array of pixels which are added on a point by point basis. The expression on the left-hand side represents the variance of a simple average. The variances of the individual images, $\sigma^2(X)$, are assumed to be equal. If the correlation coefficients between images, $\rho(X_j, X_k)$, are determined from the graph in figure 2, the effective number of independent images being summed from the four narrowband filters is 1.8. This results in a μ/σ increase of 34 percent for a composite image with equal weighting on the narrowband filters.

The discrepancy between our experiment results and the calculated SNR was somewhat disheartening, but may be partially accounted for by a number of contributing factors, the most likely of which is stationary system noise in the image due to the synchronous operation of the ultrasound imaging machine. A second contributor could be any aggregate structure in the target. Both of these factors, if present, will result in static information in the image which will not change as a function of frequency, thus creating more highly correlated images. This is reflected in our signal-to-noise calculations as a reduction in the anticipated signal-to-noise ratio increase.

In our experiments with amplitude weighting of the filters, we chose to reduce the weighting of the two center narrowband filters rather than to completely omit them, because we felt it necessary to include all of the limited receive echo information we had. By discarding the information in the center of the frequency spectrum, we would be effectively reducing the amount of target information used to create an image. Since the electrical noise of the system is a consideration, and it would increase in relative magnitude with respect to the target information, we saw very little probability of increasing the image signal-to-noise ratio by simply removing the two center narrowband filters from the summation. As was seen in our results, we did not achieve the anticipated increase in signal-to-noise ratio by increasing the weighting of the outer narrowband filters. We attribute this mainly to system noise and also look to the low transducer sensitivity as a possible contributor.

CONCLUSION

The frequency diversity process has been shown to be an effective method of reducing image speckle in real-time display format. The process is most applicable to systems with a wideband transmit pulse. While this process was implemented on a phased array system, it could be easily installed on a mechanical sector scanner. Since there is a limited amount of information available from each received echo pulse, it is obligatory to use as much of the received spectrum as possible. Maintaining a complete span of the received echo spectrum is especially important in transmission through a medium which is frequency dependent. Frequency dependent absorption will cause a downshifting of the received spectrum, thus further limiting the signal available for display. One possible application of amplitude weighting of the narrowband filters would be to compensate for this frequency dependent absorption. Although our results from amplitude weighting were clouded by system noise, we feel that it is an important avenue of investigation.

Frequency diversity filtering proves to be an easily implemented process which gives a moderate increase in image signal-to-noise ratio with no significant degradation in range resolution. By reducing the speckle contrast in ultrasound images, frequency diversity processing caused the structural information in the target to become more apparent.

ACKNOWLEDGEMENTS

This work was supported in part by National Heart, Lung and Blood Institute Grant HL12715.

REFERENCES

[1] Kozma, A., and Christensen, C.R., "Effects of Speckle on Resolution," J. Opt. Soc. Amer., Vol. 66, No. 11, pp. 1257-1260, Nov. 1976.

[2] Korpel, A., Whiteman, R.L., and Ahmed, M., "Elimination of Spurious Detail in Acoustical Images," Acoustic Holography, Vol. 5, pp. 373-390, 1975.

[3] Bartum, R.J. Jr. and Crowe, H.C., "Ultrasound Echo Averaging: A Simple Method for Improving Image Perception," J. Clinical Ultrasound, Vol. 8, pp. 63-64, 1980.

[4] Galloway, R.L., A Trimodal Parallel Processing System for Speckle Reduction in B-Mode Ultrasound Images, Thesis Dissertation, Duke University, December, 1983.

[5] Magnin, P.A., von Ramm, O.T. and Thurstone, F.L., "Frequency Compounding for Speckle Reduction in Phased Array Images," Ultrasonic

Imaging, Vol. 4, pp. 267-281, 1982.

[6] Trahey, G.E., Allison, J.W., Smith, S.W., and von Ramm, O.T., "Simultaneous Frequency and Spatial Compounding for Increased Speckle Reduction," Ultrasonic Imaging, 8, p. 68. (abstract)

[7] Entrekin, R. and Melton, H.E., "Real Time Speckle Reduction in B-Mode Images," IEEE Ultrasonics Symposium Proceedings, pp. 169-174, Sept. 1979.

[8] Gelbach, S.M., Pulse Reflection Imaging and Acoustic Speckle, Thesis Dissertation, Stanford University, March 1983.

[9] Gelbach, S.M., and Sommer, F.G., "Frequency Diversity Speckle Processing," Ultrasonic Imaging, 8, p. 67. (abstract)

[10] Yoshida, C., Nakajima, M., and Yuta, S., "Real-Time Speckle Reduction in Ultrasound Echo Imaging", Proceedings of the Fourth Meeting of the World Federation for Ultrasound in Medicine and Biology, Sydney, Australia, July, 1985. (abstract)

[11] Burckhardt, C.B., "Speckle in Ultrasound B-Mode Scans," IEEE Trans. on Sonics and Ultrasonics, SU-25, No. 1, pp. 1-6, Jan. 1978.

[12] Trahey, G.E., Smith, S.W., and von Ramm, O.T., "Speckle Pattern Correlation with Lateral Aperture Translation: Experimental Results and Implications for Spatial Compounding", IEEE Trans. Ultrasonics, Ferroelectrics, and Frequency Control, 33(3), pp. 257-264, 1986.

[13] Papoulis, A., Probability, Random Variables, and Stochastic Processes, McGraw Hill Book Co., New York, 1965.

ULTRASONIC PHASE TOMOGRAPHY FOR MEDICAL APPLICATIONS

J. A. Berry, H. W. Jones and M. Mieszkowski*

Engineering Physics Department, Technical University of
N.S., P. O. Box 1000, Halifax, N.S., B3J 2X4, and *Physics
Department, Dalhousie Univ., Halifax, N.S., B3H 3J5

ABSTRACT

In an earlier paper, we presented the data to be expected from
tomographic experiments on a phantom. The phantom contained elements with
two different sound velocities. The numerical study made three different
assumptions. The first being based on simple ray tracing, the second using
straight paths between transmitter and receiver and the third using a
diffraction solution using the Rytov approximation. None of these
approaches models the situation exactly. The ray tracing neglects
scattering and diffraction effects; the straight line path neglects
refraction as well those previously mentioned. The diffraction solution
assumes a large area coherent wavefront incident on the object being
evaluated; a wavefront which it is not practically possible to produce.

This paper reports experimental measurements on a phantom nearly
identical to that assumed in the numerical studies referred to earlier.` The
accuracy with which the various models fit the data is commented on and an
empirical hybrid model which more accurately represents the situation is
presented.

INTRODUCTION

The problems of acoustical tomography arise from the fact that sound
travels at velocities which vary with the transmission medium. Associated
with this is the related refraction and the phenomenon of scattering. These
effects make the reconstruction techniques applicable to x-rays of only
limited use in ultrasonic tomography. It will be argued in this paper that
there is no generally acceptable method of reconstruction for either phase
or amplitude acoustical tomograms. In our work, we are concerned about
conditions which exist in soft tissue so that the velocity range of the
ultrasound is relatively limited, roughly in the range of 1400 to 1600 m/s,
consequently, our comments are made with these circumstances in mind.

Our experiments, to date, have been associated with a phantom made of
gelatine in a background of water. We hope we have chosen a shape which
presents geometrical difficulties for the pixel array, in that the boundaries
of the gelatine shapes cross the pixel boundaries to enclose very variable
areas. We have been concerned to obtain the most accurate phase (or
velocity) tomograms possible and we have much concerned ourselves with the

sources of error in the tomographic reconstruction process. In order to do this, we have taken every care within the limits of our circumstances to obtain accurate tomographic data and then evaluate the errors which have appeared in the reconstruction. This work has not yet reached a stage at which we are achieving the accuracy which we are seeking but we have, we believe, made sufficient progress for it to be reasonable to report the results to date.

EXPERIMENTAL ARRANGEMENTS

Experimental work has been directed to obtaining acoustical velocity or phase tomograms for a 31 x 31 pixel array of, initially, a phantom with sound velocities ranging from about 1450 to 1600 m/s. The phantom chosen is shown in figure 1. This was made by making molded gelatine elements and

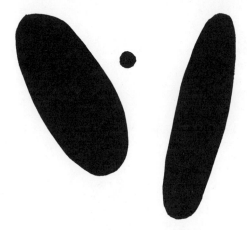

Figure 1   Gelatine phantom

mounting them on a metal supporting plate and immersing the assembly in a tank of water. This arrangement is shown in figure 2. The vertical rod holding the phantom can be rotated about its axis by a stepping motor driven mechanism and the rotation is repeatable to better than 0.01°. A pair of 4 mm diameter 2.25 MHz transducers capable of producing a short pulse in water are mounted a fixed distance apart. These transducers scan the

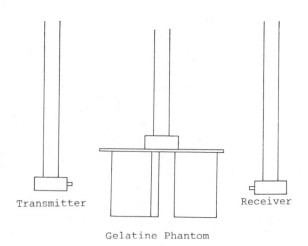

Transmitter   Receiver

Gelatine Phantom

Figure 2   Assembly in water tank

80

phantom by moving along a fixed traverse which is controlled by an accurately made mechanical assembly. Distance measurements are made by a machine tool inductive tape measuring system. A series of 30 scans of the phantom are made, advancing the phantom 6° after each scan. The data obtained from these scans is in two parts, that giving the relative position of the phantom and the traverse position of the transducers and that which can be interpreted as the time of flight. It is from this data that reconstructions are made.

As we require accurate reconstructions, it is essential that the time of flight be determined as accurately as possible. Apart from calibrating the system in distilled water at a known temperature, every effort was made to develop a method of time of flight measurement which was as accurate as our resources allowed. After some consideration, we used a system based on a 32 MHz digital sampling system (LeCroy Model TR8837 Transient Recorder).

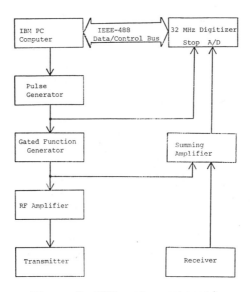

Figure 3   TOF system schematic

The process used is shown in figure 3. Essentially, the transient recorder is set running and the electronic driving and receiving pulses are fed to the digitizer and a digital record obtained. Typical signal profiles for the transmission and received signals are stored in the computer and used in a cross-correlation technique to identify the time of flight. We have spent some time investigating this system and conclude that, with the signal to noise ratios that we observe, this allows a time of flight to be determined to an accuracy of several nanoseconds. Figure 4 indicates the errors which have been determined in our time of flight studies. It should be noted that there are many factors involved in the time of flight errors - jitter and drift in the electronic sampling arrangements, and those associated with the clock which controls the digital sampling, as well as the errors arising from data processing. In practice, it is the data processing that gives the largest contribution to the final errors. It must be noted that the velocity of sound determination suffers from errors which arise due to the uncertainty in the determination of the precise distance between the transducers. One factor associated with this uncertainty in the distance is that associated with the transducer response given the need for the sound to penetrate the piezoelectric material. Fortunately, we are not primarily concerned with absolute velocities but rather with the relative velocities in the phantom. We have attempted, as mentioned earlier, a calibration

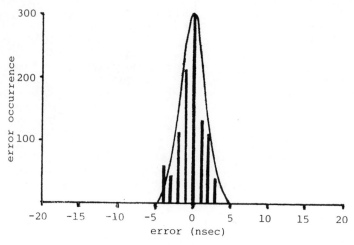

Figure 4   TOF error

based on the reported velocity of sound in distilled water[1] at a closely controlled temperature. In order to evaluate the velocity of sound in the gelatine portion of the phantom directly, slices of the phantom material were used in separate velocity of sound experiments. Some difficulties arise in such measurements in that the velocity changes with the time the gelatine elements have been immersed in water. This effect leads to gradations of velocity at the edges of the phantom. Our measurements, consequently, have an uncertainty at the outer edges of about ± 5 m/s. The mean velocity across the specimen is known to an accuracy of 2.5 m/s. Further work on the closer determination of velocities is presently in progress.

RECONSTRUCTION STUDIES

Table I

Tissue	Velocity (m/s) (± 2%)
Fat	1435
Kidney	1565
Liver	1580
Muscle	1580
Spleen	1570

Velocity of sound in various tissues at 37°C.

Questions of reconstruction are concerned with the relative effects of refraction, scattering and diffraction which take place in the phantom. The velocity range which is to be expected in our studies is shown in Table 1 and figure 5[2,3]. These quantities give definition to a basic quantity which

82

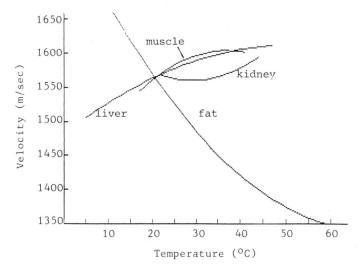

Figure 5   Velocity vs. temperature for several tissues

is used in obtaining the Rytov or Born approximation[4].   This point is demonstrated below.   Suppose we write for the wave equation:

$$\nabla^2 \psi + \frac{\omega^2}{c^2(r)} \psi = 0 \tag{1}$$

where c is the velocity of sound at some point signified by r in the image field.   If c_o is the background velocity, then (1) may be rewritten as:

$$\nabla^2 \psi + \frac{\omega^2}{c_o^2} \psi - \omega^2 (1 - (c_o^2/c^2(r)))\psi = 0 \tag{2}$$

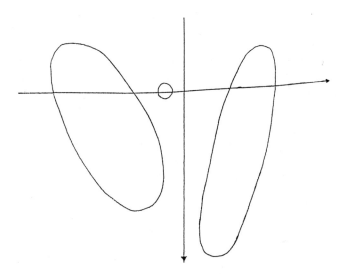

Figure 6   Refracted ray

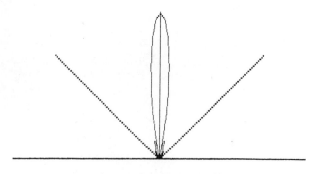

Figure 7   Beam profile

The quantity $(1 - (c_o^2/c^2(r)))$ is now significant in the approximation
referred to. In our case, this is less than 0.13 and typically has a value
in the region of about 0.09, i.e., it is a small perturbing effect. We have
traded on this fact in our attempts at reconstruction. This can be put
another way, see figure 6 in which a plot of the refracted ray is shown.
The ray is nearly a straight line. Figure 7 shows the predicted beam
profile from our transducers. The aperture of the receiving transducer
determines to a considerable extent the observed diffraction effects. A
similar comment could be made about the extent of the scattering. The point
about the smallness of the perturbing effect can perhaps be explained by the
following considerations: From equation (2) if $F(r) = k^2(1 - c_o^2/c^2(r))$,
where $k = \omega/c$. Then (2) becomes:

$$(\nabla^2 + k^2)\psi = F(r)\psi \tag{3}$$

If the object of interest is contained in a sphere of radius a, then
$F(r) = 0$, for $|r| > a$ and this is satisfied by setting the velocity to c_o
for all $|r| > a$.
Equation (3) can be transformed to a Ricatti equation by setting

$$\psi = e^u \tag{4}$$

Using this substitution in (3) we get:

$$\nabla^2 u + (\nabla u)^2 + k^2 = F(r) \tag{5}$$

If we choose to solve equation (3) by supposing that $F(r)$ to be a small
perturbation, then the solution is called Born's first approximation[5]. The
solution of (5) to a first order approximation is known as Rytov's
approximation.

Solutions of ψ and u are assumed to be developed in a power series as
below:

$$\psi = \psi_o \, (1 + \psi_1 \epsilon + \psi_2 \epsilon^2 + \ldots) \tag{6}$$

$$u = u_o + u_1 \epsilon + u_2 \epsilon^2 + \ldots \tag{7}$$

Equations (3) and (6) give:

$$(\nabla^2 + k^2) \psi_o = 0 \tag{8}$$

$$\nabla^2 \psi_1 + 2 \, \frac{\nabla \psi_o}{\psi_o} \cdot \nabla \psi_1 = F(r) \tag{9}$$

and higher order equations. Equations (5) and (7) give:

$$\nabla^2 u_o + (\nabla u_o)^2 + k^2 = 0 \tag{10}$$

$$\nabla^2 u_1 + 2 \cdot (\nabla u \cdot \nabla u_1) = F(r) \tag{11}$$

and high order equations. Equations 8 and 9 show that ψ_1 or u_1 become vanishingly small as F(r) becomes vanishingly small. This allows us to treat the reconstruction problem in the following manner:

a)   we assume that F(r) = 0. This allows us to use any method of reconstruction which is presently used with x-rays. By this assumption, we obtain an initial approximate reconstruction.

b)   next, we assume that F(r) does not equal zero but has a "small" value which can be obtained from the reconstruction already available (from a). We then generate a set of data from this reconstruction, comparable to that which has been obtained experimentally, using the Rytov approximation.

c)   we compare this data with the original experimental data and produce by, respective, subtraction "difference data". This data is used with the reconstruction method invoked in a) above to produce a reconstruction of a difference tomogram.

d)   we amend the initial reconstruction by the difference tomogram.

e)   we repeat b) through d) in an iterative routine.

Numerical studies are in hand to explore the effectiveness of this technique with increasing values of F(r); these studies will be published later.

EXPERIMENTAL RESULTS

In reviewing the experimental results, a comment is needed on the time of flight data. The time of flight data is collected from sound which traverses the phantom in approximately straight lines. Given that the velocity of the sound in the gelatine is higher than that of water, it follows that the time of flight must, apparently, be less when gelatine is traversed than it would have been had water only been the propagation medium. Figure 8 shows that this is not what is observed; times of flight longer than the equivalent water path are observed. This effect can be

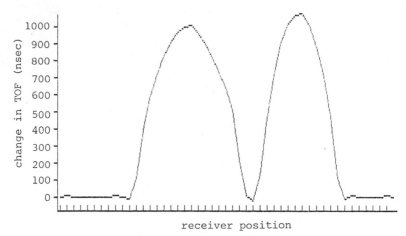

Figure 8 TOF profile

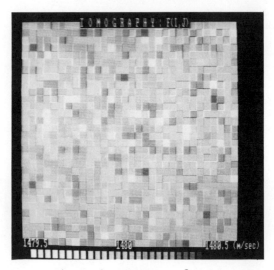

Figure 9 Tomogram of water

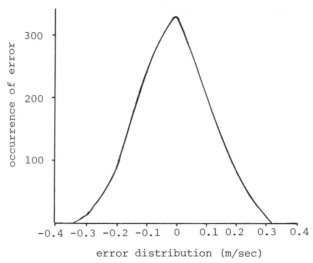

Figure 10 Error analysis of water tomogram

accounted for by noting that the net received signal integrated over all paths within the receiver aperture lead to signals which have phase changes indicating a longer time of flight. We have confirmed this finding by calculations using the Rytov approximation.

The simplest tomogram to reconstruct is one in which the velocity is everywhere constant and the data for this can be readily obtained by collecting experimental data in the tank in the absence of a phantom. The resulting tomogram is shown in figure 9. This tomogram indicates an rms error of 0.11 m/s and a maximum error of 0.35 m/s. Figure 10 shows the error analysis. Clearly, in this case, the use of iterative routines is pointless, but this test gives us confidence that the basic reconstructive program and the data collection system work satisfactorily.

Next, measurements were made with the phantom described earlier. Measurements of the time of flight were made at 30 different angles. A black and white version of the original false colour tomogram is shown in figure 11. It is essential that we must be able to obtain repeatable results when a phantom is removed and replaced. We have found that the errors involved in the repeatability tests were 0.2 m/s rms and 0.6 m/s maximum.We are of the opinion that improved mechanical arrangements can substantially reduce these figures.

Next, we compared the phantom reconstruction obtained by the recursive procedure outlined earlier, with the measurements made on the gelatinous

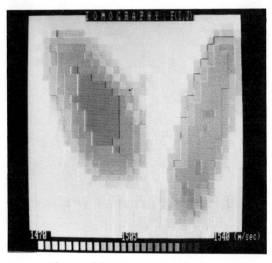

Figure 11   Tomogram of phantom

material of the phantom, within the limits of the uncertainty which were mentioned earlier. It is to be noted that the measurements of velocity in the gelatine were uncertain to 5 m/s, principally because of the uncertainties in the measurement of the length of the gelatine samples. Second, water "soaked" into the outside of the phantom elements and reduced the velocity in the gelatine by about 15 m/s, locally. Figure 12 shows the reconstruction we obtained and figure 13 the error tomogram. The rms error is 5.8 m/s. The rms errors after one and two iterations was 5.2 m/s in each case. If we are able to assume an error in our determination of the gelatine velocity, then these errors are substantially reduced and initial calculations indicate an error of ± 1 m/s rms. We do not, however, at this time, have the physical evidence to make this assumption, although detailed error analysis suggests that this assumption should be valid.

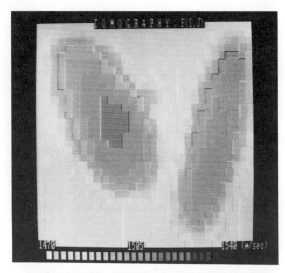

Figure 12   Tomogram after correction

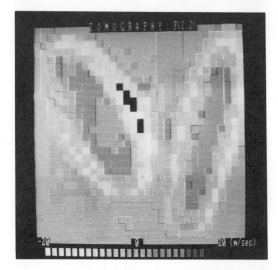

Figure 13   Error map of tomogram

CONCLUSION

This paper has discussed the process of tomographic reconstruction as
it might apply to soft tissue.   The basic mathematical and physical problems
of phase tomography relating to such circumstances have been described.
Some experimental work on phantoms has been outlined.   The accuracy of the
time of flight data collection has been discussed.   Errors in the
tomographic reconstruction have been the subject of some analysis and
discussion.   We conclude that there are good prospects in these
circumstances for obtaining tomographic reconstructions with errors of less
than 1 m/s.

REFERENCES

1. V. A. Del Grosso, Remarks on Absolute Sound Speed Measurements in Water, JASA, 45, pp. 1287, 1969.

2. S. A. Goss, R. J. Johnson and F. Dunn, Comprehensive Compilation of Empirical Ultrasonic Properties of Mammalian Tissue, JASA, Vol. 64, pp. 423, 1978.

3. R. C. Chivers and R. J. Parry, Ultrasonic Velocity and Attenuation in Mammalian Tissues, JASA, Vol. 63, pp. 940, 1978.

4. G. Wade, R. K. Mueller and M. Kaveh, Proc. IFIPTC4 Working Conference on Computer Aided Tomography and Ultrasonics in Medicine (Edited by Raviv, Greenleaf and Herman), pp. 165-215, North Holland Publishing Company, 1979.

5. M. Born and E. Wolf, Principles of Optics, Pergamon Press, 3rd ed., p. 453.

IMPROVED TISSUE CHARACTERIZATION USING SCATTERING IMAGES

P. Nauth, P. Pfannenstiel, E.-G. Loch, and
W.v. Seelen

Gessellschaft zur Förderung der Forschung an der DKD
Aukammallee 33, 6200 Wiesbaden, West Germany

The improvement of spatial resolution as well as the reduction of the noise level led to a remarkable progress in ultrasonics during the last years.

As, however, the acquisition of sound images by means of a demodulated reflected signal and its visual evaluation has been maintained, the boundaries of organs or pathological tissues are clearly visible.

As to tissue differentiation, however, many problems occur due to an insufficient evaluation of information both concerning the acquisition and the evaluation of images.

To understand the information which has been neglected in the course of image acquisition it is necessary to analyse the physical causes of the different types of sound-tissue-interaction which can be used for imaging. We distinguish between specular reflection, absorption and scattering.

Specular reflection occurs at the boundary of two media which are characterized by different acoustic impedances and diameters bigger than the wave-length λ one.

Absorption is essentially based upon friction and relaxation effects. Part of the sound energy is transformed into heat. The degree of this transformation effect depends on the chemical composition of the medium.

Scattering occurs in connection with particles which are smaller or about as big as the wave length one, i.e. in connection with cells or cell formations. Size and distance of the scattering particles as well as their fluctuation of compressibility, density and sound speed play an important role in the determination of type and intensity of the scattered parts.

When comparing the three types of sound-tissue-interaction one discovers that information about tissue contours is primarily furnished by specular reflection whereas attenuation and scattering - being correlated with the tissue structure - are likely to give information about tissue differentiation.

Reflected and backscattered signals lead to the generation of B-images which contain information about the contours and the structure of tissues. Due to the demodulation of the received sound waves it is often impossible, however, to differentiate these two parts. Furthermore B-images make no use of the angle-dependence of the signal which is necessary for the evaluation of the total scattering information. The frequency characteristics are neglected as well. Thus differential diagnosis can only make use of the so-called speckles which are produced by interference. As well it is often possible to draw indirectly conclusions from the contours as far as tissue differentiation is concerned. As to an improved differential diagnosis the deduction of physical tissue characterizing parameters from sound signals would be desirable though.

One possibility is to measure the attenuation being the energy loss caused in absorption and scattering. The impact of attenuation on tissue characterization has been examined by various research groups discovering, i.e. in liver tissue, differences between the absorption coefficients of normal and pathological organs. As however, attenuation measurements from the reflected signal are possible with a bad spatial resolution, this method is only seldom applied in clinical routine.

As scattering is correlated with the structure of tissues and is, for theoretical reasons, expected to have only minor problems as to spatial resolution, extensive studies concerning scattering depending on tissue structure have been carried out by our group.

The measurement of scattering is shown in fig. 1. The tissue or phantom probe can be fixed in the middle, the two transducers - transmitter and receiver - are grouped circularly around

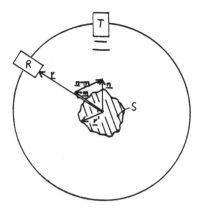

Fig. 1 Measurement equipment for ultrasonic scattering
(T: transmitter, R: receiver, S: specimen)

it. The length of vector $\underline{r}$ represents the distance between
probe and receiver.

The propagation of sound can be described by the Helmholtz
equation. If the medium is inhomogeneous and the inhomogenity
is caused by fluctuations γ_c of the sound velocity c_0, part of
the incident wave P_0 is scattered. For the scattered pressure
P_s we get

$$\vec{\nabla}^2 P_s + k^2 P_s = -2k\gamma_c P_0 .$$

If there are very small scatterers, and if the distance
$\underline{r}$ between the scattering volume and the receiver is large, the
solution of the differential equation is given by /1/

$$P_s(\omega,\beta) = P_0(\omega)\, e^{jkr}\, \frac{1}{2\pi c_0^2}\, \int \gamma_c(\underline{r}')\, e^{j\underline{K}(\omega,\beta)\,\underline{r}'}\, d^3\underline{r}'$$

with $k = \omega c_0^{-1}$
$\underline{K} = k(\underline{n}-\underline{m})$
$\beta = $ scattering angle

This equation is a product of the incident wave $P_0(\omega)$, the
delay e^{jkr} and the part which describes the scattering behav-

93

iour. This term we substitute for G_s

$$G_s = P_s(\omega,\beta)P_0^{-1}(\omega)e^{-jkr}$$

which is the so called scattering transfer function. This function depends on the frequency ω as well as on the scattering angle β. Under the assumption of very small scatterers the frequency dependence will have an exponent of 2, otherwise it will be less than 2.

We developed a special equipment to measure scattering of tissues and phantoms. In the middle of a cylindric water tank the probe is fixed, a broadband transducer is used as transmitter. The scattered waves can be received either by a second transducer or by an acoustic-optical receiver. In order to measure at each scattering angle, the receivers can be turned around the probe. For the acoustic-optical receiver we use a laser beam, which is deflected proportional to the gradient of pressure. This deflection can be measured by a photo diode. The advantages of the laser system is a broadband-frequency-characteristic and a high sensibility. Furthermore the laser beam does not disturb the wave field.

The aim of our phantom scattering measurements was to prove whether different structures were correlated to different scattering behaviour. The phantoms consisted of silicon with glass spheres in it, having diameters of 75 µm. The mean distance between the glass scatterers was 0.3mm at one phantom and 0.5mm at the other phantom, but the arrays were not regular.

Fig. 2 shows an example of the scattered pressure amplitude in dependence of the scattering angle we measured from the phantom with a lower scatterer density. Fig. 3 demonstrates the angle-dependence of the phantom with a higher concentration of scatterers. This phantom is characterized by a higher mean scattered pressure and more maxima in dependence of the scattering angle than the other one. Therefore the scattered amplitude and the angle dependence can be used to differentiate these two phantoms.

As both phantoms were equal in diameter to the scatterers, frequency dependence could not be used as a parameter to distinguish between the two samples except for the information derivable from the fluctuation of frequency.

94

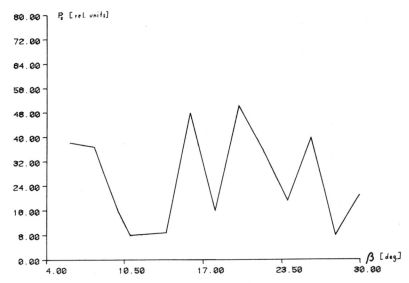

Fig. 2   Scattered pressure P_s of the phantom with lower scat-
          terer density as a function of the scattering angle ß
          (relative to the direction of backscattering).

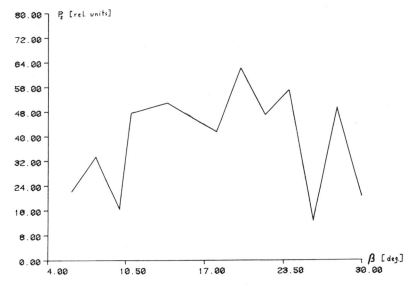

Fig. 3   Scattered pressure P_s of the phantom with higher
          scatterer density as a function of the scattering
          angle ß.

In order to get a quantitative parameter to characterize
several tissues and diseases we measured the scattering pressure and computed a scattering coefficient /2/ which is the
scattering transfer function per unit volume averaged over
the scattering angles. The scattering coefficients of muscle,
liver, uterus, uterus myoma, kidney and kidney carcinoma in
dependence of the frequency are demonstrated in fig. 4. The
datas are based on 180 experiments.

Our results show a great difference between these tissues,
i.e. at 2.7 MHz the scattering coefficient of liver is 2.6 times
higher than that of muscle tissue. The differences between
normal uterus and uterus myoma are more than 100%. The frequency
can be used as well to distinguish between normal and tumorous
uterus. The scattering coefficient of kidney is 3 times higher
than that of kidney carcinoma.

Using scattering in clinical routine, it is necessary
to visualize this information. Therefore we developed a method
to compute scattering images. Before a graphic representation
of the scattering information is possible, the lateral and
axial position of each scattering volume as well as the actual
scattering angle have to be computed.

The lateral distance was given by the displacement inter-
valls ▲d of the tissue probe perpendicular to the direction
of the transmitted sound impulse.

In a circular equipment (fig. 5) with a radius r, the
incident impulse needs the time t to pass the way x to a scatteri
volume and the way $\tilde{x}$ back to the receiver. Therefore the axail
distance of the volume is

$$x = ct - \tilde{x}$$

Using the cosinus equation x can be computed by

$$x = \sqrt{x^2 + a^2 - 2xa\cos\alpha}$$

The distance a between the transducers is given by

$$a = \sqrt{2r^2 - 2r^2\cos\tilde{\beta}}$$

for transducer, receiver and the middle of the equipment are
a symmetric triangle.

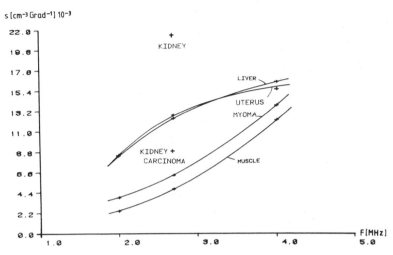

Fig. 4   Scattering parameter of various tissues as a function
of frequency

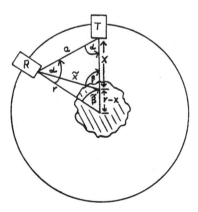

Fig. 5   Correction of the geometric shift (T: transmitter,
R: receiver)

Combining these three equations we get

$$x = ct - \sqrt{x^2 + 2r^2(1-\cos\beta) - 2xr\sqrt{2-2\cos\tilde{\beta}}\,\cos\frac{180°-\tilde{\beta}}{2}}$$

Then

$$x = \frac{(ct)^2 - 2r^2(1-\cos\tilde{\beta})}{2(ct - r\sqrt{2-2\cos\tilde{\beta}}\,\cos\frac{180°-\tilde{\beta}}{2})}$$

The scattering angle ß depends on t and ß for

$$\beta = \arccos\frac{ct - 2r^2 + 2r^2\cos\tilde{\beta}}{2x(ct-x)}$$

Therefore with the knowledge of t, ▲d and ß the position of a scattering volume and the actual scattering angle is given. The reconstruction of a scattering image is possible by this data.

A scattering image of muscle of 30 degree scattering angle is shown in fig. 6a. Fig. 6b shows muscle tissue at an angle of 50 degrees The angle dependence can be demonstrated computing the difference between the two scattering images. The difference image is shown in fig. 6c. One can see a structure which is not part of the original scattering images and which means addition- al information for tissue characterization. Fig. 6d approximates the mean scattered pressure being the mean value of both scat- tering images.

Comparing the B- and scattering images of the two phantoms, characterized by 0.3mm and 0.5mm mean scatterer distances, one gets interesting results. Using a B-image both phantoms have similar textures and grey levels (fig. 7). Measuring the scat- tering angle dependence at each point of the phantoms and gen- erating a scattering image by these datas, the phantoms can be differentiated very clearly (fig. 8). These scattering images represent the number of maxima per 100 degrees.

After the acquisition of an image, the problem of evaluation is given. This problem exists for B-images as well as for scat- tering images. Since the evaluation is insufficient in many cases, we developed a pattern recognition system. The first step after the acquisition is the image preprocessing, which can be a lin- ear and a non-linear filtering to reduce the noise-level or to improve the contrast. Then several parameters are computed from

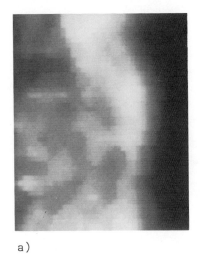

a)

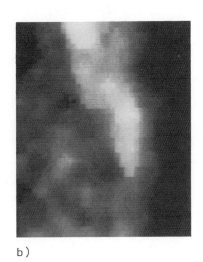

b)

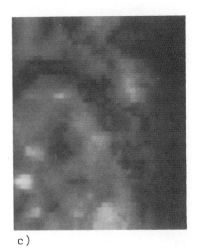

c)

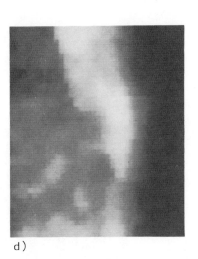

d)

Fig. 6   Scattering images of muscle

      a) amplitude   ß=30°

      b) amplitude   ß=50°

      c) difference

      d) sum

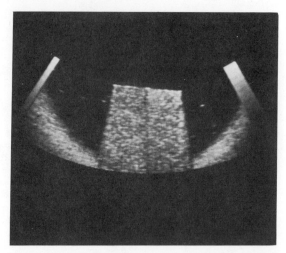

Fig. 7 B-image of phantoms with different scatterer
density

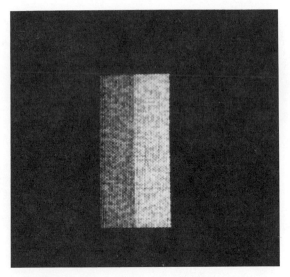

Fig. 8 Scattering angle image of phantoms with
different scatterer density

the image. In a third step this parameter vector is classified by a linear classifier.

These algorithms now are used for pattern recognition in B-images very successfully, but can also be used for the analysis of scattering images. Therefore the texture features have to be substituted for the scattering parameters or, in order to combine B- and scatter images the feature vector must be enlarged. So the total information, the specular reflection, the amplitude-, angle- and frequency-information of the scattering and, if useful, the attenuation can be used to characterize tissues.

REFERENCES

/1/ Waag, R.C.
   Theory and measurements of ultrasonic scattering for tissue characterization
   Acoustical Imaging Vol. 9
   Plenum Press, New York and London, 1980

/2/ Nauth, P.
   Entwicklung von Verfahren zur sonographischen Gewebedifferenzierung durch digitale Bildverarbeitung und Auswertung von Ultraschall-Streusignalen
   Thesis, Johannes-Gutenberg-University, Mainz, 1985

TRANSIENT ACOUSTIC SCATTERING IN DISPERSIVE SOFT TISSUE

S. Finette

Department of Biomedical Engineering
Rutgers University
Piscataway, NJ 08854 USA

ABSTRACT

A number of equations that have been used recently to describe pulse propagation and scattering in soft tissue can be solved numerically using a recently developed spectral approach. An example of transient scattering is presented for a simple system consisting of a two-dimensional curved line radiator and a circular absorbing region with frequency dependent attenuation.

INTRODUCTION

The physical basis for ultrasonic imaging in soft tissue is currently under investigation by several researchers, and a number of discrete and continuous scattering models have been introduced to describe propagation and scattering of acoustic waves in this medium. This is an important step in understanding the relationship of the gray scale sonogram to both the incident pulse shape and the acoustic properties of soft tissue.

In order to include the effects of frequency dependent attenuation, an important property of soft tissue, Leeman and coworkers (Leeman, 1980; Leeman et al., 1981, 1982; Hutchins and Leeman, 1982, Jones and Leeman, 1985) have proposed and studied several wave equations capable of describing pulse propagation and scattering in this context. Phenomenological terms in these equations can be chosen to fit attenuation and absorption data for a number of tissue types. A major assumption in the solution of these equations is that the scattering is weak (the first Born approximation): $P_s(\bar{r},t) \ll P_i(\bar{r},t)$ where $P_s(\bar{r},t)$ and $P_i(\bar{r},t)$ represent the scattered and incident acoustic fields, respectively. This simplification allows the solution for $P_s(\bar{r},t)$ to be written as an integral over the scattering volume. Unfortunately, the integral cannot be evaluated explicitly for any but the simplest spatial distributions of bulk modulus, density, etc. With regard to soft tissue acoustic imaging, the validity of the first Born approximation has recently been questioned for both the forward and inverse scattering problems (Bly et al., 1985; Azimi and Kak, 1983). It is therefore of interest to develop numerical approaches for solving such problems without invoking the weak scattering approximation.

THEORY AND IMPLEMENTATION

We wish to point out here that efficient numerical solutions can be obtained for some of the above mentioned models for arbitrary spatial distributions of tissue parameters and realistic pulse shapes. The solution includes all orders of multiple scattering because the only approximations to the original partial differential equation are those related to discretization. The approach we are using involves a generalization of a spectral method originally developed by Bojarski (1982, 1985) for nondispersive media and extended to dispersive media by Finette (1986a) and Compani-Tabrizi (1986). In the latter paper, spatial variations in density were also included. As an example, the following wave equation proposed by Leeman and Jones (1985) can be solved using the spectral approach:

$$\nabla^2 P(\bar{r},t) - \frac{1}{c^2(\bar{r})} \frac{\partial^2 P(\bar{r},t)}{\partial t^2} - 2A\frac{\partial P(\bar{r},t)}{\partial t} + B^2 P(\bar{r},t)$$

$$+ \frac{1}{\rho(\bar{r})} \bar{\nabla}\rho(\bar{r}) \cdot \bar{\nabla}P(\bar{r},t) = 0 \tag{1}$$

where $\rho(\bar{r})$, $c(\bar{r})$ represent the density and wave speed within the tissue, A and B are phenomenological constants chosen to fit the data on absorption and attenuation in soft tissue. Outside the tissue, we assume $\rho=\rho_0$, $c=c_0$, and A=B=0 so that Eq. (1) reduces to the nondispersive wave equation.

The general solution of Eq. (1) can be written as the sum of incident and scattered fields $P(\bar{r},t) = P_i(\bar{r},t) + P_s(\bar{r},t)$. The incident field may be evaluated using an impulse response approach, and it can be written as a convolution integral (Penttinen and Luukkala, 1976):

$$P_i(\bar{r},t) = -\frac{\rho_0}{2\pi} \frac{\partial v_n(t)}{\partial t} * h(\bar{r},t) \tag{2}$$

where $v_n(t)$ is the normal component of velocity of the transducer's surface and $h(\bar{r},t)$ is the impulse response of the transducer, depending only on geometric properties of the source. The scattered field at any point $\bar{r}$ outside the scattering volume can be written concisely as an integral equation

$$P_s(\bar{r},t) = \iiint f(\bar{r}',t) * \frac{\delta(t - \frac{|\bar{r}-\bar{r}'|}{c_0})}{4\pi|\bar{r}-\bar{r}'|} d^3\bar{r}' \tag{3}$$

with

$$f(\bar{r},t) = \left[\frac{1}{c_0^2} - \frac{1}{c^2(\bar{r})}\right] \frac{\partial^2 P(\bar{r},t)}{\partial t^2} - 2A\frac{\partial P(\bar{r},t)}{\partial t}$$

$$- \frac{1}{\rho(\bar{r})} \bar{\nabla}\rho(r) \cdot \bar{\nabla}P(\bar{r},t) - B^2 P(\bar{r},t) \tag{4}$$

104

The temporal convolution in the integral equation (3) is between the space-time Green's function for outgoing waves and a "source" term $f(\bar{r},t)$, which vanishes outside the tissue comprising the scattering region. Boundary conditions at the transducer surface and at infinity are accounted for in Eqs. (3) and (4), respectively, while the initial condition on the pressure distribution and its derivative limit the solution to times $t>0$.

The spectral method can be applied to Eq. (3) following the approach described recently for variable density problems (Compani-Tabrizi, 1986). Without going into details here, the basic idea is to write Eq. (3) as an equivalent set of coupled equations for the sources in real space ($\bar{r}$ space) and the fields in the spatial Fourier domain ($\bar{k}$ space). After discretization, the solution can be obtained at a given time step by determining the new source function based on the field distribution in the previous time increment, transforming to Fourier space and then calculating the new field distribution. The transient pressure field at time t is determined by an inverse Fourier transform of the scattered field at each time step.

The numerical solution of a full three-dimensional scattering problem such as described by Eqs. (1) or (3) involves a number of difficulties, regardless of the numerical method chosen (Finette, 1986b). For example, in order to form a single sector scan image from the back-scattered waves, approximately one hundred scattering problems would have to be solved, one for each transducer orientation. A huge amount of data must be stored and processed in an efficient manner for the solution to be obtained in a reasonable period of time. The size of the data base strains even the main memory of today's Class VI supercomputers. Consider transient pulse scattering from a cube of tissue 5 cm. on a side, with the transducer placed on one face of the cube. This corresponds to the contact scan mode commonly used in clinical examinations. The spatial discretization cell Δx must be less than or equal to $\dfrac{\lambda_{min}}{2}$ where λ_{min} is the minimum wavelength associated with a broadband pulse describing the incident field. The upper limit is determined by the sampling theorem and is rarely applicable in practice. A more reasonable choice is $\Delta x \cong \dfrac{\lambda_{min}}{5}$, and for an ultrasonic pulse used in medical imaging applications with a center frequency of 3 Mhz; one would require roughly 10^6 pixels to adequately resolve the scattering region. For each pixel, at least seven 32 bit words must be stored to describe the incident and scattered fields, bulk modulus, density, and other quantities necessary to compute the solution. This exceeds the main memory (4 M words, 64 bits/word) of the CYBER 205 supercomputer we are currently using for these simulations. The CYBER 205 is a virtual memory machine and efficient software design is necessary to limit the number of page faults encountered when data is shifted from virtual to main memory and vice versa. Eight-way concurrent I/O is supported on the system, and this will alleviate some of the I/O problems when we implement the full three-dimensional scheme.

For our initial work we have limited ourselves to two space dimensions. We have incorporated realistic pulse shapes in our simulations by using Eq. (2) for the incident field calculation. The impulse response for curved line radiators can be evaluated analytically (Mastey and Finette, 1985) and convolved numerically with an appropriate source excitation term to yield the incident pressure distribution. The number of CPU seconds per time step necessary to obtain a solution of the scattering problem is dominated by the speed of the fast Fourier

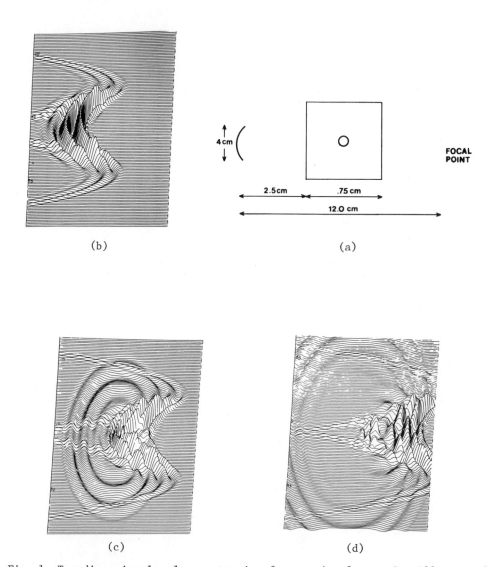

(b)

(a)

FOCAL
POINT

4 cm

2.5cm   .75 cm

12.0 cm

(c)

(d)

Fig. 1. Two-dimensional pulse scattering from a circular region illustrated
in (a). A curved line radiator of focal length 12.0 cm. from the data window
emits a pulse, calculated from Eq. (2), and enters the data window. In (b),
the pulse has just reached the left edge of the object and in (c-d) diverging
waves are clearly visible.

.transform (FFT) algorithm used to map between $\bar{r}$ and $\bar{k}$ space. The CYBER 205 supports a vectorized FFT, and timing tests show that only .2 CPU seconds per step are needed for a 256x256 spatial grid, assuming the constant density case; with variable density, an additional .2 seconds per time step is needed if only one central processor is used. This is an improvement in speed over an equivalent nonvectorized FFT algorithm by a factor of thirty.

SIMULATION EXAMPLE

In Fig. 1 we present a sequence of fixed time snapshots of two-dimensional pulse scattering for a system consisting of a single curved line radiator and a circular absorbing object with frequency dependent attenuation. The rectangular region in Fig. 1(a) (not drawn to scale) corresponds to a data window of size 128x128 pixels in which the scattering calculations are performed and displayed in Fig. 1(b-d). There are no restrictions on its placement relative to the transducer. The excitation pulse properties are described in Mastey and Finette (1985). In Fig. 1(b-d) the pulse enters the data window moving to the right. It encounters a circular inhomogeneous region centered on the transducer axis, and characterized by $c(r)=.5c_0$, A=.3 and B=.1. The density is assumed constant throughout the window, so that the gradient term in Eq. (4) does not contribute to the scattering. A complex scattering distribution is seen in the last two snapshots, as the incident pulse passes through the inhomogeneous region.

CONCLUSION

A method has been discussed which allows simulation of acoustic wave scattering in dispersive media mimicking soft biological tissue. The model is flexible in that we can choose a variety of incident pulse configurations and tissue parameter distributions. The Born approximation is not necessary in this formulation, and the only approximations introduced in the solution of the wave equation are those related to discretization. The model is not limited to pulse-echo scattering, but can be used to study angular as well as transmissive effects.

ACKNOWLEDGMENT

This work was supported in part by NSF Grant ECS-84-04786.

REFERENCES

Azimi, M., and Kak, A. C., 1983, Distortion in diffraction tomography caused by multiple scattering, IEEE Trans. Medical Imaging MI-2:4: 176-195.

Bly, S. H. P., Foster, F. S., Patterson, M. S., Foster, D. R., and Hunt, J. W., 1985, Artifactual echoes in B-mode images due to multiple scattering, Ultrasound in Med. & Biol. 11:99-111.

Bojarski, N. N., 1982, The k-space formulation of the scattering problem in the time domain, J. Acoust. Soc. Am. 72:570-584.

Bojarski, N. N., 1985, The k-space formulation of the scattering problem in the time domain: An improved single propagator formulation, J. Acoust. Soc. Am. 77:826-831.

Compani-Tabrizi, B., 1986, K-space scattering formulation of the absorptive full fluid elastic scalar wave equation in the time domain, J. Acoust. Soc. Am. 79:901-905.

Finette, S., 1986a, A computer model of acoustic wave scattering in soft tissue, IEEE Trans. Biomed. Eng., to appear.

Finette, S., 1986b, Ultrasonic scattering in soft tissue: A computer simulation approach. Submitted to IEEE Trans. UFFC.

Hutchins, L., and Leeman, S., 1982, Tissue parameter measurement and imaging, in: "Acoustical Imaging," 11, J. P. Powers, ed., Plenum Press, NY, pp. 127-137.

Jones, J. P., and Leeman, S., 1985, A new wave equation for the propagation and scattering of ultrasound in tissue, Ultrasonic Imaging 7 Abs.:105.

Leeman, S., 1980, Ultrasonic pulse propagation in dispersive media, Phys. Med. Biol. 25:481-488.

Leeman, S., Hutchins, L., and Jones, J. P., 1981, Bounded pulse propagation, in: "Acoustical Imaging," 10, P. Alais and A. Metherall, eds., Plenum Press, NY, pp. 427-435.

Leeman, S., Hutchins, L., and Jones, J. P., 1982, Pulse scattering in dispersive media, in: "Acoustical Imaging," 11, J. P. Powers, ed., Plenum Press, NY, 139-147.

Mastey, P., and Finette, S., 1985, The impulse response and transient field of a curved ultrasonic line radiator, Proc. 11th Ann. Northeast Biomed. Eng. Conf., W. S. Kuklinski and W. J. Ohley, eds., IEEE Press, pp. 189-191.

Penttinen, A., and Luukkala, M., 1976, The impulse response and pressure near field of a curved ultrasonic radiator, J. Phys. D: Appl.Phys., 1547-1557.

ESTIMATION OF ACOUSTIC ATTENUATION IN DIFFUSE LIVER DISEASE: CAN IT BE DONE

WITH THE ZERO-CROSSING TECHNIQUE?

Andre Duerinckx†, John Hoefs*, Catherine Cole-Beuglet*,
P.V. Sankar°, Dennis Fleming°, and Paul Chandler°

†Veterans Administration Medical Center, Long Beach, CA 90822
*Departments of Medicine & Radiological Sciences
University of California, Irvine
°Department of Electrical Engineering
University of California, Irvine

ABSTRACT

In-vivo attenuation measurements of the liver have been obtained in 41 patients with diffuse liver disease, 8 normal controls and a liver phantom. Using a spectral shift approach, a parameter S (in MHz/cm), the slope of zero-crossings of A-line data vs. depth was measured to estimate the slope of the attenuation coefficient with frequency, denoted by β (in dB/cm-MHz). 1 MByte of digitized data per ultrasound procedure and per liver was used to estimate the slope S. Three different acoustic transducers were used. The patients were classified by histopathological structure following blind readings of liver needle biopsies.

No correlation was found between the degree of portal fibrosis or fat and the estimate of the acoustic attenuation. The observed range of attenuation estimates in 8 normal controls was 0.23-0.73 dB/cm MHz using three different transducers. The variability in controls was similar to the variability in a liver tissue equivalent phantom. No statistical significant difference in slope of attenuation for five disease groups compared to each other and controls was found. We conclude that a spectral shift technique using small amounts of digitized data for liver is inadequate to estimate acoustic attenuation in liver.

INTRODUCTION

One approach to ultrasonic tissue characterization (TC) has been the use of a spectral-shift algorithm using the counting of zero-crossings, to estimate the slope β (in dB/cm-MHz) of change of acoustic attenuation α (f) with frequency.[1,2,3] With this technique the range of attenuation values for normal volunteers or phantoms is wide: 0.3-0.9 dB/cm MHz.[2] In addition, these studies also show an unacceptable statistical overlap in the range of acoustic attenuation for different types of liver disease. This statistical overlap could limit the use of this acoustic property for in vivo ultrasound examinations.

Ophir et al.,[4,5] taking measurements on a tissue-mimicking phantom, found that to obtain an accurate "global" estimate of acoustic attenuation over a depth of 5.5 cm, one needs over 100,000 A-lines per measurement. On the other hand, Kuc,[6] using a theoretical model to derive a lower bound for the error on the attenuation estimate for both spectral-difference and spectral-shift techniques, seems to suggest that the measurement of attenuation is possible using a smaller amount of digitized data. He and Greenleaf[7] used 25 independent A-lines over a depth of 5 cm to calculate a "global" estimate of attenuation in a homogeneous phantom. He et al.[7] showed a significant increase in the error on a "local" estimate of attenuation with decreasing number of A-lines when using the zero-crossing technique.

A double-blind prospective study of the relative range of attenuation slope (β-values) estimates obtained in phantoms, normal volunteers and patients with chronic diffuse liver disease using zero-crossing measurements was undertaken to compare the statistical spread of the estimates. No attempt was made to establish the accuracy or bias of the estimates. The ranges of the zero-crossing estimates were analyzed to determine if the spread is too large to allow the differentiation of liver pathology from normal histology.

METHOD

A modified real-time scanner (Philips SDR2500) was used to collect digitized RF data along A-lines in a region of interest (ROI) within a longitudinal view of the liver. Digitization of the reflected RF ultrasound data was done at 25 MHz using an 8-bit digitizer.

Attenuation Measurements

Phantom: Serial attenuation measurments were performed using three different transducers on a commercially available liver tissue mimicking phantom (ECOBLOC).

Eight normal volunteers with no history of disease or recent alcohol intake had three attenuation studies, each using a different ultrasound transducer.

Forty-one patients from the Liver Clinic at UCI Medical Center who had recent liver biopsies and stable liver disease had attenuation measurements in six ROI on six different longitudinal views of the liver (Fig. 1). Each ROI can contain 120 A-lines with over 4,000 samples per A-line.

Liver biopsies were read blind by a full-time histopathologist. A subjective grading system was used for portal fibrosis (0-5), fat (0-4), and sinusoidal collagen (0-3).

The number of zero-crossings was calculated over a 128 sample point window, which was shifted by 8 sample points for each calculation, giving a 93% overlap between windows for each consecutive calculation. The slope S of the change in numbers of zero-crossings with depth was estimated using a least-square straight line fit to the data. The slope S of zero-crossing versus depth (in MHz/cm) was converted to a "calculated β ", the slope of attenuation versus frequency, using the equation:

$$\beta = \frac{-S}{2\sigma^2}$$ (1)

where σ is the spectral variance, and S the measured slope. Equation 1 ignores non-linear frequency dependence of attenuation, frequency dependent diffraction filtering, and frequency dependent refraction filtering due to specular reflectors.

No diffraction corrections were made to the data prior to estimating the number of zero-crossings. Ophir[3,4] has shown that this is not essential for the zero-crossing technique. Moreover, the purpose of our study was not to determine the bias in our β estimates, but rather to evaluate the relative range of β-values.

Statistical Analysis

The attenuation, clinical and laboratory parameters in each stable etiologic group (primary biliary cirrhosis, autoimmune chronic active hepatitis, chronic viral hepatitis, and miscellaneous) were compared by Student's t-test analysis using the SPSSX statistical package. The degree of portal fibrosis was correlated by linear regression analysis in 21 stable patients with 0-1+ hepatic fat. The degree of hepatic fat was correlated with attenuation by linear regression analysis in 17 stable patients with 0-1+ portal fibrosis. A p-value less than .05 was considered statistically significant.

Data Selection

Approximately 20% of all the collected A-line data was rejected on the basis of technical B-scan inadequacies which included (1) ROI depth from the anterior abdominal wall was less than 4 cm; (2) the slope S of zero-crossing was positive or zero; (3) unacceptable noise levels in the far field.

RESULTS

Patient Population and Biopsy

Liver biopsies were adequate on 36 of the 41 patients. The majority of patients had minimal fat with varying degrees of portal fibrosis. Ten patients had minimal portal fibrosis and varying degrees of hepatic fat. The relative influence of fat and portal fibrosis on acoustic attenuation, using a narrow-band attenuation estimation technique, has been reported elsewhere.[2]

Attenuation

The range of β values for the phantom, the normal volunteers, and the 41 patients with liver pathology is shown in Figure 2. The β ranged from 0.31-0.63 dB/cm MHz for 12 measurements on the ECOBLOC, and from 0.23-0.73 dB/cm MHz for 23 measurements on 8 normal volunteer livers. If we eliminate the smallest and largest measurements in normal liver, we still have a range of 0.36-0.63 dB/cm MHz for 21 measurements on 8 volunteer patients with normal livers. If we separate the range for β by transducers, we get the following: 0.40-0.73 dB/cm MHz for transducer #3; 0.36-0.58 dB/cm MHz for transducer #5; and 0.23-0.50 dB/cm MHz for transducer #7.

The only statistical significant difference by Student's t-test analysis found between normals and the five disease categories was for autoimmune chronic active hepatitis (ACAH) (p = 0.023). No correlation was found between β and fat or fibrosis for all disease groups considered (Fig. 3).

DISCUSSION

The zero-crossing techniques for the estimation of acoustic attenuation in liver and in well-characterized phantoms did not produce reliable results under the conditions of the present study. This seems to be the case for other spectral acoustic attenuation estimation techniques when used in the liver.[1,2,9]

In the phantom experiments done by Ophir et al,[4,5] with identical ROI

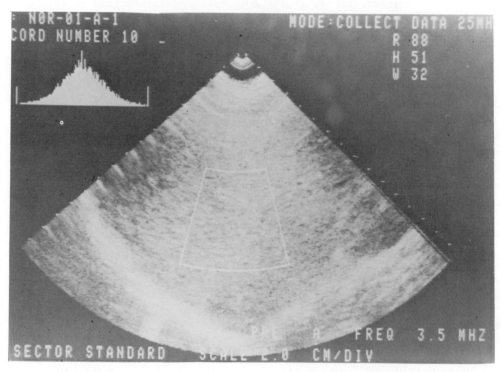

Fig. 1. Longitudinal B-scan of a liver showing a typical
Region-of-Interest (ROI) for data collection.
The parameters R, W, H refer to: R = position
(in mm; in the axial direction) of the center of
the ROI; W = width of ROI (angle, in degrees;
along lateral direction); H = height of ROI (in
mm; along the axial direction). In the upper
left corner the histogram of the distribution of
amplitudes of the digitized A-line. The shape
of the histogram is Gaussian.

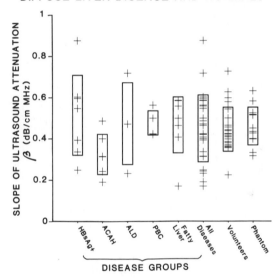

SLOPE OF ACOUSTIC ATTENUATION FOR
DIFFUSE LIVER DISEASE AND NORMALS

Fig. 2. Bar-graph showing the distribution of β for: 5
selected liver disease groups, all 37 patients
(without regard for the histologic stage of
disease), 8 normal volunteers and the ECOBLOC
phantom. The rectangular boxes enclose the
values falling between the mean plus or minus
one standard deviation.

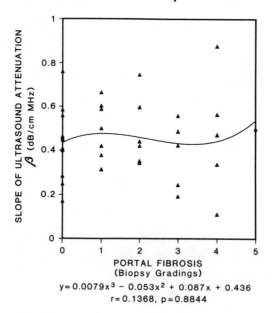

PORTAL FIBROSIS VS. β (dB/cm MHz)

y = 0.0079x³ − 0.053x² + 0.087x + 0.436
r = 0.1368, p = 0.8844

Fig. 3. Scattergram shows no correlation between calculated attenuation β and biopsy proven level of
portal fibrosis and fat for 36 patients (using
all transducers).

shape and position, with perfect temperature stabilization, and controlled scanning technique, few physical factors affected the spread on β-estimates. Diffraction, a non-Gaussian pulse shape, a non-linear frequency dependence of $\alpha(f)$, inhomogeneity of the medium will all bias the β-estimate, but they will not influence the range of β-values in the experimental setting described by Ophir.[3,4] In-vivo liver attenuation estimation will be complicated by all of the above factors.

Statistical fluctuations in reflected acoustic pulses[4,6,10] are a serious problem for tissue characterization. These fluctuations are due to scatter-induced frequency variations,[10] inhomogeneous attenuation and velocity distributions, diffractions and refraction effects. Also, purely statistical errors related to properties of statistical estimators could influence results.

It has been pointed out that the usage of a large amount of data may be necessary to obtain sufficient accuracy.[2,4]

We conclude that, within the restrictions of the current experiment, the use of the zero-crossing technique and small amounts of data is not precise enough to test for meaningful clinical correlation in phantoms, normal livers and several categories of diseased liver. For in-vivo liver attenuation estimation, other factors such as tissue characteristics (scattering, inhomogeneity of tissue absorption, and velocity) and the finite ultrasound beam size (diffraction and refraction effects) may also play a major part.

REFERENCES

1. B.S. Garra, T.H. Shawker, M. Nassi, and M.A. Russell, Ultrasound attenuation measurements of the liver in vivo using a commercial sector scanner, Ultras Imag 6(4):396 (1984).

2. A.J. Duerinckx, J.C. Hoefs, L.A. Ferrari, G.S. Lottenberg, and C. Cole-Beuglet, Attenuation of ultrasound in diffuse liver disease in-vivo using the zero-crossing technique, (Abst), Radiology 157(P):315 (1985).

3. S.W. Flax, N.J. Pelc, G.H. Glover, F.D. Dutmann, and M. McLachlan, Spectral characterization and attenuation measurements in ultrasound, Ultras Imag 5(2):95 (1983).

4. J. Ophir, M.A. Ghouse, and L.A. Ferrari, Tradeoffs in attenuation estimation using the zero-crossing technique. Ultras Med Biol, in press, (1986).

5. J. Ophir, M.A. Ghouse, and L.A. Ferrari, Attenuation estimation with the zero-crossing technique: phantom studies. Ultras Imag 7(2):122 (1985).

6. R. Kuc, Bounds on estimating the acoustic attenuation of small tissue regions from reflected ultrasound, Proc IEEE 73(7):1159 (1985).

7. P. He and J.F. Greenleaf, Attenuation estimation of phantoms – a stability test. Ultras Imag 8(1):1 (1986).

8. J. Ophir, T.H. Shawker, N.F. Maklad, J.G. Miller, S.W. Flax, P.A. Narayana, and J.P. Jones, Attenuation estimation in reflection: progress and prospects, Ultras Imag 6(4):349 (1984).

9. R. Kuc, Estimating the acoustic attenuation from reflected ultrasound signals: comparison of spectral-shift and spectral-difference approaches, IEEE Trans Acoust Speech Signal Process, ASSP-32(1):1 (1984).

10. S.M. Gehlbach, F.G. Sommer and R.A. Stern, Scatterer-induced frequency variations in reflected acoustic pulses: implications for tissue characterization, Ultras Imag 7(2):172 (1985).

CALCULATION OF TRANSIENT RADIATION FIELDS FROM AXIAL SYMMETRIC SOURCES

Daniel Guyomar and John Powers

Department of Electrical and Computer Engineering
Naval Postgraduate School
Monterey, California 93943

ABSTRACT

Proper understanding of the results of acoustic imaging, tissue characterization, and tomography utilizing pulsed ultrasound requires inclusion of the diffraction effects of the pulsed wave. A method is presented for the efficient calculation of pulsed ultrasonic waves from an axially symmetric source mounted in a rigid baffle and excited with an arbitrary time excitation. The technique uses a spatial modal analysis based on a series expansion of the source velocity term in either of two sets of basis functions. The choice of basis functions is arbitrary. The expansion is equivalent to a decomposition of the excitation into a set of propagation modes. Each mode is then simply propagated by the technique with rapid convergence of the solution that requires evaluation of approximately thirty (or less) terms of a series, allowing rapid computer-based solutions of the field at an object plane or at a receiver plane. Several numerical solutions are given.

INTRODUCTION

Different methods now exist to compute the transient radiation or diffraction of a rigidly baffled planar source in linear, homogeneous media (Stepanishen, 1971 and 1981; Harris, 1981a and 1981b; Guyomar and Powers, 1985 and 1986; Meideros and Stepanishen, 1984; Greenspan, 1979). These techniques typically require the use of fast Fourier transforms (FFTs) or the evaluation of difficult integrals. A large fraction of transducers used in acoustical applications possess radial symmetry. Such symmetry allows techniques to be developed that increase the the calculation efficiency of these techniques. Stepanishen (1981), Meideros and Stepanishen (1984), and Greenspan (1979) have developed series expansions of the solutions for axial symmetric sources that require evaluation of integrals over limits with geometrical interpretations. The method presented in this paper is also based on the expansion of the source excitation into an infinite series over a set of orthogonal basis functions where each of these basis functions corresponds to a vibrational mode of a circular transducer. By using the spatial frequency domain, however, a simpler expression can be found that allows rapid evaluation of the fields with a digital computer. The basic effect of propagation is to redistribute the amplitudes of the different modes. Through the development of a time-varying transfer function, it is possible to show that the redistribution is from the higher-order modes into the lower-order modes. As a consequence, the field can be simply calculated by summing the significant lower order modes after calculation of their amplitudes (as affected by propagation).

THEORY

Using the result of diffraction theory, one can express the acoustic velocity potential, $\phi(x, y, z, t)$, in terms of the normal velocity, $v_z(x, y, 0, t)$, on a planar emitting surface imbedded in a rigid baffle as (Stepanishen, 1971; Harris, 1981a)

$$\phi(x, y, z, t) = v_z(x, y, 0, t)^{***}_{xyt} \frac{\delta(ct - R)}{2\pi R} \tag{1}$$

where * indicates convolution over the indicated variable and $R = \sqrt{x^2 + y^2 + z^2}$.

For a separable velocity given by

$$v_z(x, y, 0, t) = \tau(t)s(x, y) \tag{2}$$

we have

$$\phi(x, y, z, t) = \tau(t)^*_t \left[s(x, y)^{**}_{xy} \frac{\delta(ct - R)}{2\pi R} \right] \tag{3}$$

This latter expression is the convolution of the time excitation with the 'spatial impulse response' (Stepanishen, 1971; Harris, 1981a), h(x,y,z,t), given as

$$h(x, y, z, t) = s(x, y)^{**}_{xy} \frac{\delta(ct - R)}{2\pi R} \tag{4}$$

The term on the right side of the convolution is the Green's function for lossless propagation (Stepanishen, 1981) from a planar source in a rigid baffle.

To perform field calculations it is more efficient to work in the spatial frequency domain using f_x and f_y to express the spatial frequencies. To do so, we will decompose the Green's function by using the properties of the Dirac delta function. Recalling that

$$\delta(f(r)) = \sum_{i=1}^{N} \frac{\delta(r - r_i)}{|df/dr||_{r=r_i}} \tag{5}$$

where $r = \sqrt{x^2 + y^2}$ and r_i are the N zeros of f(r), we can write an expression for the outward-traveling wave (neglecting multiplicative constants) as

$$\frac{\delta(ct - R)}{R} = \frac{\delta(r - \sqrt{c^2t^2 - z^2})}{|R\sqrt{c^2t^2 - z^2}/ct|} \tag{6}$$

Taking the two-dimensional spatial transform (and recognizing that it reduces to the Hankel transform due to the radial symmetry), we have (Erdelyi et al., 1954)

$$B\left\{ \frac{\delta(ct - R)}{R} \right\} = J_0(\rho\sqrt{c^2t^2 - z^2})H(ct - z) \tag{7}$$

where $B[\cdot]$ is the Hankel transform operator, J_0 is the zero-order Bessel function, and $\rho = \sqrt{f_x^2 + f_y^2}$. This transform of the Green's function is the 'propagation transfer function'.

The spatial transform, $\tilde{h}(f_x, f_y, t)$, of the spatial impulse response (Eq. 4) can be written after substitution of Eq. 7 as

$$\tilde{h}(f_x, f_y, z, t) = \tilde{s}(f_x, f_y)J_0(\rho\sqrt{c^2t^2 - z^2})H(ct - z) \tag{8}$$

where the multiplicative constant of $1/2\pi$ has been dropped for simplicity. (All computer-simulated fields shown in the results will be normalized to the maximum value of the field.) The transfer function, $J_0(\rho\sqrt{c^2t^2 - z^2})H(ct - z)$, is now seen to be a time-varying spatial filter acting on the modulus of the source spectrum. As time increases, the J_0 function decreases, thereby enhancing the lower spatial frequencies. This will cause the field to become smoother as time advances (Guyomar and Powers, 1985 and 1986).

For a radial distribution of source velocity, $s(r)$, Eq. 8 can be written as

$$\tilde{h}(\rho, z, t) = \tilde{s}(\rho) J_0(\rho \sqrt{c^2 t^2 - z^2}) H(ct - z) \tag{9}$$

Computing the spatial impulse response from Eq. 8 or Eq. 9 normally requires performing a transform of the source velocity, multiplication by the transfer function, and an inverse transform of the product to obtain the field. For radially symmetric sources, however, the number of operations can be reduced and the field can be obtained without any Fourier or Hankel transform evaluations.

It is true, mathematically speaking, that a spatially bounded function can always be decomposed into a series expansion over a set of orthogonal basis functions. The wave that arrives at a plane located a distance z from the source plane will be spatially bounded. Due to causality, we know that the wave will not reach a point on the observation plane located a distance r_0 from the center of the observation plane before a time t_0 given by

$$t_0 = \frac{\sqrt{z^2 + (r_0 - A)^2}}{c} \tag{10}$$

where A is the radius of the source and c is the sound velocity. For any given time t, this equation tells us that the spatial domain of the wave in the observation plane located a distance z away from the source will be between $-r_0$ and r_0 where

$$r_0 = \sqrt{c^2 t^2 - z^2} + A \tag{11}$$

For any given z and t, we need an expansion of the wave over the interval $[0, r_0]$. Since circular symmetry is present, the expansion is over Bessel functions and we can find a series that represents the spatial impulse response of the wave, $h(r, z, t)$, as

$$h(r, z, t) = \sum_{i=1}^{\infty} h_i J_0(\alpha_i r) \qquad \text{for } 0 \le r \le r_0 \tag{12}$$

where the coefficients h_i are functions of z and t. The values of α_i depend on the particular orthogonal basis functions chosen.

Two sets of orthogonal basis functions can be profitably considered for circular symmetry (Erdelyi et al., 1954; Guyomar et al., 1983). They correspond to the roots of the following equations,

$$J_0(\alpha_i r_0) = 0 \tag{13}$$

and

$$\beta_i r_0 J_0'(\beta_i r_0) + \xi J_0(\beta_i r_0) = 0 \tag{14}$$

where J_0' is the derivative of J_0 and ξ is an arbitrary constant. The first set of eigenvalues leads to a Bessel expansion, and the second leads to a Dini expansion. Both sets are considered below.

1) Bessel expansion

The series expansion of the spatial impulse response is given by

$$h(r, 0, t) = \sum_{i=1}^{\infty} h_i J_0(\alpha_i r) \qquad \text{for } 0 \le r \le r_0 \tag{15}$$

where the evaluation of the series coefficients is

$$h_i = \frac{2 \int_0^{r_0} r h(r) J_0(\alpha_i r) \, dr}{r_0^2 J_1^2(\alpha_i r_0)} \tag{16}$$

and α_i satisfies the relation,

$$J_0(\alpha_i r_0) = 0 \qquad (17)$$

A similar expansion can be found for the radial velocity distribution at the source. Expanding again over the same interval $[0, r_0]$, we have

$$s(r) = \sum_{i=1}^{\infty} s_i J_0(\alpha_i r) \qquad \text{for } 0 \le r \le r_0 \qquad (18)$$

where s_i are the weighting constants given by

$$s_i = \frac{2 \int_0^A r s(r) J_0(\alpha_i r)\, dr}{r_0^2 J_1^2(\alpha_i r_0)} \qquad (19)$$

2) Dini expansion

Different sets of eigenfunctions can be generated for the eigenvalues of Eq. 14, depending on the value of ξ. For simplicity, we will assume that $\xi = 0$. Hence, Eq. 14 will reduce to

$$J_1(\beta_i r_0) = 0 \qquad (20)$$

The expansion of the spatial impulse response is

$$h(r, z, t) = \sum_{i=1}^{\infty} h_i J_0(\beta_i r) \qquad (21)$$

with

$$h_i = \frac{2 \int_0^{r_0} r h(r) J_0(\beta_i r)\, dr}{r_0^2 J_0^2(\beta_i r_0)} \qquad (22)$$

A similar expansion is obtained for the input velocity distribution,

$$s(r, 0, t) = \sum_{i=1}^{\infty} s_i J_0(\beta_i r) \qquad (23)$$

with

$$s_i = \frac{2 \int_0^A r s(r) J_0(\beta_i r)\, dr}{r_0^2 J_0^2(\beta_i r_0)} \qquad (24)$$

EFFICIENT FIELD CALCULATIONS

We now want to find a series expansion for the spatial impulse response in terms of the series coefficients s_i of the spatial excitation $s(r)$. The derivation is done in terms of the Bessel expansion. The Dini expansion would be similar except that β_i would appear insread of α_i. The Bessel series expansion of the spatial impulse response is given by Eq. 15,

$$h(r, 0, t) = \sum_{i=1}^{\infty} h_i J_0(\alpha_i r) \qquad \text{for } 0 \le r \le r_0 \qquad (25)$$

with expansion coefficients given by Eq. 16,

$$h_i = \frac{2 \int_0^{r_0} r h(r) J_0(\alpha_i r)\, dr}{r_0^2 J_1^2(\alpha_i r_0)} \qquad (26)$$

Since h(r) is zero for $r > r_0$, we can replace the upper limit by ∞. Equation 26 becomes

$$h_i = \frac{2 \int_0^{\infty} r h(r) J_0(\alpha_i r)\, dr}{r_0^2 J_1^2(\alpha_i r_0)}. \qquad (27)$$

The Hankel transform $\tilde{f}(\rho)$ of a function $f(r)$ is defined by the integral,

$$\tilde{f}(\rho) = \int_0^\infty rf(r)J_0(\rho r)\, dr \qquad (28)$$

and, so we can write Eq. 27 as

$$h_i = \frac{2\tilde{h}(\alpha_i)}{r_0^2 J_1^2(\alpha_i r_0)} \qquad (29)$$

Similarly since $s(r)$ is zero for $r > A$ and since $r_0 \geq A$, we can write the series coefficients s_i as

$$s_i = \frac{2\tilde{s}(\alpha_i)}{r_0^2 J_1^2(\alpha_i r_0)} \qquad (30)$$

We can solve this equation for $\tilde{s}(\alpha_i)$ as

$$\tilde{s}(\alpha_i) = \frac{s_i r_0^2 J_1^2(\alpha_i r_0)}{2} \qquad (31)$$

From Eq. 9, we have the expression for the Hankel transform of the spatial impulse response,

$$\tilde{h}(\rho, z, t) = \tilde{s}(\rho)J_0(\rho\sqrt{c^2 t^2 - z^2})H(ct - z) \qquad (32)$$

Substituting Eq. 32 into Eq. 29 and letting $\rho = \alpha_i$, as indicated, Eq. 29 becomes

$$h_i = \frac{2\tilde{s}(\alpha_i)J_0(\alpha_i\sqrt{c^2 t^2 - z^2}H(ct - z)}{r_0^2 J_1^2(\alpha_i r_0)} \qquad (33)$$

Substituting Eq. 31 we get

$$h_i = s_i J_0(\alpha_i \sqrt{c^2 t^2 - z^2})H(ct - z) \qquad (34)$$

and Eq. 25 becomes

$$h(r, z, t) = \sum_{i=1}^\infty s_i J_0(\gamma_i \sqrt{c^2 t^2 - z^2})J_0(\gamma_i r)H(ct - z) \qquad (35)$$

where γ_i is α_i for this Bessel expansion or β_i for the Dini expansion.

Equation 35 is the desired result that shows how each mode of the source is propagated. The $J_0(\gamma_i\sqrt{c^2 t^2 - z^2})J_0(\gamma_i r)$ term is a time-varying propagator that decreases the amplitude of the i-th mode of the expansion. (The $H(ct - z)$ term ensures causality.) The filter, therefore, serves to enhance the lower order modes. As time increases, the argument of the filtering function increases, favoring the lower order modes.

Two special cases can be identified (Greenspan, 1979; Stepanishen, 1981). For $ct = z$, the spatial impulse response becomes

$$h(r, z, t) = \sum_{i=1}^\infty s_i J_0(\gamma_i r) \qquad \text{for } ct = z \qquad (36)$$

which is an exact replica of the spatial distribution of the source. On-axis ($r = 0$), the spatial impulse response is

$$h(0, z, t) = \sum_{i=1}^\infty s_i J_0(\gamma_i\sqrt{c^2 t^2 - z^2})H(ct - z) \qquad \text{when } r = 0 \qquad (37)$$

which is also a replica of the source spatial distribution but it is obtained along the time axis.

NUMERICAL SIMULATIONS

Using Eq. 35, the spatial impulse response is easily computed. For each value of z, one finds the value of r_0 for each time of interest from Eq. 11. One then finds N zeros of Eqs. 17 or 20. The number N required depends on the convergence of the field. Thirty values were arbitrarily chosen as adequate for these computations. (The choice was borne out by comparison with known exact solutions.) Calculation of s_i is done from either Eq. 19 or Eq. 24 and then the sum of the products in Eq. 35 is found to produce the spatial impulse response. While the summation is theoretically infinite, the fast convergence of the series ensures that only a few terms of the series are required to evaluate the fields with sufficient accuracy. The solution to the field with a nonimpulse temporal excitation requires evaluation of the temporal convolution of Eq. 3.

The following plots have been evaluated using thirty-two points along the radial axis, r, and fifty points along the time axis. The plots are normalized to unit amplitude and the axes are expressed in terms of the source diameter, A. All of the field patterns are observed in a plane at a distance of 10 cm from the source plane. The source radius is assumed to be 1.7 cm. The time axis begins at $t = z/c$ (i.e., when the first portion of the excited waveform arrives at the observation plane). The average CPU time was about 6 seconds on an IBM 3033 mainframe computer.

To compare the fields obtained by the two expansions, Figs. 1 and 2 show the field calculated for the spatial impulse response of a circular uniformly-excited transducer using the Bessel and Dini expansions. There is no apparent difference between the representations. Despite the high spatial frequency content of the circular step wave at $t = z/c$, we note that the limited series of thirty terms still describes the field very well. The effect of the truncation of the series is apparent at that location in the form of 'ringing' of the field in the regions of discontinuity (due to the Gibbs phenomenon). As time progresses and the high-order modes are filtered out, the convergence becomes better. The fields of Figs. 1 and 2 compare well with closed-form solutions for the uniform piston (Stepanishen, 1971 and 1981; Harris, 1981b; Greenspan, 1979; Guyomar et al., 1983; Oberheltinger, 1961; Tupholme, 1969; Weight and Hayman, 1978).

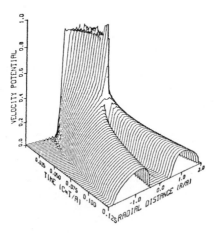

Figure 1 Spatial impulse response for a circular piston transducer using the Bessel expansion (A=3.4 cm, z=10 cm)

Figure 3, 4, and 5 illustrate the convergence of the Dini series for ten, fifteen, and twenty terms, respectively. More terms are required near $ct = 0$ due to the higher spatial frequencies there. As time progresses and the spatial frequency content is less due to the filtering action of the propagation, fewer terms are required to reach an accurate representation of the field.

Figure 6 gives the spatial impulse response for a truncated Gaussian source excitation as calculated with a Dini expansion. The $1/e$ point is located at r=0.981 cm from the center.

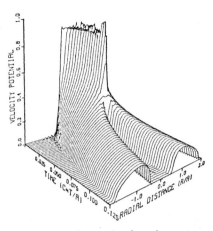

Figure 2 Spatial impulse response for a circular piston transducer using the Dini expansion (A=3.4 cm, z=10 cm)

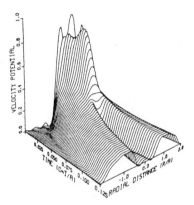

Figure 3 Ten-term Dini series impulse response for a square transducer (A=3.4 cm, z=10 cm)

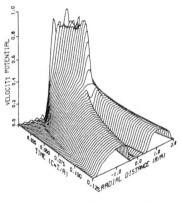

Figure 4 Fifteen-term Dini series impulse response for a square transducer (A=3.4 cm, z=10 cm)

Since the excitation consists of primarily low spatial frequencies, the effect of propagation spatial filter on the field shape is small.

While the velocity potential is a useful quantity, it has little physical significance. One can obtain the acoustic pressure, $p(x, y, z, t)$, from the potential by the relation,

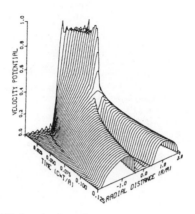

Figure 5 Twenty-term Dini series impulse response for a square transducer (A=3.4 cm, z=10 cm)

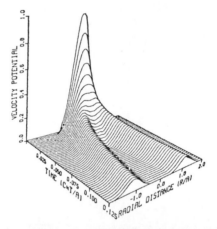

Figure 6 Spatial impulse response for a circular transducer with a truncated Gaussian spatial excitation $e^{-12(r/A)^2}$ using a Bessel expansion (A=3.4 cm, z=10 cm)

$$p(x, y, z, t) = \rho_0 \frac{\partial \phi}{\partial t} \tag{38}$$

where ρ_0 is the density of the medium. Assuming axial symmetry, the acoustic pressure at an observation point will be

$$p(r, z, t) = \frac{c^2 \rho_0}{\sqrt{c^2 t^2 - z^2}} \sum_{i=1}^{\infty} s_i J_1 \left(\gamma_i \sqrt{c^2 t^2 - z^2} \right) J_0(\gamma_i r) \tag{39}$$

This equation provides a direct way to compute the pressure spatial impulse response from the input velocity distribution. The computations are as easy and fast as the computation of the potential.

For a time excitation other than an impulse, one must convolve (in the time domain) the spatial impulse response with the time-varying excitation function as in Eq. 3. The convolution can be done either in the space-time domain or in the spatial frequency domain as the order of the inverse spatial transform and the temporal convolution is interchangeable.

Figure 7 represents the transient pressure response of a uniform circular piston excited by a positive pulse excitation of time duration equal to 0.02A seconds. The noticeable difference between this response and the spatial impulse response for the same geometric source (Fig. 1 or 2) is due to the time derivative of Eq. 38 followed by the smoothing of the convolution of Eq. 3.

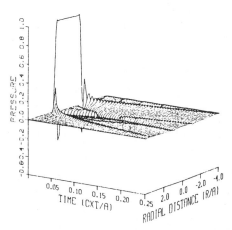

Figure 7 Transient pressure wave from a uniform circular piston excited by a pulse using the Bessel expansion (A=3.4 cm, z=10 cm)

SUMMARY

A method for rapidly calculating the acoustic potential field or the acoustic pressure field from an axially symmetric source has been presented . The method is based on two possible series expansions of the source velocity spatial distribution. The expansions are rapidly convergent, and, therefore, are efficient in calculation. The method does not use any Fourier or Hankel transforms, nor does it require evaluations of integrals (other than to obtain the s_i coefficients). All operations are carried out in the space domain. The sampling intervals in time and space are independent of each other and the field solutions can be represented as desired.

ACKNOWLEDGMENTS

This work was partially sponsored by the Foundation Research Program of the Naval Postgraduate School. Daniel Guyomar was a Research Associate of the National Research Council and is currently with Schlumberger-EPS in Clamart, France.

REFERENCES

Erdelyi, A.; Magnus, W.; Oberhettinger, F.; and Triconi, F.G.; **Tables of Integral Transforms, Vols. 1 and 2**, (McGraw-Hill, New York, 1954)

Greenspan, M., "Piston radiator: Some extensions of the theory", J. Acous. Soc. Am., **65**(3), pp. 608-621, 1979

Guyomar, D.; Fink, M.; and Coursant, R.; "Acoustical displacement reconstruction of axisymmmetric transducers", Presented at the 1983 IEEE Ultrasonics Symposium, Atlanta, 1983

Guyomar, D., and Powers, J., "Boundary effects on transient radiation fields from vibrating surfaces", J. Acous. Soc. Am., **77**(3), pp. 907-915, 1985

Guyomar, D., and Powers, J., "A Fourier approach to diffraction of pulsed ultrasonic waves in lossless media", submitted for publication, 1986

Harris, G.R., "Review of transient field theory for a baffled planar piston", J. Acous. Soc. Am., **70**(1), pp. 10-20, 1981a

Harris, G.R., "Transient field of a baffled piston having an arbitrary vibration amplitude distribution", J. Acous. Soc. Am., **70**(1), pp. 186-204, 1981b

Meideros, A.F., and Stepanishen, P.R., "The forward and backward propagation of acoustic fields from axisymmetric ultrasonic radiators using the impulse response and Hankel transform techniques", J. Acous. Soc. Am., **75**(6), pp. 1732-1740, 1984

Oberheltinger, F., "On transient solutions of the baffled piston problem", J. Natl. Bur. Standards, **65B**, pp. 1-6, 1961

Stepanishen, P.R, "Transient radiation from pistons in an infinite planar baffle", J. Acous. Soc. Am., **49**(5), pp. 1629-1637, 1971

Stepanishen, P.R., "Acoustic transients from planar axisymmetric vibrators using the impulse response approach", J. Acous. Soc. Am., **70**(4), pp. 1176-1181, 1981

Tupholme, G.E., "Generation of acoustic pulses by baffled plane pistons", Mathematika, **16**, pp. 209-226, 1969

Weight, J., and Hayman, A., "Observation of the propagation of very short ultrasonic pulses and their reflection by small targets", J. Acous. Soc. Am., **63**(2), pp. 96-404, 1978

PULSED PVDF TRANSDUCER FIELDS - COMPARISON OF

THEORY AND EXPERIMENT

D.A. Hutchins and H.D. Mair

Physics Department, Queen's University
Kingston, Ontario
Canada K7L 3N6

ABSTRACT

A series of theoretical programs have been developed for the prediction of the radiated pressure fields of transient radiators in the form of discs and annuli. Such transducers have been constructed using polyvinylidene difluoride (PVDF) polymer film, and their pressure fields sampled in two-dimensional planes following transient excitation. It is shown that good agreement is possible between theory and experiment for such transducers.

INTRODUCTION

PVDF has been used extensively for the construction of ultrasonic transducers[1], with attention being paid to its use as a hydrophone receiver[2]. In the work to be described, we have investigated its use as an ultrasonic transmitter. Certain geometries of specific interest to acoustical imaging are examined below, namely disc and annular transducers. PVDF is also convenient for use in transducers with curved geometries, in that in the form of 90μm thick sheets it can conform to curved surfaces. Further, at frequencies <10MHz, resonance of the film does not present a problem.

In earlier work[3], the authors found that PVDF was a reasonable material for CW work, in that transducers could be fabricated with a reasonably uniform amplitude and phase across their front face. Thus, if a transient disc radiator were to be formed from such a material, it would be expected to behave as a plane piston source, the theoretical field from which is well known[4-8]. This paper will thus compare the fields of disc radiators to theory for transient excitation, and will use the approach outlined by Lockwood and Willette[4]. As will be demonstrated below, this method may also be extended to other geometries, such as annuli. Although curved geometries (such as conical and spherical radiators) will not be treated here, it should be noted that the theoretical technique may be applied to such transducers also[9].

THEORY

The impulse respose h(x,t) of a circular piston source may be expressed in terms of radial (ρ) and axial (z) coordinates at any point P in the radiated field[6]. The value of h(x,t) depends on whether P is inside or outside $\rho = a$, where a is the transducer radius. If $\rho < a$, $h(x,t)$ is given by

$$h(x,t) = -\frac{cUa}{\pi} \begin{cases} 0 & t < t_1 \text{ and } t > t_3 \\ 1 & t_1 < t < t_2 \\ \cos^{-1}\left[\frac{c^2 t^2 - z^2 + \rho^2 - a^2}{2\rho(c^2 t^2 - z^2)^{1/2}}\right] & t_2 < t < t_3 \end{cases} \tag{1}$$

whereas if $\rho > a$,

$$h(x,t) = -\frac{cUa}{\pi} \begin{cases} 0 & \\ \cos^{-1}\left[\frac{\rho^2 + c^2 t^2 - z^2 - a^2}{2\rho(c^2 t^2 - z^2)^{1/2}}\right] & t_2 < t < t_3 \end{cases} \tag{2}$$

Here, c is the acoustic velocity and U is the normalized particle velocity of the front face. The times t_1, t_2 and t_3 correspond to travel times of signals from the nearest point on the disc to the point P, and from the nearest and farthest edges respectively. They may be written as

$$t_1 = z/c \tag{3a}$$

$$t_2 = \frac{\left(z^2 + (\rho-a)^2\right)^{1/2}}{c} \tag{3b}$$

$$t_3 = \left(z^2 + (\rho+a)^2\right)^{1/2} \tag{3c}$$

The result, $h(x,t)$, is the scalar velocity potential field for an impulse, which may be differentiated to find the pressure field. The pressure field $P(x,t)$ for any other transient form of excitation ($f(t)$) is then obtained by a convolution of the form

$$P(x,t) = -\rho_o \frac{\partial(h(x,t))}{\partial t} * f(t) \tag{4}$$

Hence, the pressure amplitude at any point is dependent upon $f(t)$. As an example of two extreme cases, consider excitation by (a) one cycle and (b) CW waveforms, at a wavelength λ such that $a \approx 8\lambda$ (in fact, for ease of comparison to later experiments in water, a disc of 25 mm radius is to be assumed, where the excitation frequency is 470kHz). The two fields are shown in Fig. 1, and there are several features of interest. For CW excitation the well-known interference maxima and minima lead to a compli-cated nearfield variation; for single-cycle excitation, however, only one axial maximum is predicted due to constructive interference between plane and edge waves form the disc. Destructive interference cannot take place in this case as the two pulse-length is not sufficiently long for appreciable overlap of the two contributions.

The pressure field of an annulus may also be predicted theoretically, in that it may be considered as the difference between the fields of two plane pistons. For instance, the field of an annulus of outer diameter 2a, with a width of a/2, is equivalent to the difference between the fields of two plane pistons of radii a and a/2 respectively. Assuming a = 25mm, and an excitation frequency of 400kHz, the pressure field radiated by such a transducer into water is presented in Fig. 2 for (a) single cycle and (b) CW excitation. Note that again the CW field is more complicated, with side-lobe levels being more prominent than in the transient case.

The aim of the current investigation was to compare theory and experi-ment for PVDF transducers, and the apparatus used will now be described.

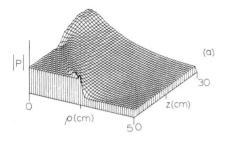

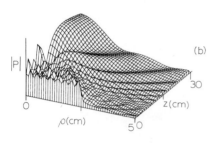

Fig. 1 Theoretical predictions of the pressure amplitude distribution from a plane piston of 50 mm diameter, excited at 470 kHz in water. (a) single cycle of excitation, (b) CW excitation.

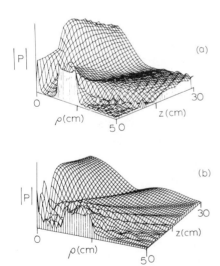

Fig. 2 Theoretical predictions of the pressure amplitude distribution in water of an annulus of outside diameter 2a and width a/2, with a = 25 mm. (a) Single cycle and (b) CW excitation at 400 kHz.

APPARATUS AND EXPERIMENT

The apparatus used to record the pressure fields of PVDF discs and annuli is presented in Fig. 3.

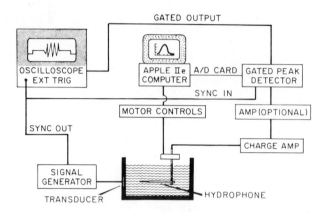

Fig. 3 Schematic diagram of computer-controlled scanning hydrophone and water tank used in this investigation.

A 1mm PZT hydrophone was scanned in two-dimensional planes throughout a water tank, into which the transducer under test radiated. The hydrophone scanning was under computer control, and data was collected in the form of peak pressure using a gated peak detector and 12-bit digitization by the same computer. Note that at excitation frequencies less than 500 kHz, the hydrophone diameter was always $<\lambda/3$. The input voltage waveform to the transducer could also be digitized using a Data 6000 Waveform Analyzer, for later comparison to theory. In a typical scan, the hydrophone sampled horizontal sections of the field, which were replotted as three-dimensional graphs.

The PVDF transducers were fabricated by cementing the piezoelectric film to an aluminum backing in a pressure cell. Silver paint and insulating varnish were used to ensure a continuous ground plane on the water side, with the signal being applied to the aluminum backing plate.

RESULTS AND DISCUSSION

The first PVDF transducer examined experimentally was a 50 mm diameter disc, excited with various durations of tone burst at 470 kHz. The resultant pressure fields are presented in Figs. 4(a)-(e) for each duration of excitation signal. For a single cycle of excitation, Fig. 4(a), excellent agreement exists with that predicted theoretically for a plane piston radiator (Fig. 1(a)), evaluated for the same frequency and radius. In both cases, a reasonably uniform axial nearfield exists, together with higher amplitude ridges, which converge onto the axis to form a single axial maximum. Greater complexity is introduced experimentally, as the number of cycles in the drive signals increases (Figs. 4(b)-(e)). In the extreme case of CW excitation, Fig. 4(e), the nearfield axial region has become complicated, with sidelobe levels also being high. This again agrees well with theory (Fig. 1(b) assuming a plane piston radiator.

Comparison to theory may also be undertaken for Figs. 4(b)-(d), generated by excitation with 2,5 and 10 cycles of excitation. Theoretical predictions for this case are shown in Figs. 5(a)-(c), where the pulse shape $(f(t))$ used for the convolution of Eq. (4) was the actual digitized drive waveform. There are several interesting features. The axial minima are not zero, but are constant at some finite value for each type of excitation, a

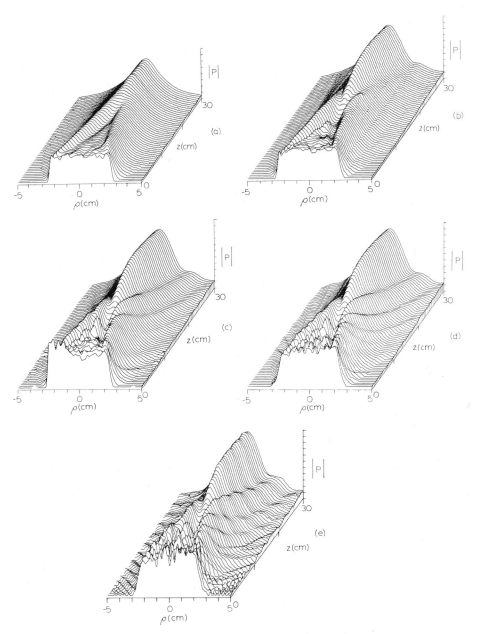

Fig. 4 Experimental pressure fields in water of a
PVDF disc transducer excited at 470 kHz. The tone
burst duration was (a) 1 cycle, (b) 2 cycles, (c) 5
cycles, (d) 10 cycles and (e) CW. The disc diameter
was 50 mm.

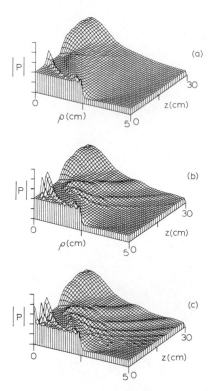

Fig. 5 Theoretical predictions of the pressure
field in water of a 50 mm diameter plane piston
radiator, excited with (a) 2 cycles, (b) 5 cycles
and (c) 10 cycles at 470 kHz.

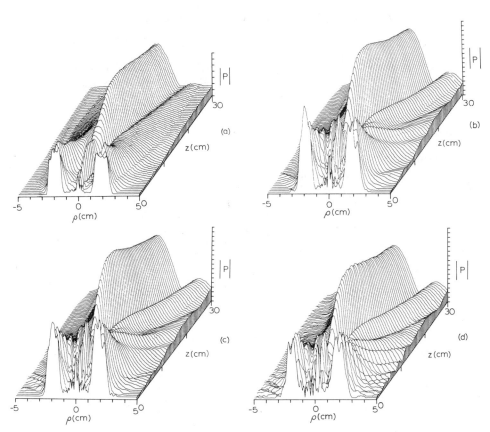

Fig. 6 Experimental pressure variations
in the field of a PVDF annulus, of outside
diameter 50 mm and inside diameter 25 mm.
(a) 1 cycle, (b) 5 cycles, (c) 10 cycles
and (d) CW excitation at 400 kHz was used.

trend observed in our experimental measurements. The increased complexity of the fields with an increase in tone burst length is due to the interference processes occurring within the nearfield. These may be visualized as being due to the interaction of plane and edge waves, with the latter being an inverted version of the former. In the extreme case of CW excitation, perfect destructive interference can occur between the two, whereas at shorter, finite pulse lengths the region of overlap decreases, leading to a less complicated field.

A second set of experiments was undertaken using a PVDF annulus, of 25mm outside radius and width 12.5mm. This was excited with various lengths of tone burst at 400kHz, and the experimental pressure fields that resulted from 1,5,10 cycle and CW excitation are presented in Figs. 6(a)-(d). As will be seen, a region of high pressure is present on-axis, as expected from an annulus. In common with the disc radiator, side lobe amplitudes and the overall complexity of the pressure field increased with the number of cycles within the excitation tone burst. Comparison to theory may also be made for this case. Referring to theoretical fields already presented in Fig. 2, it will be observed that good correlation again exists between theory and experiment, in this case for single cycle and CW excitation.

CONCLUSIONS

From the above comparison, it will be seen that the PVDF transducers examined could be modelled successfully as uniform radiators, and provided a good method for examining the correlation between theory and experiment for axisymmetric transducers. We are currently extending this analysis to treat non-planar sources such as spherical bowl and conical geometries, and the results of this extended work are to be published elsewhere[9].

ACKNOWLEDGEMENT

This work was funded via grants from NSERC and Queen's University.

REFERENCES

1. J.W. Hunt, M. Arditi and F.S. Foster, Ultrasound transducers for for pulse-echo medical imaging, IEEE Trans. Biomed. Eng. BME-30:453 (1983).

2. P.A. Lewin, Miniature piezoelectric polymer ultrasonic hydrophone probe, Ultrasonics 19:213 (1981).

3. D.A. Hutchins, H.D. Mair, P.A. Puhach and A. Osei, Continuous wave pressure fields of ultrasonic transducers, to be published in J. Acoust. Soc. Am. (1986).

4. J.C. Lockwood and J.G. Willette, High speed method for computing the exact solution for the pressure variations in the near field of a baffled piston, J. Acoust. Soc. Am. 53:735 (1973).

5. P.R. Stepanishen, Asymptotic behaviour of a circular piston, J. Acoust. Soc. Am. 59:749 (1976).

6. G.R. Harris, Review of transient field theory for a baffled planar piston, J. Acoust. Soc. Am. 70:10 (1981).

7. G.R. Harris, Transient field of a baffled planar piston having an arbitrary vibration amplitude distibution, J. Acoust. Soc. Am. 70:186 (1981).

8. D. Guyomar and J. Powers, Transient fields radiated by curved surfaces-application to focusing, J. Acoust. Soc. Am. 76:1564 (1984).

9. D.A. Hutchins, H.D. Mair and R.G. Taylor, Transient fields of PVDF transducers, submitted for publication to J. Acoust. Soc. Am.

A NEW TECHNIQUE FOR CHARACTERIZING ULTRASONIC

TRANSDUCERS IN INHOMOGENEOUS MEDIA

Mark E. Schafer*, Peter A. Lewin, and John M. Reid

Department of Electrical and Computer Engineering and
Biomedical Engineering and Science Institute
Drexel University, Philadelphia, Pa. 19104

*Interspec, Inc., Conshohocken, Pa. 19428

ABSTRACT

This work describes several extensions to the angular spectrum method
of acoustic field analysis in order to account for wave propagation in
inhomogeneous media. The method provides three dimensional prediction of
both near- and farfield complex pressure distributions for differently
shaped ultrasonic radiators, both planar and focussed. In addition, the
method also models a layered inhomogeneous medium, concurrently accounting
for several media properties. The approach is based on a systematic
extension of the angular spectrum method; this involves modifying the
phase factor to account for refraction, dispersion, attenuation and the
effects of weak inhomogeneities. A computer simulation has been
developed, and results for various transducer geometries and media
properties are discussed. Specifically, the field patterns from focused
and phase steered apertures are modelled, and propagation in media which
have refractive and phase distorting properties is examined.

1. INTRODUCTION

Ultrasonic transducer design has gradually evolved over the last
three decades (Wild and Reid, 1952) to the point that there are standard
design approaches for producing a transducer with given imaging
characteristics (Schafer and Lewin, 1985). These characteristics,
however, are generally determined on the basis of imaging resolution
obtained in a homogeneous medium such as water. Tissue, on the other
hand, is not homogeneous and both attenuates the sound beam and distorts
its phase coherence, reducing penetration and resolution performance.
Additional tissue properties such as refraction and dispersion also
contribute to reduced resolution. The main goal of this research is to
develop a technique which will model tissue propagation properties in a
way which is both suitable and convenient for the design and analysis of
various types of transducer configurations, including phased linear
arrays. In homogeneous media, one of the most powerful techniques used to
predict transducer fields is based on the angular spectrum or Fourier

decomposition method (Goodman, 1968). With this method, the spatial pressure distribution over a plane surface is decomposed into a two-dimensional spectrum of plane waves. Acoustic wave propagation through the medium is modelled by applying the appropriate phase factor to each term in the Fourier spectrum. The angular spectrum method has the advantages of high computational efficiency using the FFT algorithm, high spatial resolution even in the nearfield of acoustic sources, and the capability to predict sound fields over an entire plane surface with a single two-dimensional FFT operation. The method has already been used to analyze transducer performance (Higgins, Norton, and Linzer, 1980), to predict transducer beam patterns (Stepanishen and Benjamin, 1982), and to image scattering objects (Sondhi, 1969), all in homogeneous media.

Since one of the underlying assumptions of the angular spectrum method is that wave propagation occurs in a homogeneous medium, the technique cannot properly account for tissue properties such as refraction, dispersion, and phase distortion. The work presented here describes several extensions to the angular spectrum method to account for wave propagation in inhomogeneous media. The extensions are based on certain modifications to the phase propagation factor used in the angular spectrum method; with these modifications, it is possible to model an inhomogeneous medium as a series of layers, each with its own sound speed, attenuation, and phase properties. For the sake of completeness, and to provide a better insight into the modifications that have been introduced as a result of this research, the basic derivation of the angular spectrum method is presented in Section 2. Section 3 presents the details of the modifications which were introduced to model a layered (tissue-like) medium.

One of the most important aspects of using the angular spectrum approach is that not only is it capable of predicting the radiated field from a source velocity distribution, but also it is equally useful in finding the source function from measurements of a transducer's radiated field. This was clearly demonstrated in the work of Higgins, Norton and Linzer (1980). It is therefore possible to measure the field of a transducer radiating into water and backpropagate the field to the source plane. Subsequently, this source distribution can be used as the input to a forward propagation model which includes the appropriate tissue characteristics. Thus the performance of new transducers can be predicted in various imaging situations. For example, the effects of a refractive layer (fat or bone) on the focusing of a phased linear array could be predicted and accounted for by correctively rephasing the beam. The simulation results which illustrate this approach are shown in Section 4.

2. ANGULAR SPECTRUM METHOD IN HOMOGENEOUS MEDIA

The following derivation of the angular spectrum method is largely based on the approach outlined in Powers (1977), and is summarized here partly to provide some insight into the technique, and partly to form the basis for the description of the extensions to be given in the next section.

Originally developed in the study of optical diffraction phenomena, the angular spectrum, or plane wave decomposition technique, decomposes the acoustic field at a plane surface into an equivalent set of plane waves, each with unique amplitude and direction cosines. Propagation is modelled by multiplying each plane wave component by a free-space transfer function, which accounts for the phase change caused by propagation over a known distance. The transfer function can be considered a space-invariant filter, and can be derived from the free-space Green's function.

Summation of the individual Fourier components allows the diffracted field to be reconstructed.

Consider a pressure wave field, travelling in the +Z direction, generated by a set of monochromatic sources. Consider further the complex pressure field that exists on a plane passing through the point Z_0 and parallel to the X-Y plane. This pressure field is characterized by a three-dimensional fuction $u(X,Y,Z_0)$, and the ultimate goal is to determine the field at a parallel plane passing through Z_1, where $Z_1 \neq Z_0$. Across the plane of interest, the function $u(X,Y,Z_0)$ has a two-dimensional Fourier Transform given by

$$U(\omega_x,\omega_y,Z_0) = \int\int_{-\infty}^{+\infty} u(X,Y,Z_0) e^{-j(\omega_x x + \omega_y y)} \, dxdy \qquad (1)$$

The individual Fourier components can be considered as simple complex-exponential functions which form the more complicated function $u(X,Y,Z_0)$. The inverse transform which reconstructs $u(X,Y,Z_0)$ is

$$U(X,Y,Z_0) = \frac{1}{4\pi^2} \int\int_{-\infty}^{+\infty} u(\omega_x,\omega_y,Z_0) e^{j(\omega_x x + \omega_y y)} \, d\omega_x d\omega_y \qquad (2)$$

The Fourier decomposition results in a two-dimensional spectrum of plane wave components. Each (ω_x,ω_y) spatial frequency represents a plane wave travelling with direction cosines $(n_x = \omega_x/k, \; n_y = \omega_y/k)$. In order to model the propagation of the angular spectrum, each (ω_x,ω_y) component is multiplied by a phase propagation factor which accounts for the plane wave propagation in the (n_x,n_y) direction. This change is expressed as (Stepanishen and Benjamin, 1982):

$$G(\omega_x,\omega_y,Z_0,Z_1) = e^{j(Z_1-Z_0)\{k^2-\omega_x^2-\omega_y^2\}^{\frac{1}{2}}} = \Phi(\omega_x,\omega_y,Z_0,Z_1) \qquad (3)$$

Thus $G(\omega_x,\omega_y,Z_0,Z_1)$ is a propagation factor, which introduces a phase change $\Phi(\omega_x,\omega_y,Z_0,Z_1)$ to account for the propagation from Z_0 to Z_1. If each term in the Fourier expansion is propagated to a new Z_1 using the appropriate phase factor Φ, the complex pressure field at the plane Z_1 can be found by inverse transforming the resultant set of two-dimensional components.

One important aspect of this method is the treatment of propagating and non-propagating (evanescent) waves. It can be seen that for $n_x^2 + n_y^2 < 1$, the phase propagation factor in Eq. (3) is purely imaginary, indicating unattenuated harmonic wave propagation. If $n_x^2 + n_y^2 > 1$, then there will be a strong attenuation of the waves in the +Z direction. In backpropagation, on the other hand, their positive exponential Z dependence can lead to a divergent wave integral (Williams and Maynard, 1980).

With the background outlined above, the primary goal of this work was to modify the phase factor Φ to account for propagation in a layered medium. The next Section details the modifications, and describes the simulation used to examine the effects of various propagation parameters.

3. EXTENSIONS TO THE ANGULAR SPECTRUM METHOD

One property of the angular spectrum method is that it precludes the modelling of any variations in the X or Y directions. This is due to the fact that the angular spectrum method involves planar measurement and reconstruction surfaces, and considers wave propagation in the Z direction only. Therefore, tissue is modelled as a layered medium, with variations in attenuation, dispersion, and refraction occuring in the Z-direction (depth) only. These parameters are considered constant within each layer, so that the medium is described as a series of homogeneous layers. In addition to this, the inhomogeneous nature of tissue is modelled by a random index of refraction distribution. The following paragraphs detail the way in which each tissue propagation parameter is included in the model.

Attenuation is perhaps the most dominant tissue property affecting ultrasound transmission. The value of attenuation (a) in different tissue is usually calculated from

$$a = A \times f^q \tag{4}$$

where A ranges from 0.015 to 0.56 and q ranges from 0.763 to 1.18 (Edmonds and Dunn, 1981). To a first approximation, the value of attenuation can be considered constant (space-invariant) for a given tissue layer. This is included in the phase propagation factor $\Phi(\omega_x, \omega_y, Z_0, Z_1)$, Eq. (6), as a perturbation of the unattenuated form, using a wave number (k) with both real and imaginary components. Although the overall attenuation is frequency dependent, the forward or backward propagation algorithm is performed at a single discrete frequency at a time, so the corresponding value of attenuation can be used. Nikoonahad and Ash (1982) have presented a detailed theory on the inclusion of attenuation in the derivation of the angular spectrum technique, and concluded that the perturbation approach is valid for the values of attenuation typical of tissue.

The effects of refraction can be examined in the following way. Assume that a wave field is propagating from layer 1 to layer 2, which have sound speeds c_1 and c_2 respectively. At the interface between layers, the sound beam refracts due to the change in velocity, and both the wave number and the direction cosines of each plane wave component in the field will change. The wave then propagates in medium 2 with new wave number and direction cosines. Within the angular spectrum formulation, this effect is implemented by varying the wave number from layer to layer. One complication of this approach is due to the spatial sampling requirements which must be met in each layer. More specifically, it arises from the requirement that the field be sampled at half-wavelength intervals, in order to minimize spatial aliasing. Hence, the sampling requirements become dependent upon the medium with the shortest wavelength (for a given frequency), and the field in other layers will then be oversampled, reducing computational efficiency. This effect has been considered in the development of the simulation described in Section 4.

Dispersion, the change in sound velocity with frequency, leads to resolution degradation in pulsed field propagation, as each frequency component travels at a slightly different speed. This can be accounted for in the model in a way similar to refraction. At any given frequency, there is a unique sound speed associated with each layer. Because the model is, at present, fully developed only for the monochromatic case, it is not possible to demonstrate the effects of dispersion. This is a topic of the ongoing work aiming at further development of the model, and is mentioned here for the sake of completeness.

138

The technique for introducing phase distortion (weak inhomogeneities) into the angular spectrum technique follows that suggested by Lasota, Delannoy and Moriamez (1982). They modelled phase distortion in propagation by adding a random phase term to the free-space Green's function, which was then incorporated into a Rayleigh-Sommerfield diffraction integral (Goodman, 1968). Similarly, weak inhomogeneities in the medium can be introduced into the angular spectrum by modifying each Fourier-space component by a phase distortion term, using a normalized random function that describes the inhomogeneities in the medium (Frisch, 1968). Since the algorithm for propagating the angular spectrum involves computation of the total distance that each plane wave element must travel in propagating from plane Z to Z , given the direction cosine, (See Eq. (3)), inhomogeneities have been represented as errors in the calculation of $\Phi(\omega_x, \omega_y, Z_0, Z_1)$ for each (ω_x, ω_y). The errors are thus distributed over the spatial frequency domain with reduced phase coherence of the spatial components, resulting in a defocussing effect.

A simulation procedure has been developed which models a complex pressure wavefield over a 64 by 64 point grid. The size of the grid influences both the frequency of the transducer which can be modelled, and its physical dimensions. This is due to the fact that spatial sampling is performed at half wavelength intervals. Thus higher frequency transducers require finer spatial sampling, reducing the area that can be represented by the grid. The procedure developed also allows for the shading of the field using Hanning, Hamming, or Kaiser-Bessel weightings. These weighting functions can further be applied in the spatial frequency domain, thus reducing the influence of high spatial frequency components and smoothing the reconstructed wavefields.

Evanescent waves are included in the forward propagation case, because they do contribute to the accurate modelling of the nearfield structure, even though the waves generally die out within a few wavelengths of the source. When backpropagating, the effect of evanescent waves can either be included, or their contribution can be set to zero, for the reason discussed in Section 2.

This next section describes the simulation results obtained to date, using a single frequency model, with the effects of refraction and phase distortion included. Results showing the effects of attenuation were omitted because these have previously been discussed in the literature (Nikoonahad and Ash, 1982)

4. RESULTS OF THE SIMULATION

All simulations were performed by means of a PDP-11/73 computer, using a 64 by 64 point grid. This is the largest grid which can be implemented on this computer, due to its memory management structure. This had an influence on the simulations which could be performed. Therefore the results presented here show simulations carried out using a frequency of 1 MHz, and using a maximimum transducer diameter of 10 mm. It should be emphasized that these frequency and size limitations are due to the computer available, and are not a fundamental limitation of the technique.

The first series of plots show the backpropagation of a complex pressure field. The field was generated using the technique described by Lockwood and Willette (1980) for a circular aperture. The field was sampled at one-half wavelength spacing, assuming propagation in water at 21^0 C. Figure 1 shows the reconstruction of the field in the plane of the source, from an axial distance of 20 mm, without the inclusion of evanescent waves. The accentuation of the edge of the radiator, characteristic of Gibbs phenomena, (Stepanishen and Benjamin, 1982), can clearly be identified here. This is caused by the abrupt cut-off of the spatial frequency components at the edges of the 64 by 64 point grid. Filtering the wave field in the spatial frequency domain using a Hanning-type weighting smoothes the cut-off in the frequency domain, reducing the ringing phenomena, as shown in Figure (2).

The next plot shows the forward propagated field from a simulated focussed 10 mm diameter radiator. Phase variations were introduced across the face of the source to simulate focussing at an axial distance of 10 mm. The field in the focal plane is shown in Figure (3). Backpropagating to the source plane allowed reconstruction of the phase of the radiator in the source plane, as shown in Figure (4).

The fields from similar radiators were then examined in the X-Z plane, by iteratively propagating and reconstructing at small (approximately one third of a wavelength) intervals. The results for a focussed 10 mm square radiator which was phase steered to 30 degrees, are shown as a three-dimensional plot and as a contour plot in Figures (5) and (6). Phase steering was implemented to mimic a phased linear array. Thirty degree steering was chosen in order to keep the main lobe of the beam within the confines of the sampling grid as the field was forward propagated. The field was propagated to a distance of 20 mm along the Z axis, taking slices every 0.5 mm. The width of these plots is approximately 24 mm (32 points spaced at half-wavelength intervals).

The final series of plots show the effects of refraction and phase distortion. Figure (7) shows the same radiator as Figures (5) and (6), except that a 10 mm layer with 30 percent higher sound speed was introduced at 5 mm axial distance from the source. This resulted in a bending of the beam, and a smearing out of the peak focal zone. Similarly, a 10 mm layer which produced a random phase error of 30 percent was placed at 5 mm axial distance from the source. This field is shown in Figure (8); again the defocussing effects are worthwhile to note.

5. CONCLUSIONS

The extension of the angular spectrum method which has been developed and implemented on the PDP-11/73 computer is now being used to examine differently shaped radiators and various layered media. The simulations described here have demonstrated the technique to be a useful tool for the three-dimensional analysis of transducer fields. Experiments are in progress in which ultrasound transducers are measured in water; the data are then used in the backpropagation model. These calculated backpropagated source fields will subsequently be used to predict the fields produced by the actual transducers operated in layered, inhomogeneous media. Additionally, the computer facilities are being upgraded by the acquisition of a DEC MicroVax II, which will allow larger grids than those achievable with the PDP-11/73. The MicroVax II will allow the frequency and transducer size capabilities of the model to be significantly improved. It will also facilitate extension of the model to the pulsed radiator case, as described by Higgins, Norton, and Linzer (1980). This extension will further allow a closer investigation of dispersion, and of the wideband focussing properties of phased linear arrays in inhomogeneous media. With these improvements, the model will provide a powerful tool in the design and analysis of ultrasonic transducers for medical imaging and non-destructive testing.

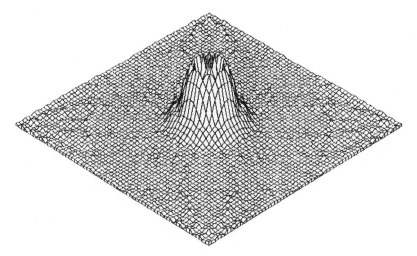

Figure 1. Magnitude of the reconstructed source plane field backpropagated from a distance of 20 mm. Source: 10 mm circular, unfocussed, operating at 1 MHz. Plot shows 64 x 64 points at half-wavelength spacing.

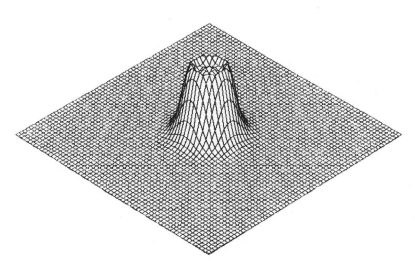

Figure 2. Same conditions as Figure (1), except a Hanning weighting was applied in the spatial frequency domain.

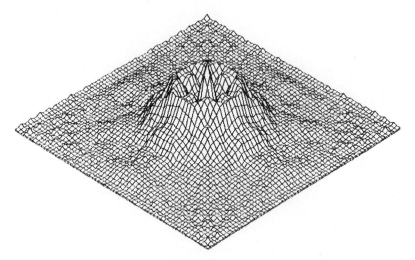

Figure 3. Magnitude of the pressure field forward propagated to the focal plane. Source: 10 mm circular, focussed at 10mm. Spacing of grid is the same as Figure (1).

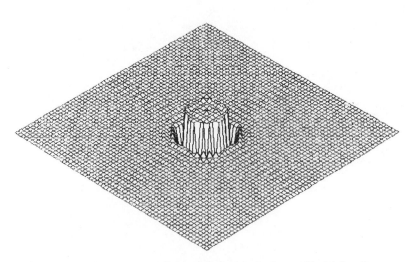

Figure 4. Phase of the reconstructed source plane field backpropagated from the field shown in Figure (3).

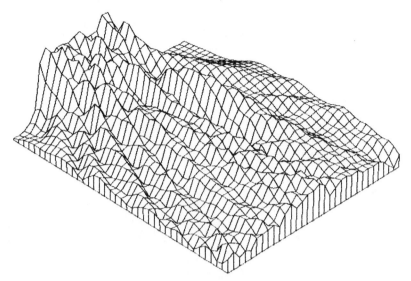

Figure 5. Magnitude of the pressure field calculated in the X-Z plane. Source: 10 mm square, focussed at 10mm, phase steered to 30 degrees. Z (axial) axis dimension is 20 mm; X (lateral) axis dimension is 24 mm.

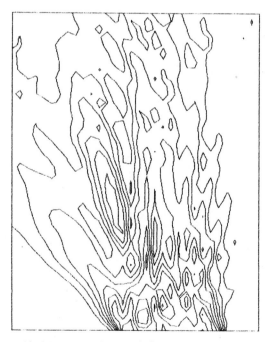

Figure 6. Same conditions as Figure (5), except shown as a contour plot.

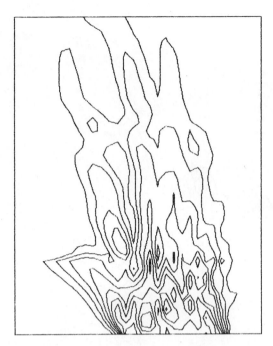

Figure 7. Same source as Figures (5) and (6), except a 10 mm thick layer with 30 percent higher sound speed was introduced, at 5 mm axial distance from the source.

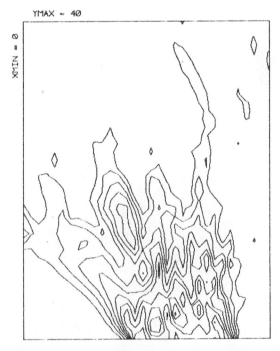

Figure 8. Same source as Figures (5) and (6), except a 10 mm thick layer with 30 percent random phase properties (See Section 3) was introduced, at 5 mm axial distance from the source

6. ACKNOWLEDGEMENTS

This work was supported by Research Grants from the National Science Foundation, Grant ECE-8504602, and the National Institutes of Health, Grant HL30045. Additionally, the authors would like to express their thanks to Dr. Tat-Jin Teo, and Mr. Frank W. West, for their helpful discussions and assistance with computer graphics techniques.

7. REFERENCES

Edmonds, P.D. and Dunn, F., 1981, Physical description of ultrasonic fields, in "Methods of Experimental Physics," P.D. Edmonds, ed., Academic Press, New York, Vol. 19, "Ultrasonics".

Frisch, U., 1968, Wave propagation in random media, in "Probabilistic Methods in Applied Mathematics," A.T. Bharucha-Reid, ed. Academic Press, New York, Vol. 1.

Goodman, J.W., 1968, "Introduction to Fourier Optics," McGraw-Hill, New York.

Higgins, F.P., Norton, S.J., and Linzer, M., 1980, Optical interferometric visualization and computerized reconstruction of ultrasonic fields, J. Acoust. Soc. Am., 68:1169.

Lasota, H., DeLannoy, B., and Moriamez, M., 1982, Directivity patterns in inhomogeneous media, in "Acoustical Imaging," E.A. Ash and C.R. Hill eds. Plenum Press, New York, Vol. 12.

Lockwood, J.C., and Willette, J.G., 1980, High speed solution for computing the exact solution for the pressure variations in the nearfield of a baffled piston, J. Acoust. Soc. Am., 53:735.

Nikoonahad, M. and Ash, E.A., 1982, Ultrasonic focussing in absorptive fluids, in "Acoustical Imaging," E.A. Ash and C.R. Hill eds. Plenum Press, New York, Vol. 12.

Powers, J.P., (1977), Computer simulation of linear acoustic diffraction, in "Acoustical Holography," L.W. Kessler, ed. Plenum Press, New York, Vol. 7.

Schafer, M.E. and Lewin, P.A., 1985, The influence of front-end hardware on digital ultrasonic imaging, IEEE Trans. Son. Ultrason., SU-31(4):295.

Stepanishen, P.R. and Benjamin, K.C., 1982, Forward and backward projection of acoustic fields using FFT methods, J. Acoust. Soc. Am., 71:803.

Sondhi, M.M., 1969, Reconstruction of objects from their sound diffraction patterns, J. Acoust. Soc. Am., 46:1158.

Wild, J.J., and Reid, J.M., 1952, The application of echo ranging techniques to the determination of structure of biological tissues, Science,15:226.

Williams, E.G., and Maynard, J.D., 1980, Holographic imaging without the wavelength resolution limit, Phys. Rev. Lett., 45:544.

DEVELOPMENT OF AN ELECTROMAGNETIC ACOUSTIC TRANSDUCER

FOR INSPECTING THE WALL THICKNESS OF OFFSHORE RISERS FROM THE INSIDE

W.H. van den Berg, M.H. Homs and A.B.M. Hoff

Koninklijke/Shell-Laboratorium, Amsterdam
(Shell Research B.V.)
Postbus 3003, 1003 AA   Amsterdam, The Netherlands

ABSTRACT

The design requirements for an electromagnetic acoustic transducer to determine remaining wall thickness of offshore gas risers from the inside are presented, together with the results of evaluation of a prototype. A specially designed configuration of high-energy-density permanent magnets, the choice of dedicated emitter/receiver coils and impedance matching between coils and electronics have resulted in optimum ultrasonic performance. Aspects related to implementation in an inspection vehicle, such as mechanical protection and negotiation of local obstructions inside a riser pipe, have received special attention and will be discussed.

INTRODUCTION

In offshore production the inspection of some riser pipes, in particular those inaccessible from the outside, requires a special approach. A feasibility study has been carried out to determine the best technique to measure quantitatively a decrease in wall thickness due to external corrosion. This feasibility study revealed that the most appropriate technique would be wall thickness measurement based on ultrasonics. Ultrasonic sensors can be built into a vehicle that is propelled by the medium in the pipe, known as an inspection pig (pipeline inspection gauge). A general layout of such a vehicle, consisting of a sensor module, a data collection module and a power supply module, is shown in Fig. 1.

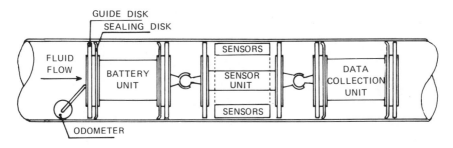

Fig. 1. A schematic diagram of the riser-pipe inspection vehicle.

If the riser to be inspected is an oil-carrying riser, conventional, piezoelectric transducers can be used as the oil will act as a perfect coupling medium. In a gas-carrying riser, however, no coupling medium is present, but use can be made of electromagnetic excitation of ultrasonic waves. Electromagnetic acoustic transducers (EMATs) have been used before (Maxfield and Fortunko, 1982; Alers, 1981), mostly based on large electromagnets. For this specific application, however, no adequate EMAT was available. Therefore, Shell and Röntgen Technische Dienst (RTD, Rotterdam) started a joint development programme. The generation efficiency of an EMAT is very low compared to that of conventional piezoelectric transducers, so the optimization of the ultrasonic performance is of major importance. Optimization had to be realized with regard to several conflicting requirements:

- in view of the space and energy available in the inspection vehicle, use had to be made of permanent magnets rather than electromagnets;
- measurement of thin wall sections had to be possible, which could be achieved by excitement of short, relatively high-frequency pulses; i.e. a short dead zone was required.

Efficient excitation of ultrasonic waves by electromagnetic means requires, however, as high a magnetic induction and as low a frequency as possible. In this paper an optimal solution to the problem of coping with these conflicting requirements is described. Constructional aspects in relation to the use of the EMAT sensor in an inspection vehicle, such as mechanical protection and negotiation of local obstructions, will also be addressed.

THEORY OF 'NORMAL-INCIDENT' EMAT

Lorentz Force Mechanism

An acoustic wave of normal incidence is frequently used for measurement of the remaining wall thickness. The generation of such a wave by electromagnetic means is based on the Lorentz force mechanism and/or magnetostriction. The generation of a normal-incident shear wave in low-carbon steel, the material normally used for riser pipes, is dominated by the Lorentz force mechanism. The efficiency with which the Lorentz force mechanism is generated increases monotonically with the static magnetization applied, Fig. 2.

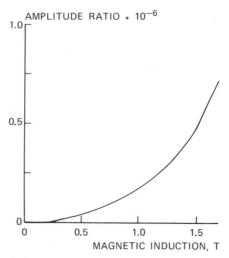

Fig. 2. Generation efficiency versus static magnetic induction.

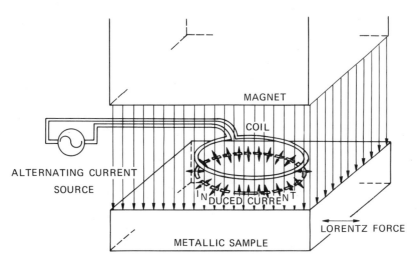

Fig. 3. Principle of the Lorentz mechanism.

The use of the Lorentz force mechanism to generate ultrasound in metals
is well understood (Beissner, 1976; Dobbs, 1973). An emitter coil carrying a
radiofrequency current in the proximity of a metallic sample induces eddy
currents in the skin layer of the surface of this sample. If at the same time
a static, normal-incident, magnetic field is present, a Lorentz force acts on
these eddy currrents, Fig. 3. At ambient temperature the mean free path of the
electrons in the metal is of the order of 10 nm, so the change of the
momentum of the eddy currents due to this force is readily transferred to a
shear stress in the surface of the metal:

$$\underline{\tau} = \underline{J} \times \underline{B} \tag{1}$$

where: $\underline{\tau}$ = shear stress,
$\underline{J}$ = eddy current density,
$\underline{B}$ = static magnetic induction.
This shear stress forms the source of the acoustic wave that propagates in
the material, reflects at the far side and is received by a receiver coil
via the inverse Lorentz mechanism.

The energy conversion efficiency, at frequencies of a few megahertz,
from a plane, normal-incident electromagnetic wave to an acoustic wave in
a plate of low-carbon steel, is given by:

$$\eta = \left[\frac{2\sigma}{\mu\omega}\right]^{\frac{1}{2}} \cdot \frac{1}{\rho c} \cdot B^2 \tag{2}$$

where: η = energy conversion efficiency,
σ = electrical conductivity of the metal,
μ = magnetic permeability of the metal,
ρ = density of the metal,
c = velocity of the acoustic wave,
ω = angular frequency of the wave,
B = normal component of static magnetic induction.
The conversion efficiency depends on material properties, the frequency and
the static magnetic induction. To maximize the efficiency, only frequency
and static magnetic induction can be used. The frequency, however, cannot be

varied over a wide range, as the selected centre frequency of the emitted pulse has to be a compromise between maximum conversion efficiency and minimum remaining wall thickness that has to be measured. The latter determines the acceptable 'dead zone', which is the length of time after the beginning of the pulse excitation during which no acoustic reflection can be detected. In spatial terms, the dead zone is required to be less than 8 mm for the application concerned, which resulted in the use of a broad-band emitter pulse with a centre frequency of 2 MHz. At this frequency the energy conversion efficiency on low-carbon steel is $10^{-5} \cdot B^2$.

Receiving the signal requires conversion of acoustic to electromagnetic energy, of which the efficiency is also given by eq. (2). The overall energy conversion efficiency then becomes $10^{-10} \cdot B^4$.

Maximization of the Signal to Noise Ratio

As the energy conversion efficiency in low-carbon steel is very low, first priority in the design of the sensor is given to the maximization of the signal to noise ratio. The signal to noise ratio is defined as the ratio of the amplitude of the ultrasonic back wall reflection to the highest level of disturbing signals received in the time interval following the emitted pulse.

The overall signal to noise ratio that is obtained depends on:
- the electromagnetic energy radiated by the emitter coil,
- the electromagnetic coupling between the emitter coil and the material under inspection,
- the conversion of electromagnetic to acoustic energy,
- the attenuation of the reflected acoustic wave and reflection at the far side,
- the conversion of acoustic to electromagnetic energy,
- the electromagnetic coupling between the receiver coil and the surface of the material,
- the disturbing signals and thermal noise received, and the electric noise added by the receiver circuitry.

The basic circuit for generation of the emitted pulse is a second-order series resonance circuit, see Fig. 4. The charged capacitor is discharged through the emitter coil as soon as the switch is closed. The frequency of the oscillation is given by the capacitance and inductance, while the resistance determines the damping. The inductance and resistance in the circuit are mainly formed by the emitter coil in the proximity of the material under inspection. For a given oscillation frequency the energy of the pulse is inversely proportional to the magnitude of the inductance. Therefore the impedance of the emitter coil is chosen to be as low as is acceptable, but significantly exceeding the parasitic impedances of the wiring of the transmitter circuitry and the cable to the coil. That a low-inductance coil requires only a few windings is considered an additional advantage.

The electromagnetic coupling of the emitter and receiver coils with the material is a function of the ratio of the diameter of the coil to the distance between coil and material, called lift-off. A theoretical calculation of the induction of eddy currents by a circular coil in the surface of a ferromagnetic sample is given by Hammond, 1962. The average diameters of the emitter and receiver coils are selected to be 8 and 5 mm respectively,

The disturbing signals detected above the thermal electric noise level can originate from several sources. Sources that were encountered are:
- Unwanted ultrasonic reflections from the magnet pole. These are suppressed by laminating this magnet pole, so as to decrease the ultrasonic waves

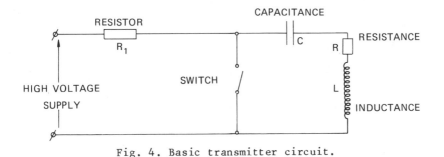

Fig. 4. Basic transmitter circuit.

generated parasitically. The remainder of these signals is shifted in time out of the measurement interval by increasing the length of the magnet pole.
- Mechanical vibration of the receiver coil in the static magnetic field, which is overcome by minimization of the coupling between emitter and receiver coils, in combination with increased mechanical damping of the coils.
- Pick-up of electromagnetic interference, which can be eliminated by proper design of the electronic circuitry and cabling.

After these disturbing signals had been successfully suppressed, see Fig. 5, the electric noise was addressed. The electric noise at the input

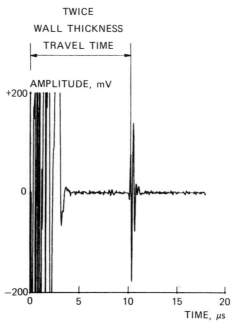

Fig. 5. Amplitude scan of an EMAT on low-carbon steel sample with a wall thickness of 16 mm.

of the receiver originates primarily from random thermal motions of the electrons in the surface of the material, which are sensed by the receiver coil. The power of the thermal noise is proportional to the absolute temperature and the bandwidth of the frequency spectrum. As both noise and signal are sensed by the same coil the number of turns of the receiver coil does not affect the signal to noise ratio. The impedance of the coil is matched to the input impedance of the receiver in order to minimize the noise added by this receiver. A low-noise receiver with a low-input impedance is used, so that the impedance and consequently the number of turns of the receiver coil can be kept small.

REALIZATION OF THE EMAT AND ITS SUSPENSION

Optimal signal to noise ratio requires a high static magnetic induction and a minimum distance between coils and pipe wall. As the EMAT is to be contained in an inspection vehicle other essential aspects for the design of the sensor have been addressed, viz.:
- protection of the coils, located in a gap between the magnet pole and the pipe, against mechanical damage when the sensor passes a penetrating circumferential weld,
- flexible mounting of the sensor to the body of the inspection vehicle, in order to pass diameter reductions and bends,
- minimal energy consumption, as the total energy supply is limited by the space available in the vehicle,
- a facility to enable it to pass barred T-joints.

Static Magnetic Circuits

In order to minimize the power consumption of the sensor, the magnetic circuit is designed with permanent magnets of high energy density, instead of electromagnets. The magnetic induction achieved in the gap under the magnet pole, where the coils are located, depends on:
- the cross section of the magnets with respect to the cross section of the tip of the pole,
- the amount of leakage of magnetic flux from the circuit,
- the length of the magnets in relation to the gap,
- the loss in the circuit due to the reluctance of the circuit elements in relation to the reluctance of the gap.
The dimensions, length and cross section, of the magnets are selected with the aim of operating the magnets at the point of maximum energy density. Via focussing of the magnetic field lines, a static magnetic induction of 1.8 T under the tip of the magnet pole has been achieved.

Configuration of the Emitter and Receiver Coils

The emitter and receiver coils selected for implementation in the EMAT are concentric coils mounted in the same plane. These coils combine optimal ultrasonic performance with a minimal space requirement. The latter is of importance, as space is then available for the protection of the coils.

The emitter coil generates a radially polarized shear wave with an acoustic beam profile as shown in Fig. 6; see also Fig. 3 for the reason for this. The radius of the receiver coil should be such that on a sample of nominal wall thickness the coil projects on the maxima locus of the reflected beam. The optimum average diameters of the coils can be estimated using:

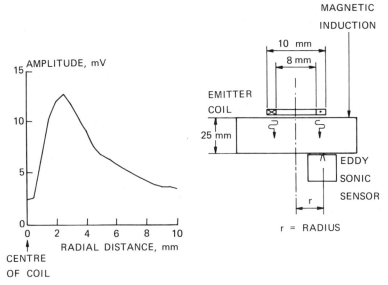

Fig. 6. Radially polarized beam profile of a circular coil.

$$\langle d_r \rangle . \langle d_e \rangle = 2.W.\lambda_c \qquad\qquad (3)$$

where: $\langle d_r \rangle$ = average diameter of the receiver coil,
$\langle d_e \rangle$ = average diameter of the emitter coil,
W = nominal wall thickness,
λ_c = centre wavelength of the acoustic pulse.

For a wall thickness of nominal 0.5 inch and a 2 MHz centre frequency of the emitted acoustic pulse, the product of average diameters of the coils is 40 mm^2. To be able to mount both coils in the same plane, the average diameters for the emitter and receiver coils are chosen to be 8 and 5 mm respectively. For coils of these dimensions the electromagnetic coupling is found to decrease by 10 dB/mm at increasing lift-off.

Constructional Aspects

The main objectives in the mechanical design are to keep the coils within close proximity of the pipe wall and to protect them against damage.

Suspension mechanism. The prototype suspension developed for mechanical tests and tests in a 16-inch test loop is shown in Fig. 7. This suspension provides the radial flexibility required to pass bends and diameter reductions. A cardan joint between the suspension and the sensor is required to allow the sensor to follow the contour of the pipe in case the inspection vehicle is excentric, e.g. in a bend, or when minor buckles have to be passed.

Protection of coils. Protection of the coils is essential as the coils are mounted under the magnet pole and the speed of the sensor relative to the pipe wall may be as high as several metres per second. Consequently the coils have to be protected against mechanical damage by local obstructions, e.g. penetrations of the circumferential welds. The protection should not have ferromagnetic or conductive properties as these will degrade the electromagnetic coupling between coils and pipe wall. In addition, high-strength

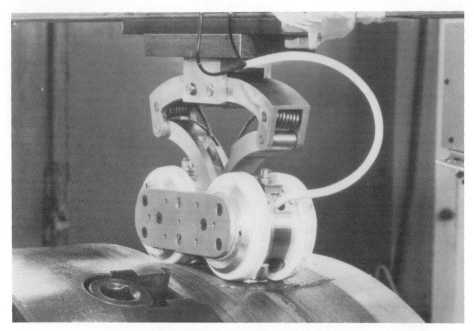

Fig. 7. Sensor and suspension on the mechanical test bench.

material should be used as the space available between coils and pipe wall
is only approx. 0.8 mm. The protection adopted consists of a ceramic cap to
provide high strength, surrounded by a nylon bumper to absorb the impact of
local obstructions. The impact force is reduced by using a pendulum-like
magnet pole, such that only the mass of the pole has to be accelerated during
an impact.

TEST RESULTS

Ultrasonic Performance

The minimum ultrasonic performance required for the sensor to be implemented in the inspection vehicle is specified as:
- a spherical reflector with 10 mm surface diameter and a depth of 2.5 mm
  should be detectable,
- the minimum detectable wall thickness should be at least 8 mm.
The ultrasonic performance has been evaluated under static conditions in the
laboratory, see Fig. 8. As can be seen in Fig. 8,a, measurement of wall
thicknesses (WTs) between 7 and 30 mm can easily be performed. In Fig. 8,b,
the decrease in amplitude with decreasing diameter (D) of a spherical reflec
tor, located at the far side wall, is shown. The spherical reflector with th
specified 2.5 mm depth can be detected in a 16 mm nominal wall thickness, bu
is only 2 dB above the threshold level to be exceeded in order to perform a
wall thickness measurement. The threshold level is selected at 2 dB above th
maximum noise level determined from 256 amplitude recordings in the time
interval of interest. One should bear in mind that the detectability of smal
pits decreases with increasing wall thickness, see Fig. 8,c. From Fig. 8,d
a decrease of 20 dB/mm lift-off (LO) can be derived. This 20 dB/mm is due to
a fall in electromagnetic coupling (10 dB/mm) and static magnetic induction
(10 dB/mm).

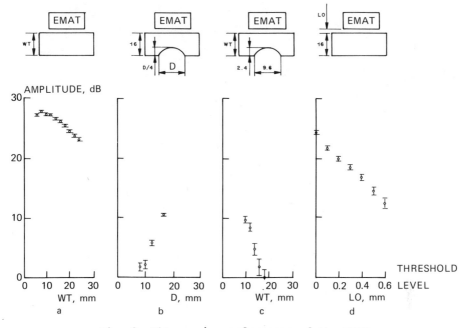

Fig. 8. Ultrasonic performance of the EMAT.

The sensor has been subjected to a combined temperature and pressure test under static conditions. The sensor was placed in an autoclave filled with helium; first, the pressure was raised to 150 bar, then the temperature was raised from 20 to 60 °C over a period of 2 h. The pressurization did not measurably affect the ultrasonic performance, but the increase of temperature caused a 1 dB decrease of the signal to noise ratio. Further, during the rapid (2 min) depressurization the noise level increased temporarily (for 5 min) as the pressure dropped below 40 bar.

Further tests have shown that neither collection of magnetic fouling at the magnet pole nor the velocity with which the sensor moves relative to the sample (up to 18 m/s) affects the ultrasonic performance.

Mechanical Performance

The mechanical performance of the sensor has been evaluated under conditions equivalent to 50 km of pipeline or riser operation. First, the sensor was placed on a rotating pipe in a lathe, see Fig. 7. After 50 km, the wear of the wheel of the sensor was found to be less than the measurement accuracy of 0.05 mm. After the wear test a weld seam was made on the pipe in order to simulate a circumferential penetration. This simulated penetration was passed 5000 times at a speed of 1.9 m/s, without any significant damage occurring to the sensor.

155

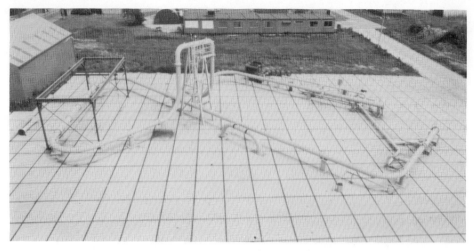

Fig. 9. Test loop (16-inch).

Test in Test Loop

After the test on a lathe the sensor was tested in a 16-inch test loop, which has a length of 110 m and comprises vertical parts, several bends with a radius of three to five times the pipe diameter, a 6 % buckle and two full-bore barred T-joints: see Fig. 9.

The EMAT sensor and transmitter/receiver electronics were mounted on a single-body vehicle with polyurethane guide and sealing disks. The receiver output was connected to the instrumentation located in a cabin near the loop by means of a 100 m long cable. Part of a wall thickness record obtained during a run at a speed of 0.8 m/s through the test loop is shown in Fig. 10.

During testing it was found that the moving parts of the sensor were liable to fouling, especially by magnetic dust that is attracted by the permanent magnets. During the test, therefore, the pendulum-like magnet pole was surrounded by silicone rubber compound, which proved to be a successful way of preventing excessive fouling and subsequent lifting of the pole.

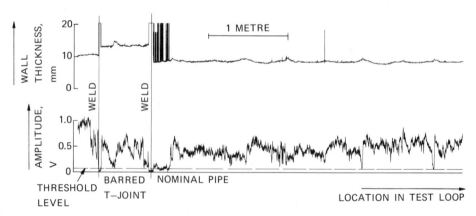

Fig. 10. Wall thickness and amplitude records obtained during a test in the 16-inch loop at a speed of 0.8 m/s.

CONCLUSIONS

The ultrasonic performance of the sensor that has been designed is such that:
- a spherical reflector of 10 mm in diameter and a depth of 2.5 mm, in a sample of 16 mm wall thickness, is detected at 2 dB above the threshold level,
- the minimum wall thickness that can be measured is 7 mm.

The EMAT sensor can be used in an inspection vehicle provided that the internal bore of the pipe is clean and not corroded, as an increase in lift-off will degrade the ultrasonic performance.

In a 50-km wear test followed by 5000 passes of a simulated penetration at 1.9 m/s, the mechanical performance of the sensor was satisfactory.

The sensor is capable of negotiating barred T-joints and bends with a radius of three to five times the diameter of a 16-inch pipe while providing a virtually complete record of the pipeline wall thickness.

Prevention of fouling of the moving parts of the sensor, in particular by magnetic particles, is something that requires special attention. Surrounding the magnet pole by silicone rubber proved effective.

REFERENCES

Alers, G.A., 1981, Application of electromagnetic acoustic transducers (EMATs), Proceedings of the 26th National SAMPE Symposium, 28-30 April 1981, pp. 34-44.
Beissner, R.E., 1976, Electromagnetic acoustic transducers, a survey of the state of the art, South-West Research Institute, San Antonio, Texas, NTIAC-76-1.
Dobbs, E.R., 1973, Electromagnetic generation of ultrasonic waves, in: "Physical acoustics; principles and methods", Vol. 10, W.P. Mason and R.N. Thurston, eds., Academic press, New York, Chapter 10, p. 127.
Hammond, P., 1962, The calculation of the magnetic field of rotating machines, part 3. - Eddy currents induced in a solid slab by a circular current loop, The Institution of Electrical Engineers, Monograph No. 514S.
Maxfield, B.W. and Fortunko, C.M., 1983, The design and use of electromagnetic acoustic wave transducers (EMATs), Materials Evaluation, 41: 1399.

TRANSDUCER ARRAY FOR ULTRASOUND HOLOGRAPHIC B-SCAN IMAGING

Veijo Suorsa, Esko Alasaarela and Antti Tauriainen

Department of Electrical Engineering
University of Oulu
90570 Oulu, Finland

ABSTRACT

A 128 element transducer array with 64 PZT ceramic transmitter elements and 64 PVDF polymer receiver elements is described. The array is working at a frequency of 4 MHz and it has been constructed with the requirements of the ultrasound holographic B-scan (UHB) imaging in mind. The most important of these requirements are high sensitivity and a wide angular response in the azimuth plane. The sensitivity of the PVDF receiver elements of the prototype array, however, was found to be nearly 7 dB less when the response from an electrically tuned PVDF element was compared to the response from an untuned PZT element of the same array as a receiver.

INTRODUCTION

Acoustic transducers and imaging arrays using piezoelectric ceramics as the active elements have been widely explored and a wide range of these transducers is commercially available. However, the high acoustic impedance of piezoelectric ceramics, like lead zirconate titanate (PZT) compounds, greatly complicates the construction of efficient wideband transducers. This is the case especially in the field of medical applications of ultrasound, where the transducer face is loaded by waterlike, mostly liquid body constituents.

A good acoustic impedance match between the ceramic ($Z \approx 30$ MRayl) and the tissue ($Z \approx 1.5$ MRayl) is not easily achieved. Matching layers are both difficult to fabricate and the materials from which they are to be constructed have to be carefully selected. Because of the great impedance step to be bridged by the matching, the allowable tolerances in the thickness and the acoustic impedance of the matching layer are narrow. Matching layers also tend to affect the bandwidth and the impulse response of the transducer since each layer increases the efficiency only over a limited frequency band. Despite these problems piezoelectric ceramic materials are widely used because of the high value of the electromechanical coupling factor ($k \approx 0.5$).

Piezoelectric polyvinylidene difluoride (PVDF) offers a low value of acoustic impedance (Z ≤ 4 MRayl) which simplifies broadband coupling to the tissue. PVDF, however, suffers from a low value of the electromechanical coupling factor (k ≤ 0.3) and the large dielectric loss. Generally this means that PVDF will not be as efficient as a transmitting material as PZT. Despite the low piezoelectric activity of PVDF, the low dielectric constant ($\epsilon \approx 10$) and the high value of the piezoelectric voltage constant g_{33} make it attractive to be used as the receiving element material. Especially when a broadband response and a short ringdown time of the impulse response together with good sensitivity are of prime importance PVDF may be an effective substitute for PZT.

The ultrasound holographic B–scan (UHB) imaging method sets some special requirements for the performance of the transducer array. The UHB imaging method is a combination of conventional B–scan imaging and one dimensional ultrasonic holography. The theory of UHB imaging has been described more precisely in previous papers[1,2]. The main advantage offered by the UHB imaging method when compared to the conventional B–scan imaging is the improved lateral resolution. In the sense of array construction requirements this means a wide angular response in the azimuth plane and a narrow response in the elevation plane. To keep up with the longitudinal resolution and the imaging depth offered by conventional B–scan systems the short impulse response and high sensitivity of the array are of prime importance. We have fabricated a prototype array utilizing PZT as the transmitting element material and PVDF as the receiver element material. The design and performance of the prototype array will be described in this paper.

WORKING PRINCIPLE

The UHB array consists of 64 transmitter elements and 64 receiver elements. A short pulse is transmitted from the addressed transmitter element. The returning echoes are received by the neighbouring receiver element and digitized and stored. This process, measuring both the amplitude and the phase of the returning echoes, is repeated until all the elements are scanned. The working principle of the UHB transducer is illustrated in figure 1.

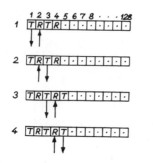

A short pulse is transmitted from the addressed transmitter element (T) and the returning echoes are received by the neighbouring receiver element (R).

Fig. 1. Shematic of UHB array working principle.

SPECIFIC DESIGN CRITERIA

According to the theory of holography[2] the resolution in lateral direction is

$$d = \frac{\lambda z}{2a} \qquad (1)$$

where   z = the distance between the hologram plane and the object
         a = the aperture of the hologram plane.

The resolution in the depth direction (z) is restricted by the pulse response of the receiver element and the receiver electronics.

Following the equation (1) an angular response as wide as possible would be desirable. However, in practise there is a compromise between the wideness of the angular response and sensitivity to be made. The wider the angular response, the less power is radiated back from a single object point. Then the usable imaging depth is restricted by the sensitivity of the receiver elements of the array. Inadequate sensitivity can be compensated to a certain degree by narrowing the beam pattern by the means of focusing in the elevation plane, perpendicular to the scanning plane. As a result of this action acoustic power in the imaging area is increased.

CONSTRUCTION AND FABRICATION TECHNIQUES

Figure 2 shows the construction of the prototype UHB array which utilizes both PZT and PVDF. The backing element was fabricated by mixing tungsten powder with epoxy and centrifuging the mixture. A mixture ratio of one part epoxy to four parts tungsten powder by weight was chosen for the high backing impedance. According to electron microscope analysis of the equally fabricated backing element, the highest concentration of tungsten powder was found as a 0.3 mm wide belt just behind the ceramic plate.

A configuration ratio near 0.6 with a working frequency near 4 MHz for PZT was chosen. Ratios less than unity have been proposed by Selfridge et al.[3] for a wide angular response and by Sato et al.[4] for high efficiency. The cuts between the PZT elements were made extending well into the backing in order to suppress acoustic cross coupling through the tungsten powder belt.

Focusing in the elevation plane was achieved with an acoustic lens made from epoxy. Epoxy was chosen for the lens material because of its relative low acoustic impedance ($Z \approx 3$ MRayl), maintaining the wide angular response conditions in the azimuth plane for both PZT and PVDF. This is due to attenuation of lateral resonances of PZT elements in epoxy. In the case of a higher impedance filler between the elements, these resonances would be more pronounced resulting in peaks in the angular response as shown by Kino and DeSilets[5]. On the other hand, epoxy serves as a lower impedance backing for PVDF receivers. This condition applies if an angular response without peaks for PVDF working below its mechanical resonance is desired as shown by Weinstein[6] and Granz[7]. However, as shown by Nguyen et al.[8], higher efficiency for PVDF could have been achievable with a quarter wavelength resonance mode with a high impedance backing.

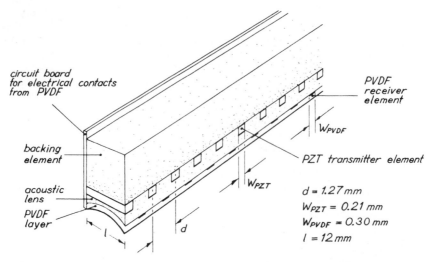

Fig. 2. Construction of UHB array using both PZT and PVDF.

The signal electrodes of 0 3 mm × 12 mm for the PVDF elements were evaporated on the lens surface first a chrome layer of 20 nm for good adhesion and then a copper layer of 300 nm. The electrical contacts could be made simultaneously on the 0.35 μm thick (or wide as seen from the lens surface) copper layer on the circuit board glued on the side of the backing element. The only crucial alignment was to be made when the mask for the signal electrodes was positioned on the lens. After the evaporation process a non-metallised, uniaxially drawn and poled PVDF film of 110 μm thickness was glued on the lens surface. A non-uniform pressure was applied using a cylindrically shaped jig thereby avoiding the problem of having trapped glue. Granz[7] has shown that capacitive coupling through the suitable thin glue layer does not produce remarkable signal reduction. A common ground electrode for the PVDF elements was made with the same procedure as described. Only a layer of gold with a thickness of 20 nm was added on the surface.

EXPERIMENTAL RESULTS

Angular response

For the measurement of the angular response the UHB array was insonified in the water tank in the far field of a 4 MHz, self made PZT hydrophone. Bursts of 10 cycles with a center frequency of 4 MHz were produced to excite the hydrophone. The amplitudes of the received bursts were maximized by optimum placement of the array. The amplitudes of the received bursts were then registered at 2 degree intervals of the hydrophone movements. The setup for this measurements is illustrated in figure 3.

The angular responses are shown in figure 4. The measurement distance is 55 mm for the PVDF elements and 80 mm for the PZT elements. The resultant -6 dB beamwidth for PZT is 37 degrees, with minima at 28 degrees and secondary peaks at 34 degrees. The appearance of the minima was expected due to the use of epoxy between the elements. However, the result is acceptable and indicates relatively low cross coupling between the elements. The measurement

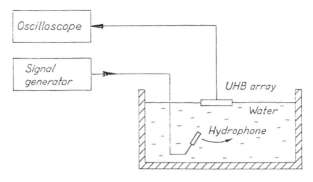

Fig.3. Setup for measurement of the angular response

was also done for PZT with the reversed setup a Medisonics Mk II PVDF
hydrophone as a receiver. A good agreement between the shown results
was found . The PVDF elements were found to be extremely sensitive to
cross coupling. With all the neighbouring elements open circuited a
very peaky response was observed (figure 4, curve a). With the first
PVDF neighbours short circuited a smoother response was obtained
(figure 4, curve b). The resultant -6 dB beamwidth in the latter case
is 33 degrees. Slight asymmetry in the beamform indicates an error
with the metallisation mask alignment.

<u>Focusing</u>

The measurement of the focusing effect was performed by insonifying
the UHB array with a 4 MHz, self made hydrophone. The hydrophone was
placed at a fixed axial distance from the UHB array and the placement
of the hydrophone was adjusted for maximum responses. The amplitudes
of the received bursts of 10 cycles were then registered at the
intervals of 1 mm hydrophone steps. The process was repeated for
several axial distances. The measurement was also done for PZT with
the reversed setup using Medisonics Mk II hydrophone as a receiver. A
good agreement was found between the results shown. However, the same
could not be done for the PVDF elements because of their low
efficiency as transmitters.

Figure 5 shows the focusing effect of the UHB array in the
elevation plane. A typical -6 dB beam width for a PZT element is less
than 4 mm at an axial distance of 70 mm. The narrowest -6 dB beam for
a typical PVDF element of 2 mm was measured at a distance of 40 mm.
The difference in the depth of the focusing field is due to a
compromise between the focusing of the PZT and PVDF elements.

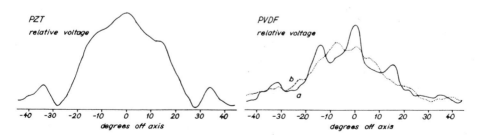

Fig.4. Typical angular responses for UHB array in the azimuth plane

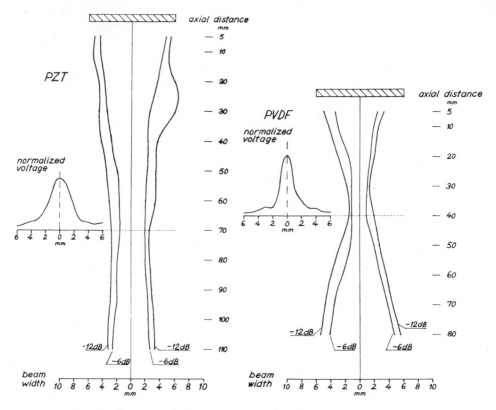

Fig.5. Beam profile variation in the elevation plane.

Cross coupling

For the cross coupling measurement an untuned array element was excited with one cycle of 4 MHz from a signal generator. The voltages across the neighbouring elements without electrical tuning were observed with a high impedance oscilloscope probe. During the measurement all the other elements besides the excited and the measured one were open circuited. The array face was loaded by water. The highest degree of cross coupling between the excited PZT element and its first neighbouring element was -30 dB. Between the excited PVDF element and its first neighbouring element the corresponding figure was -25 dB. Following the same technique the cross coupling between the PVDF and PZT elements was found to be -47 dB (a PZT element excited) and -55 dB (a PVDF element excited). In all cases the cross coupling was found to decrease with the increasing distance between the excited and measured element. The results are also shown in table 1.

Relative sensitivity and pulse response waveforms

The performance of the PVDF elements was compared to that of PZT elements by using a self made, 4 MHz PZT hydrophone as a transmitter and receiving the transmitted pulses both by a PVDF and a PZT element. The hydrophone was placed in the water tank at an axial distance of 55 mm from the UHB array and was excited with one cycle of 4 MHz. The received pulses were peaked by the proper orientation of the UHB transducer. Slight adjustments for peak response were also

Table 1. Cross coupling in the UHB array. Results in dB for one cycle of 4 MHz.

excitation	neighbour	1st	2nd	3rd
PZT	PZT	-30	-41	-50
	PVDF	-47	-48	-49
PVDF	PVDF	-25	-31	-36
	PZT	-55	-59	-62

made when the probe was moved from one element to the other thus to compensate the 0.635 mm center-to-center distance of neighbouring elements. All neighbouring elements were open circuited.

The received waveforms for the different tuning arrangements are shown in figure 6. The impedance measurements for the tuning were made with a Rohde Schwarz ZPV vector analyzer. Also the load due to the probe capacitance of 25 pF nominal value was compensated in the case of the tuned responses. The values for the shunt inductances were selected on the basis of the phase angle zero crossing of the electrical impedance near 4 MHz.

The waveform for an untuned PVDF element shows some ringing likely due to the transmitted waveform from the hydrophone and to the reflections from the boundary between the acoustic lens and the backing element. In addition the signal is decreased through the capacitive loading caused by the probe. When the untuned response from a PVDF element is compared to the response from a PZT element, the maximum amplitude is approximately 16 dB less than that of the untuned PZT element and 22 dB less than that of the tuned PZT element. When tuned the corresponding figures are nearly 7 dB and about 12 dB. The parallel tuning, however, not only increased the amplitude by about 10 dB but also clearly affected the bandwith of the PVDF response. This effect can be seen as ringing due to a reduced bandwith. For the PZT response the same effect was not as pronounced as in the case of the PVDF response. The increase in the amplitude of the PZT response was nearly 6 dB.

DISCUSSION AND CONCLUSIONS

A 128 element transducer array with 64 PZT ceramic transmitter elements and 64 PVDF polymer receiver elements was constructed. The sensitivity of the PVDF receiver elements was nearly 7 dB less than that of the PZT elements of the same array as receivers. This figure was achieved when the pulse response signal level of a shunt inductance tuned PVDF element was compared to that of an electrically untuned PZT element. The most promising property of the PVDF part was the ease of construction when compared to the PZT part.

A large lateral distance between the individual PZT elements of the prototype array produces acceptable beam forming properties although epoxy between the elements apparently causes cross coupling with resultant peaks in the angular response[5]. However, the cross coupling was even higher for the PVDF elements than for the PZT ones. If the

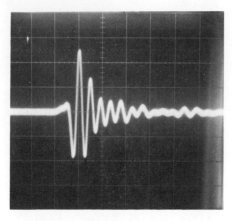
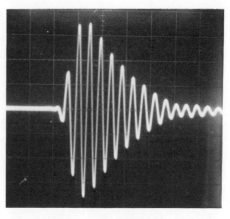

a) Untuned PVDF
(scales 5 mV/div, 0,5 µs/div).

b) Parallel tuned PVDF
(scales 10 mV/div, 0,5 µs/div).

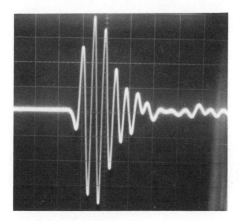
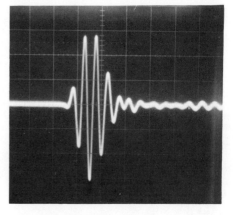

c) Untuned PZT
(scales 20 mV/div, 0,5 µs/div).

d) Parallel tuned PZT
(scales 50 mV/div, 0,5 µs/div).

Fig.6. Received waveforms.

cross coupling were not a problem the angular response of the PVDF elements could be widened by narrowing the element width[6]. On the other hand, this would decrease the sensitivity through the decreased element area. The difference in the focusing effect of the PZT and PVDF elements remains in the present construction.

The sensitivity of the PVDF elements can be increased through the introduction of a high impedance backing and thus a quarter wave resonance mode for PVDF[7]. Simultaneously, however, the cross coupling level between the PZT elements should not be increased. The sensitivity can also be raised by increasing the PVDF film thickness[8] At the same time, this solution would lead to a decreased value of the element capacitance and thus extra stress should be placed on the receiver electronics.

ACKNOWLEDGEMENTS

We wish to express our thankfulness to the Semiconductor Laboratory
of the Research Centre of Finland (VTT) for the assistance in the PVDF
processing. We also wish to thank Ms. Tarja Hentilä and Mr. Jussi
Kaleva for the practical construction work with the arrays, Mr. Sakari
Annala and Mr. Seppo Noponen for assisting in the measurements and
finally Ms. Ritva Lahtinen and Ms. Riitta Piirainen for their
assistance in the manuscript preparation.

The financial support from the Academy of Finland, TEKES, Alfred
Kordelinin Säätiö, Emil Aaltosen Säätiö and Oulun Yliopiston
Tukisäätiö is also gratefully acknowledged.

REFERENCES

1. E.Alasaarela, K. Tervola, J. Ylitalo and J. Koivukangas, UHB
    imaging, in: "Acoustical Imaging, Vol. 12," E.A. Ash et al.,
    ed., Plenum Press, New York, 1982.

2. E.Alasaarela, "Ultrasound holographic B (UHB) imaging,"
    doctoral thesis, University of Oulu, 1983.

3. A.R. Selfridge, G.S. Kino and B.T. Khuri-Yakub," A theory for
    the radiation pattern of a narrow strip acoustic transducer,"
    Appl. Phys. Lett. 37 (1), July 1980.

4. J. Sato, M. Kawabuchi and A. Fukumoto,"Depedence of the
    electromechanical coupling on the width-to-thickness ratio of
    plank-shaped piezoelectric transducers used for electronically
    scanned ultrasound diagnostic systems, "J.Acoust. Soc. Am. 66
    (6), December 1979.

5. G.S. Kino and C.S. DeSilets," Design of slotted transducer
    arrays with matched backings," Ultrasonic Imaging 1, 1979.

6. D.G. Weinstein," Polyvinylidine fluoride acoustic transducers
    and imaging arrays," doctoral thesis, Stanford University,
    October 1982.

7. B. Granz, A linear monolithic receiving array of PVDF
    transducers for transmission cameras, in: "Acoustical
    Imaging,Vol.12," E.A. Ash et al., ed., Plenum Press, New York
    1982.

8. H.G. Nguyen, P. Hartemann and D. Broussoux, Single element
    and array PVF2 transducers for acoustic imaging, in: "1982
    Ultrasonics Symposium Proc.," B.R. McAvoy, ed., IEEE, New
    York 1982.

ACCURATE RECONSTRUCTION OF FLAWS IN MATERIALS

USING A SYNTHETIC APERTURE ULTRASONIC IMAGING SYSTEM

Junichi Ishii, Souji Sasaki, and Jun Kubota

Hitachi Research Laboratory
Hitachi Ltd.
Hitachi-shi, Ibaraki-ken 319-12 Japan

ABSTRACT

A compact synthetic aperture ultrasonic imaging system, which rapidly reconstructs precise sectional images of flaws in steel, has been developed. Two side-drilled holes, 1 mm in diameter, at an interval of 1 mm were separately reconstructed when tested with a pulsed 5 MHz transmitted wave (wavelength:1.2 mm) and with a transducer whose aperture angle was 90°. Round profiles of larger diameter holes (4 - 8 mm) were also clearly reconstructed. Simulation studies have been carried out in order to predict the lateral and range resolutions of the imaging system. Most specifications of the imaging system have been determined by these simulation studies. Acquisitions of echo signals and calculations for synthetic aperture processing were carried out with a 16 bit microcomputer and the distance calculation between the transducer and reflectors were performed by a specially designed echo location calculator (5 microseconds per distance calculation). The transducer was scanned linearly along the tested blocks, and the received echoes were processed into a sectional image after each echo acquisition. It took 20 seconds to get a full image display. Another application to evaluate the crack size of the disk plates was also carried out. In this case, circular scanning was applied, and an error of ±0.5 mm in crack depth was obtained. From the viewpoint of fracture mechanics, a more accurate evaluation is required in nondestructive testing than that obtained by the conventional B-scan system. By using the developed system, the accuracy of flaw evaluation was improved.

INTRODUCTION

Nondestructive testing has become important in order to ensure the safety and reliability of structural materials. Progress in fracture mechanics has made it necessary to evaluate flaw sizes exactly to predict the remaininglife of material. A focused beam type transducer[1] is useful to examine flaws exactly. But it is difficult to get a precise image of a flaw far from the transducer, when we reconstruct images of flaws using the transducer and a conventional B—scope system. If the examined part is far from the transducer, for example over 200 mm, the beam width increases because of ultrasound diffraction. And the area of the image, except in the focused zone cannot be examined exactly. Many testing trials with transducers of various focal lengths are needed to get a fully focused image.

Synthetic aperture imaging is one of the high resolution imaging techniqueS using signal processing. High resolution images can be obtained using a small size transducer scanning and aperture synthesis. Even though the examined part is far from the transducer, the flaw image is focused because of its large effective aperture, and as the focusing is achieved via signal processing, a fully focused image is obtained at once, making the technique convenient. The technique of synthetic aperture imaging was first developed for radar[2]. Since then, it has been applied to acoustical imaging for sonar[3,4,5], medical diagnosis[6], and nondestructive testing[7]. However synthetic aperture ultrasonic imaging systems developed so far do not have sufficiently high capability for nondestructive testing, even if the lateral resolution is one wavelength. For this use, the imaging equipment must be compact and a image must be obtained quickly as with a conventional B—scope system.

This paper describes a compact synthetic aperture ultrasonic imaging system which reconstructs a precise sectional image of flaws in steel. The system uses a single probe or a pair of probes, which move along the surface of a test block. The system offers easy handling and adaptability to various test surfaces. A specially designed compact echo location calculator and a microcomputer controller were developed to shorten the execution time. Experiments with test blocks were carried out, and flaw images with resolution superior to that of the conventional B—scope system were obtained.

PRINCIPLE OF IMAGING

Figure 1 shows the fundamental principle of a synthetic aperture ultrasonic imaging system. The transmitted wave St(t) is radiated from a probe at $r_{s,n}$ (n=1,2,3,...), which is mechanically scanned in a straight line along the specimen surface. A spreading beam transducer is used to get a large aperture. Assume a point reflector is in the specimen shown in the figure. An echo from the point reflector is detected after the time needed for a round trip between the probe at $r_{s,1}$ and the point reflector at r_o'. The image is reconstructed using the sum of each echo locus for which the center and radius correspond to the probe position and beam path distance for every probe position $r_{s,1}, r_{s,2}, r_{s,3}, \ldots$ respectively . The image of the point reflector is formed at the intersection of the echo loci.

The formulation of image reconstruction can be discussed as follows. The transmitted signal, which is radiated from the probe at r_s, can be written as the pulsed wave form with amplitude So(t) and center frequency f, as follows:

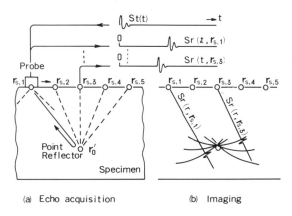

(a) Echo acquisition   (b) Imaging

Fig. 1. Principle of synthetic aperture ultrasonic imaging
using mechanical probe scanning.

$$St(t)=So(t)\exp(j2\pi ft) \tag{1}$$

The received signal $Sr(t,r_s)$, which is detected by the probe at r_s and is formed as follows:

$$Sr(t,r_s)=\int\rho(r')St(t-2/v|r'-r_s|)/|r'-r_s|dr' \ , \tag{2}$$

where r' is the coordinate of the object, r_s is the coordinate of the probe, $\rho(r')$ is the coefficient of the reflection of the position r', and v is the velocity of waves in the specimen. In this representation some factors such as attenuation are compensated for mathematical simplicity.

The reconstruction of the image $I(r)$ at r is performed according to the following operation.

$$I(r)=\left|\int Sr(2/v|r-r_s|,r_s)dr_s\right|^2 \tag{3}$$

Using relation (2), Equation (3) is represented as follows:

$$I(r)=\left|\int\int\rho(r')St(2/v|r-r_s|-2/v|r'-r_s|)/|r'-r_s|dr'dr_s\right|^2 \tag{4}$$

Changing $r_s'=r_s-r'$ and considering the effective aperture, we can obtain a new two-dimensional point spread function as follows:

$$H(r)=\int St(2/v|r-r_s'|-2/v|-r_s'|)/|-rs'|dr_s' \tag{5}$$

This formulation is approximately valid for almost all positions of r'.

Using the above equations, equation (4) is reduced as follows:

$$I(\mathbf{r})=\left|\int\rho(\mathbf{r'})H(\mathbf{r-r'})d\mathbf{r'}\right|^2 \qquad (6)$$

This relation means that the reconstructed image is performed as the convolution of $\rho(\mathbf{r'})$ and a two-dimensional point spread function $H(\mathbf{r'})$. The resolution of the synthetic aperture ultrasonic imaging system is determined by $H(\mathbf{r'})$ which is independent of the location of $\mathbf{r'}$. The waveform of the transmitted pulse determines the distribution of $H(\mathbf{r})$.

IMAGING SIMULATIONS

As described above, the point spread function is important to examine the resolution of this system. So we investigated the images of one point reflector and two point reflectors using computer simulations.

Figure 2 shows the geometry for the simulations. We consider a sectional image involving the x and z axes. The probe at $S(x_s,0)$ is scanned along the x axis, and its scanning distance is indicated as D. The reconstructed point $P(x,R)$ is on a line which is parallel to the x axis with a distance R. The angle ϕ is referred to as aperture angle which is an index of an aperture size, in this paper.

Amplitude distribution on the x axis $H(x)$ is plotted in fig. 3 when the scanning distance D is 100 wavelengths, the reconstructed distance R is 50 wavelengths, and the aperture angle is 90°. Four types of transmitting waveforms are plotted. (1) C.W. denotes a continuous

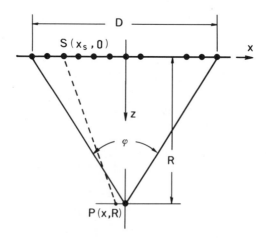

Fig. 2. Geometry of simulation. Aperture size:D=100λ, distance of
reconstructed line:R=50λ, aperture angle:ϕ=90°,
probe position:S(xs,0), reconstructed point P(x,R).

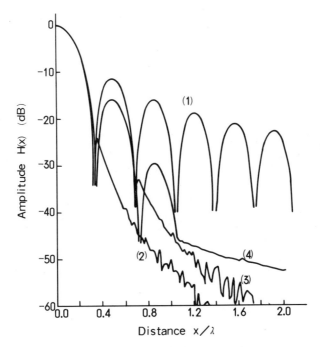

Fig. 3. Point spread functions for four types of transmitted
waveforms. (1) Continuous wave, (2) one cycle sinusoidal wave,
(3) two cycle sinusoidal wave, (4) three cycle sinusoidal
wave with Gaussian weighting.

sinusoidal wave, (2) 1 cycle denotes a burst wave with a one cycle
sinusoidal wave, (3) 2 cycle denotes a burst wave with a two cycle
sinusoidal wave, and (4) Gaussian denotes a burst wave with a 3 cycle
sinusoidal wave and Gaussian weighting as follows:

$$St(t)=u(t)exp(-(ft)^2)exp(j2\pi ft) \tag{7}$$

where u(t)= 1 when $|t| < 1.5/f$
              0 for all other values

As described by Equation (5), amplitude H(x) depends on the waveform
St(t). For case (1) C.W., the main lobe is sharp, but the first side-lobe
level is -11.6dB, and many side-lobes exist because of its coherency. In
cases (2) and (3) coherence lengths are shorter than a continuous wave,
and the side-lobe level is smaller than for (1). Each of the side-lobe
levels using the Gaussian wave(4), which is most likely to be the actual
transmitted wave, is less than that of the continuous wave(1). But the

173

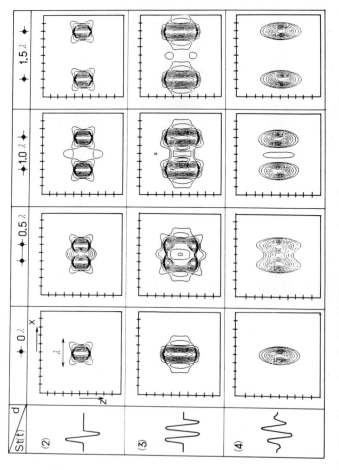

Fig. 4. Two-dimensional image reconstruction of two point reflectors using computer simulation. Transmitted waves are (2) one cycle sinusoidal wave, (3) two cycle sinusoidal wave and (4) three cycle sinusoidal wave with Gaussian weighting. And d is the distance between the two points.

174

half width of the main lobe is a little wider than that of a continuous wave. As a result of these simulations, each side-lobe level obtained using the pulsed waves (2),(3), and (4) is less than the one using a continuous wave (1). Based on the side-lobe level, an actual transmitted wave like (4) is better than one like (1). It is desirable in a imaging system to decrease the side-lobe level.

The width of the main lobe xl is expected as follows:

$$xl=\lambda/2/\sin(\phi/2) \tag{8}$$

This equation suggests that the lateral resolution is sufficiently small at any depth if the aperture angle is wide. When the aperture angle is 90°, the width of the main lobe is expected to be 0.71 wavelengths. From figure 3, the widths of the main lobe of (1) C.W., (2) 1 cycle and (3) 2 cycle are 0.66 wavelengths. But the width of the main lobe of (4) is 0.70 wavelengths.

The point spread function H(r) has two dimensional distribution. To investigate H(r) further, we reconstructed images of two point reflectors using computer simulations. Figure 4 shows the reconstructed images of two point reflectors. Images are plotted as 10 contour lines, 5,10,20,30, ... ,90%, where 100% is the maximum intensity of the image. The distance d, which is the distance between two points, is 0.0, 0.5, 1.0, 1.5 wavelengths.

The point spread functions are shown as the condition d=0.0. The distributions in the lateral direction for (2) one cycle and (3) two cycle cases resemble each other. The lateral distribution of (4) is smooth because of the amplitude modulation. The range distribution depends on the duration and the form of the envelope of the transmitted wave. The Gaussian waveform (4) has smooth distributions laterally and longitudinally. In the case of d=0.5 wavelengths, there are some spurious images at the center between the two points. As d is increased to 1.0 wavelength, the level of the spurious images is less than 10%. From these images, a pulsed waveform is useful to get good resolution image. When the Gaussian waveform, which resembles the actual transmitted wave, is used, it is good enough to get one wavelength lateral resolution.

CONSTRUCTION OF THE SYSTEM

The compact synthetic aperture ultrasonic imaging system rapidly reconstructs precise sectional images of flaws in steel. From the simulation studies described above, the aperture angle of this system is determined to be 90° to get less than one wavelength of lateral resolution. Acquisitions of echo signals and calculations for synthetic aperture processing are carried out with a 16 bit microcomputer and the distance calculation between the transducer and reflectors is performed by a specially designed echo location calculator (5 microseconds per distance calculation).

A block diagram and flow chart of the system are shown in figs. 5 and 6. This system uses a sequential signal processing algorithm. After echo acquisition, synthetic aperture signal processing is immediately started and finished before the next echo acquisition. It is possible to perform these calculations quickly by means of the echo location calculator. The

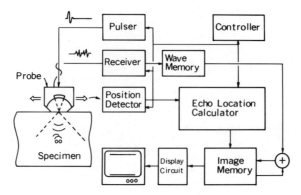

Fig. 5. Block diagram of synthetic aperture ultrasonic imaging system.

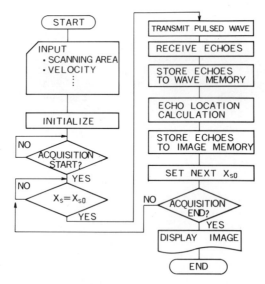

Fig. 6. Flow chart of synthetic aperture ultrasonic imaging system.

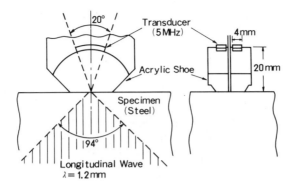

Fig. 7. Construction of the probe.

spreading beam type probe(frequency:5MHz) transmits and receives
ultrasound at every point along the surface of the specimen where the
probe is scanned. The received signals and the probe position obtained
from the receiver and position detector, respectively, are digitally
processed through the wave memory and echo location calculator to form an
ultrasonic tomographic image of the specimen in the image memory. Once
stored in the image memory, the data are read by display circuits and
displayed on a CRT(cathoderay tube). An image can be built up in about 20
seconds.

    The echo location calculator consists of three printed circuit
boards, 230mm wide and 200mm high. Probe position data and echo path are
fed to the echo location calculator, and calculation of echo location for
the image memory is carried out automatically. The distance calculation is
done in 5 microseconds, and a locus of the echo is calculated in 1.28
milliseconds. This imaging system has two image memories, for which there
are 256 x 256 pixels with 16 bit data length.

    Figure 7 shows the construction of the probe. The transducer is a
line focused type with an acrylic shoe and its focus is on the specimen
surface. The transmitter and receiver are electrically independent and
acoustically independent of each other. The center frequency of the probe
is 5 MHz. In the steel specimen, a longitudinal wave is used with an
aperture angle of about 90°.

EXPERIMENTAL EXAMINATIONS

    Figures 8, 9, and 10 show reconstructed images of side-drilled holes
using the synthetic aperture ultrasonic imaging system. The probe (5MHz,
φ:90°) was used as illustrated in fig. 7. The aperture angle is about 90°,
and a scanned pitch is 0.5 mm.

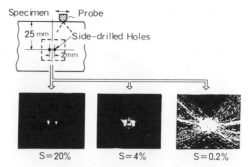

Fig. 8. Experimental results of two side-drilled holes (diameter:1mm)
in steel, threshold levels S=20,4,0.2%. The distance between
them is 2 mm, and their depth is 25 mm. The white parts of the
image indicate that the intensity level is higher than the
threshold level, where S=100% means the maximum intensity
level of the image.

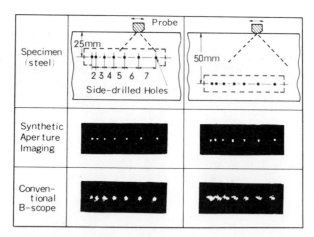

Fig. 9. Reconstructed images of side-drilled holes at depths of 25
and 50 mm. The conventional images are obtained by a focused
and angled beam transducer (45° shear wave, 30mm in diameter)

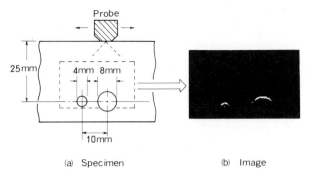

(a) Specimen   (b) Image

Fig. 10. Reconstructed image of bigger holes.

Figure 8 shows the image of two side-drilled holes in steel. The distance between them is 2 mm, and their depth is 25 mm. The white parts of the image indicate that the intensity level is higher than the threshold level, where S=100% means the maximum intensity level of the image. In the case of S=20%, the two images are separately reconstructed. In the case of S=4%, spurious images appear in the center between the two objects. And in the case of 0.2%, echo loci become visible. We can select the optimum threshold level in the range from 20 to 30% as desired, while the half maximum amplitude level corresponds to 25%.

Figure 9 shows images of two groups of side-drilled holes. One set is located at a depth of 25 mm. The other is at 50 mm. The conventional B-scope images are shown in the lower part of the figure. The conventional images are obtained by a focused and angled beam transducer (45° shear wave, 30mm in diameter), which focused at a depth of 25 mm. In using synthetic aperture imaging, the images of the holes at both depths show sufficient separation, while the images in using conventional B-scope imaging are insufficient to distinguish two holes 2 mm apart at the 50 mm depth. As a result of these experiments, the synthetic aperture ultrasonic method is seen to be effective to reconstruct fine images of objects.

Figure 10 shows the image of two large side-drilled holes with contours. The hole diameters are 4 and 8 mm. The image shows a circular arc profile for the objects. From these image data, the size and the shape of a flaw in the material can be measured which allows us to evaluate the effect of flaws on material strength.

CIRCULAR SCANNING

Figure 11 shows the geometry for another application of the synthetic aperture ultrasonic imaging system. A disk plate involving a key way was used as a test specimen. A notch, as an artificial flaw, was machined on the key way, where height h is to be measured. As described in the

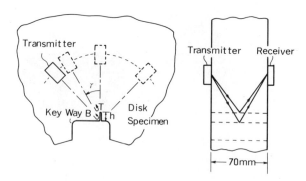

Fig. 11. Geometry of circular scanning for measuring the notch height.

previous section, a spreading beam transducer is needed in the usual synthetic aperture ultrasonic imaging system. However, to detect weak echo signals from remote sources, a narrow beam-width transducer is suitable here, if the examined area can be directly irradiated by the beam from the transducer. In this case, a pitch and catch combination of transmitter and

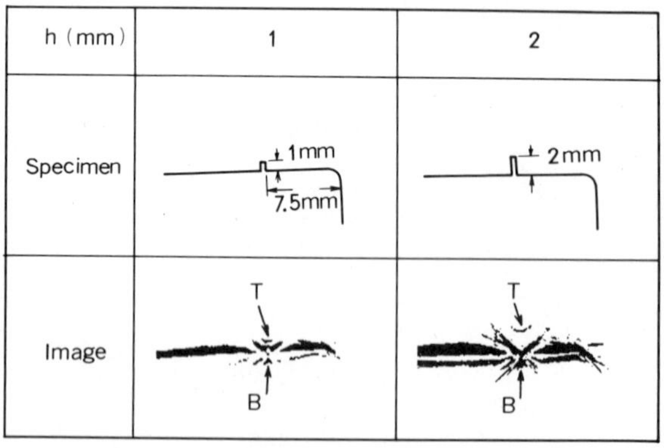

h (mm)	1	2
Specimen	± 1mm 7.5mm	± 2mm
Image	T B	T B

Fig. 12. Reconstructed images of notches on the key way.

receiver are used. These transducers are 70° angled-beam shear wave type. In order to measure the height h of the notch, the probes are simultaneouly scanned along the circular arc loci on the respective opposite disk surface, which are perpendicular to the key way. The flaw image reconstruction is performed by using the echo signals from the corner and the tip of the notch. The values of γ (the projected angle of beam incidence) are -45, -30, -15, 0, 15, 30, 45°. In this use the transmitter and receiver are always directed to the object area, and the aperture angle of this geometry is 90°. Fortunately, in this application it is convenient to obtain a large aperture angle even using a conventional probe.

Figure 12 shows the images of notches for which heights are 1 and 2 mm. The tip echoes T of the notches are indicated above the corner echo indications B and the height of notches can be measured. From the figure, it is possible to evaluate flaw sizes more exactly using synthetic aperture ultrasonic imaging system than with the conventional ultrasonic pulse echo method.

CONCLUSION

A synthetic aperture ultrasonic imaging system for nondestructive testing was developed. The probe used in this system transmits pulsed sinusoidal waves into a steel specimen with a 90° aperture angle. Using linear scanning of a probe, two side-drilled holes spaced 2 mm apart were separately observed. The profile of bigger side-drilled holes, for which diameters were 4 and 8 mm, were reconstructed as circular arc images.

Using a specially designed echo location calculator, which is able to carry out a distance calculation within 5 microseconds, it took 20 seconds to get a complete image in this system.

This system was adapted to another application for evaluating the height of some notch-like flaws. A pair of conventional narrow beam width transducers were scanned around the examined area, with the aperture angle of 90°. Heights of notches of 1 and 2 mm high were measured through the images reconstructed by the tip and the corner echo signals.

As a result of the experimental examinations, the synthetic aperture ultrasonic imaging system was proven effective to evaluate sizes and profiles of material flaws. Accordingly it is expected that development of a compact synthetic aperture ultrasonic imaging system will contribute to improving the accuracy of flaw evaluation and to ensure the safety and the reliability of plants and their components in various industrial fields.

REFERENCES

1. J. Kubota, J. Ishii and S. Sasaki, High Resolution Ultrasonic Testing Using Dynamic Focusing and Signal Correlation, in:"Acoustical Imaging Vol.11", J. P. Powers, ed., Plenum Press, New York (1982)
2. L. J. Cutrona, Synthetic Aperture Radar, in:"Radar Handbook," M. Skolnik, ed., McGraw-Hill, New York (1970)
3. T. Sato, M. Ueda and S. Fukuda, Synthetic Aperture Sonar, J. Acoust. Soc. Am., 54:799(1973)
4. T. Sato and O. Ikeda, Sequential Synthetic Aperture Sonar System, IEEE Trans. on Sonics and Ultrasonics, SU-24:253(1977)

5. K. Nitadori, K. Mano and H. Kamata, An Experimental Underwater
   Acoustic Imaging System Using Multibeam Scanning, in:"Acoustical
   Imaging Vol.8," A. F. Metherell, ed., Plenum Press, New York (1980)
6. F. Duck, S. Johnson, J. Greenleaf and W. Samayoa, Digital Image
   Focussing in the Near Field of a Sampled Acoustic Aperture,
   Ultrasonics, March:83(1977)
7. G. S. Kino, Acoustical Imaging for Nondestructive Evaluation, Proc.
   IEEE, 67:510(1979)

PARAMETRIC APPROACH ON FIELD PROPAGATION

Sun I. Kim, and John M. Reid

Biomedical Engineering and Science Institute

Drexel University, Philadelphia, PA. 19104

ABSTRACT

Conventional Fourier transform method of angular spectrum propagation to estimate field distribution at planes distant from the measuring plane has several problems. These are wrap-around arror, replicated sources problem and side-lobe leakage effects due to windowing the data. These effects are inevitable as far as the discrete Fourier transform is concerned. One suggestion to eliminate these effects is to apply a parametric modelling approach to estimate the Fourier transform pair.

We have found that the auto-regressive (AR) modelling approach has better resolution than the Fourier transform method when used to estimate source field distributions. The modelling method produces even better results when it is applied to the new Fresnel integral to get a direct spatial source property distribution, rather than using the angular spectrum propagation approach.

INTRODUCTION

Because of the computational advantage in using the Fourier transform, angular spectrum propagation approach was used commonly to reconstruct field distributions. In this case, a field distribution over a plane can be reconstructed from a forward or backward angular spectrum propagation of measured complex field at a plane parallel to the reconstruction plane [1]. The angular spectrum is usually obtained by the discrete Fourier transform. However, if the data collecting aperture size is finite, the angular spectrum is a distorted version of the true spectrum due to the side-lobe leakage of the window. Windowing of data makes the implicit assumption that the unobserved data outside window are zero, which is normally an unrealistic assumption. A smeared spectral estimation is a consequence of the window.

Other problems of the conventional Fourier transform method are wrap-around error resulting from the convolution of a repeated function with a non-bandlimited function [2] and replicated sources problem because DFT assumes that the input sequence is periodic [3]. Also, resolution is limited by the available data length [4]. Thus, the resulting reconstructed field from the distorted angular spectrum shows limited resolution and fluctuations.

Parametric modelling is an alternative method for spectral estimation. It is usually possible to obtain better results based on the auto-regression (AR) model from the finite set of measured data. This modelling provides good spectral information with relatively good noise rejection from short data records with no windowing effect. Thus this modelling approach gives better reconstruction than the conventional direct Fourier transform method, in terms of improved resolution and reduced fluctuation. We applied AR modelling approach to the Fresnel integral, which is a simplified version of the Rayleigh-Sommerfeld diffraction formula.

In this paper, an ultrasound source intensity distribution is reconstructed by two methods from a computer simulated field, and compared. Also a new Fresnel approximation is tested from an angular data collecting configuration.

THEORY

Although the field reconstruction methods have been referred to by several names, like forward-backward angular spectrum propagation, inverse scattering and holographic reconstruction [5], all of these techniques originate from the same phenomenon of diffraction. There are two conventional formulations of diffraction theory. The angular spectrum formulation and the Rayleigh-Sommerfeld diffraction formula.

If we assume the propagating medium is linear and homogeneous, a propagation phenomenon between the complex acoustic field distribution of two parallel planes can be thought of as a linear space-invariant system with a field of one plane as an input and another plane as an output. So the output field $u(x,y,z1)$ across X-Y plane at $z1$ can be represented by convolution integral of input field $u(x,y,z0)$ at $z0$ and impulse response $h(x,y;z0,z1)$ [6];

$$u(x,y,z1) = A \iint u(x',y',z0) \ h(x-x',y-y',d) \ dx'dy' \qquad (1)$$

where A is a constant and the distance $d = z1-z0$. Define $u(x,y,z0)$ as a 2-dimensional inverse Fourier transform of its angular spectrum;

$$u(x,y,z0) = 1/2\pi \iint U(fx,fy,z0) \ Exp[\ 2\pi j \ (fx \ x + fy \ y)] \ dfxdfy \qquad (2)$$

where the angular spectrum $U(fx,fy,z0)$ is given by;

$$U(fx,fy,z0) = \iint u(x,y,z0) \ Exp[\ -2\pi j \ (fx \ x + fy \ y)] \ dxdy \qquad (3)$$

then by convolution theorem we have from Eq. (1);

$$U(fx,fy,z1) = H(fx,fy,d) \ U(fx,fy,z0) \qquad (4)$$

where the transfer function is given by;

$$H(fx,fy,d) = \begin{cases} Exp[\ jkd \ (1 -(\lambda fx)^2 -(\lambda fy)^2 \ )^{\frac{1}{2}} \ ] & fx^2 +fy^2 < 1/\lambda^2 \\ 0 & \text{otherwise} \end{cases} \qquad (5)$$

Here $k =2\pi/\lambda$ and the distance d is assumed at least several wavelengths long so the evanescent waves can be neglected. So in order to reconstruct source field distribution from the measured comlex field away from the source, first Fourier transform u(x,y,z1) to get U(fx,fy,z1) and multiply by the inverse transfer function H(fx,fy,-d) to get U(fx,fy,z0). After that, inverse Fourier transform U(fx,fy,z0) to u(x´,y´,z0). This is called the angular spectrum propagation method, because the angular spectrum can be propagated by multiplying the transfer function H(fx,fy,d) which is a function of distance.

To obtain computational efficiency and reasonable results, fast Fourier transform (FFT) is commonly used to estimate angular spectrum. But there are several sources of errors and limitations to using FFT in conjunction with angular spectrum propagation approach. First, the frequency resolution is inversely proportional to the available data points and the side-lobe leakage from data window obscures and distorts the true spectrum. The FFT approach is particularly troublesome when analyzing short data records. Practically, the date collecting aperture size is finite, and the data size are usually small in most ultrasound measurements. Thus the resulting reconstruction from the smeared angular spectrum shows limited resolution and fluctuations. In order to improve the quality of the reconstruction, some kind of tapered window can be used, but it always has to compromise with the loss of resolution [7].

There is also a limitation of maximum propagation distance for which the angular spectrum approach can be used. Because the DFT assumes the input sequence is periodic, at some propagation distance the other object will overlap the reconstruction of the original object. The error of this replicated source problem can be reduced by attaching a guard band (zeros) to the measured data. Another source of error is wrap around error resulting from the convolution of a repeated function with a nonband-limited function. The function H(fx,fy,d) in Eq. 5 is inevitably undersampled and only frequencies which satisfy the criterion $fx^2 + fy^2 < 1/\lambda^2$ were utilized.

One suggestion to eliminate these unwanted side effects is to apply a parametric modelling approach to estimate spectrum. One of the promising aspects of the modelling approach to spectral estimation is that one can make more realistic assumptions concerning the nature of the measured process outside measurement interval, other than to assume it is zero or periodic. Thus the need for windows can be eliminated along with their distorting impact. As a result, the improvement over the conventional FFT spectral estimate can be very good, especially for short data records [4].

We would like to apply the auto-regressive (AR) model to fit the complex ultrasonic field distribution and estimate the spectrum. However AR spectrum estimation only gives power spectral density function, not phase information, thus we can not apply AR spectrum to the preceeding angular spectrum propagation approach at this moment.

There is another way to reconstruct u(x´,y´,z0) from u(x,y,z1) by using the Fresnel approximation. Fresnel diffraction formula is a simplified version of the Rayleigh-Sommerfeld diffraction formula with the aid of the paraxial approximation. Then in Eq. 1, the impulse response will be;

$$h(x,y;d) = Exp\{[jk/(2d)] [(x-x´)^2 + (y-y´)^2]\} \qquad (6)$$

The quadratic terms in Eq. 6 can be expanded to yield;

$$u(x,y,z1) = B \iint \{ u(x´,y´,z0) \, Exp[\, jk/(2d)(x´^2+y´^2)] \}$$

$$Exp[\, -2\pi j/(\lambda d) \, (xx´+yy´)] \, dx´dy´ \qquad (7)$$

As seen in Eq. 7, $u(x,y,z1)$ may be found from a single Fourier transform of $u(x´,y´,z0) \, Exp[\, jk/(2d) \, (x´^2+y´^2)]$, where the transform must be evaluated at frequencies $fx = x/\lambda d$, $fy = y/\lambda d$ to assure correct space scaling in the reconstruction plane. In the same way, the inverse relation can be derived from the inverse Fourier transform of Eq. 7;

$$u(x´,y´,z0) = B´ \iint \{ u(x,y,z1) \, Exp[\, -jk/(2d) \, (x^2+y^2)] \}$$

$$Exp[\, 2\pi j/(\lambda d) \, (xx´+yy´)] \, dxdy \qquad (8)$$

We applied AR modelling to Eq. 8 to reconstruct the amplitude distribution $|u(x,y,z0)|$, and compared the estimation with the result of the angular frequency domain approach.

COMPUTER SIMULATION

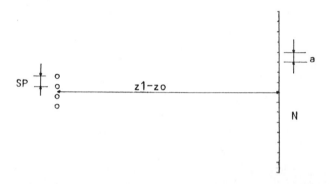

Fig.1. Source and data collecting aperture geometry.

For simplicity, we simulate 1-dimensional reconstruction of 4 point sources located at 4 cm away from the data collecting aperture as in Fig. 1. For the first test of reconstruction, the complex field distribution is calculated from the radiation of a single point source located at 8 cm, oscillating· at 1 MHz. The separation of data collecting elements is a = 0.1 cm and number of elements N = 65. In Fig. 2, the left side shows the result of angular frequency domain approach and the right side, the Fresnel approximation using AR modelling. Frequency domain approach shows side-lobe leakage and fluctuation. Bottom graphs are dB plots of each case. Notice the side-lobe of the left is about -12 dB while the right side has virtually no side-lobe effect.

The next simulation is of 4 simple sources, oscillating at 1 MHz located at 4 cm, the sample spacing is sp = 0.4 cm. The number of data collecting elements is 2^M +1 for convenience of calculation and symmetric where M is an integer. In Fig. 3, the left side shows the reconstruction of frequency domain approach and the right is AR modelling reconstruction. For the upper, N = 17 and for the lower N = 33. Although the frequency domain approach can not resolve 4 points with N = 17, it resolves with N = 33. The modelling approach can resolve 4 points clearly with 17 elements, and even better with N = 33 elements without any side-lobes.

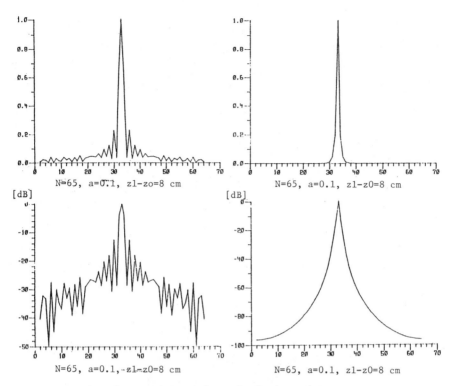

Fiq. 2. Reconstruction of single point source.
A distance is 8 cm.

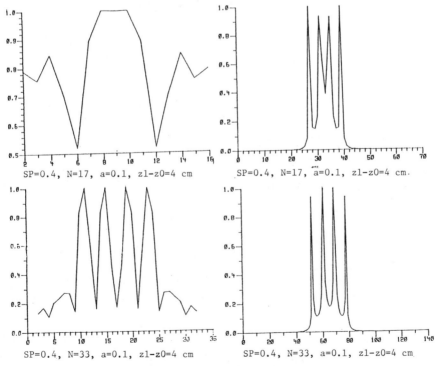

Fig. 3. Reconstruction of 4 point sources.
Spacing of sources is 0.4 cm at a distance of 4 cm.

A second test was done under more difficult conditions, using half the source spacing (sp = 0.2 cm) but other conditions are the same. In this case, frequency domain approach can not resolve 4 points until the number of elements reaches 129, as shown in Fig. 4, while the AR modelling can resolve even with 33 elements. However, when the aperture size becomes larger, the aliasing phenomenon occurs, because wave length is about 0.15 cm so the Nyquist rate becomes 0.075 cm. Here sampling separation a = 0.1 cm. When we decrease sampling separation to a = 0.05 cm with N = 257, which is the same aperture size, then as seen in lower left of Fig. 5, the aliasing effect disappears. The right side shows poor reconstruction and failure to reconstruct when N = 257 with 0.05 cm separation. This is because of the nature of the Fresnel approximation. This Fresnel approximation is valid only for small angles. This effect starts to appear when aperture size is 6.4 cm, and is worse when it is 12.8 cm (at 4 cm of distance).

NEW FRESNEL APPROXIMATION

The Fresnel approximation has generally been represented by the small angle approximation, which was presented in the previous section, and the general Fresnel approximation. As we noticed in the previous section, for large angle data collecting apertures, the small angle approximation was not valid, so the general approximation should be used.

Recently a new Fresnel approximation was derived for angular field patterns of linear source apertures [8]. This new Fresnel approximation is a simplified general approximation and gives a Fourier transform relation between the angular field pattern of Fresnel region and a simple function of the source aperture distribution. So, we can also apply FFT as well as AR modelling approach to reconstruct source distributions from the angular data collecting configuration.

A new Fresnel approximation is given by;

$$U(z,v) = \text{Exp}\{[-jk(L/2)^2 v^2]/(2z)\}$$

$$\int_{-L/2}^{L/2} u(x) \, \text{Exp}[jk \, x^2/(2z)] \, \text{Exp}[-jkxv] \, dx \qquad (9)$$

where L is source aperture length at v = sin θ and z is distance from source to angular data collecting elements. The inverse relation derived from Eq. 9 is;

$$u(x) = k/2\pi \, \text{Exp}\{-jkx^2/(2z)\}$$

$$\int U(z,v) \, \text{Exp}\{jk(L/2)^2 v^2/(2z)\} \, \text{Exp}[jkxv] \, dv \qquad (10)$$

We applied Eq. 10 to reconstruct 5 point sources at a distance z = 4 cm and data collecting elements N = 65. In Fig. 6, upper pictures are the reconstructions of source spacing sp = 0.2 cm, and the lower are for sp = 0.5 cm. Again left is FFT and right is AR modelling reconstruction.

DISCUSSION

Even though AR modelling approach improves resolution and reduces fluctuations when reconstructing source distributions, there are several drawbacks. First, the computational requirement of AR modelling approach dramatically increases over the FFT method depending

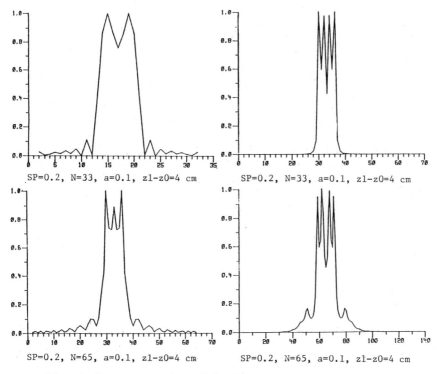

Fig. 4. Reconstruction of 4 point sources.
Spacing of sources is 0.2 cm at a distance of 4 cm.

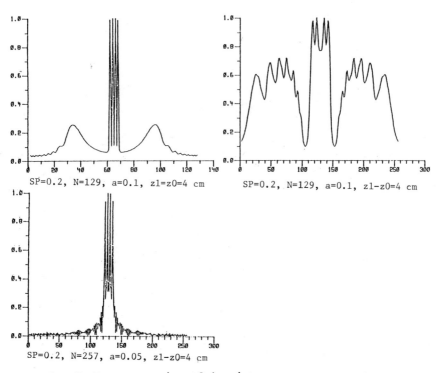

Fig. 5. Reconstruction of 4 point sources.
Spacing of sources is 0.2 cm at a distance of 4 cm.

upon the model order and number of plot points. The shape of reconstruction can vary as the model order changes. It is another big problem to select optimal model order to properly fit the measured data. We found that computational time is not prohibitive, and unless the order is too large or too small, the reconstruction is not affected much by the model order. Ulrych and Bishop suggested in the case of short data segments that an order selection between N/3 to N/2 often produce satisfactory results [10].

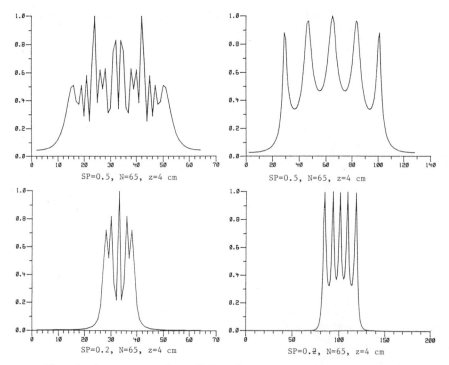

Fig. 6. Reconstruction of 5 point sources by new Fresnel
approximation. Spacing of sources is 0.2 cm at a
distance of 4 cm.

Here we used Burg algorithm for AR spectrum estimation, and tried several other algorithms like Marple's algorithm [9]. However, we couldn't find significant differences between the diffent algorithms. Also unlike FFT method, AR modelling does not need a guard-band or any special kind of window to reduce replicated source effect or side-lobe leakage.

One thing to be noticed is the scaling. The data spacing on the reconstruction plane is $x = \lambda d/Na$, which is a function of number of data collecting elements and sampling separation with fixed wave length and distance. So care should be taken to avoid serious scaling problems by adjusting N, depending upon distance. Scaling occurs in new Fresnel approximation, too. But it is not a function of distance.

CONCLUSION

These results show that, in this case, the AR approach gives results that are more free from artifact than the angular spectrum approach. This is anomalous, since the Fresnel integral is only an approximate diffraction formula, while the angular spectrum propagation formulation gives exact solution. The AR modelling based upon the Fresnel approximation appears to yields better results, we believe, because of the intrinsic problems of using DFT in conjunction with the angular spectrum approach.

ACKNOWLEDGEMENT

We wish to thank Dr. O. Tretiak for helpful discussion. This work was supported by NIH Grant HL-30045.

REFERENCES

[1] E.G. Williams, J.D. Maynard and E. Skudrzyk, "Sound source reconstruction using microphone array," J. Acoust. Soc. Am., vol. 68(1), pp. 340-344, July 1980.

[2] E.G. Williams and J.D. Maynard, "Numerical evaluation of the Rayleigh integral for planar radiation using FFT," J. Acoust. Soc. Am. vol. 72(6), pp. 2020-2030, Dec. 1982.

[3] J.P. Powers, "computer simulation of linear acoustic diffraction," in Acoustic Holograph, edited by A. Metherell (Plenum, New York, 1974), vol. 7, pp. 193-205.

[4] S.M. Kay and S.L. Marple, "Spectrum analysis - A modern perspective," proc. IEEE, vol. 69, No. 11, pp. 1380-1419, Nov. 1981.

[5] F.P. Higgins, S.J. Norton and M. Linzer, "Optical interferometric visualization and computerized reconstruction of ultrasonic field," J. Acoust. Soc. Am. vol. 68(4), pp.1169-1176, oct. 1980.

[6] J.W. Goodman, "Introduction to Fourier optics," Ch. 3 and Ch. 4., Mcgraw-Hill, New York, 1968.

[7] P.R. Stepanishen and K.C. Benjamin, "Forward and backward projection of acoustic fields using FFT methods," J. Acoust. Soc. Am. vol. 71(4), pp. 803-812, Apr. 1982.

[8] W.J. Graham, "A new Fresnel region approximation," Proc, Int. IEEE AP-S Symposium, Vancouver, BC. Jun. 1985.

[9] S. L. Marple, "A new autoregressive spectrum analysis algorithm," IEEE Trans. Acoust., Speech, Signal Process., vol. ASSP-28, pp. 441-454, Aug. 1980.

[10] T.J. Ulrych and T.N. Bishop, "Maximum Entripy analysis and Autoregressive decomposition," Rev. Geophysics and Space Phys., vol. 13, pp. 183-200, Feb. 1975.

PERFORMANCE OF FAST INVERSE SCATTERING
SOLUTIONS FOR THE EXACT HELMHOLTZ EQUATION
USING MULTIPLE FREQUENCIES AND LIMITED VIEWS

M. J. Berggren[1], S. A. Johnson[1,2,3], B. L. Carruth[2], W. W. Kim[2],
F. Stenger[4] and P.L. Kuhn[2],

[1]Department of Bioengineering
[2]Department of Electrical Engineering
[3]Department of Radiology and
[4]Department of Mathematics

University of Utah, Salt Lake City, UT 84112

ABSTRACT

We have previously reported fast algorithms for imaging by acoustical inverse scattering using the exact (not linearized) Helmholtz wave equation [1]. We now report numerical implementations of these algorithms which allow the reconstruction of quantitative images of speed of sound, density, and absorption from either transmission or reflection data. We also demonstrate the application of our results to larger grids (up to 64 x 64 pixels) and compare our results with analytically derived data, which are known to be highly accurate, for scattering from right circular cylindrical objects. We report on the performance of our algorithms for both transmission and reflection data and for the simultaneous solution of scattering components corresponding to speed of sound and absorption. We have further examined the performance of our methods with various amounts of random noise added to the simulated data. We also report on the performance of one technique we have devised to extract quantitative density images from our algorithms.
(*Acoustical Imaging 15*, Halifax, Nova Scotia, July 1986).

INTRODUCTION

We start with a model for the propagation of an ultrasonic pressure wave p(x) in tissue which includes both compressibility and density fluctuations and may be described with the following scalar wave equation [2,3]:

$$\nabla^2 p(x) + k^2(x)\, p(x) - \nabla \ln \rho(x) \cdot \nabla\, p(x) = 0 \tag{1}$$

We have previously shown [3] how this equation may be transformed into the more familiar inhomogenous Helmholtz equation with the substitution $p(x) = f(x)(\rho(x))^{1/2}$, where ρ is the density. In order to determine the unknown object distribution from a knowledge of the incident field and the measured field on a set of detectors (a process called inverse scattering) we transform the differential equation into a system of algebraic equations which we can solve numerically. This process is described for single frequencies in our papers in [3-5], with the extension to multiple frequencies given in [6], and will be summarized here. The Helmholtz wave equation in f(x) is transformed to the Lippmann-Schwinger integral equation (which allows the scattered field measurement data to be treated as boundary conditions and thus be formally and easily incorporated into the solution) which may be written as follows:

$$f_{\omega\phi}^{(sc)}(x) \equiv f_{\omega\phi}(x) - f_{\omega\phi}^{(in)}(x) = -\int k_o^2 \gamma_\omega(x') f_{\omega\phi}(x') g_\omega (|x - x'|) d^Q x' \quad (2)$$

Here, $f_{\omega\phi}^{(sc)}(x)$ is the scattered field, $f_{\omega\phi}^{(in)}(x)$ is the incident field, ω is the frequency, ϕ is source location, $g_\omega(|\bullet|)$ is the outward-going free space Green's function, Q is the dimension of the space containing the body to be imaged, and $\gamma(x)$ is the scattering potential. $\gamma_\omega(x)$ (which in general is frequency dependent) may be written as

$$\gamma_\omega(x) = 1 - [c_o^2/c^2(x)] + [c_o^2/\omega^2] \rho^{1/2}(x) \nabla^2 [\rho^{-1/2}(x)] -$$
$$2 i \{c_o^2/[\omega c(x)]\} \alpha(x) \quad (3)$$

where $\alpha(x)$ is the imaginary part of k and is essentially equal to one-half the linear power absorption coefficient. We take $\gamma = 0$ in a homogenous (here, water) medium outside a finite region of support. Here $k_o = \omega/c_o$ is the wave number in the homogenous medium surrounding the scattering potential and $\lambda_o = 2 \pi c_o/\omega$ is the wavelength in this medium. For two-dimensional problems Q = 2 and $g(|\bullet|) = (i/4) H_o^{(1)}(k_o|\bullet|)$, where $H_o^{(1)}$ is the zero order Hankel function. We have described in reference [3,4] how Eq. (2) may be transformed into a system of algebraic equations by expanding the product $k_o^2 \gamma_\omega(x') f_{\omega\phi}(x')$ with a set of basis functions. The result is a set of detector or measurement equations given by

$$f_{\omega\phi m}^{(sc)} = \sum_{j=1}^{N} D_{\omega mj} \gamma_{\omega j} f_{\omega j\phi}, \qquad \begin{aligned} m &= 1, \ldots, M \\ \phi &= 1, \ldots, \Phi \\ j &= 1, \ldots, N \\ \omega &= 1, \ldots, \Omega \end{aligned} \quad (4)$$

and a set of field constraint equations (also called the forward inverse problem equations) given by

$$f_{\omega\phi l} = f_{\omega\phi l}^{(in)} + \sum_{j=1}^{N} C_{\omega l j} \gamma_{\omega j} f_{\omega j\phi}, \qquad \begin{aligned} j &= 1, \ldots, N \\ l &= 1, \ldots, N \\ \phi &= 1, \ldots, \Phi \\ \omega &= 1, \ldots, \Omega \end{aligned} \quad (5)$$

where $f_{\omega\phi l} \equiv f_{\omega\phi}(x_l)$ and $f_{\omega\phi l}^{(in)} \equiv f_{\omega\phi}^{(in)}(x_l)$ are the internal field and incident field respectively. Also $f_{\omega\phi m}^{(sc)} \equiv f_{\omega\phi}^{(sc)}(x_m)$ are the measured values of the scattered field on detector points x_m. Note that the matrix elements $D_{\omega mj}$ and $C_{\omega lj}$ have the same definitions (which are given in [3,4] for a sinc basis set), but we use a separate symbol $D_{\omega mj}$ to correspond to a measurement point x_m on a detector.

ANALYSIS OF OUR INVERSE SCATTERING METHODS

Equations (4) and (5) constitute a nonlinear system which must be solved for $\gamma_{\omega j}$ and $f_{\omega \phi j}$. We have investigated several methods for solving these nonlinear equations (such as a a generalization of the Kaczmarz method [3,4] or descent procedures [7] which minimize the appropriate residual functions). However, we have had considerable success using an alternating variable approach with linear solution methods. For example, we would first hold the field ($f_{\omega \phi j}$) fixed in Eq. (4) and solve for the scattering potential ($\gamma_{\omega j}$) using linear methods, and then we hold the scattering potential ($\gamma_{\omega j}$) fixed in Eq. (5) and use linear methods to solve for the field variable ($f_{\omega \phi j}$). We previously listed four methods for solving these linear equations [3]. Although our earlier methods required on the order of n^5 operations per iteration (using an n by n pixel grid with approximately n views and n detectors per view and only one frequency), our more recent methods, such as the one demonstrated in [5] make use of Fast Fourier Transforms to reduce the number of operations to $n^3 \log(n)$ per iterations for the same size problem.

With these methods we have been able to extend our inverse scattering simulations to a more practically useful 64 x 64 pixel grid. Figure 1(a) shows a digitized representation of the real part of a test object which was composed of a Gaussian distribution of speed of sound and absorption (with a linear frequency dependence) for which the peak values of $\gamma(x)$ were (.01 − .001 j). Forward scattering data was simulated for a single incident frequency (the width of each pixel is $\lambda_o/4$) for 64 incident directions (uniformly spaced around 360°) using 126 detectors. Figure 1(b) shows a reconstruction of the real part of $\gamma(x)$ (which corresponds to the speed of sound) after 8 iterations of our algorithm, which took about 4.5 minutes on a Cray XMP/48 computer. The reconstructed values agree with the test object to within .3% at the peak. The reconstructions of the imaginary part of $\gamma(x)$, which corresponds to the absorption, are very similar (except for a scale factor) and are omitted for brevity.

We have also tested our algorithm using data calculated from the analytic, closed form series expansion, solutions to the forward scattering problem, which are known to be highly accurate [8], for a right circular cylinder. Figure 2(a) shows a representation of a 64 x 64 digitized right circular cylinder whose diameter is $8 \lambda_o$ and the pixel width is $\lambda_o/4$. A reconstruction of the scattering potential $\gamma(x)$ for this object (note that we assumed no absorption was present) is given in Figure 2(b) using exactly the same amount of data and number of iterations as in the first example. A more detailed comparison of the line profiles through the center of the grid for both the test object and its reconstruction are shown in Figure 3. Note that the assumption that our cylinder has infinitely sharp edges violates the assumption that the scattering potential is band limited (which was used in expanding our functions on a set of sinc basis functions). This causes the ripples seen in the image (which is known as the Gibbs phenomena). Otherwise the reconstructions are of the same accuracy as the example in Fig. 1.

We have also further examined the tolerance of our algorithms to noisy data. A simple numcrical test experiment data was conducted whereby we started off with perfect data for a

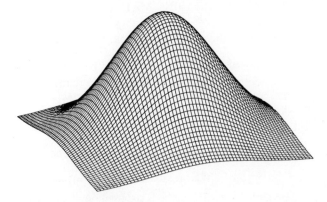

Fig. 1(a)   An isometric plot of the real part of a scattering potential with a peak value of $\gamma = (.01 - .001\,j)$ and a Gaussian shape. Note that this function is represented on a 64 x 64 pixel grid and the width of each pixel is $\lambda_o/4$.

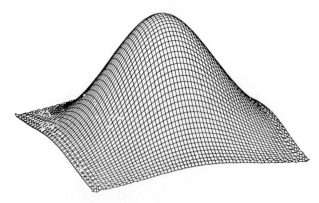

Fig. 1(b)   An isometric plot of a reconstruction of the test object shown in part (a) after 8 iterations. The peak values of the reconstruction agree with the actual object to within .3%.

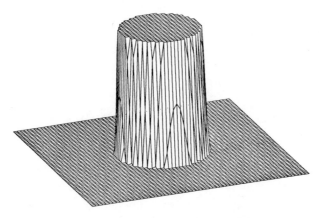

Fig. 2(a)   An isometric plot of the scattering potential of a cylindrical object ($\gamma = .01$ in the center). Again we use a 64 x 64 pixel grid and the width of each pixel is $\lambda_o/4$.

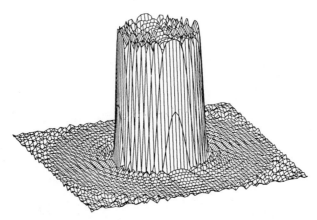

Fig. 2(b)   An isometric plot of a reconstruction from analytically generated data for the object shown in Fig. 2(a) using 64 uniformly spaced views with 126 uniformly spaced detectors per view.

Gaussian test object ,whose peak value of $\gamma(x)$ was $(.1 - .01 \text{ j})$, for 16 views using 30 detectors uniformly distributed around the perimeter of the grid. The reconstruction of this object was compared with an actual digitized representation of the object on a 16 x 16 pixel grid for the first five iterations. Then various amounts of random noise (with an assumed normal distribution) were added to the data, and the reconstructions were repeated. Figure 4 shows a plot of the relative noise in the reconstructions for data with rms noise from 0.0 to 10.0%. One can readily see that our methods are indeed quite stable and have reasonable signal to noise ratios for these amounts of noise present in each case, but the potential exists to reduce the noise in the images still further. We have noted that for 64 x 64 pixel grids the rate of convergence of the alternating variable algorithms with higher object contrast ratios (e.g. on the order of $\gamma = .1 - .01 \text{ j}$) is very slow or absent even with no noise present.

MULTIPLE FREQUENCIES AND REFLECTION MODE IMAGES

It is clear from Eq. (3) that in general we will need multiple frequency data to separate the frequency independent material properties c, ρ, and α from the frequency dependent terms of $\gamma(x)$. However, in those situations where we have no (or very limited) frequency dependence for $\gamma(x)$ (e.g., where there is no density fluctuation or absorption present) we can use an over-determined set of frequency measurements to substitute for some (possibly unavailable) source angles or to obtain more accurate (less noisy) images. This will allow us to apply our methods to data from a limited set of angles, and, in particular, to reflection mode only data. We shall report on the preliminary success that we have had on this topic.

We created an 8 x 8 pixel test object to represent the speed of sound variations in an artery filled with blood and imbedded within soft tissue as shown in Figure 5(a). We then performed two numerical experiments. First we simulated the scattering from 8 frequencies and 8 source directions (uniformly spaced over 180°) that would be received by 15 detectors located on the same side of the object as the sources at uniformly spaced fixed points along 1/2 of the outer border of the grid. A reconstruction from this data after 10 iterations is shown in Fig. 5(b). We also simulated the scattering for the same 8 frequencies with 8 source directions (uniformly spaced over a full 360°) into 28 detectors uniformly spaced around the entire outer border of the grid. A reconstruction from this data after 5 iterations is shown in Fig. 5(c). We note that while the reconstruction in Fig. 5(b) is very promising it is not as good as that in Fig. 5(c). We are investigating ways to improve the reconstruction from the data used for Fig. 5(b).

IMPROVED DENSITY IMAGES

We have previously [9] demonstrated one technique for solving for density with our methods. Basically the procedure was to first use multiple frequency scattering to solve for the density component of Eq. (3) , i.e., $V(x) = -[\rho^{1/2}(x)] \nabla^2[\rho^{-1/2}(x)]$. Then we used a sinc-Galerkin method to transform the corresponding differential equation (with known boundary conditions—i.e., the density of water) into a set of linear equations which may be solved numerically. However our test examples shown [9] may have given the false impression that there was some difficulty in reconstructing two or more Gaussian objects. The actual problem with those images [9] was that we choose a Gaussian with too sharp of a peak (a FWHM of 1.43 pixels or .35 λ_0 using a pixel width of 1/4 λ_0), which thereby severely violated our band limiting assumptions and produced errors as large as 30% in the image. Figure 6 compares the center line of the reconstruction with the initial test object for a density distribution consisting of two Gaussian peaks separated by four pixels with each peak having a FWHM = 1.72 pixels. One can readily see, with a test object that is nearly spatially band limited, that this method works very well with noise free data.

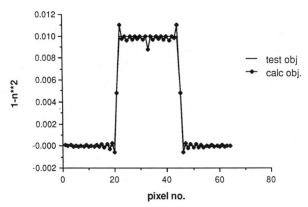

Fig. 3   A comparison of the center line profiles of the test object and its reconstruction as given in Fig. 2. The oscillations are due to the violation of band limiting assumptions by the sharp edges of the cylinder which is the well-known Gibbs phenomena.

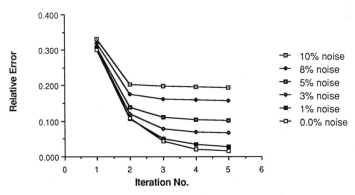

Fig. 4   A plot of the relative one-norm error, i.e. $\| \gamma_{true} - \gamma_{calc} \|_1 / \| \gamma_{true} \|_1$, vs. the number of iterations for various amounts of random noise (an rms value) added to the scattering data. The reconstructions were of Gaussian test objects with a peak value of $\gamma = (.1 - .01\, j)$ and were done on a 16 x 16 pixel grid using 16 views (equally spaced around 360°) and 16 detectors per view.

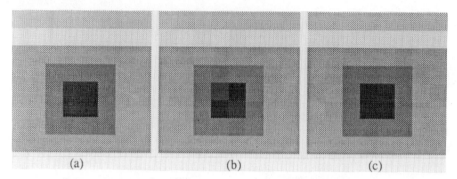

Fig. 5   Gray scale representations of the scattering potential $\{1 - c_o^2/c(\mathbf{x})^2\}$ for a test object simulating a blood filled artery in soft tissue. (a) Original Test Object, (b) Reconstruction from 180°, (c) Reconstruction from 360°. The simulation in (a) represents a top layer of water, a layer of fat, then a background layer of soft tissue surrounding the arterial wall with the blood in the very center. These images use an 8 x 8 pixel grid with the pixel width equal to 1/4 of the wavelength in water of the highest incident frequency. The reconstruction in Panel (b) is after 10 iterations using the reflection data for 8 frequencies and 8 source directions (uniformly spaced over 180°) into 14 detectors. The reconstruction in Panel (c) is after 5 iterations from scattering data for 8 frequencies and 8 source directions (uniformly spaced over 360°) and 28 detectors.

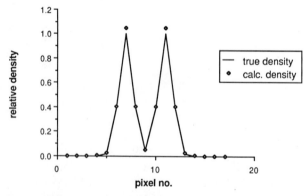

Fig. 6   A plot of the center line profile of the actual and calculated density distributions. The test object was a 17 x 17 pixel representation of a density distribution consisting of two Gaussian peaks separated by 4 pixels and with a FWHM = 1.72 pixels. The calculated values are obtained from a sinc-Galerkin solution to the differential equation for density.

SUMMARY

We have demonstrated that our methods for inverse scattering of ultrasound can actually be applied to practical sized (at least 64 x 64 pixel) grids, can tolerate reasonable amounts of random noise, can simultaneously solve for several of the major components of the scattering potential, can use multiple frequency data to solve for the scattering potential with reflection only data, and have the capability of solving for density fluctuations. Now that we have shown these basic imaging capabilities with numerical simulations we next intend to improve their performance in several critical areas such as contrast range, limited angle response, etc. We also intend to test them with laboratory data.

ACKNOWLEDGMENTS

We wish to thank Professor Calvin H. Wilcox, Department of Mathematics, University of Utah, for his advice and stimulating discussions. We wish to thank David Borup of the Department of Electrical Engineering, University of Utah, for his advice and for assisting us in getting very fast FFT algorithms for the Cray–XMP. This work supported in part by PHS Contract No. N43-CM-57805 and Grant No. 2 R01 CA29728-04 from NCI, and PHS Grant No. 1 R01 HL34995-01 from NHLBI.

REFERENCES

1. S. A. Johnson, Y. Zhou, M. L. Tracy, M. J. Berggren, and F. Stenger, "Fast Iterative Algorithms for Inverse Scattering of the Helmholtz and Riccati Wave Equations," *Acoustical Imaging 13,* Plenum Press, pp. 75–87 (1984).
2. S. A. Johnson, F. Stenger, C. Wilcox, J. Ball, and M. J. Berggren, "Wave Equations and Inverse Scattering Solutions for Soft Tissue," *Acoustical Imaging 11,* pp. 409-424 (1982).
3. S. A. Johnson and M. L. Tracy, "Inverse Scattering Solutions by a Sinc Basis, Multiple Source, Moment Method -- Part I: Theory", *Ultrasonic Imaging 5,* pp. 361-375 (1983).
4. M. L. Tracy, and S. A. Johnson, "Inverse Scattering Solutions by a Sinc Basis, Multiple Source, Moment Method -- Part II: Numerical Evaluations", *Ultrasonic Imaging 5,* Academic Press, pp. 376-392 (1983).
5. S. A. Johnson, Y. Zhou, M. L. Tracy, M. J. Berggren, and F. Stenger, "Inverse Scattering Solutions by a Sinc Basis, Multiple Source, Moment Method -- Part III: Fast Algorithms", *Ultrasonic Imaging 6,* pp. 103-116 (1984).
6. S. A. Johnson, Y. Zhou, M. J. Berggren, M. L. Tracy, " Acoustic Inverse Scattering by Moment Methods and Backpropagation,", in *Conference on Inverse Scattering: Theory and Application,* ed. by J. B. Bednar, R. Redner, E. Robinson, and A. Weglin, SIAM, pp. 144–155 (1983).
7. R. D. Fletcher, *Practical Methods of Optimization, Vol.. 1, Unconstrained Optimization,* John Wiley and Sons, New York, (1980).
8. B. S. Robinson and J. F. Greenleaf, "Measurement and Simulation of the Scattering of Ultrasound by Penetrable Cylinders," *Acoustical Imaging 13,* Plenum Press, pp. 163–178 (1984).
9. M. J. Berggren, S. A. Johnson, B. L. Carruth, W. W. Kim, F. Stenger, and P. L. Kuhn, "Ultrasound inverse scattering solutions from transmission and/or reflection data," presented at the Intern. Workshop on Physics and Engineering of Computerized Multidimensional Imaging and Processing, Newport Beach, Calif, April 2–4, 1986 and to be published by SPIE as volume 671.

AN ECG-GATED COLOR DOPPLER IMAGING SYSTEM FOR

DETERMINATION OF CORONARY BYPASS GRAFT PATENCY

John R. Klepper, Richard Ferraro, Donald L. Davis,
and Rosario Nasca

Institute of Applied Physiology and Medicine
701 16th Avenue
Seattle, Washington 98122,

ABSTRACT

A computer based pulsed Doppler imaging system designed for the
noninvasive assessment of coronary and cardiac dynamics has been
constructed. A multigate pulsed Doppler of the moving target indicator
type is implemented using CCD delay lines. Doppler sector scan images of
flow, gated on the ECG, allow on-line direct imaging of flow in blood
vessels within the body. Our display is gated on the electrocardiogram so
that the heart cycle is divided into 16 time segments. Information is
recorded and displayed in real time along the direction of current
interrogation along with previously recorded information along other
sector lines during the same portion of the heart cycle. In addition, a
real time Doppler M-mode display at 210 lines per second provides a method
for displaying Doppler flow information with better time resolution. A
simultaneous echo image of surrounding tissues is also possible.
Experimental trials on flow-through phantoms and human volunteers
indicates the ability to directly image flow in the vessels as small as 3
mm diameter. It is anticipated the device will be used to image flow in
coronary bypass grafts, followed by real time spectrum analysis of a
conventional single gate pulsed Doppler in order to quantify the velocity
of flow in such vessels.

INTRODUCTION

Coronary artery disease is a major health problem of epidemic
proportions in the United States. A variety of interventions have been
developed to ease the symptoms and prolong the lives of those suffering
from coronary artery disease. Coronary bypass grafting has become a
widespread procedure since the 1970's; with an estimated 159,000 patients
in the United States alone having bypass surgery in 1981. In recent
years, percutaneous transluminal angioplasty (PTCA) and direct
streptokinase infusion have also become significant procedures for
treatment of the symptoms of coronary artery disease. Unfortunately, all
of these treatments are means to ameliorate the symptoms of the disease,
but they do not cure the atherosclerosis which produces the stenoses being
treated. Thus, a significant reoccurrence of the disease results in a

This work supported by NIH Grant HL 30642.

typical patency rate for bypass grafts of only 85% after 8 months.[2] A noninvasive means to determine patency of grafted vessels and the reoccurrence of stenosis in native coronaries subjected to transluminal angioplasty would be of great significance to the medical management of these patients.

Doppler ultrasound holds promise for providing a noninvasive means that would allow regular follow-up of patients who have undergone one of these treatments for coronary artery disease. A number of investigators[2-6] have reported the ability to detect flow in bypass grafts using various types of Doppler. In the hands of experts, current Doppler measurement techniques combined with standard echocardiography can provide excellent diagnostic results. A few reports of the detection of native coronary arteries have been made via echocardiography[7] and Doppler,[8] although these exams can be described as difficult at best. Standard echocardiography provides a road map clearly delineating the chambers and valves of the heart but it does not immediately show the operator any information of hemodynamic significance. Range-gated Doppler, in conjunction with echocardiography, can be used to individually interrogate flow through valves and in flow channels to understand the hemodynamic significance and thereby aid in the diagnosis.[9,10] Detection of small vessels such as coronaries or bypass grafts in the vicinity of the heart is not readily apparent in standard echocardiography nor commonly found by current Doppler techniques. What is needed is a road map to allow the examiner to better understand the location and direction of flow channels within and around the heart in relation to the phase of the heart. The ECG-gated Doppler sector scanner under development in this project aims to provide such a road map, thereby allowing the examiner to quickly choose regions of interest for more detailed examination using either single-gate pulse Doppler or CW Doppler techniques with spectrum analysis.

Color coded Doppler imaging of flow in the heart in real time duplex format has recently become commercially available. These units have provided the first glimpse of the future capabilities of Doppler flow imaging. An atlas of images has been published[11] showing applications primarily in adult acquired valvular disease and some pediatric applications to determination of congenital malformations. The only substantial published results so far are applications for imaging of the flow in the chambers of the heart. The information content is high but the spatial resolution is low with significant gaps sometimes occurring in the images. An inherent limitation in a real time Doppler imaging device is the amount of signal averaging that can be done to improve the quality of Doppler signal. In cardiology applications, a typical such scanner can only average signals from 8 to 10 pulse repetition periods before moving on to the next interrogation angle.[12] In our device a significantly greater amount of signal averaging can and does occur. Although such averaging certainly is not necessary to produce good images of flow in major vessels and chambers of the heart, we feel that significant signal averaging is necessary in order to positively identify flow signals from smaller vessels, particularly those with low flow rates. By ECG gating our signal, we have the possibility to average over more than 400 pulse repetition periods thereby greatly increasing the signal-to-noise ratio of the resultant image.

METHODS

The Doppler system developed here was specifically designed for use in detection of coronary bypass grafts. The Doppler modes of operation are as follows: (1) a 295 gate multigate pulse Doppler is used to form the Doppler flow image and can operate at a carrier frequency of either 4 MHz or 2 MHz; (2) a simultaneous single gate pulse Doppler that can be located at the depth of particular interest--this module outputs a quadrature pair of audio signals which can be used for directional audio analysis and real time spectrum analysis; (3) an ECG module for gating of the Doppler image, and (4) a CW mode of operation.

The 4 MHz pulse Doppler uses a transmit tone burst length of one microsecond, corresponding to a depth resolution of 0.8 mm. The 2 MHz pulse Doppler uses a tone burst of 1.6 microseconds corresponding to a range resolution of 1.3 mm. Either 2 or 4 MHz Doppler can be operated in CW mode if an appropriate 2 element transducer is used. In imaging mode, the PRF is 6.8 kHz resulting in a depth of penetration of 11 cm for either frequency. The maximum spatial-peak temporal-average intensity in situ is estimated at 25 mW/cm^2 which is well within FDA guidelines for ultrasound devices with cardiac applications. Operation at 2 MHz is chosen only if the depth of penetration is insufficient due to the higher attenuation at 4 MHz. In either case, Doppler aliasing occurs at 3.4 kHz. Optimum signal is obtained from the multigate pulse Doppler in the frequency range of 1 to 2.5 kHz. From catheter measurements,[13] typical native coronary flow should produce a Doppler shift of 2 kHz at 4 MHz or 1 kHz at 2 MHz assuming zero Doppler angle.

The basic Doppler design is patterned after the so-called "Infinite Gate Pulse Doppler" (IGPD) developed by Nowicki and Reid.[14] The term "infinite gate" came from the method of Doppler target detection, which in its original form, used a quartz crystal delay line to provide a continuous analog output (therefore an "infinite" number of gates). Although this device was functional, it had severe limitations; particularly, that the operating frequency was fixed at 4.3 MHz and a limited penetration depth of only 4.5 cm resulted from the quartz delay line. The next generation of IGPD was dubbed the "Imaging Gate Pulse Doppler" and still forms the basis for the Doppler used in our current device. Instead of analog quartz crystal delay lines, this device uses CCD delay lines with 295 cells corresponding to 295 range gates along the line of interrogation.

This Doppler is patterned after the moving target indicator (MTI) type of radar, first adapted to ultrasonic use by Grandchamp[15] and Brandestini[16] and refined by Hoeks.[17] Two types of signals must be dealt with in developing an image from a pulse Doppler device. First, there are echos from stationary targets along the path of interrogation, such as tissue interfaces and scattering from motionless targets which form the standard ultrasonic echo image. Then there are also the low amplitude Doppler shifted signals reflected from moving targets along the beam. In an MTI arrangement, all of the data from one repetition period is stored, in this case, in 295 individual range gates in the CCD delay lines. On the following pulse repetition, the incoming data is subtracted from the stored data with the result that perfectly stationary targets are cancelled by the subtraction process, however moving targets produce a signal related to the phase shift that has occurred from one pulse repetition to the next. At this point, the signal from moving targets has been detected, however the relative rate of motion remains unknown. In order to extract the frequency of the Doppler shift, further processing is necessary. In our case, two channels of signals are generated: an in-phase (I) and quadrature (Q) baseband signal demodulated from the RF. These signals have retained approximately 1 MHz of bandwidth in each channel and thereby form the analytic signal representation of the complex envelope of the 4 MHz tone burst that was transmitted and received.

If the dynamic range of the input signals exceed the dynamic range of the CCD delay line, then incomplete stationary echo cancellation can occur. Because of the low signal level of the Doppler signals of interest compared to specular reflectors, this frequently occurs. To overcome this limitation, a double delay line canceller is used. This arrangement places two delay line-subtractor pairs in series, thereby providing further cancellation of unwanted echoes. The only drawbacks of this arrangement are further complexity of electronics, degraded frequency response for low frequency Doppler shifts, and some loss of range resolution. Detailed block[18] diagrams and further description of this apparatus are given elsewhere.

Mathematically, the incoming signals can be represented as $I(T,z)$ and $Q(T,z)$ and the output of the canceller can be represented as $dI(T,z)$ and $dQ(T,z)$ respectively, where the capital T represents time measured in steps of the pulse repetition period and z represents depth in the body. It has been shown that the time rate of change of the arctangent (dQ/dI) is equal to the instantaneous frequency or centroid frequency of the signal relative to the carrier demodulation frequency.[19] In our case, that is equal to the Doppler shift frequency, or

$$d/dT \ (\tan^{-1} dQ/dI) = f_d \tag{1}$$

It turns out that the $\tan^{-1}(dQ/dI)$ is a reasonably difficult function to calculate at the speeds required to display Doppler flow images in real time. A variety of approximations to this function have been used in pulse Doppler MTI phase detectors.[18] The functional form of the phase detector, as developed by Nowicki,[18] was mathematically equivalent to differentiating one channel with time and cross-multiplying it with the other, that is,

$$f_d \sim [d/dT(dQ)] \ dI \tag{2}$$

It turns out that this is a rather noisy and incomplete approximation. We have shown[19] that

$$d/dT[\tan^{-1} (dQ/dI)] = (d\dot{Q}dI - d\dot{I}dQ) \ / \ (dI^2 + dQ^2) \tag{3}$$

where the superscript dots represent time derivatives.

A new phase detector corresponding to the above equation has been developed and implemented. Comparison of old and new phase detectors is shown in figure 1. In figure 1 the upper trace is the output of the new phase detector and the lower traces the output of the previous phase detector simultaneously displayed for the same input frequency shifted signal. The new phase detector corresponds only to the numerator of equation (3) and the old phase detector corresponds to the second term of the numerator. As can be seen, the subtraction of the other cross-multiplied term in equation (3), has resulted in a signal with significantly less noise, as well as an increase in amplitude on the same scale. Overall the new phase detector has produced an increased signal noise ratio of approximately 3:1. An additional advantage of the new phase detector is that it produces a stable output independent of the phase of the signal relative to the PRF. This is not the case for the old detector which oscillates between zero output and the maximum as is shown in figure 1. An analog sweep integrator was necessary with the old detector in order to produce a stable output, with some confusion in directionality occurring for frequency shifts greater than 2 kHz. A comparison of the frequency response of the old and new phase detectors is shown in figure 2. Both show a frequency dependence to the third power

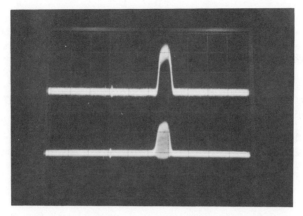

Fig. 1. Comparison of old and new phase detectors.
The upper trace is the output of the new
phase detector and the lower trace is the
simultaneous output of the old phase detector.

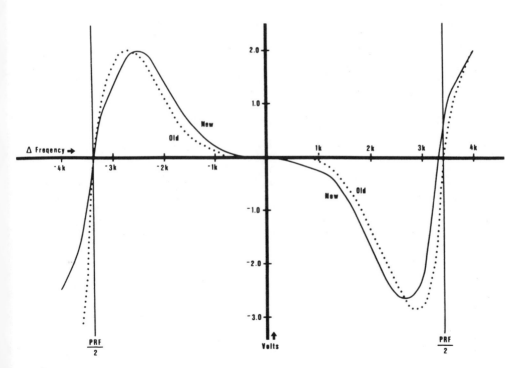

Fig. 2. Comparison of measured frequency response of old and new phase
detectors.

207

around zero frequency which could be made linear by division by the denominator in equation (3).

The division required to fully implement a linear phase detector and thereby produce a linear frequency response is very difficult to implement in a stable fashion in analog electronics. We have built and tested such a circuit which provides some improvement in reducing the amplitude dependence of the signals. However, we feel that the division can better be done digitally at this point where the use of some logic with respect to the denominator signal strength can be useful in improving the image.

A block diagram of the current system is shown in figure 3. The Doppler provides four inputs to the signal averager. These are the PRF synchronization pulse, the Doppler A-mode flow data, the depth position of a single gate used for audio listening and spectrum analysis, and the ECG-gating signal. The PRF pulse synchronizes the averager to acquire one Doppler line every 148 microseconds.

The averager digitizes the Doppler A-mode at a 2 MHz rate using a TRW 1008 8 bit A-D converter and averages over three time bins producing 97 gates in depth. Each gate represents a sample length of 1.5 microseconds which corresponds to 1.2 mm in depth. These gates are then averaged over a selectable number of PRFs before the averaged data is sent to the 11/73 processor through a DMA port. Currently this system is sending 211 Doppler lines per second to the 11/73. Single gate position and the ECG signal are also sent to the 11/73 for additional processing. The used Unirad B-arm has been modified for the purpose of position sensing to allow us to do the scan conversion for the Doppler sector scan. The scan arm monitors the X and Y position as well as the dX/dY slope of the Doppler transducer. This information is digitized separately by a 12 bit A-D converter on the 11/73. The 11/73 processor uses this data to calculate a color Doppler M-mode type display as well as a color 2-D sector scan type display. The ECG signal is generated on an auxiliary board internal to the Doppler using a three lead ECG. The ECG signal is processed with an R-wave detector and an R-wave synchronization pulse is sent to the signal averager to synchronize the sector scan.

The sector scan is gated to begin on the R-wave and divide the heart cycle up into 16 equal time intervals. A manual pot adjustment is currently used to set the time bin lengths to insure that a full heart cycle is being used. The ECG R-wave detector has been fully tested using an ECG simulator and performs well under all conditions except for an extremely damped, low amplitude R-wave. Operation of the R-wave detector has proven reliable on all human subjects tested so far, although none of the test subjects had an abnormal ECG.

A 2-dimensional type of display of the Doppler information in a sector-type format is developed in shades of red and blue corresponding to flow towards the transducer and flow away from the transducer, respectively. This image is created in pseudo-real time by accumulating across multiple heart cycles as the transducer on the B-arm is slowly scanned manually. The 211 Doppler lines per second are then further averaged from 6 to 52 lines per second before being entered into the "2D" display buffer. The display buffer is actually 16 display buffers, each corresponding to 1/16th of the heart cycle. When the new Doppler line is ready for display, its position vector is calculated and it is entered into one of the 16 buffers, depending on the amount of time that has passed since last R-wave. These 16 buffers are built within the raster graphics memory. The resolution of this graphics memory is 512 X 512 which allows each of the 16 buffers to have a resolution of 128 X 128.

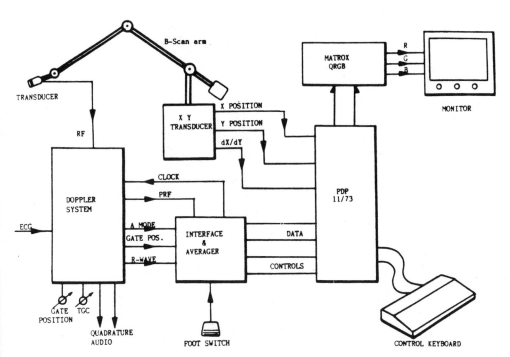

Fig. 3. Block diagram of the Doppler imaging system.

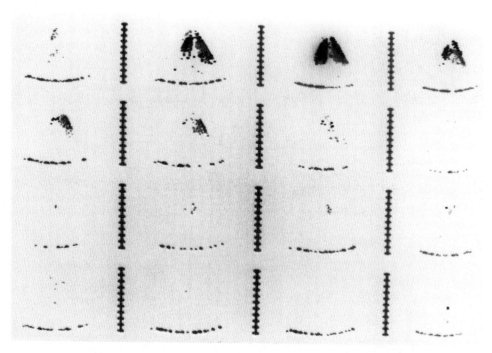

Fig. 4. A sixteen frame image of flow during the heart cycle. Systole
begins with the R-wave in the upper left hand corner and ends
with frame six. Normally the display is in color, however, for
publication we show flow away from the transducer in black and
flow towards the transducer in gray.

The "2D" display is then recreated in real time by zooming each of the 128 X 128 buffers to full screen, displaying one buffer at a time. The buffer displayed corresponds to the current time relative to the last R-wave. A non-real time display is also available which allows redisplay of any portion of the heart cycle at a variable rate selectable by the operator.

An alternative imaging mode displays either a standard M-mode or an ECG gated echo sector image which is accumulated in the same way as the Doppler image. This image is quite crude compared to modern ultrasonic imaging systems because its range resolution is only 1.2 mm (the same as the Doppler image) and only a 3 bit gray scale is used. These limitations arise solely from the limited display memory currently being used. Despite the low resolution, the images produced have been quite useful in understanding the morphology, thereby improving our ability to interpret the Doppler images.

RESULTS

To really appreciate in vivo images generated on this system, a dynamic playback of the entire heart cycle is needed. We can do that in our laboratory but it is difficult to put it on a single sheet of paper. Figure 4 shows all 16 frames of the heart cycle image of a 25-year old male with Marfan's Syndrome. In figure 4, the R-wave trigger occurs with the upper left hand frame, and time proceeds in 60 msec intervals to the right, then down one row, etc. This image sequence was generated in a parasternal short axis view about 45° from parallel to the ribs through the third intercostal space at the pulmonary artery/right ventricular outflow tract level. In this image sequence, the subject's head is towards the left. Almost all of the activity in this image sequence occurs during systole, as would be expected in the pulmonary artery. The time required to acquire this image sequence was less than one minute and required no special effort to limit patient motion.

CONCLUSIONS

Although we have successfully completed the prototype development of the ECG-gated pulse Doppler sector scanner, a number of improvements are necessary before the device is truly ready for serious clinical trials. The current system is limited to 16 frames/heart cycle of 128 X 128 resolution. We intend to expand to a 256 X 256 matrix at 16 frames/heart cycle with a simultaneous echo image format or to provide a format at 32 frames/heart cycle without the echo image. Other combinations between these two extremes are also possible, such as 25 frames/heart cycle at 200 X 200 with simultaneous Doppler and echo images.

Our preliminary experiments indicate that a simultaneous echo/Doppler capability is highly desirable for interpretation of the resulting image. The system should be incorporated into a real time sector scanner which can be switched to a slow scan, ECG-gated mode to provide the increased signal averaging undoubtedly necessary to reliably image coronary bypass grafts.

REFERENCES

1. Kolata, G: Some bypass surgery unnecessary, Science, 605 (1983).
2. Fabian, J, Vojacek, J, Eng., AG, Prerovsky, I, Belan, A, Hejhal, L: Noninvasive Doppler ultrasound evaluation of aortocoronary bypass, Jap Heart J, 20(6):823-830, Nov (1979).

3. Diebold, B, Theroux, P, Bourassa, MG, Peronneau, P, Guermonprez, JL: Noninvasive assessment of aortocoronary bypass graft patency using pulsed Doppler echocardiography, Amer J of Cardiology, 43:10-16, Jan (1979).

4. Gould, KL, Mozersky, DJ, Hokanson, DE, Baker, DW, Kennedy, JW, Sumner, DS, Strandness, DE: A noninvasive technique for determining patency of saphenous vein coronary bypass grafts, Circ 46:595-600, Sep (1972).

5. Theroux, P, Bourassa, MG, Diebold, B, Peronneau, P, Barbet, A, Guermonprez, JL: Noninvasive assessment of aortocoronary graft patency by pulsed Doppler flowmeter, Circ 55-56, Supl III, pp 25, Sep (1977).

6. Benchimol, A, Reyns, P, Alvarez, S, Desser, KB, McCoullough, K: Noninvasive assessment of left internal mammary-coronary bypass patency using the external Doppler probe, Am Heart J, 96(3):347-349, Sep (1978).

7. Weyman, A, Feigenbaum, H, Dillon JC, Johnston, KW, Eggleston, RC: Noninvasive visualization of the left main coronary artery by cross-sectional echocardiography, Circ 54(2):169-174 (1976).

8. Gramiak, R, Holen, J, Moss, AJ, Gatierrez, OH, Roe, SA: Coronary artery flow: noninvasive detection by Doppler Ultrasound, presented at RSNA (1984).

9. Hatle, L, Angelsen, B: Physical Principles and Clinical Applications of Doppler Ultrasound in Cardiology, Lea & Febiger, Phila (1985), 2nd Ed.

10. Spencer, MP, ed: Cardiac Doppler Diagnosis, Vol 1, Martinus Nijhoff, Dordrecht (1984).

11. Omoto, R, ed: Color Atlas of Real Time Two-Dimensional Doppler Echocardiography, Shindan-To-Chiryo, Tokyo (1984).

12. Kasai, C, Namekawa, K, Koyano, A, Omoto, R: Real time two-dimensional blood flow imaging using an auto correlation technique, IEEE Trans Sonics and Ultrasonics, 32(3):458-464 (1985).

13. Benchimol, A, and Dresser, K: Coronary artery blood flow velocity in man, in Cardiovascular Applications of Ultrasound, R. Reneman, ed. 193-200, North Holland, Amsterdam (1974).

14. Nowicki, A, and Reid, J.M.: An Infinite Gate Pulse Doppler, Ultrasound in Med and Biol, 7, 44-50 (1981).

15. Grandchamp, P.A: A novel pulsed directional Doppler velocimeter, Proc Second European Cong on Ultrasonics in Med (Kazner, E., ed), pp 122-132, Excerpta Medica, Amsterdam, Oxford (1975).

16. Brandestini, M: Topoflow--a digital full range Doppler velocity meter, IEEE Trans on Sonics and Ultrasonics, SU-25:287 (1978).

17. Hoeks, APG, Reneman, RS, Peronneau, PA: A multigate pulsed Doppler system with serial data processing, IEEE Trans on Sonics and Ultrasonics, SU-28: 242-247 (1981).

18. Nowicki, A, Klepper, JR, Reid, JM, Spencer, MP: An Imaging Gate Pulse Doppler for Examination of Coronary Bypass Graft Patency, in Cardiac Doppler Diagnosis, Vol 1, Spencer, MP, ed, Martinus Nijhoff, Dordrecht, 51-60 (1984).

19. Miwa, H, Murakami, K, Reid, JM, Klepper, JR: Attenuation Extraction from Quadrature-Detected Phase of an Ultrasonic Echo in Bio-tissue Characterization. FUJITSU Scientific and Technical Journal, Vol 21 (2), 165-181 (1985).

A TWO DIMENSIONAL PVDF TRANSDUCER MATRIX

AS A RECEIVER IN AN ULTRASONIC TRANSMISSION CAMERA

B. Granz, and R. Oppelt

Forschungslaboratorien der Siemens AG
8520 Erlangen, FRG

ABSTRACT

A two dimensional ultrasonic receiver matrix with the piezoelectric polymer PVDF has been developed and tested in an ultrasonic transmission camera. The major advantage of this matrix over known receiver devices for ultrasonic cameras is its high sensitivity along with high bandwidth, its large number of small receiver elements and its pure electronic read-out. No mechanical moving of either the image or the receiver array is needed. The matrix read - out is realized by a stack of 29 thin film substrates with 128 switchable preamplifiers each. One side of the stack forms a contact matrix with 29 * 128 metal contacts of the size 0.75 mm * 0.65 mm, covering a total area of 26 mm * 96 mm. The contact matrix is pressed against a common 25 um PVDF foil as a common transducer. A parallel signal procession results in a homogenous image presentation. Transmission images of technical and biological objects with a frame rate of 25 Hz and a sensitivity of $6 * 10^{-6}$ V/Pa are shown. The intrinsic resolution of the camera - 1.7 mm at 2 MHz is reproduced in the image.

1. INTRODUCTION

An ultrasonic transmission camera produces medical images which are substantially different from common B-scan images. The image plane lies normal to the direction of propagation of the ultrasound and the transmitted part of the ultrasound contains other information about the structure of the human body than the reflected one. Transmission cameras with linear arrays working in the field of medical research are used to examine hip-joints of babies [1] or the extremities [2]. In both camera systems additional expense has to be introduced for the mechanical movement of either the ultrasonic image or the receiver array. This mechanical movement results in a limited frame rate.

This limitation can be overcome by means of a receiver matrix with a high number of densely packed receiver elements. Each of these elements (and their number can be up to 10,000) has to be distinguished from any other by an electronic switch. Because the area of one element is usually very small, this switch has to be a preamplifier as well. There are strict constraints on the size of these switches: they have to fit into the geometric shadow of the area of the receiver element [3] . Otherwise no multiple production technique could be used and the volume of the electronics would become bulky.

The principle that helps deal with this geometric constraint is demonstrated by Gelly[4] and Papallardo[5]. Their matrices are joined together by a stack of very flat linear arrays. The material sensitive to ultrasound is piezoelectric ceramics diced to single elements which work either in the 33 or the 31 mode. Their bandwidths are relatively small. The switching is done by a multiplexer chip or by other means of hybrid electronics concentrated on one area on the flat side of every linear array.

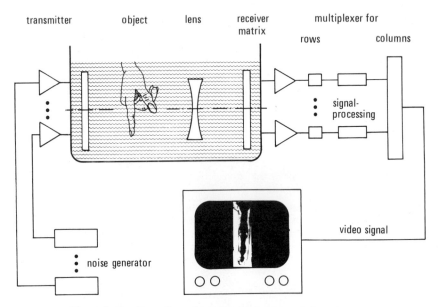

Figure 1: Configuration of an ultrasonic transmission camera

An ultrasonic camera is shown schematically in figure 1. A transmitter matrix of piezoelectric transducers, each excited by a signal generator, transmits ultrasound which insonates an object field. The portion of the ultrasound which is not absorbed or reflected by the object, e.g. a finger, is collimated by an acoustic lens into the image plane. The piezoelectric receiver matrix in the image plane converts the pressure image into a charge image. The charge image is then electronically read out and finally converted into a video signal.

Magnification of the image is achieved by moving the lens along the axis of propagation of the ultrasound. All calculations here are made with a 1 : 1 representation.

The construction parameters of the camera define their physical performance and thus their medical usefulness. In our construction a 100 element transmitter matrix insonates the object plane with ultrasound of a mid-frequency of 2 MHz and a bandwidth of 1 MHz. A crude estimation of the lateral resolution Δx of a biconcave polystyrene lens with focal length f is given in equation (1):

$$\Delta x = 1.22 * \lambda * d/A \qquad (1)$$

with a wavelength $\lambda = 0.75$ mm, an image distance of d = 2*f = 320 mm (for a 1 : 1 representation) and a lens aperture A = 190 mm we get in this idealized model a resolution

$$\Delta x = 1.55 \text{ mm} \qquad (2)$$

A more realistic calculation of Δx is demonstrated in part 5.1. To reproduce the intrinsic resolution of 1.7 mm the image must be scanned by single receiver elements each smaller than 0.8 mm. On the other hand, for more detailed examinations of biological structures higher frequencies have to be used, so a bandwidth up to 10 MHz of the receiver system is desirable.

For a 1 : 1 representation of a part of a hand or a foot an image size of approximately 100 mm * 100 mm is necessary. By comparing this area to the area of a single receiver element we get an estimation of $1.5 * 10^4$ receiver elements each to be connected and separately switchable.

3. CONSTRUCTION OF THE MATRIX

An electronic device like the receiver matrix with such a large number of elements cannot be made monolithic. Considering that an ordinary 4 inch wafer with MOSFETs has a yield of less than 90 %, a construction of the matrix out of smaller pieces, each separately tested, is the method of choice.

Our way of constructing a receiver matrix which satisfies the condition of fitting the electronics into the geometric shadows of the receiver elements, as well as the condition of the built up in separable parts, is shown in figure 2.

As basis material we used ceramic substrates as they are common in thin-film techniques. On the front side of the substrate are 128 contact areas of the size 0.65 mm * 0.75 mm and a raster step of 0.75 mm. On the flat side there are 128 signal leads, resistors and the contact pads for the 128 dual-gate MOSFETs. All leads are of equal length for the transistors. So the signal reduction by parallel capacitances is homogeneous. Additionally there are two leads for the signal out and the common ground for all 128 MOSFETs. The dual-gate MOSFETs are glued to the substrates and wire bonded.

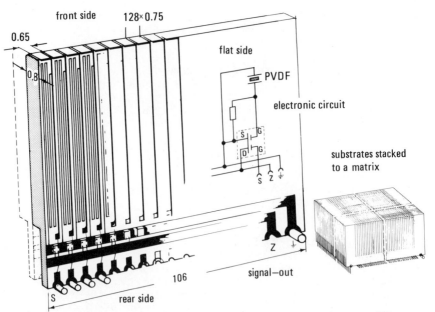

Figure 2: Substrate with 128 contact areas and 128 switchable preamplifiers and a complete matrix in the right corner

On the rear side there are 128 switch leads. With these leads one of the 128 transistors per substrate can be selected. This one alone amplifies the signal from the contact area and feeds the signal into the signal-out lead.

All leads and the contact area are produced by aphotoetching technique. Every substrate behaves like a 128 : 1 amplifing analog multiplexer. With a strip of piezoelectric material connected to the front side, every substrate would behave like a linear receiving array.

Near the rear side a part of the substrate is ground off; thus there is enough space for the transistor chips when the substrates are stacked to a block. A stacked block of substrates is shown on the lower right side of figure 2. The front side of the block forms a n * 128 contact matrix, where n is the number of substrates. In our construction we finally used 29 substrates; Thus leading to a 29 * 128 = 3.712 element contact matrix covering an area of 26 mm * 96 mm.

The contact matrix is pressed against a polarized PVDF foil of 25 um thickness. This foil acts simultaneously as a window for the water bath shown in figure 1. The foil is metallized only on the inner side which contacts the water and forms the common ground. On this side the ultrasonic image is formed. The outer side of the PVDF foil is not metallized; it contains the ac charge pattern of the ultrasonic image which is then capacitively connected to the contact matrix. In this schema the receiver matrix consists of a common transducer foil and a contact matrix, both representing a transducer matrix with 3.712 elements.

PVDF on metal contacts on a hard backing exhibits high sensitivity and an excellent angle of acceptance[6].

The contact matrix is easily mounted and dismounted to the common transducer foil, and all the electronics are outside the water and easily accessible without the need of additional protection.

4. ELECTRONIC SIGNAL READ-OUT AND SIGNAL PROCESSING

4.1 Analog Signal Processing

Figure 3 shows a schematic diagram of the electronic signal read-out and signal processing. Each matrix element consists of an ultrasonic transducer connected to a switchable amplifier. By means of a ring shift register each of the 128 matrix columns is sequentially addressed for about 300 us. Within this time interval the amplified signals of all 29 receiver elements of one column being addressed appear at their respective 29 signal output terminals. Consequently, the same number of signal processing channels has to be installed. This rather expensive parallel signal processing is necessary to obtain real-time frame rates.

The output levels of the signal processing channels represent the average values of the ultrasonic pressure amplitudes which have been detected by the respectively addressed matrix column. These output levels are multiplexed by a 29 : 1 multiplexer to form the final video signal. After each of the 128 matrix columns has been addressed, one complete image is read-out. Note that the timing for the ring shift register and the multiplexer is chosen for real-time read-out of matrices up to 128 * 128 elements.

The electronic part of the receiver matrix is shown in figure 4 in more detail. The switchable amplifiers are realized by dual-gate MOSFETs.

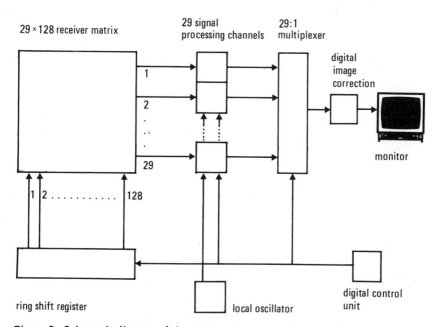

Figure 3: Schematic diagram of the electronic signal read—out and signal processing

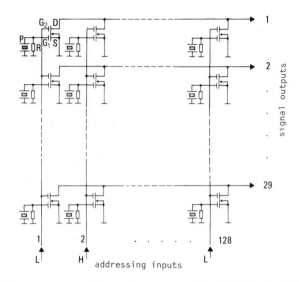

Figure 4: Electronic part of the receiver matrix with 29×128 switchable amplifiers realized by dual—gate MOSFETs

Their gate-1-terminals are connected to the respective transducer electrodes and biased by high-ohmic resistors to ground. All gate-2-terminals of each column are connected in parallel for addressing. Similarly, all drain terminals of each line are connected in parallel to the signal-out leads. To address a particular matrix column, its address input level is set to a positive voltage, all other input levels being negative.

Besides the power-less switching capability there are dual-gate MOSFETs available which combine further advantageous features like low input capacitance (<2 pF), high forward transmittance (>14 mmho), excellent switching insulation, and low output capacitance. However, the last feature still means a parasitic capacitance of about 250 pF parallel to each signal output path caused by the drain-source terminals of the 127 unaddressed MOSFETs. Only with a succesive amplifier stage with very low input impedance can one avoid signal reduction by leakage currents into these parasitic capacitances. An appropriate circuit is represented by a base-grounded bipolar transistor which forms together with the adressed MOSFET, the so-called cascode amplifier. These amplifiers are well known for their broad frequency bandwidths.

The usable bandwidth of the PVDF transducer in connection with the cascode amplifier is more than 8 MHz.

One of the 29 signal processing channels is shown in more detail in figure 5. The received ultrasonic signal (1.5 to 2.5 MHz) is amplified and converted down to a range of 0 to 0.5 MHz by a fully balanced mixer.

As figure 5 shows, each of the 29 mixers is injected by a common local oscillator frequency (in this example 2 MHz). The following 500 kHz low pass filter eliminates noise and unwanted mixing products at higher frequencies. This superheterodyne receiving principle combines two essential advantages: First, the whole receiver can work at other frequency ranges by simply changing the local oscillator frequency (e.g. a local oscillator frequency of 3 MHz causes a frequency range from 2.5 to 3.5 MHz

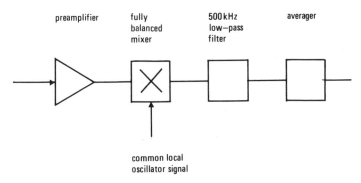

preamplifier   fully   500 kHz   averager
                 balanced   low—pass
                 mixer   filter

common local
oscillator signal

Figure 5: Schematic diagram of one of the 29 signal processing channels

to be received) and second, the upper frequency limit of the following signal processing stage need not exceed half of the ultrasound bandwidth, which is a rather low freqency of 500 kHz.

The above mentioned signal processing stage may be denoted as "averager". It forms the amplitude mean value of the low pass filter output signal within the 300 us addressing period and holds this for the time of the next addressing period. So all the 29 mean values, which represent the average ultrasonic pressure amplitudes of a complete matrix column, can be multiplexed within the following addressing period to form the final video signal. The images on the video screen are presented with a frame rate of 25 Hz in the interlaced line method.

4.2 Digital Image Correction

Of course, some of the 29 * 128 receiver elements will show unequal sensitivities, also the object plane cannot be insonated fully homogeneously.Furthermore some of the receiver elements may fail totally. These effects can best be studied with an image without object (zero image): Instead of a uniform bright area there will appear pixels and also whole regions of different brightness on the monitor. Complete dark pixels will show that some receiver elements are failing fully.

This drawback can be eliminated by a digital image correction unit shown in figure 6., inserted between the 29 : 1 multiplexer and the monitor. (See also figure 3.) Before imaging an object, a zero image is stored digitally in a RAM. All following images (with arbitrary object) are then divided pixel by pixel by the zero image. Thus, the background will appear of homogeneous brightness. The digital division operations are performed by an EPROM look-up-table. All digital operations are done with 8 bit.

Totally failing receiver elements, however, cannot be corrected in this way for the division by zero is undefined. Therefore an additional unit called "dead pixel averager" is used between the digital divider and the final D/A converter. This module detects failed pixels in the stored zero image by comparing the contents of each of the RAM storage elements with an adjustable minimum threshold level. The "dead pixel averager" assigns the mean value of the surrounding intact pixels to those elements which are below threshold.

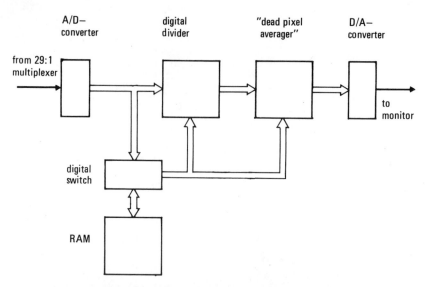

A/D–converter   digital divider   "dead pixel averager"   D/A–converter

from 29:1 multiplexer

to monitor

digital switch

RAM

Figure 6: Schematic diagram of the digital image correction unit

5. MEASUREMENTS

5.1 Resolution

To determine the lateral resolution of an imaging system the well known formulas from the optical regime can be applied to the ultrasonic transmission camera. A common resolution criterion is the coherent lens impulse response, also called the point spread function $h(r_i)$. For a 1 : 1 imaging system it is found to be [7].

$$h(r_i) = \frac{1}{2\pi} \int_0^{\omega\kappa} \omega_r J_0(\omega_r r_i) d\omega_r = \frac{(\omega\kappa)^2}{2\pi} \frac{J_1(r_i \omega\kappa)}{r_i \omega\kappa} \qquad (3)$$

where $\kappa = R_1 / (cd)$
with
         R_1 radius of the ultrasonic lens aperture
         ω ultrasonic angular frequency
         c   wave propagation velocity of ultrasound in water
         d   distance between lens and image plane
         ω_r radial spatial frequency
         r_i radial coordinate in the image plane
      J_0, J_1 Bessel functions of the order 0 and 1, respectively

Because wave propagation in the lense medium polystyrene is faster than in the surrounding water, an appropriate imaging lens is biconcave. Because of the attenuating material of the biconcave lens, the waves through the lens will be more attenuated the more they are off axis. Further we have to consider the convolution effect caused by the finite transducer aperture of the receiver element. Eq (3) has to be extended, see [8,9]

$$h(r_i) \sim \int_0^{\omega\kappa} J_1(\omega_r R_t) J_0(\omega_r r_i) \exp\left\{-[\frac{\omega_r}{\omega\kappa'(\omega).}]^2\right\} d\omega_r \qquad (4)$$

where $\qquad \kappa'(\omega)= \sqrt{R_c/.\alpha(\omega)} / (cd)$

with
$\qquad R_c \qquad$ curvature radius of the symmetric biconcave lens
$\qquad R_t \qquad$ transducer aperture radius
$\qquad \alpha(\omega) \qquad$ frequency dependent attenuation coefficient of
$\qquad\qquad\qquad$ the lens medium.

For simplicity a circular transducer aperture has been assumed, where the quantity R_t is given by the criterion of equal aperture sizes compared to the real quadratic transducers.

Figure 7 shows two plots of impulse responses. The *-marked curve is calculated according to Eq. (4) while the other one has been measured. The calculation has been made with the following parameters:

R_1 = 85 mm, R_c = 110 mm, R_t = 0.45 mm, d = 2*f = 320 mm, c = 1480 m/s,
ω = 2* π *2 MHz, $\alpha(\omega)$ = 7.33 * 10^{-7} * ω s/m, (f = focal length).

The point object used in the measurement was well approximated by a pin hole of 0.8 mm diameter. Its finite extension can be neglected. As figure 7 shows, there is a - 3 dB width of 1.7 mm in good agreement with the calculated resolution. The deviations in the side lobes may be assigned to multiple reflections inside the lens, because they vary strongly with freqency.

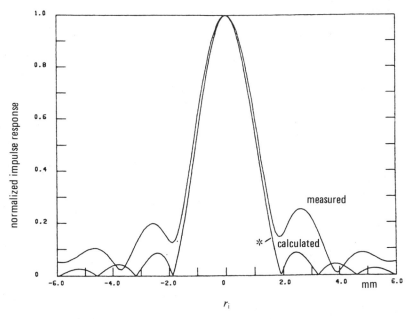

Figure 7: Impulse response of the ultrasonic transmission camera at 2 MHz

5.2 Sensitivity

The sensitivity of a piezoelectric receiver is composed of the output voltage per input pressure and the noise limited minimum detectable signal. We measured the sensitivity by comparing the pressure at the inside of the PVDF foil to the output voltage of the cascode amplifier. The pressure was measured with a calibrated hydrophone over a frequency range from 1.5 to 2.5 MHz. The sensitivity was determined to

$$S = 6 * 10^{-6} \text{ V/Pa} \tag{5}$$

By comparing this number to a noise level at the same electrical point of 144 μV, the minimum detectable signal (mds) will have an intensity of

$$mds = 1.9 * 10^{-8} \text{ W/cm}^2 \tag{6}$$

5.3 Homogeneous Image Representation

The function of the digital image correction is shown in figure 8. On the left side there is the original image; one of the 29 substrates is totally missing (black vertical line). The other black dots demonstrate that about 5 % of the pixels are not working. The stored image after the "dead pixel averaging" is shown in the middle of figure 8. To the right side the corrected image is shown with homogeneous background without an object in the object plane.

5.4 Transmission Images of Technical Objects

All following images are made with the corrected homogeneous background. Figure 9 shows the transmission image of silicon rubber balls embedded in a silicon rubber block, the smallest ball being 10 mm in diameter. Note that these balls are clearly seen, though their acoustical impedances differ only by 1 % against the surrounding medium. We found that especially round or cylindrical objects always contrast very well with their surroundings. This is also true for biological objects, e.g. tendons in tissue.

An interesting consequence of the finite bandwidth is demonstrated in figure 9 b and 9 c with the transmission image of a sheet of aluminium dense perforated with holes of 2 mm diameter. In figure 9 b the sheet is located in the object plane. The holes in the center are clearly imaged; at the edges they are blurred because of the curvature of the focal plane. The images of the holes are light, because the ultrasound is easily transmitted there.

Moving the sheet some millimeters off the lens, another clear image appears, but with the holes now dark (figure 9 c). This is a diffraction effect, where the waves from different Fresnel zones of the holes interfere to zero at certain distances from the holes. If these results of interference are in the object plane they are imaged by the lens like an object.

5.5 Transmission Images of Biological Objects

Our first experiments in vivo are done with human extremities. The extremities are easy to introduce into the water bath and they are well matched to the size of the receiver matrix. The object plane of interest is found by moving the 3-dimensional object along the beam axis. By moving the lens with respect to the receiver matrix more detailed structures of the object can be presented in magnification. Figure 10 a

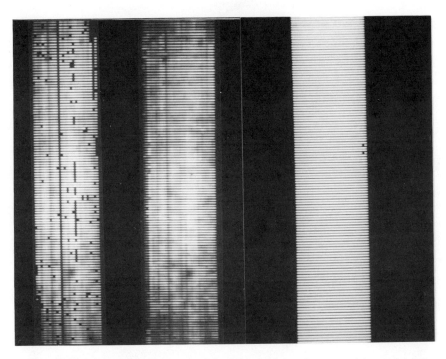

Figure 8: Original image (left), stored image (middle) and corrected image (right) by the digital image correction

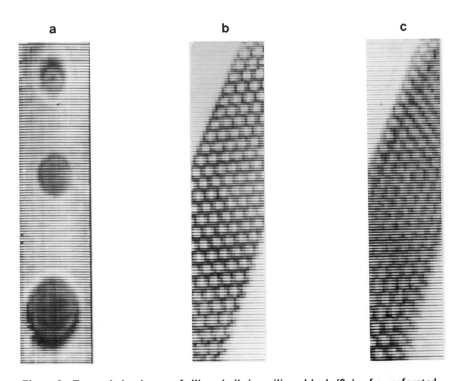

Figure 9: Transmission image of silicon balls in a silicon block (9a), of a perforated aluminium sheet in the object plane (9b) and outside the object plane (9c)

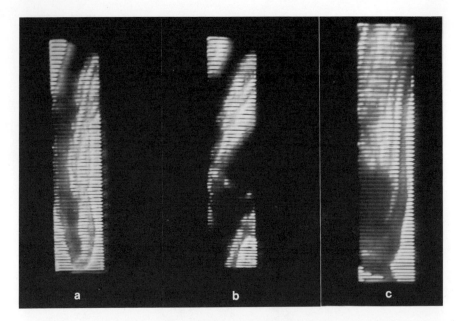

Figure 10: Transmission images of human extremities: finger lateral (10a),
hand dorsal (10b) and achilles heel (10c)

shows a transmission image of a finger. Its bones and tendons are clearly
distinguished, as well as the ligaments in figure 10 b with a part of the
human hand. The Achilles' heel in figure 10 c presents the tendons in
connection with the bone. Because of the 25 Hz frame rate, the function of
these human extremities can be controlled during their natural movement.

6. RESULTS

With the 2-dimensional PVDF receiver matrix, transmission images in an
ultrasonic camera can be presented with large bandwidth and high sensitivity.

Biological objects, especially tendons in their coherence with the
bones in human extremities are seen in vivo. Because of the real time
frame rate of 25 Hz not only the structure but also the function of such
internals of the human body can be controlled under unaffected conditions.

ACKNOWLEDGEMENTS

The authors wish to thank Herrn B. Sachs and his team from the Siemens
technical laboratory, especially Frau B. Bittel, for their never ending
patience during the construction of such a sophisticated device.

REFERENCES

1. P.S. Green, L.F. Schaefer, E.D. Jones and J.R. Suarez
   A New High-Performance Ultrasonic Camera, in "Acoustical
   Holography", Vol. 5, Plenum Press, New York, 1973.
   H.H. Mathias, H. Woltering and V. Guth
   Die Ultraschalltransmissionskamera bei der Diagnostik von
   instabilen dysplastischen und dislozierten Hüftgelenken bei
   Neugeborenen und Kindern im 1. Lebensjahr, Klinische Pedia-
   trie, 196 (1984)
2. H. Brettel, U. Roeder and C. Scherg
   Ultrasonic Transmission Camera for Medical Diagnoses,
   Biomed. Tech., Ergänzungsband, 26, (1981), 63.
3. J.D. Plummer, R.G. Swartz, M.G. Maginnes, J.R. Beaudouin
   and J.D. Meindl
   Two-Dimensional Transmit/Receive Ceramic Piezoelectric
   Arrays: Construction and Performance, IEEE Trans. on Son.
   and Ultrason., 25, (1978), 273
4. J.F. Gelly and C. Maerfeld
   Properties for a 2 D Multiplexed Array for Acoustic Imaging,
   Proc. of the IEEE Us. Symp. (1981), 685
5. M. Papallardo
   Hybrid Linear and Matrix Acoustic Arrays, Ultrasonics, 19,
   (1981), 81
6. B. Granz
   A Linear Monolithic Receiving Array of PVDF Transducers for
   Transmission Cameras, in "Acoustical Imaging", Vol. 12,
   Plenum Press, New York, 1982
7. J.W. Goodman
   "Introduction to Fourier Optics", Mc Graw Hill, New York,
   1968
8. R. Oppelt and H. Ermert
   Transfer Function Analysis of a Quasioptical Ultrasonic
   Imaging System, Ultrasonic Imaging, 6, (1984), 324
9. R. Oppelt
   Theoretische und experimentelle Untersuchung zur quasi-
   optischen Abbildung mit einer Ultraschall-Transmissions-
   kamera, Dissertation, Institut für HF-Technik, Universi-
   tät Erlangen-Nürnberg, 1985

A NEW DIGITAL SCAN PROCESSOR FOR ULTRASONIC IMAGING

Bruno Richard, Jean-Claude Roucayrol, and Jean Perrin

Laboratoire de Biophysique
Faculté de Médecine Cochin
F-75014 Paris, France

INTRODUCTION

Digital scan converters were introduced some ten years ago in manual B-scan units and are now currently used in all kinds of real time ultrasound scanners for medical imaging[1].

Digital processing of ultrasonic images is used primarily for freeze frame capability and video scan conversion. Another interesting feature of digital processing is that it makes possible interpolation[2] and spatial or temporal filtering which give a better visual comfort. However, what can be done to modify frozen images is limited: gray scale modification and magnification by a simple factor (x2., x4.).

We present here a new digital processor (processeur d'images ultrasonores: "PIU"), the main interest of which is, besides the above mentioned characteristics of DSC, the extension of post processing capabilities to such adjustments as:
- depth gain compensation

- choice of any section depth and magnification

PREVIOUS WORK

Nowadays, a digital scan converter is able to transform in real time polar into rectangular coordinates, to make interpolation between pixels[3], to accomplish some kind of post processing (mainly contrast modifications).

The fast data acquisition of real time ultrasound requires a fast digital processing, more difficult to achieve in sector than in linear scanning[4]. One solution that is used to simplify conversion processes is to sample ecoes of one scan line at a frequency depending on the angle θ of the line:

$$f = f_o . \cos \theta$$

where f_o is the sampling frequency of the center line. Thus, the i_{th} sample of each echo line will be displayed on the i_{th} horizontal line of the video screen[5].

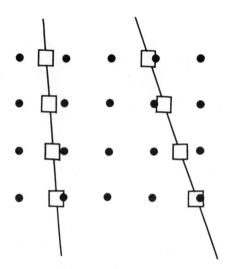

Fig. 1: Echo signals are sampled at a frequency
$f_0 \cos\theta$ so that samples of different scan
lines will be aligned on a horizontal line
of the picture (▢).
As a consequence, pixels of the display
matrix (●) may be derived from these data
by a one dimensional horizontal interpolation.

Then, spacing of data pixels along the i_{th} line depends on the number i
(vertical position) and the horizontal position j, measured from the center,
according to the function:

$$\theta = \tan^{-1}(j/i)$$

When a data pixel does not correspond exactly to a pixel of the display
matrix, one can take either the nearest neighbour value or an interpolated
value from surrounding neighbours[6]. As i_{th} samples are on the i_{th} line, a
one dimensional horizontal interpolation is sufficient which simplifies
electronic design (fig. 1).

An example of results that we obtained with such a DSC has been shown
in a previous paper[7]. Moiré artifacts are avoided by this technique but a
digitized pattern ("steppy appearance") may be seen on echoes located on
the side of a sector image (fig. 5).

Another approach has been proposed by Leavitt et al.[8]. In this case
sampling frequency is the same for all scan lines so that the i_{th} pixels
of all scan lines are disposed along a circle. To place echo data into a
rectangular matrix therefore requires a two dimensional interpolation.
Memory matrix is progressively filled after computing interpolated values
from adjacent pairs of scan lines (fig. 2).

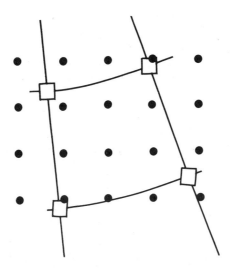

Fig. 2: When sampling frequency is the same for
all scan lines, data samples are disposed
along concentric rings (□).
A two dimensional interpolation must be
performed to fill correctly the display
matrix pixels (●) which are not on the
same horizontal nor vertical lines as
data samples.

This technique is more complicated but gives a better reconstruction
as the sampling procedure is better adapted to echoes which often appear
like small curvilinear segments perpendicular to scan lines (fig. 5).

In these different scan converters, magnification of the displayed image
is predetermined by the sampling frequency and interpolation applied before
memorization.

Taking into account the experience acquired in scan conversion, we have
developed the PIU which includes, in addition, new possibilities by introducing the main controls (gain, magnification) in the post processing field.

DESCRIPTION OF THE PIU (fig. 3)

Scan conversion

Conversion from polar to Cartesian coordinates is an important part of
the processor but, unlike previously described converters, the whole conversion is made after memorization (post conversion).

Echo signals, after logarithmic compression, are digitized with 7 or 8
bits. As the full dynamic range of echoes is about 120 dB, this gives at
least one digital level per dB. Sampling frequency is the same for all scan
lines which are stored in successive columns of the memory.

This memory contains direct data information, which is different from
displayed image. The conversion operator is applied while memory reading,
resulting in a reconstructed image.

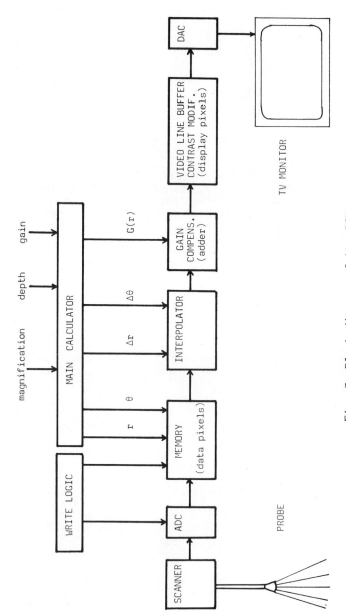

Fig. 3: Block diagram of the PIU

230

Correspondence between a data pixel (r, θ) and an image pixel (x, y) is given by the classical formulae:

$$r = \sqrt{x^2 + y^2}$$

$$\theta = \tan^{-1} (x/y)$$

But post conversion requires a faster computation because image pixel rate is approximately four times higher than data pixel rate.

Interpolation

Each displayed pixel is the result of a two dimensional interpolation between the four nearest surrounding data pixels. A calculator gives addresses of the four data pixels as well as weighting interpolation coefficients. A special circuitry is devoted to interpolation calculation and its "pipe line" structure allows a new image pixel to be delivered every 125 ns, which is necessary to produce a 512 x 512 image.

One important point of PIU is that the main calculator is programmed to give conversion values as well as interpolation weightings as a function of display magnification, data matrix being unchanged. So, any magnification factor may be introduced after memorization and acts even on a frozen image: images of various sizes are always presented with a precise reconstruction which differs from usual "post zooms" where pixels are often duplicated.

Gain correction

Once these operations are accomplished, image pixel values are corrected for depth attenuation.

As pixel value is the logarithmic value of echo amplitude, applying a "gain" results simply in adding to the pixel the logarithmic value of gain (dB). Gain is a function of depth, which is known for each pixel as "r" given by the main calculator.

Resulting values of pixels are stored in a line buffer and displayed at the appropriate time of the next TV line.

Classical "post processing", i.e. contrast modifications, is of course included in the PIU, as well as different smoothing functions.

Applying the PIU to linear scanning

Linear array images can be treated by the PIU as a particular case of sector scanning. Post magnification is also possible for these rectangular images and offers a new interesting feature compared to current digital converters for linear scanning: instead of the few simple magnification factors usually available (x1. ,x1.5,x2.), any factor may be introduced in the PIU. In our prototype, for instance, we can choose sixteen values between x1. and x2..

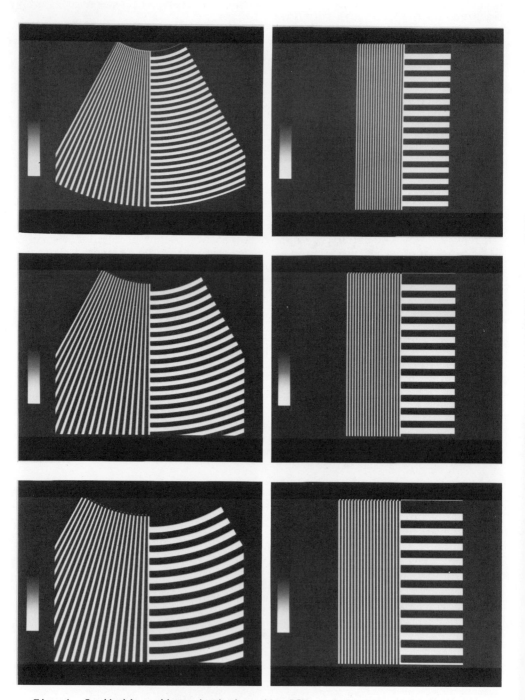

Fig. 4: Synthetic pattern tested on the PIU.
On the left a sector image with different magnifications shows
quality of image conversion with no evidence of digitizing
artifacts.
On the right, the same kind of pattern is applied to linear
scanning with demonstration of magnification by non integer
numbers (x1.16, x1.32).

RESULTS

Test pattern

A synthetic pattern has first been tested. It consists of half an image
with radial lines and half with concentric rings in order to emphasize ability of the processor to correctly map data in any direction. Although this
test is hard because "information" changes abruptly from white to black, the
image shows no evidence of quantization, no steps, neither in the lateral
nor in the azimuthal direction (fig. 4).

Clinical results

Up to now, physicians had to adjust gain and image size before freezing:
post zoom capabilities were limited and usual "post processing" did not
concern fundamental adjustments.

It is possible to get a freeze frame picture here without being worried
about the different settings (real time moving pictures may be understood
without optimization of adjustments). When a picture is frozen and a photograph is to be taken, this optimization can now be done.

Clinical tests were made with the electronic sector scanner using curved
arrays (here a probe with an angle of 60° and a radius of curvature of 60mm)
that we also developed in our laboratory[7].

Illustrations (fig. 6, 7 and 8) give examples of a sequence of post
adjustments:

- first, gain setting is improved -any gain control: slope,near gain,
  general gain;

- then, depth of presented image is chosen and

- finally image is magnified by any factor.

Such possibilities will facilitate sonographers' work, permitting the
best documentation to be obtained from all examinations. It will also lower
examination time: when a frozen image is not good enough, it can be corrected and has not to be re-made in better conditions. It will be an important
feature of ultrasonic instruments for students learning ultrasonography:
it is easier to optimize settings on a still frame.

CONCLUSION

When digital scan converters replaced analog ones for manual B-scanners,
zooming became essentially a "write" procedure (pre processing). This was
still true for real time scanners.

The PIU brings back the "old" function of post zoom which was available
on analog scan converters, and the exact reconstruction with 2D-interpolation
in all magnifications ensures even better results than analog systems.

Introduction of the "post gain" will expand the post processing field
to all important controls of ultrasonic scanners and makes   good use of the
knowledge of the depth corresponding to each memorized pixel.

Last but not least, the relatively simple electronic design with low
power consumption (25 W) makes the PIU an interesting alternative to other
lower performance scan converters.

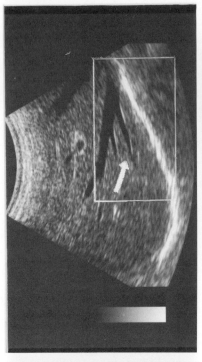
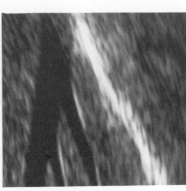
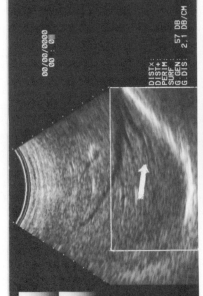
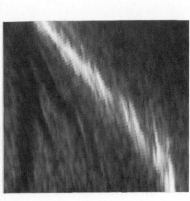

Fig. 5:   Comparison between one dimensional (left) and two dimensional (right) interpolation exhibiting a digitized pattern on oblique lines in the first case, well seen on the enlarged portion.

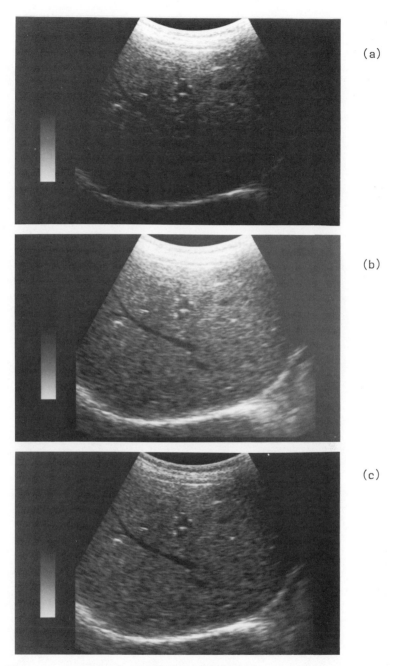

(a)

(b)

(c)

Fig. 6: Action of the "post gain":
the top image (a) has been frozen with
a bad gain compensation curve;
by increasing far gain (b) and reducing
near gain (c) on this same frozen image
a good result is obtained.

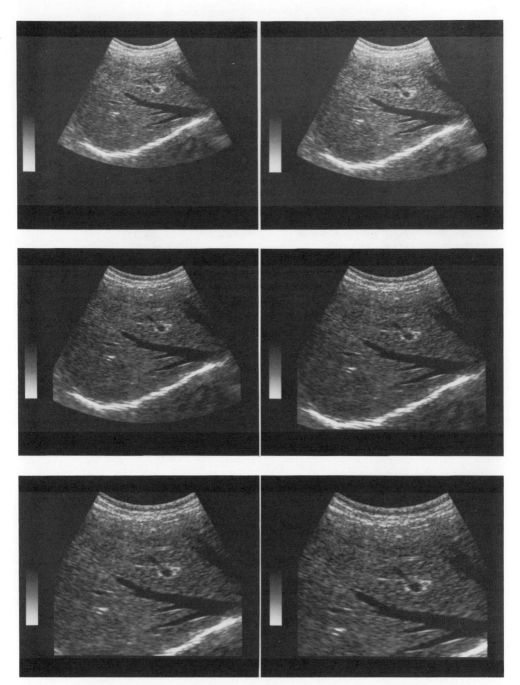

Fig. 7: Example of "post zoom": on a frozen image, any magnification factor
may be applied. The exact reconstruction with 2D interpolation
in all cases avoids image degradation when zooming.

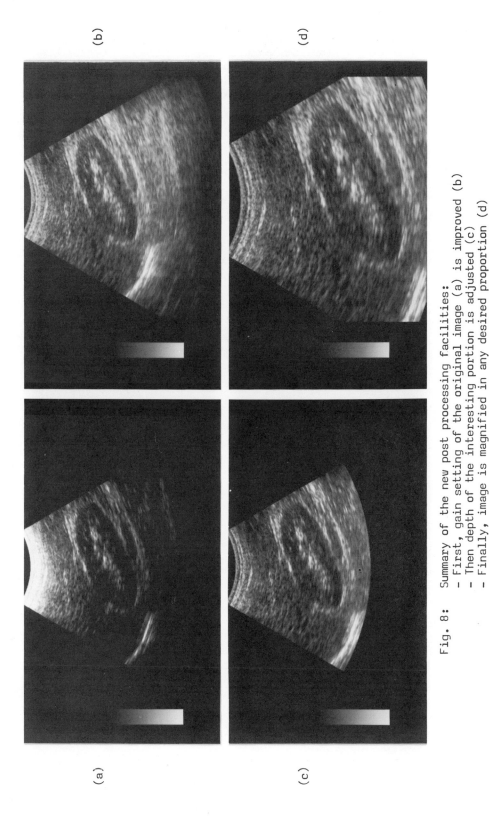

Fig. 8: Summary of the new post processing facilities:
         – First, gain setting of the original image (a) is improved (b)
         – Then depth of the interesting portion is adjusted (c)
         – Finally, image is magnified in any desired proportion (d)

(a)   (b)   (c)   (d)

REFERENCES

1. J. Ophir and N. F. Maklad, "Digital scan converters in diagnostic ultra-sound imaging", Proc. IEEE, 67(4): 654-664, 1979.
2. J. T. Walker, "Digital scan conversion and smoothing for a real time linear array imaging system", in: "Acoustical Imaging", vol.8, 1-14 A. F. Metherell ed., Plenum Press, NY 1980.
3. D. E. Robinson and P. C. Knight, "Interpolation scan conversion in pulse echo ultrasound", Ultrasonic Imaging, 4:297-310, 1982.
4. J. Ophir and J. M. Brinch, "Moiré undersampling artifacts in digital ultrasound images", Ultrasonic Imaging, 4:311-320, 1982.
5. M. H. Lee, J. H. Kim and S. B. Park, "Analysis of a scan conversion algorithm for a real time sector scanner", IEEE Trans. Med. Im., MI-5 (2): 96-105, 1986.
6. R. Lütolf, A. Vieli, M. Kesselring and M. Anliker, "A versatile digital scan converter for high quality imaging", in: "Acoustical Imaging", vol. 14, 671-674, A. J. Berkhout, J. Ridder and L. F. Van Der Wal ed., Plenum Press, NY 1985.
7. B. Richard, J. C. Roucayrol and J. Perrin, "Wide angle electronic sector scanning with curved arrays", in: "Acoustical Imaging", vol. 14, 685-688, A. J. Berkhout, J. Ridder and L. F. Van Der Wal ed., Plenum Press, NY 1985.
8. S. C. Leavitt, B. H. Hunt and H. G. Larsen, "A scan conversion algorithm for displaying ultrasound images", HP Journal, 30-34, oct 1983.

A REAL-TIME IMAGING SYSTEM FOR NON-DESTRUCTIVE EVALUATION

P. Alais*, P. Kummer*, B. Nouailhas** and F. Pons**

* Institut de Mécanique Théorique et Appliquée
  Université Pierre et Marie Curie
  Paris, France

** Direction des Etudes et Recherches
   Electricité de France
   Saint-Denis, France

INTRODUCTION

In non destructive evaluation, most ultrasonic devices operate in the A-echographic mode. Imaging systems are now proposed, which give B or C echograms using ordinary focusing techniques or holography or a synthetic aperture reconstruction technique [1][2][3].

Most of them are slow techniques using the mechanical scanning of a single transducer. Although one may think that in N.D.E. a real-time imaging technique is not required, it appears that for many industrial controls, fast operating may be a very important characteristic of the system.

We have developed such a technique inspired from a medical echographic experience, trying to keep the complexity of the system reasonable. The necessity of launching oblique beams in most cases has led us to use a linear array made of transducers obliquely oriented, which limits the possibilities of the system but reduces considerably the number of transducers. As very large delays are required for focusing obliquely, we have also chosen to focus only at emission, the reception being done through a non focusing relatively small aperture. Several shots are used with different focal lengths to obtain a good lateral resolution over a reasonable depth of field. The ultrasonic information is written in an electronic memory which is read according to an ordinary T.V. scanning, which permits easy storing of the information.

THE LINEAR ARRAY

Different authors have proposed, for N.D.E., arrays very similar to those used in medical applications for making sectorial scanning, usually called "phased arrays" [4][5][6][7][8]. These arrays should permit both sectorial and translational scannings but require a basic pitch for the elementary transducers smaller than the acoustical wavelength in the material.

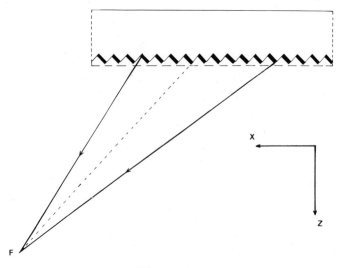

Figure 1

The linear array.

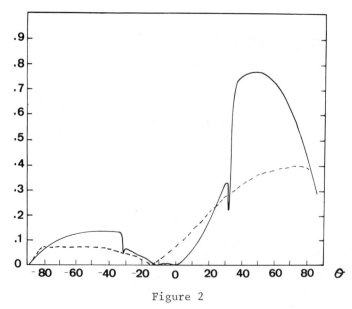

Figure 2

Theoretical directivity in steel of one single elementary transducer.

———— : transverse waves,

----- : longitudinal waves.

Such arrays, with high angular acceptance transducers, are difficult to elaborate and require a correspondingly complex electronic circuitry.

Deliberately choosing simplicity, we have decided to limit our focusing technique to a focused beam of transversal waves at the vicinity of an angle of incidence of 45° in steel, with an angular aperture which should permit reasonable lateral resolutions.

In such accepted conditions, we may use an array of transducers oriented at 45° in a staircase shape (Fig. 1). The acoustical link with steel is ensured by a front plate mouldered from a silica charged epoxy resin, with a longitudinal wave sonic celerity of 3100 m/s, which permits a relatively good conversion of the ultrasonic energy into transverse waves in steel. We have fixed our choice to a pitch along the array equal to 2 mm, i.e. a 128 mm long array of 64 transducers.

This geometry imposes a numerical aperture of nearly 1.4 mm for each transducer, which represents 1.3λ in steel for a mean frequency of 2.9 MHz and a sonic celerity in steel of 3200 m/s.

In a crude model, we may figure the obtained directivity in steel of such a transducer assuming the directivity of a piston-like transducer in the epoxy resin and transmission in steel for plane waves at an interface separating two infinite mediums, i.e. deliberately not taking in account the back and forth complicated reflections in the front plate.

The figure 2 shows the result obtained with this simple model. Of course, using transverse waves at the incidence of 45° is interesting, because most of the related longitudinal waves remain evanescent, but as we use a large angular aperture, some energy is launched into the material with longitudinal waves. We should emphasize that while it is important to keep a sufficient angular acceptance (or emittance) around 45°, it is necessary to reduce at the lowest level the ultrasonic energy launched at normal incidence into the steel because of the enormous specular reflection coming from the bottom of the steel block which is, in most cases, parallel to the face used for exploration.

We may say this from experience : having built a first array working at 2.5 MHz, we have obtained an image blurred by artefacts due to this specular reflection and associated with a quasi-secondary array lobe of longitudinal waves oriented not far from zero incidence. A new array, achieved with a shift of frequency to 2.9 MHz, permitted us to reduce very substantially this phenomenon.

The theoretical directivity shown by the figure 2 has allowed us to predict the lateral resolution obtained from 2-D punctual targets (holes parallel to the interface) while operating the ideal delays on a retained aperture of up to 16 transducers, i.e. 32 mm long, with a mean incidence of 45°.

The figure 3 shows the result obtained at a depth of 27 mm with an aperture of 20 mm (10 transducers).

As for medical arrays, the resolution in the direction normal to the tomographic plane is ensured only by a fixed focusing imposed by the geometry of the array. In our case, we have kept a flat face with a width of 16.6 mm, which leads to a natural Fresnel focusing at a depth of about 35 mm in steel.

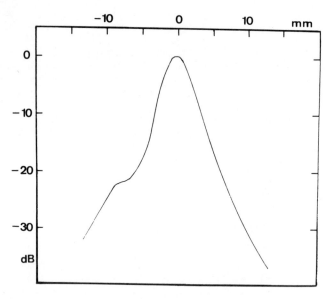

Figure 3

Theoretical lateral resolution obtained at a depth of 27 mm focusing with an aperture of 20 mm.

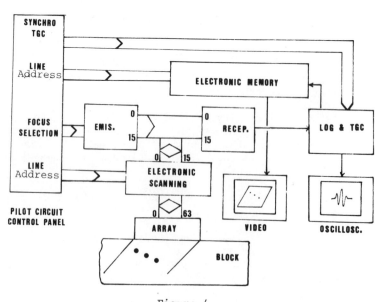

Figure 4

Architecture of the imaging device.

THE SYSTEM ARCHITECTURE

The over-all device is very similar to a medical B echographic system using a linear array : it operates electronically the translation of a focusing aperture made of 16 transducers. The figure 4 shows the adopted architecture.

A substantial difference from a medical device comes from the fact that delays associated with an oblique focused beam are much longer and more difficult to control, so that we have preferred to limit the focusing operation during emission for which delays are easier to achieve. The sixteen emitting pulses are triggered with an accuracy of less than 16 ns, which corresponds to a fraction 1/20 of the mean period of the signal.

In the present device, delay instructions are programmed in a PROM circuit for a mean incidence of 45° in steel (sonic transverse celerity is 3200 m/s), four different depths of focus, with an aperture of 16 transducers centered between two transducers, or centered in the middle of one transducer. These instructions permit us to obtain information from 512 shots contributing to build an image of 128 lines oriented at 45°.

The local information delivered by each shot is stored in an electronic memory of 128×256 pixels of 16 levels (4 bits) after a classical echographic treatment, i.e. a time-gain control of the echographic signal, detection and logarithmic compression. The image is read and delivered with a classical T.V. scanning (Fig. 6).

It should be remarked that there is no electronic focusing at reception. Only the numerical aperture is reduced to optimize the natural Fresnel focusing for the examined depth.

The figure 5 shows results obtained from a steel block with holes observed at different depths. Unhappily, we have been unable to reduce the duration of the noise observed at the interface less than an equivalent depth of 9 mm. This duration is not associated with delays between emitting pulses, because for these depths only one or two transducers may be used, but results most probably from reflections inside the complicate front plate.

CLASSICAL IMAGING VERSUS SYNTHETIC APERTURE TECHNIQUE

The state of the art in electronic circuitry now allows development of a real time imaging technique using synthetic aperture reconstruction algorithms. The mechanical scanning of a single transducer must obviously be replaced by an electronic scanning obtained from a linear (or matricial) array.

While developing our relatively simple ordinary imaging technique, we have tried to evaluate the potential characteristics of a synthetic aperture technique using our array or a similar one.

This evaluation was carried out experimentally with one transducer of the array and a mechanical translation of the array.

Advantages offered by the synthetic aperture reconstruction technique are well known : the lateral resolution is optimized at any depth and should be equivalent to a frequency double the one effectively used. On the other hand, the signal to noise ratio and the level of side lobes of the reconstructed signal may not be very encouraging.

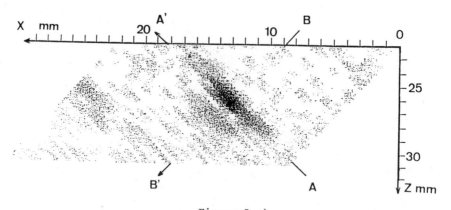

Figure 5-a)

Image of one hole at a depth of 27 mm obtained with a Synthetic Aperture Technique. The grey scale corresponds to a 24 dB dynamic.

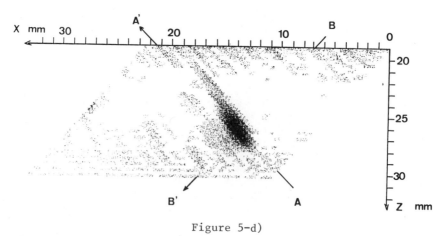

Figure 5-d)

Image of the same hole obtained with the real-time imaging device and delivered with a computer in the same grey scale the fig. 5 -z).

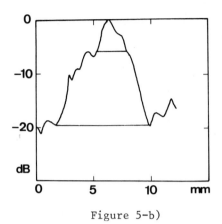

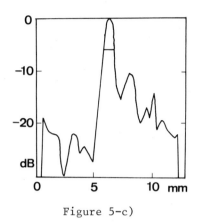

Figure 5-b)   Figure 5-c)

Lateral resolution, Profile A-A'   Logitudinal resolution, Profile B-B'

obtained in the S.A.R. technique (Image Fig. 5-a).

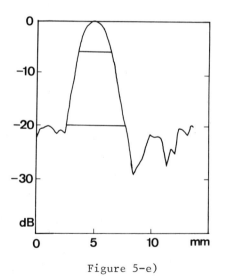

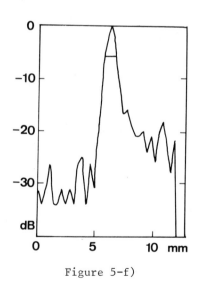

Figure 5-e)   Figure 5-f)

Lateral resolution, Profile A-A'   Longitudinal resolution, Profile B-B'

obtained with our real-time imaging technique.

Our experiment has been carried out with the following parameters :

- the mechanical scanning pitch was equal to 1 mm ;
- the temporal sampling pitch of the signal was 20 ns (50 MHz) ;
- the reconstruction was operated from the stored signals with pixels of 0.25 mm in the z direction (depth) and 0.5 mm in the x direction (scanning). It was carried out for each pixel by superimposing the stored signals adequately translated coming from an angular aperture limited by the acceptance of the used transducer.

The figure 5-a) shows the result obtained from a hole of 0.3 mm at a depth of 27 mm in steel. The figures 5-b) and c) give the corresponding lateral and longitudinal resolution.

To ensure a valid comparison with our classical imaging technique, we have built an image of the same hole with our imager and processed the information through a computer to obtain a grey scale, in the same conditions as in Fig. 5-a).
The figures 5-b), c), e) and f) allow us to compare quantitatively the lateral and longitudinal resolutions in both techniques.

The main result is that while the −6dB lateral resolution is a little better for the synthetic aperture technique, which it should be, the apodisation is better in the classical technique, at least up to −20dB.

Of course, these experiments cannot be used to draw final conclusions in favour or not of the Synthetic Aperture Technique. Our aim is only to emphasize here that operating such a technique in real time, with a limited spatio-temporal sampling, is not necessarily the best thing to do.

FIRST PRACTICAL RESULTS

As mentioned above, we carried out our first experiments with punctual defects, i.e. holes drilled in a steel block, parallel to the face of investigation.

We used a first block with 0.3 mm diameter holes set at different depths up to 70 mm . The figures 6-a) and b) show images obtained from holes set near the surface and deeper.

It may be checked that, for imaging defects at depths less than 10 mm, it is necessary to use another block with flat parallel faces as a delay line.

Our system permits us to visualize on an oscilloscope the temporal echogram of any of the 512 shots used for building the image, i.e. any one of the 128 lines with any of the four focusing depths. This visualization is obtained without stopping the real-time image formation, so that it is very easy to use this information in conjunction with the image, where the selected line appears as a bright line, to study a defect.

The figure 7 shows the typical echogram of one hole, and the figure 8 gives the lateral resolution measured in such a way from different holes at different depths using the same focusing depth around 25 mm . The limits of the −6 dB and −15 dB lateral resolutions have been drawn and show a good depth of field between 15 and 35 mm, so that the total depth is very well covered with only four focusing depths.

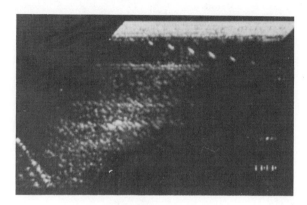

Figure 6-a)

Image of 7 holes located at depths of 10 mm to 30 mm .

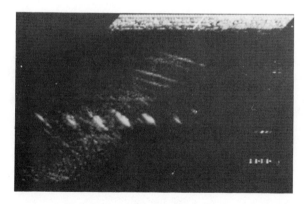

Figure 6-b)

Image of holes drilled at depths of 65 to 70 mm.

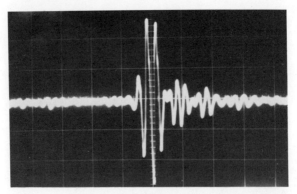

Figure 7

Echographic signal of a hole.

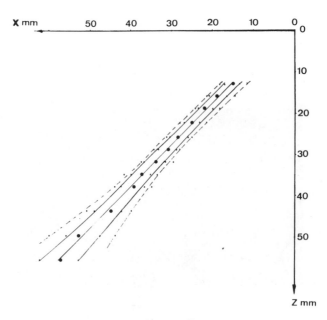

Figure 8

Lateral resolution obtained experimentally
when focusing at a depth of 25 mm.

――― : - 6dB limits,
---- : -15dB limits.

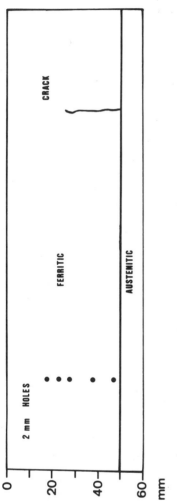

Figure 9-a) : Sketch of the composite austenitic-ferritic block.

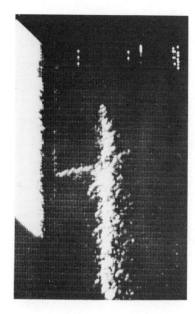

Figure 9-c) : Image of the crack.

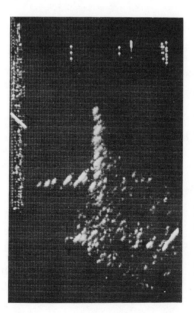

Figure 9-b) : Image of the 5 holes.

A second set of experiments was carried out with another block of ferritic steel coated with austenitic steel, typical of the technology used in nuclear vessels.

In this block, five 2 mm-diameter holes have been drilled, as shown on the figure 9-a).

There is also a fatigue crack located in the ferritic steel from the austenitic-ferritic interface up to a depth which varies between 22 and 25 mm along the width of the block.

We got good images of the five holes (Fig. 9-b) and of the crack (Fig 9-c).

The image of the crack was obtained from the uncladded face and is made of a quasi-continuous succession of bright spots.

Of course, the corner at the junction of the crack and the austenitic-ferritic interface gives a very strong echo.

Although it is possible to evaluate the depth of the crack from the image, we found that it was easy to obtain a better measurement, with an error less than 0.5 mm , using the temporal echograms obtained from the lines that correspond to the ends of the crack.

The artefacts related to the specular reflection of longitudinal waves by the flat bottom of the blocks may be seen more or less on the images but remain at an acceptable level.

On the other hand, a strong echo appears on the figures 9-b) and 9-c) due to the reflection of transverse waves at the rough austenitic-ferritic interface.

CONCLUSION

Results obtained from this imaging device seem competitive in comparison with other techniques. The quality of the image is guaranteed by a lateral resolution which remains nearly as low as 3 mm , at 6 dB for any depth.

The real-time imaging technique appears specially useful to discriminate easily artefacts from echos associated to real defects.

On the other hand, the possibility of visualizing simultaneously the echogram relative to a selected line of the image, permits very accurate measurements and the use of various signal treatments for implementing the analysis of defects.

REFERENCES

1. H. ERMERT, J.O. SCHAEFER, "Flaw Detection and Imaging by High Resolution Synthetic Pulse", Acoustical Imaging, 10, 629-642 (1980).

2. S. BENNETT, D.K. PETERSON, D. CORL, G.S. KINO, "A Real Time Synthetic Aperture Digital Acoustic Imaging System", Acoustical Imaging, 10, 669-692 (1980).

3. V. SCHMITZ, W. MÜLLER, G. SCHÄFER, "Imaging with Holosaft", Acoustical Imaging, 14, 237-245 (1985).

4. J.M. SMITH, "A Practical Linear Array Imaging System for N.D.T. Applications", Acoustical Imaging, 8, 641-650 (1978).

5. R.C. ADDISON, "Multi-element Arrays for N.D.E. Applications", Acoustical Imaging, 11, 505-519 (1981).

6. R.C. ADDISON, K.A. MARSA, J.M. RICHARDSON, C.C. RUCKANGAS, "N.D.E. Imaging with Multi-element Arrays", Acoustical Imaging, 12, 643-663 (1982).

7. P. BARDOUILLET, "Application des systèmes de focalisation et de balayage électronique ultrasonore au Contrôle Non Destructif", Proc. 5th Intern. Conf. on N.D.T. Methods, Bordeaux (1983).

8. A. McNAB, I. STUMPF, "Monolithic Phased Array for the Transmission of Ultrasound in N.D.T. Ultrasonics", Ultrasonics, 24, 148-155 (1986).

IMPLEMENTATION OF A REAL-TIME ULTRASONIC SAFT SYSTEM

FOR INSPECTION OF NUCLEAR REACTOR COMPONENTS[a]

T. E. Hall, S. R. Doctor, L. D. Reid,
R. J. Littlefield, and R. W. Gilbert

Pacific Northwest Laboratory
P. O. Box 999
Richland, WA

ABSTRACT

In recent years, the Pacific Northwest Laboratory has been developing the Synthetic Aperture Focusing Technique for Ultrasonic Testing (SAFT-UT) for the U.S. Nuclear Regulatory Commission (NRC). The program objective has been to develop and validate the SAFT-UT technology for inservice inspection of nuclear power plant components. This technique utilizes the full three-dimensional SAFT algorithm computed in the time domain. The project has included development of a field-usable, real-time SAFT-UT imaging system, and also enhancement of the SAFT-UT algorithm to achieve real-time rates. This paper discusses techniques that have been employed to achieve these goals, including a description of the system, system performance data, and a discussion of a real-time SAFT processor peripheral device for performing the computer-intensive SAFT algorithm computations. An overall view of the SAFT-UT system itself will also be discussed.

INTRODUCTION

In the mid 1970s, the NRC began funding research at the University of Michigan for the investigation and development of SAFT technology for ultrasonic testing. The Synthetic Aperture Focusing Technique (SAFT) had been implemented previously in other areas (such as sonar and radar) and looked promising for ultrasonic applications as well. The NRC perceived the need to develop improved inspection methods for the primary components of nuclear reactors, such as piping and pressure vessels. The University of Michigan performed extensive laboratory research related to developing the algorithm and evaluating methods to expedite the highly computational intensive coherent summation SAFT algorithm (Ganapathy et al, 1985; Busse, Collins, and Doctor, 1984).

In 1982 the project was transferred to PNL as a shift in emphasis occurred in the project. It became important to produce a fieldable system

---

[a]Work supported by the U.S. Nuclear Regulatory Commission under Contract DE-AC06-76RLO 1830; Dr. J. Muscara, NRC Program Monitor.

that would collect, process, and display SAFT-UT information at the reactor site. This effort proved to be an ambitious challenge in a number of ways. The hardware previously utilized included a large VAX 11/780, and obviously, a field system must be reduced in size to allow transportability to the field site. A scanner and data acquisition system needed to be developed to accommodate SAFT inspection in the nuclear reactor environment. The algorithm needed to be accelerated to provide real-time three-dimensional SAFT processing. And finally, graphics software needed to be developed to display the resultant image in a clear and interpretable manner.

The hardware components incorporated in the SAFT-UT field system are commercially available whenever possible. The purpose for this was to improve the final system reliability and facilitate technology transfer to the commercial realm. Also, it allowed internal PNL engineering resources to be focused on developing the SAFT field system algorithm and related software rather than developing uniquely tailored hardware.

The final field system, consisting of three 19-inch racks, is shown in Fig. 1 and may be viewed graphically in the block diagram shown in Fig. 2. The left-most rack in Fig. 1 consists of the data acquisition system that utilizes a Digital Equipment Corporation (DEC) PDP 11/23 for scanner control, pulse synchronization, and controls the signal digitization. A Lecroy digitizer located in a CAMAC crate is used to sample the unprocessed signal at rates up to 32 MHz. The unprocessed ultrasonic data is then transferred in block form to the host processor, a DEC VAX 11/730, located in the center rack. A disk drive and video display are also located in this rack. The host processor receives the data and transports it to the real-time SAFT processor located in the right-most rack. This processor serves as a peripheral to the VAX and accelerates the SAFT processing to achieve real-time operation. The processed resultant data array is transferred to the host computer for subsequent display on the Ramtek graphics monitor.

SAFT-UT THEORETICAL OVERVIEW

"Synthetic aperture focusing" refers to a process in which the focal properties of a large-aperture focused transducer are generated from an orderly series of measurements over a large area using a small-aperture

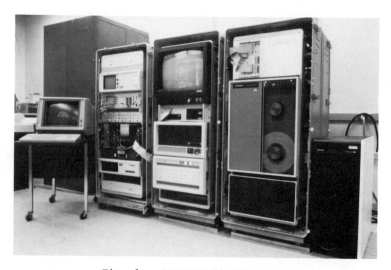

Fig. 1. SAFT-UT field system

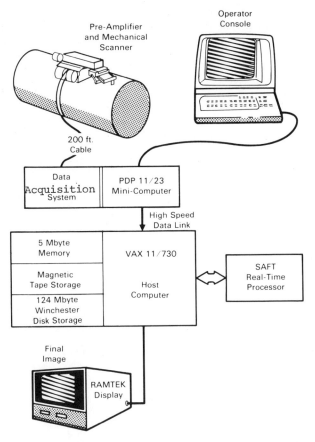

Fig. 2. Block diagram of the SAFT-UT field system hardware

transducer. The processing required to focus this collection of data has been called beam forming, coherent summation, or synthetic aperture processing.

Inherently, SAFT has an advantage over physical focusing techniques in that it provides a full-volume focused characterization of the inspected area; where traditional physical focusing techniques provide focused data only at the depth of focus of the lens. For the typical data collection scheme used with SAFT-UT, a focused transducer is positioned with the focal point located at the surface of the part to be inspected. This configuration is used to produce a broad, divergent ultrasonic beam in the object under test. As the transducer is scanned over the surface of the object, a series of A-scan lines (rf waveforms) are digitally recorded for each position of the transducer. Each reflector produces a collection of echoes in the A-scan records. If the reflector is a single-point reflector, then the collection of echoes will lie on a hyperbolic curve. The shape of the hyperboloid is determined by the depth of the reflector within the test object and the velocity of sound in the material under test. This relationship between echo location in the series of A-scans and the actual location of the reflectors within the test object makes it possible to reconstruct a processed image from the acquired signals.

If the scanning and surface geometries are well known, it is possible to accurately predict the shape of the locus of echoes for each point within the test object. The process of coherent summation involves shifting of the A-scans by a predicted time delay and summing the shifted A-scans. This process may also be viewed as performing a spatial-temporal matched filter operation for each point within the volume to be imaged. Each element is then averaged by the number of points that were summed to produce the final processed value. If the particular location correlates with a locus of A-scan echoes, then all of the values summed will be in phase and produce a high-amplitude result. If the location does not correlate with a locus of predicted echoes, then destructive interference will take place, and the spatial average will result in a low amplitude.

Figure 3 shows a diagram of an aluminum test specimen. Seven flat-bottom holes were placed in the part such that the flat tops are coplanar at an angle of 45° relative to the scanned surface. Assuming a transducer center frequency of 2.25 MHz, the diameter of the holes was 3.5 wave-

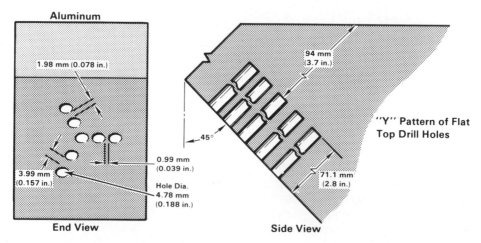

Fig. 3. "Y" pattern resolution block including seven flat bottom holes placed at 45 degrees.

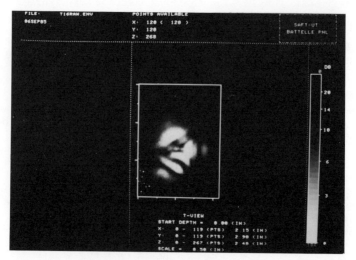

Fig. 4. Unprocessed data collected of "Y" pattern (2.25 MHz, 45 degree shear wave)

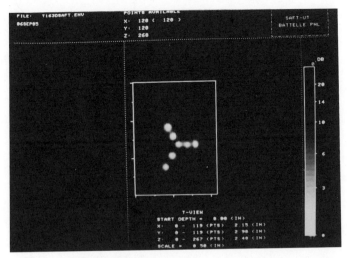

Fig. 5. Three-dimensional full SAFT-UT processed
image of "Y" pattern

lengths, and the edge-to-edge spacing varied from 0.72 wavelengths to 2.9
wavelengths. Figure 4 shows an image of the unprocessed data collected on
this specimen. The scan utilized 2.25-MHz shear-wave illumination with a
0.25-inch-diameter transducer operated in the contact mode. Figure 5
shows the focusing effects of three-dimensional SAFT processing on this
data as each reflector is clearly distinguishable.

The computer reconstruction algorithm consists of a large number of
fetch-and-sum operations. The number of operations for a given inspection
volume is related to the transducer aperture shape, lateral sample
spacing, and temporal sample rate. This varies from test to test; but for
a typical large-volume inspection, there may be as many as 2.8×10^6
summations per cubic inch of material inspected. This number becomes very
significant when considering 300 to 400 cubic inches in an inspection
volume. A major task has been undertaken to increase the computation rate
of the SAFT algorithm through signal processing techniques and through
development of a special-purpose SAFT processor.

SIGNAL PROCESSING METHODS

Selective Processing

Through analysis of the SAFT-UT pulse-echo algorithm, one may acquire
some insights as to how to more efficiently execute the SAFT algorithm
without sacrificing system integrity. If we analyze deep section material
such as echoes that would be expected from pressure vessel material, it is
noted that the data sets generally are much larger than thin section data
sets; and the apertures are much larger due to the divergence of the
ultrasonic cone. One other characteristic of this type of data set is that
the background noise may be less since the return echo is typically well
separated from the large front surface signal. There tends to be a vast
quantity of data points that are very low in intensity. With this in mind,
a method has been devised, in which a selection process is introduced with
respect to signal amplitude, in order to minimize the quantity of off-
center A-scan summations necessary to process the data set. This method
has been termed SAFT-UT selective processing.

When one observes the SAFT algorithm as a hyperbolic matched filter, it can be seen that, for every elementary point object that provides an echo sufficient to be recorded, a hyperboloid is drawn that is weighted in amplitude. It has a high-amplitude center point with the amplitude trailing off in lateral directions. This amplitude weighting is due to the variance of the distance of the transducer to the point reflector, to the attenuation of the material, and to the directivity pattern of the transducer itself. If the tangent plane to the high-amplitude point can be assumed to be very close to perpendicular to the center beam angle, then we should be able to know something about the amplitude distribution around the center point simply by knowing the amplitude of that point.

One can make the previous assumption and then make a very simple observation: if a single center A-scan element in the SAFT algorithm is at the location of the object point, then the amplitude at that center A-scan element will be larger than any of its corresponding off-center A-scans in the hyperboloid. And conversely, the observation can be stated that if the given center A-scan element is not at the location of the object point, then its amplitude will be much less than the element that is at the

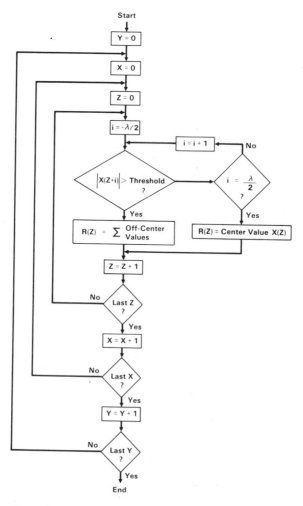

Fig. 6.   Flow chart of SAFT-UT selective processing

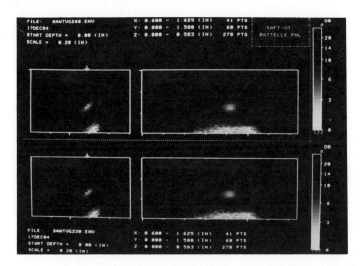

Fig. 7. Comparison view of SAFT-UT images of semi-circular
         notch in stainless steel coupon showing effects of
         SAFT-UT selective processing. Upper image was pro-
         cessed with no selective processing, while the lower
         image implemented -20 dB selective processing.

location of the object. So SAFT-UT selective processing makes the
assumption that, within the SAFT summation iteration loop, if the
amplitude of the center A-scan value is very low, then it is not at an
object location and there is not a need to sum the off-center values to
obtain its final value. Rather, if the point has this condition, then its
own amplitude is retained for the final result since it is assumed the off-
center values will not contribute.

Figure 6 shows a flow chart of the logic of SAFT-UT selective
processing. For each element in the center A-scan, its amplitude is
determined by observing a window of adjacent points one wavelength in
width. This value is then compared with a preselected noise level. If the
value is greater than the level, then all off-center A-scans are summed to
form the result. If the value is less than the level, then the algorithm
does not sum off-center values, but places the element's value in the
resultant array. In this manner no data values are discarded, but rather
off-center A-scans that do not significantly contribute to the result are
not summed.

A comparison presentation may be viewed in Fig. 7. This photograph
shows two images (B-scan side view and B-scan end view) of the same data
file. The data was collected utilizing a 2.25-MHz, 45° shear-wave, single
transducer (pulse-echo) configuration on a 0.585-inch-thick stainless
steel specimen. A semi-circular notch was introduced into the far surface
of the test coupon with a penetration of 0.3 inches and a lateral extent of
0.6 inches. One may easily see the tip-diffracted signal and the strong
corner reflection located at the far surface of the part. The top image in
Fig. 7 shows the results of full SAFT processing with no selective
processing implemented. The lower image shows the results with a -20 dB
selective processing threshold selected. One can see immediately in this
typical example that there is no image information lost when implementing
this technique on this data file. Significant processing speed improvements are realized when implementing this feature, particularly in thick
sections. Computation rate increases by as much as a factor of 40 have been

observed. However, the user may elect not to employ this technique, simply by selecting a very low threshold level. Specifically, if very low-level reflectors in the noise region are of interest in the image, then the operator would not elect to implement this technique.

Envelope Detection of Processed Data

Following the summation sequence in the SAFT processing algorithm, the amplitude of the resultant signal needs to be calculated prior to graphic presentation. This has normally been termed as demodulation or envelope detection, since the result of this is effectively the low-frequency envelope component of the output of the coherent summation algorithm. Traditionally this has been performed by generating a complimentary data set that is identical in amplitude, but shifted in phase by 90°. If F(wt) is the data set result of the processing as follows:

$$F(wt) = A(t) \sin (wt) \tag{1}$$

and, since a 90° phase shift of a cosine function generates a sine function, and the square of a cosine function added to the square of the sine function is unity, then the complete amplitude description may be extracted by summing the squares of the two data bases:

$$A^2(t) = [A(t) \sin(wt)]^2 + [A(t) \cos(wt)]^2 \tag{2}$$

The complimentary phase-shifted data set is generated by performing the Hilbert transform on the unshifted data set. The Hilbert transform has been well described by Bracewell (1978). In the time domain, the Hilbert transform is defined as the convolution of the original signal with the kernal -1/(pi*t) or

$$V_{HIL}(t) = \frac{1}{\pi} \int \frac{v(t')}{(t'-t)} \, dt \tag{3}$$

In the frequency domain the Hilbert transform can be expressed as a multiplicative filter where positive frequency components are multiplied by +i and negative frequency components are multiplied by -i. The Hilbert transform is equivalent to an all-pass filter where the amplitudes of spectral components are left unchanged, but their phases are altered by 90°. The mathematical representation of this filter is [i sgn(w)]. In effect then,

$$V_{HIL}(t) = e(t) \sin(wt+90) = e(t) \cos(wt) \tag{4}$$

where we have phase shifted the carrier by 90°, which is exactly what is desired to produce the complement data set previously described.

This envelope detection (demodulation) algorithm can be explained clearly in a flow diagram as shown in Fig. 8. The data set produced by the SAFT coherent summation algorithm is operated on by the Hilbert transform, then squared, summed with the square of the original, and then a square root is performed. The result is the low-frequency data set consisting of amplitude information only.

A drawback with the Hilbert transform approach is the amount of computational effort necessary to extract this amplitude information. In the interest of developing a field-usable SAFT-UT system without adding additional hardware components (such as an array processor), a simpler alternate envelope detection scheme was developed.

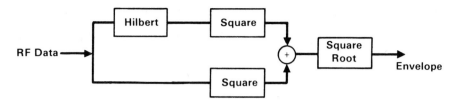

Fig. 8. Block diagram of Hilbert transform algorithm

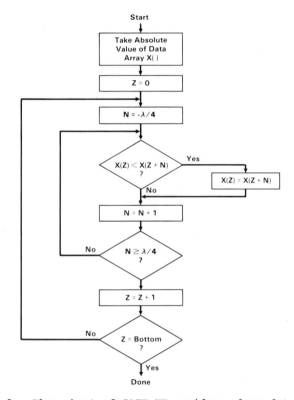

Fig. 9. Flow chart of SAFT-UT rapid envelope detection

The SAFT alternative envelope detection algorithm assumes that the peak value in the vicinity of a given data point is equivalent to the instantaneous amplitude at that time. This can be thought of as a form of a digital sliding window method for extracting amplitude information.

Figure 9 shows a flow diagram of the developed algorithm. This diagram shows the operation that occurs on each processed A-scan produced by the coherent summation SAFT algorithm. The sign of each resultant data element is first discarded. Then for each depth (z) of the A-scan, a vicinity region, defined as half a wavelength in width, is searched. The largest value in this vicinity is then assumed to be the amplitude of the signal at that depth. The effect of this technique is simply to "fill in the valleys" of the rf signal supplied by the SAFT algorithm.

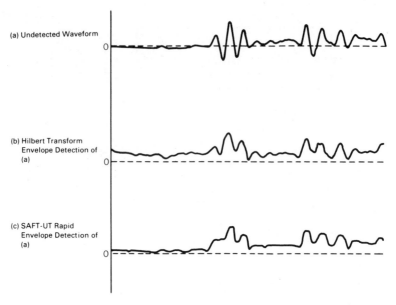

(a) Undetected Waveform

(b) Hilbert Transform
Envelope Detection of
(a)

(c) SAFT-UT Rapid
Envelope Detection of
(a)

Fig. 10.   Comparison of envelope detection techniques

Figure 10 graphically shows the envelope detection process. The top waveform is a typical processed A-scan that is the output of the SAFT processing.   The high frequencies (2.25-MHz center frequency) in this waveform are retained. The second waveform in this figure is the result of performing the Hilbert transform algorithm on this A-scan, and the final waveform is the result of performing the rapid envelope detection scheme.

Intuitively, the accuracy of this technique increases as the temporal increment, dz, goes to zero. A flattening effect occurs as the rf sampling becomes coarse relative to the wavelength of the return echo. This occurs because the accuracy is dependent on the maximum amplitude of the waveform being present in the time domain.   Happily though, the results of this technique have proved to be favorable and have been used extensively.

Sampling Adjustments in Processed Data

The result of the envelope detection operation is a slow varying demodulated function relative to the original rf data set.   The requirements, therefore, on the temporal sampling are somewhat relaxed and one would expect that fewer data points are necessary to accurately describe the envelope detected signal.   It is important to be sure these requirements are understood in order that an adjustment in data set size may be made to ensure that unneeded data handling is not being performed.

The resulting demodulated pulse shape can be associated directly to the system bandwidth (Skilling, 1957) as follows:

$$v(t) = 2 g_ow \left(\frac{\sin(wt)}{wt} \right) \tag{5}$$

where g_o is the linear gain of the system and w is half the bandwidth expressed in radians.   This assumes the system has a perfect bandpass response with constant gain throughout the bandwidth and zero response outside of the bandwidth.

262

The process of demodulation can be described simply in the frequency domain: the spectral response is shifted such that the center frequency is at zero. Thus the highest frequency contained in the demodulated signal is equal to half the bandwidth of the system. If the system has a bandwidth of w_O, then we know that the highest frequency component of the demodulated signal is $w_O/2$.

If it can be assumed that the original data was sufficiently sampled, then it can now be determined what the relative data sampling of the demodulated signal should be. If the system has a bandwidth of 100% [this is a worst-case number; usually SAFT systems have a bandwidth of about 50% (Busse, Collins, and Doctor, 1984, p. 33)], then the maximum component in the demodulated signal is one third the maximum component of the rf signal. The sampling in the output file needs only be one third of that of the input rf data file. This is a significant result in that the output file can now be tailored to satisfy its frequency content with no information loss and yet the data set, which the graphics module must subsequently manipulate, has become significantly smaller.

REAL-TIME SAFT PROCESSOR

A significant level of effort has been directed toward improving the SAFT computation time. It was at one time common to experience CPU time, during SAFT processing, of 30 hours on a DEC VAX 11/780 for a single large data file (327 cubic inches in carbon steel). In order to present SAFT-UT as a viable tool for inservice inspection, it was determined that the processing efficiency had to be significantly improved. A target processing speed of 10 A-scans/sec (or an elapsed processing time of 5 minutes for the above sample) was set as the goal. This was determined as the rate at which real-time would be achieved. The goal was to process and display the SAFT-UT image as fast as the data acquisition system collected the ultrasonic waveforms. This would give the operator nearly instant feedback concerning the inspection area during the actual scanning operation.

Initially a search was performed to locate a device that would accelerate the SAFT computations such as an array processor. A cost-effective unit was not located. It was then decided to design a peripheral device in-house that would serve as the accelerator mechanism or real-time SAFT processor.

The final design of the real-time SAFT processor is shown in general terms in Fig. 11. As with the design of the complete field system, the components implemented are commercially available wherever possible. The real-time SAFT processor serves as a peripheral to the VAX host computer and communicates via a high-speed 16-bit parallel interface. The processor is configured to achieve the rapid computation rates by utilizing parallel processing techniques. A Motorola VME bus system was chosen with multiple 68000-family single-board computer cards. One of the CPU elements is designated as the processor executive and as such communicates with the host computer and supervises the computations performed by the "slave" CPU cards on the VME bus. The data is transferred to the processor plane-by-plane and is then distributed to each slave CPU on the bus. Each slave performs a partial summation of the overall coherent summation algorithm and upon completion returns the result to a global memory. The executive CPU then performs the final summation and envelope detection operation, and transmits the resulting image plane to the host.

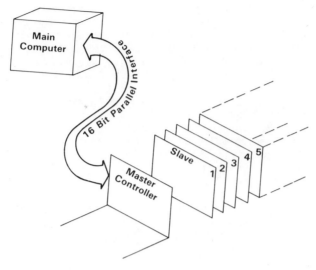

Fig. 11. Generalized block diagram of SAFT-UT real-time processor

The current configuration implemented uses two 68000 CPU cards for the slave processors. This provides a performance improvement such that rates equivalent to   VAX 11/780 rates are achievable in the field system even though a much slower host computer (VAX 11/730) is used for this portable system. This acceleration, in addition to the previously described signal processing techniques, allows for real-time operation in thin materials (up to 1.0 inch). Addition of more slave cards will increase the parallel performance and should significantly improve the expected throughput.

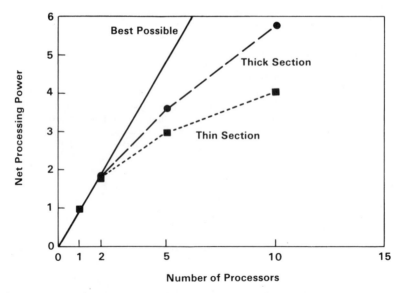

Fig. 12. Estimated real-time SAFT processor performance as a function of the number of slave processors

264

Figure 12 indicates the expected performance curves due to the number of slave cards. Ideally, if there is no executive overhead involved, there would be a linear relationship as indicated by the straight line. The thicker material case (larger aperture size) experiences the more favorable improvement from adding slave processors because more relative time is spent performing parallel operations in the slave cards. The percentage of overhead time, time spent computing by the executive only, is thus reduced.

Another method of improving the real-time SAFT processor performance is to implement faster slave CPU cards. With the rapid expansion of today's computer industry, this has become realizable. Implementation of the 68020 CPU is expected to increase the computation rate by a factor of 2.5.

Tables 1 and 2 show the performance improvements achieved by implementing various methods. These tables indicate the evolution of performance during the development process of the SAFT-UT field system. The values are given in elapsed time in minutes and A-scans per second. There are two cases presented here. The first case is representative of thin material (piping). This is a data file collected on 1.25-inch-thick stainless steel material at 2.25 MHz with shear-wave illumination. The second case was collected in thick-section material with a sampling gate from 4.0 to 11.3 inches in the specimen. This material was carbon steel and was scanned with a 2.25-MHz transducer with 45° shear illumination. The performance goal of the real-time SAFT processor is 10 A-scans per second as previously described. Table 1 shows that the thin-section processing time with a full complement of slave processors (10) will easily achieve this target, and processing data acquired from the thicker material will also achieve real-time speeds.

Table 1. SAFT-UT Speed Performance of Data Collected on a
1.25-inch-thick Stainless Steel Pipe Section

	Elapsed Processing Time (min)	A-Scans/ Sec.
VAX 11/780 Full Processing	6.0	6.9
VAX 11/780 -20 dB Selective Processing	5.2	7.9
Current Real-Time SAFT Processing Implementation	11.2	3.72
Projected Configuration Real-Time SAFT Processor	1.8*	23*

*estimated value

Table 2. SAFT-UT Speed Performance of Data Collected on a
10-inch-thick Carbon Steel Block

	Elapsed Processing Time (min)	A-Scans/ Sec.
VAX 11/780 Full Processing	134	0.39
VAX 11/780 -20 dB Selective Processing	44	1.2
Current Real-Time SAFT Processing Implementation	25*	2.1*
Projected Configuration Real-Time SAFT Processor	5*	10.2*

*estimated value

SUMMARY

Successful development of a field-viable SAFT-UT inspection system
has been dependent on implementation of signal processing techniques and
acceleration hardware that facilitate real-time operation. This gives the
operator the nearly instant feedback necessary to make defect detection
and sizing judgments at the reactor site utilizing an automated system.
With the full complement of slave processors implemented in the dedicated
processor, these real-time SAFT processing speeds are achievable.

REFERENCES

Bracewell, R. N., "The Fourier Transform and Its Application," Academic
    Press (1978).
Busse, L. J., H. D. Collins, and S. R. Doctor, Review and Discussion of the
    Development of SAFT-UT, U.S. Nuclear Regulatory Commission Report
    NUREG/CR-3625 (1984).
Doctor, S. R., L. J. Busse, S. L. Crawford, T. E. Hall, R. P. Gribble, A.
    J. Baldwin, and L. P. Van Houten, Development and Validation of a
    Real-Time SAFT-UT System for the Inspection of Light Water Reactor
    Components, U.S. Nuclear Regulatory Commission Report NUREG/CR-4583,
    Semi-annual Report April-September 1984.
Ganapathy, S., B. Schmult, W. S. Wu, T. G. Dennehy, N. Moayeri, and P.
    Kelly, Design and Development of a Special Purpose SAFT System for
    Nondestructive Evaluation of Nuclear Reactor Vessels and Piping
    Components, U.S. Nuclear Regulatory Commission Report NUREG/CR-4365
    (1985).
Green, A. J., The Interpretation of B-Scan Images, Central Electricity
    Generating Board, Technology Planning and Research Division, Berkeley
    Nuclear Laboratories, Report No. TPRD/B/0167/R82 (1982).
Skilling, H. H., "Electrical Engineering Circuits," John Wiley and Sons
    (1957).

266

FLAW IDENTIFICATION IN ALOK IMAGING SYSTEMS

Yu Wei and Xing-quen Zhao

Department of Biomedical Engineering
Nanjing Institute of Technology
Nanjing, China

ABSTRACT

In this paper the theoretical study and experimental work to improve
the ability of flaw identification in an ALOK imaging system are presented.
After flaws have reliably been detected by TTLC method, the migration imaging
can be executed with lesser computation time only for a determined small
space. Then two methods, ALC method and instantaneous phase correlations,
are introduced to decide the features of pattern recognition. The experimental results of two kinds of artificial defects, holes and cracks, show that
the improvement on flaw identification has been obtained.

INTRODUCTION

In recent years many ultrasonic imaging systems used for NDT have been
developed quickly. The ALOK imaging method proposed by Barbian et al.[1,2,3]
is one of the most useful methods and can easily be put into practice. ALOK
which is Amplitude-Laufzeit Orts Kurven in German, means amplitude-transit
time locus curves.

An ultrasonic imaging system with the ALOK imaging method has been developed in our institute, including hardware and software. The theoretical
study and experimental work are made and it has been demonstrated that this
imaging system has at least two obvious advantages: Firstly, the signal to
noise ratio may be enhanced, so that the flaw detection is more reliable.
Furthermore, it can provide the exact positions of flaws on line.On the other
hand it has also been found that the ALOK imaging system has difficulties
in flaw identification and display of defect details. However, both these
requirements are very important for the failure prediction of tested objects.

In order to improve the ability of flaw identification in the ALOK imaging system, some possibilities of combining other ultrasonic testing methods with the ALOK imaging method are investigated, for example, the migration imaging method, the utilization of the amplitude locus curves (ALC)
and in particular using the instantaneous phase correlations for pattern
recognition, other than amplitude spectrum analysis as usual. Since the application of these methods is realized in the case that the noise of received signals has been removed successfully by transit time locus curves(TTLC)
and the range in which defects exist is already restricted to a small space,
some new aspects are presented.

In this paper, in the first place, an ALOK imaging system is described and the experimental results of flaw detection are shown, and then the theoretical study based on the application of ray method in elastic solids[4] and experimental work to improve the ability of flaw identification in an ALOK imaging system are presented. The experimental results of two kinds of artificial defects, holes and cracks, show that the improvement on flaw identification has been obtained.

ALOK IMAGING SYSTEM AND FLAW DETECTION

Fig.1 shows the frame of an ALOK imaging system set up in our institute. It consists of an ultrasonic pulse generator, a receiver with a time gate, a high speed A/D set of the sampling frequency 1 MHz - 32 MHz in six stages, and an interface connected with a microcomputer. A wedge transducer (or two for tandem technique) controlled by a microcomputer moves along the surface of a metal block being tested. The centre frequency of transducer set at 5 MHz or 2.5 MHz, while it moves, the ultrasonic pulses are transmitted and the echoes are received at different positions in the same stepping interval. The echo amplitude, the transit time and the corresponding coordinate of the wedge transducer are recorded respectively and stored in computer memory in the form of trinity.

The program diagram of the ALOK imaging system is shown in Fig.2. The following steps should be implemented:
1. Setting the threshold of the echo amplitude
2. Determination of the echo peaks by i-k value method or Hilbert transform
3. Noise elimination by TTLC
4. Curve polynomial fitting
5. Triangular of arc reconstruction
6. B - type or C - type display.

The most important step is noise elimination. For a fixed reflecting point in a tested object the locus curve of transit time (t) to position of transducer (x) is hyperbolae. We can write as follows:

$$(\frac{c\,t}{2})^2 - x^2 = h^2 \tag{1}$$

In above equation, c is the sound velocity, h is the depth of the reflecting point from the surface of the metal block.

Based on above equation, a movable filter frame runs through the recorded data of t-x and automatically seeks. The points on the t-x curves, which are in accordance with the hyperbolic rule will remain, and the rest points are treated as noise and will be eliminated. The choice of the filter frame width is a key to ensure the noise elimination in a correct form. The width of filter frame is dependant not only on the properties of transducer, but also on the characters of flaws. Therefore, at executing the iterative reconstruction, the results of identification of flaws by pattern recognition, which will be described in the next sections, should be fed back in order to choose the suitable type of filter frame which has been stored in computer memory already. Since the step of eliminating noise is included in signal processing, not only can the signal to noise ratio be enhanced but the setting of the threshold is not critical as well. The threshold can be chosen lower, so that the lack of flaw detection can be avoided and reliable detection of defects may be ensured. At right of Fig.3, B - type image of two artifitial defects, two holes and cracks, are illustrated.

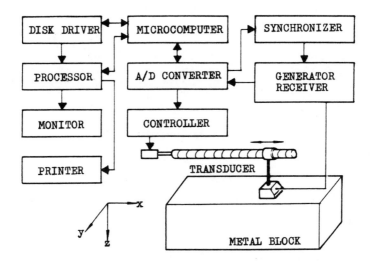

Fig.1. A hardware frame of ALOK imaging system

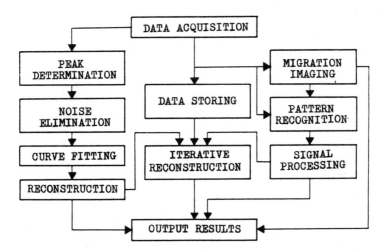

Fig.2. A program diagram of ALOK imaging system

For comparing, the original sizes of both defects are also shown by the line of the same figure. The crosses of short lines point out the existing range of cracks. The experimental results demonstrate that the exact positoins of flaws may be given by ALOK system.

MIGRATION IMAGING

Wave migration imaging has widely been applied to geophysics[5], and can also be used in radar, sonar, medical diagnosis and material NDT with almost similar principle but different names, such as the synthetic aperture technique, the Sommerfeld holography, the multifrequency holography etc..

Generally the migration imaging includes three steps:

Phase reconstruction. In the case of a monochromatic source operating at one or multifrequency, the phase and the amplitude can be recorded simultaneously by using a suitable phase meter. If the pulse signal is used, the recorded echo E(t) can be given as follows:

$$E(t) = A(t) \exp[j\phi(t)] \tag{2}$$

In this case we can only get the amplitude sequence E(t) as a function of time. It is necessary to reconstruct a phase function $\phi(t)$ from E(t). One way to implement the phase reconstruction is to utilize the Hilbert transform:

$$E^*(\tau) = \frac{1}{\pi} \int_{-\infty}^{\infty} \frac{E(t)}{\tau - t} \, dt \tag{3}$$

to execute the Hilbert transform by computer, its discrete form is used:

$$E^*(t) = \frac{2}{\pi} \sum_{n=-\infty}^{\infty} f(t - n \cdot \Delta t) \frac{\text{Sin}^2(n \cdot \pi / 2)}{n} \qquad n \neq 0 \tag{4}$$

The value of singularity at the original point will be set to zero.

Wave migration. Usually the second Rayleich-Sommerfeld equation may be used for the wave migration in frequency domain. For the scalar wave migration we get:

$$P(x, y, z_i, \omega) = \frac{1}{2\pi} \iint_{S_1} P(x_1, y_1, z_{i+1}, w) \frac{1 + jkr}{r^2} \text{Cos}(\vec{n}, \vec{r}) e^{-jkr} \, ds_1$$

$$r = [(x - x_1)^2 + (y - y_1)^2 + (z_{i+1} - z_i)^2]^{\frac{1}{2}} \tag{5}$$

The wave propagates from the plane $(x_1, y_1, z = z_{i+1})$ to the aperture plane $(x, y, z = z_i)$. Using the measured field crossing the aperture, the wave extrapolation from the surface of testing objects towards the range near the flaws is a backpropagation. Following the concept of matching filter or the least square approximation, Eq.(5) can be rewritten to get the formula for backpropagation:

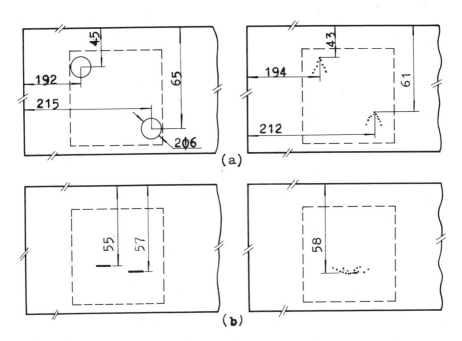

Fig.3. Defects (left) and their B-type images
by ALOK method (right)
(a) holes, (b) cracks
(real dimension within dashed line frame)

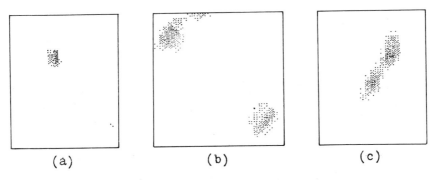

(a)   (b)   (c)

Fig.4. B-type images by superposition of diffraction
(a) a hole, (b) two holes, (c) cracks

$$P(x_1, y_1, z_{i+1}, \omega) = \frac{\Delta z}{2\pi} \iint P(x,y,z_i,\omega) \frac{1-jkr}{r^3} e^{jkr} \, ds$$

$$\Delta z = z_{i+1} - z_i \tag{6}$$

For the case of pulse echo signals, using the wave migration in the time domain, that is a superposition of the diffracted field, is more convenient. If the approximations of single scattering and the point scatter model are introduced, we find

$$A(x_1, z_1) = \int_{Xmin}^{Xmax} \int_{-\infty}^{\infty} [A(t,x) * W(t)] \, \delta \, (t - t_a) \, dx \, dt \tag{7}$$

Here δ is Dirac delta function, t_a is the corresponding transit time determined by TTLC. $W(t)$ is a convolution function concerned with properties of transducer and receiver. Some experimental results are shown in Fig. 4. Usually the computational time is too long, if the imaging range is the whole body of the tested object and a reasonable resolution is needed. In our case, the problem can be solved, because before executing the wave migration the imaging range may be restricted to a determined small range by the ALOK imaging method. The computational time can be saved obviously, so that a on-line display of the outline of flaws is possible with the specific hardware

In the above process of wave migration the noise was ignored and the scalar wave propagation was supposed. This procedure is also called inverse of diffration.

Inverse scattering. In this step the scatters would be given from the wave field near them. This is a difficult problem, because in essence the ill-posed problem is always existing. Without prior knowledge, the inverse scattering could not be implemented. Various methods have been proposed[6], but none of general methods has been obtained and no clear conclusions have been drawn. In different cases the corresponding method should be suitable.

In our case, the application of the echo amplitude and signal processing as mentioned in the next section may give the prior knowledge, then the pattern recognition can be combined with an inverse process.

PATTERN RECOGNITION

Pattern recognition seems a good way for resolving the inverse problem of scattering. The essential difficulties are which features should be chosen as the identification objects of pattern recognition. The amplitude spectrum analysis for specific artificial flaws has been studied[7], but there are still many further works which we must do until this method can be put into the QNDT practices. Here, two other methods to decide the features of pattern recognition are introduced.

One method is the application of ALC. As well known, the echo amplitude is easily affected by many factors, such as the properties of transducers, the transfer function of receiver system, contacting condition of transducers at the surface of tested metal etc. For this reason the ALC can not be found in a similar way as TTLC. Using the relation of the trinity in the computer memory, the ALC may be found out by means of the TTLC. Such amplitude locus curves carry the characteristic information which can further be treated with different processing methods[8].

If flaws are carried into a space of an isotropic, homogenous, linear elastic solid, the total displacement field may be expressed as follows:

$$u_t = u_i + u_s \tag{8}$$

where u_i is the incident wave, and u_s is the scattered wave. According to the ray theory, the total wave field may also be represented in the form:

$$u_t = u_{ge} + u_d = u_i + u_{rr} + u_{rf} + u_d \tag{9}$$

Here u_{ge} and u_d are the geometrical elastodynamic field and the diffracted field respectively. u_{ge} consists of the incident wave u_i, reflection wave u_{rf} and refraction wave u_{rr}. The correction introduced by the diffracted field to the geometrical elastodynamic field is proportional to the dimension of $(ka)^{-\frac{1}{2}}$. It means that for a sufficiently large frequency the diffraction wave may be ignored, i.e. the scattering phenomenon can be entirely dominated by geometrical elastodynamics. This is the case for backscattering from smoothly curved surfaces of holes with radii very large as compared to the wavelength. On the other hand, for crack-like flaws which have sharp edges, the effect of edge diffraction may be quite pronounced. This is the essential difference between the scattering from holes or cracks. Edge diffraction is particularly relevant to backscattering, because the echo signals come from the discontinuous boundary of the shadow zone and the bundles of reflected rays which are given by geometrical elastodynamic approximation. The diffraction coefficients for the canonical problems have been calculated by the geometrical theory of diffraction (GTD).

Based on above statement, we can determine the echo peak amplitude dependence on the incline angle of incident ray (see Fig.5) in the normalized form:

$$A_n(\partial) = F_1(\partial)F_2(\partial)[F_3(\partial) + F_4(\partial)] \tag{10}$$

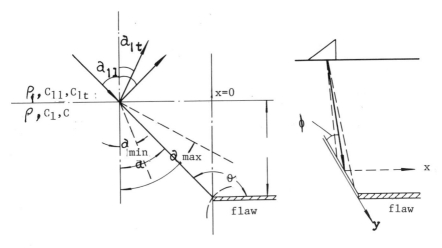

Fig.5. Ray path and interfaces

Using $x = h \cdot tg\,\partial$, the function $A_n(\partial)$ may be changed to a function of the position of wedge transducer x. The length of the receiving aperture can approximately be given by the maximun and the minimum impinging angles:

$$\Delta x = h(tg\partial_{max} - tg\partial_{min}) \tag{11}$$

In Eq.10 $F_1(\partial)$ represented the direction diagram of transducers is measurable. $F_2(\partial)$ describes the transmitting coefficient crossing the surface between the wedge transducer and the tested metal block. In case where the incline angle of the incident wave is greater than the critical angle of the longitudinal wave, the longitudinal wave will be converted into a TV transverse wave which only transmits and propagates in the metal block. $F_2(\partial)$ may be expressed in the form[9]:

$$F_2(\partial) = \frac{c^2_{11}\, c_1\, \cos^3(2\partial_{1t})\, \cos\partial}{c^2_{1t}\, c\, \sin(2\partial_{11})\, \sin(2\partial_1)\, N_1 N_2}$$

$$N_1 = 2Ctg\partial_{1t} + \frac{c_{11}\cos^2(2\partial_{1t})}{2c_{1t}\cos\partial_{11}} + \frac{2\rho c^4 Ctg\partial}{\rho_1 c_{1t}^4} + \frac{\rho\, c_{11} c^3\, \cos^2(2\partial)}{2\rho c_{1t}^4\, \cos\partial_{11}} \tag{12}$$

Here ρ_1, c_{11} and c_{1t} are the density, velocities of longitudinal and transverse waves respectively in the medium of a wedge transducer, ρ, c_1 and c are the corresponding parameters for metal block. N_2 has same expression as N_1 with exchanging indices. It simplifies the notation to omit all indices t concerning the TV transverse wave in the metal block. The relations between ∂_{11}, ∂_{1t}, ∂ and ∂_1 are determined by Snell's law.

$F_3(\partial)$ related the wave couple is determined by conditions on the boundaries of flaws. It is only concerned with the geometrical elastodynamics. Suppose the boundary condition of zero surface tractions; a plane incident wave which impinging the surface of flaws will generate reflection waves. Function $F_3(\partial)$ may be written as follows[4]:

$$F_3(\partial) = \frac{c^2\, \sin(2\Theta_1)\, \sin(2\Theta) - c_1^2\, \cos^2(2\Theta)}{c^2\, \sin(2\Theta_1)\, \sin(2\Theta) + c_1^2\, \cos^2(2\Theta)} \tag{13}$$

For holes, $\Theta \doteq 90°$, $\Theta_1 = 0$, $F_3(\partial) = 1$, for horizontal cracks along the direction x, $\Theta = 90° + \partial$, the Θ_1 is defined by $c^2\cos\Theta_1 = c_1^2\cos\Theta$.

$F_4(\partial)$ is introduced for considering the diffraction wave depending upon the impinging angles. It is complicated to calculate the exact value of $F_4(\partial)$. Here the approximate estimation of function $F_4(\partial)$ is implemented by considering only the amplitude of the first diffracted wave[10]. For the far field we find

$$F_4(\partial) = \frac{D(2kh\,\cos^2\Theta/\cos\partial)}{(8\pi\, kh/\cos\partial)^{\frac{1}{2}}\, \cos\Theta} \tag{14}$$

Here function D(x) is the corrected Fresnel integral:

$$D(x) = 2jx^{\frac{1}{2}}\, e^{jx} \int_{x^{\frac{1}{2}}}^{\infty} e^{-jt^2}\, dt \tag{15}$$

274

Comparision of the theoretical prediction with the experimental results
in Fig. 6 shows that a good coincidence appears for ALC of holes, but in
some cases of cracks there are substantial deviations. This is probably
due to the roughtness at the surface of cracks and the estimating errors
at angle Θ. In the case of thick tested bodies, the effect of diffraction
field becomes less compared to other factors. It may be noted that the ALC
is one possible way using in pattern recognition, but not sensible enough.
Furthermore, it is necessary to perform this experiment very carefully,
otherwise, the echo amplitude is seriously affected by contact condition and
incline angle of transducers.

Therefore, another method using the phase information than amplitude
is proposed. At a fixed position of transducers, changing the incline angle
ϕ (Fig.5) about 2°- 5° symmetrically to the axis x. The echo signals at
three incline angles are recorded. Using Hilbert transform the instantaeous
phase may be calculated by Eq. 4 and plotted in Fig. 7a-7d. Then the autocorrelation functions S(t) and the cross correlation function C(t) are calculated respectively:

$$C(\tau) = \lim_{T \to \infty} \frac{1}{T} \int_{-T/2}^{T/2} \phi_1(t)\, \phi_2(t+\tau)\, dt \qquad (16)$$

when $\phi_1(t)$ and $\phi_2(t)$ are identical, above equation gives S(t).

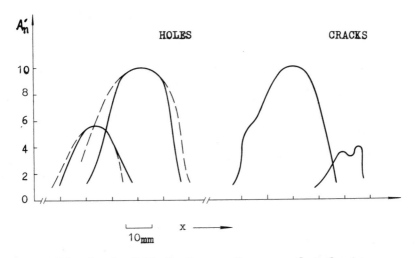

Fig.6. Amplitude Locus Curves of defects
------ Theoretical value
——— Experimental value

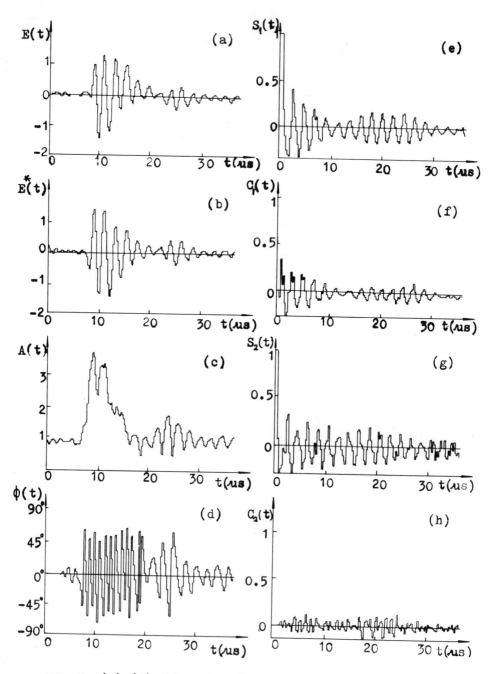

Fig.7. (a)-(d) Echo signals and their Hilbert
transform
(e)-(h) Auto- and cross correlation functions for holes (index 1) or cracks (index 2)

It has been found that the considerable difference occurs between holes and cracks. Results drawn in Fig. 7e - 7h illustrate that the value of the cross correlation function for holes are about 0.4-0.5 which are essentially larger than the value about 0.2 for cracks. This fact may be due to the complicate superposition of the reflected fields and also the diffracted waves and the second diffracted transverse wave converted from Rayleich surface wave generated by the edge diffraction. Such phase features are more useful than ALC. Moreover, using the correlation function can avoid difficulties to keep the identical experimental conditions. This method gives good hope of finding new features for pattern recognition.

CONCLUSION

For ultrasonic testing of NDT, it is the first task to detect the flaws reliably and to determine the positions of such defects. This can be implemented with the ALOK imaging method.

In order to correctly predict the failure of tested objects, the flaw identification and the display of flaw details are also required for QNDT. To meet the need, some methods combined with the ALOK imaging method have been studied and some results are obtained. The most difficulties come from the ill-posed nature of the inverse scattering problem. There is no a unique optimum method up to now. The combination of multiple methods, including pattern recognition, would be a useful way to overcome this barrier. In this case the ALOK imaging method can be considered as a good base.

Utilization of phase correlation shows an interesting way to obtain the feature of pattern recognition. In this direction more work will be done in the future.

REFERENCES

1. O.A.Barbian, B. Grohs and R.Licht, Signalanhebung durch Enststoerung von Laufzeit-Messwerten aus Ultraschallpruefungen von ferritischen und austenitischen Werkstoffen--ALOK (Amplitude-Laufzeit-Ortskurve)-Teil 1, Materialpruef. 23:379(1981)
2. B.Grohs, O.A.Barbian, W.Kappes and H.Paul, Fehlerbeschreibung nach Art, Lage und Dimension mit Hilfe von Laufzeit-Ortskurven aus Ultraschall-pruefungen-ALOK-Teil 2, Materialpruef. 23:427(1981)
3. W.Kappes, B.Grohs and O.A.Barbian, Berechnung von Laufzeif-Ortskurven fuer die Tandempruefung mit Ultraschall und Fehlerlage-Rekonstruktion aus Tandem-Laufzeit-Ortskurven beim ALOK-Verfahren-ALOK-Teil 3, Materialpruef. 24:161(1982)
4. J.D.Achenbach, A.K.Gautesen and H.McMaken, "Ray Methods for Waves in Elastic Solids," PITMAN PUBLISHING INC, Boston-London-Melbourne(1982)
5. A.J.Berkhout, "Seismic Migration," ELSEVIER SCIENTIFIC PUBLISHING COMPANY, Amsterdam-Oxford-New York(1980)
6. Yu Wei, Inverse Problem in Imaging, Lecture in the Seminar on Ultrasonic Testing, Nanjing(1985)
7. J.D.Achenbach, L. Adler, D.K.Lewis and H.McMaken, Diffraction of Ultrasonic Waves by Penny-Shaped Cracks in Metals: Theory and Experiment, J.Acoust. Soc. Amer. 66:1848(1979)
8. Yu Wei, Ming Shen and Xing-Quen Zhao, "A Study of ALOK Method," Proceeding of the Second NDT Conference, China(1984)
9. J.Krautkraemer and H.Krautkraemer, Werkstoffpruefung mit Ultraschall, translated in Chinese(1984)
10. Wang Shuo-Zhong, The Diffracted Acoustic Field around a Wedge, ACTA ACUSTICA 10:247(1985)

A NEW SURFACE ACOUSTIC WAVE IMAGING TECHNIQUE

Abdullah Atalar and Hayrettin Koymen

Electrical and Electronics Engineering Department
Middle East Technical University
Ankara, Turkey

ABSTRACT

A new type of imaging technique is presented which incorporates focussed surface acoustic waves. Surface acoustic waves are generated on the surface to be imaged by use of conical wavefronts. The conical wavefronts are obtained through the reflection of planar wavefronts from a parabolic cylindrical mirror. An imaging system is built which uses focussed surface acoustic waves in a mechanical scanning arrangement controlled by a computer. The resulting images show subsurface features with diffraction limited resolution.

INTRODUCTION

Acoustic imaging systems for nondestructive evaluation purposes are becoming popular and widely used after commercialization of several such instruments. The scanning acoustic microscope is widely accepted as a scientific instrument finding applications in areas such as thin film technology, metallurgy, material science and biology[1]. It produces acoustic images of plane surfaces of materials by a spherically converging bulk wave obtained by an acoustic lens in the form of a spherical cavity. These images result in a diffraction limited resolution determined by the frequency of acoustic waves. Images are sensitive to acoustic parameters of the surface material as well as to the thicknesses of the layers close to the surface. When the acoustic beam is focussed below the surface, it is possible to get subsurface information on acoustic images, because the acoustic waves can penetrate most materials. If the images are taken at that position, a high contrast is obtained in acoustic micrographs. The principal mechanism for material dependence of acoustic microscope response is the interference of nonspecular leaky surface acoustic waves (SAW) with specularly reflected bulk waves[2].

In acoustic microscopy, the penetration depth of acoustic waves into the object material is limited by SAW wavelength if the object has acoustically high impedance[3]. The obtained images are superposition of two types of information: surface data as produced by bulk waves in the liquid and subsurface data as produced by SAW. The relative contribution of SAW is small, because only a small fraction of available power is converted into this mode. On the other hand, for low impedance materials it is possible to increase the penetration if bulk waves are used in focussing[4].

To increase the sensitivity to subsurface properties, one may try to increase the contribution of the SAW in the imaging system. Smith et. al.[5] tried to obtain focussed SAW on the surface to be examined by defocussing a spherical acoustic microscope lens. Nongaillard et. al.[6] proposed to use cylindrically focussed waves to generate focussed SAW. Jen et.al.[7] used optical excitation techniques to generate it. But these techniques suffer from low conversion efficiency or from aberrations.

In this paper, we describe a new acoustic imaging mode, which could be used with acoustic microscopes. With this novel method, conical wavefronts are produced by reflection of plane waves from a cylindrical mirror and conical wavefronts generate the surface acoustic waves on the surface of the material, focussed on a diffraction limited size[8]. When this focussing technique is used in pulse-echo mode with suitable scan and display mechanisms, it is possible to obtain acoustic images. We will present SAW images using this technique demonstrating the subsurface capabilities and the predicted resolution.

DESCRIPTION OF THE IMAGING SYSTEM

First we will explain how a conical phasefront can be generated. Then we will show how a conical phasefront can be used to obtain focussed surface acoustic waves.

Let us first define what we mean by a conical surface and a conical phasefront: A smooth surface in space is said to be conical surface with respect to an axis (called cone axis), if the the following two conditions are satisfied:

Condition 1. The intersection of this surface with any plane containing the cone axis is a straight line.

Condition 2. The intersection of this surface with any plane perpendicular to the cone axis is circular.

A wave is said to have a conical phasefront if the equal phase surfaces are conical.

With these definitions in mind, we may now proceed to prove that a conical phasefront can be generated if a planar wavefront is obliquely incident on a parabolic cylindrical mirror. Consider the geometry shown in Fig.1. Let the parabolic cylindrical mirror be placed such that its focal axis is coincident with y axis and the vertex of the parabola be on the z axis. Hence y-z plane intersects the mirror into two symmetrical parts. Let the incident plane wavefront (plane A) be perpendicular to the y-z plane and make an angle δ with the focal axis (y-axis). Let AA' be a straight line in this plane and parallel to the y-z plane. The acoustic rays emanating from AA' intersect the mirror surface at BB'. BB' is parallel to the focal axis. The acoustic rays, after reflection from the mirror will travel toward the focal axis. Therefore, they lie in a plane, B that contains the focal axis and BB'. Because the AA' wavefront is reflected from the straight line BB', the equal phasefront in plane B is a straight line, CC'. This meets the condition 1.

Now we will show that a line in A plane that is parallel to x-axis (perpendicular to the y-z plane), AD, upon reflection is mapped onto a circular arc which is in a plane parallel to x-z plane. All the acoustic

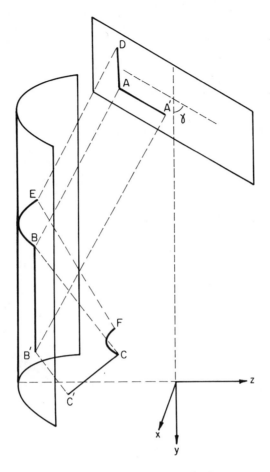

Fig.1. Three dimensional view of the geometry

rays emanating from AD make an angle 90-γ with y-axis. After reflection from the mirror surface which is perpendicular to the x-z plane, they preserve their angle of approach to x-z plane. This fact can be proven easily using vector analysis for these rays. Let an incident ray before reflection be the vector a=(0,sin(γ),cos(γ)). The mirror surface (or a normal to this surface) at the reflection point can be represented by the vector b=(-sin(β),0,cos(β)), where β is the angle between this surface and the z-axis. Let the reflected ray be represented by the vector c=(u,v,w). a, b and c vectors must lie in the same plane. This condition can be written as a x b = c x b. Expansion of the cross product gives v=sin(γ). The direction cosines of rays in y direction are preserved upon reflection. Therefore, the y components can be separated and the remaining x-z components can be analysed independently. Consider the top view of the geometry as in Fig.2. It is clear from the figure that AD maps onto CF arc upon reflection from the parabolic surface. Since AB+BC is equal to DE+EF, the total y displacement from A to C is equal to that from D to F. Hence, DF arc lies in a plane perpendicular to y-axis and condition 2 is also met. With the above arguments, the reflected wavefront is shown to be a conical wavefront with its cone axis coincident with the focal axis.

Let us suppose that we place a planar object surface perpendicular to the cone axis (or parallel to x-z plane). The intersection of this surface and the conical phasefront is a circular arc. If the size of the parabolic cylinder is finite, the reflected wave will be a section of the conical surface, and hence the intersection with the material surface will be a circular arc rather than a complete circle.

It is well known[8] that a beam incident on a liquid-solid interface excites surface waves strongly, provided that the incidence angle is equal to the Rayleigh critical angle. This phenomenon has been used to build highly efficient wedge transducers which convert bulk waves to SAW[9]. In a similar arrangement, if bulk waves with conical phasefronts are used, focussed SAW can be obtained: Referring to Fig.3, the object surface is placed perpendicular to the cone axis and the cone angle of the conical wave is adjusted so that the waves hit the surface at the Rayleigh critical angle ($\gamma = 90 - \theta_R$). As the conical wavefront propagates towards the interface (at time t_2, t_3 and t_4 in Fig.3), the intersection with the material surface will be a circular arc with diminishing radius. The center of curvature of all the arcs will be the same and they will converge to this center which is the SAW focus (at time t_5). The excited surface wave will reinforce the surface wavefront previously excited when the arc radius was larger. This is because of the fact that the incidence angle selected matches the k vector components along the interface. Notice that by this process all the energy in a conical wavefront is converted into a single circularly converging wavefront of the surface wave.

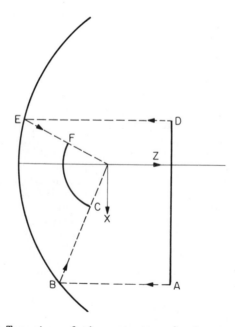

Fig.2.Top view of the geometry showing two rays

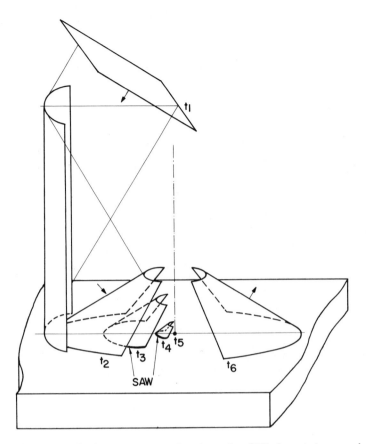

Fig.3. 3-D view of the geometry showing the SAW focussing mechanism

It may be shown[10] that there is an optimum focal length to optimize the conversion efficiency into SAW. This optimal focal length depends on factors like Schoch displacement and the attenuation constant of surface waves on the surface under investigation, and the openning angle of the parabolic cylindrical mirror. For example, the optimal focal length for a mirror involving an opening angle of 77 degrees is given by

$$f_{OPT}=1.1/(\alpha_L+\alpha_D)$$

where $\alpha_L=2/\Delta_S$, α_D is the attenuation constant of SAW and Δ_S is the Schoch displacement[12]. The conversion efficiency under this condition is approximately 70%.

EXPERIMENTAL WORK

The experimental acoustic imaging system is realized by using a planar ultrasonic transducer, in pulse-echo mode with a resonance frequency of 1.5 MHz. The parabolic cylindrical mirror is approximated by a circular cylindrical surface. This approximation is very good[10] if the lateral extent of the mirror is not too big. It has been shown[10] that the f-number of the imaging system can be as low as 0.47 (for aluminum) if the maximum phase error is to be kept less than a quarter wavelength. The transducer and mirror assembly is mounted on a mechanical X-Y stage (oriented on x-z plane in Fig.1.) which is driven by two stepper motors. The step size is 10 micrometers in either direction. The X-Y stage scans the surface of the test material under the control of an IBM-XT personal computer. The speed of the scan is limited by the maximum speed of the stepper motors and it is not particularly fast. A 10 mm by 10 mm area scan is completed in about 5 minutes.

The signal is produced and received by simple electronics. As depicted in Fig.4., a short base-band pulse is applied to the transducer through a transformer-type power divider. The output arm of the power divider is connected to the receiver amplifier. The power divider provides some degree of isolation between pulse generator and the receiver. The output of amplifier is fed to a sample and hold circuit to generate the video signal. The bandwidth of the video signal is rather low and it is determined by the scan speed. The video data is acquired by the computer through an ordinary A/D converter add-on card. The 12 bit A/D converter has a conversion time of 30 microseconds. Once the data is stored in the computer, the signal processing operations can be performed with ease.

The images can be produced on a computer graphic screen in several

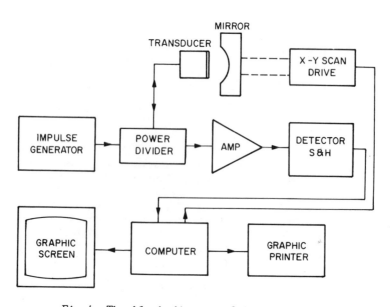

Fig.4. The block diagram of imaging system

ways. The video signal obtained for each scan line can be plotted on the screen with a little displacement each time. With the hidden line blanking, the resulting picture has a three dimensional impression, but it is hard to recognize and identify structures in such images. Another imaging mode that can be used is to define pixels with varying intensity, and assign these pixels to varying acoustic signal intensity. Both techniques are suitable to get hard-copies with ordinary dot-matrix printers. If a computer color graphic screen is used, the acoustic intensity can be mapped to colors to obtain false-color acoustic images. Fig.5.(a) and (b) show acoustic images of a test piece using the techniques described above as obtained with a dot-matrix printer. The test piece is an aluminum block with holes drilled from the side of the block as shown in Fig.5.(c). In the acoustic image only the ends of the holes are delineated, since these are the only places where a SAW backscatter can occur. Note that, the presence of holes also modifies the edge reflection through a complex process[13] at the points where the holes start. If the mirror had been aligned such that the z-axis in Fig.1 is perpendicular to the axis of the holes rather than parallel to them, the image would have shown the holes in their entirety. The focussing system does not receive all the scattered signals at a discontinuity, but rather those falling within the coverage angle of the mirror.

To test the system we have fabricated other phantoms made of drawn aluminum. The first piece contains holes of 2 mm diameter drilled from the backside arranged in 3 by 3 matrix as shown in Fig.6(a). The holes stay clear of the front surface by 0.5 mm in the first matrix and 1.5 mm in the second. The SAW image of the test piece is displayed in Fig.6(b). The holes are clearly resolved and the received signals are well above the noise. Although round holes are involved, the images of holes are not quite circular. This is most likely due to the non-circular point spread function of the focussed SAW. It is evident that the resolution in z-axis (see Fig.1) direction is less than that in x-axis. The image also shows some structures which may have to do with the microscopic properties of the aluminum surface, such as differing porosity, grain structure or residual stress.

The second piece contains a line of holes of varying separation drilled from the back side to test the resolution of the system. The end of the holes are 0.5 mm from the front surface. The image obtained by scanning the line of 2 mm and 2.5 mm spaced holes is depicted in Fig.7. The z-axis of Fig.1. is perpendicular to the line of holes. This grating structure made of holes, with a periodicity equal to the SAW wavelength, is well resolved. The resolution of the system is less than a wavelength. On the other hand, the resolution along the z-axis is not as good as this, but 2 mm spaced holes can still be resolved in that direction.

DISCUSSION

The imaging system described above is different from popular imaging systems like the scanning acoustic microscope[1] or the scanning laser acoustic microscope, in that it is a "zero-background" system. When the SAW focus is at a point where there are no inhomogeneities or surface irregularities, no signal will reflect, and hence the response of the imaging system will be zero. There will be signal only if there is something different on the focal point that will cause a reflection of SAW. In the scanning acoustic microscope, there will be a signal even when the surface under consideration is perfect. To find defects one needs to measure the minute changes on top of a large signal. This requires an extremely stable mechanical scan system.

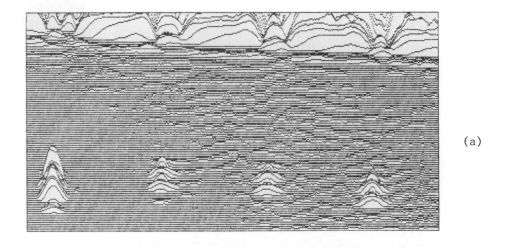

(a)

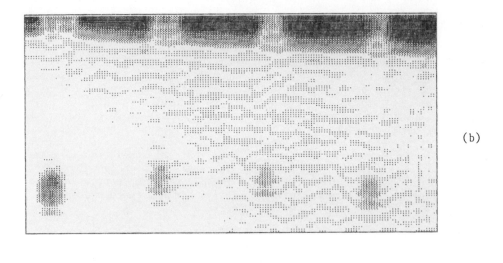

(b)

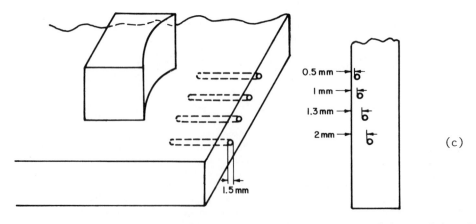

(c)

Fig.5. SAW images using two different display techniques, (a) and (b), of the aluminum phantom shown in (c).

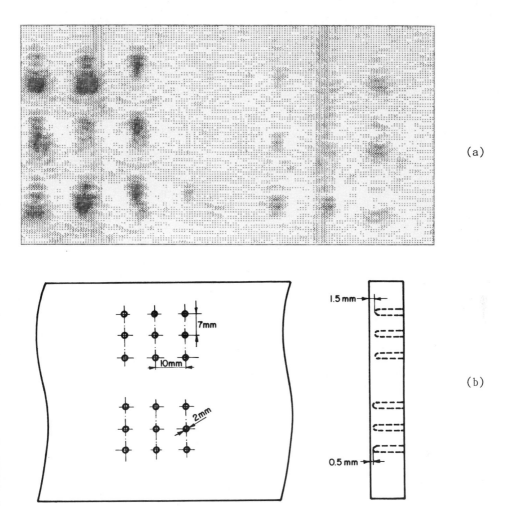

Fig.6. SAW image (a) of an aluminum phantom surface (b).

On the other hand, using focussed SAW, one may expect to get images full of artifacts, if the surface under consideration is rich in structures (e.g. surfaces of integrated circuits). Such surfaces are more appropriate for a bulk wave focussing lens. SAW images will be meaningful and easily interpreted if the object surface is mainly smooth (e.g. a coated surface of a magnetic disk) and has defects (cracks, etc) below the surface. In this case, any presence of signal will indicate a defect. The magnitude of the signal can be related to the size or depth of the defect.

The detection of flaws in metals which are very close to surface is difficult by acoustic techniques using bulk waves, due to the presence of strong reflection at the interface. In such systems, the acoustic mismatch at the interface causes most of the incident energy be reflected. Only a small fraction of the energy is coupled into the medium. The interface reflection invades any reflection of flaws close to the surface. In our imaging technique almost all the energy is converted into SAW and is used for imaging. Since there is no significant background, the system is inherently sensitive to flaws close to the surface. When flaws which are away from the surface are to be detected, our imaging system is not very appropriate and in that case bulk wave imaging systems must be preferred.

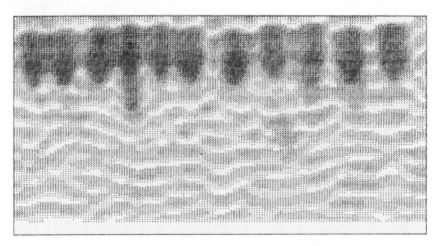

Fig.7. SAW image of 2 mm and 2.5 mm spaced subsurface holes.

It is possible to increase the resolution of the imaging system by increasing the operation frequency. Initial experiments at 20 MHz indicate that it is possible to use this technique at least up to 100 MHz. When used in this frequency range, it can be employed as a new type of lens in acoustic microscopy.

ACKNOWLEDGEMENTS

This work is supported by TUBITAK. We acknowledge Hüseyin Yavuz, Tolga Çiloglu and Bülent Mutlugil who built the imaging system. We thank Ernst Leitz Wetzlar GmbH, W.Germany for donating us the scan mechanics used in the experimental system.

REFERENCES

1. C.F.Quate, A.Atalar, K.Wickramasinghe, "Acoustic microscopy with mechanical scanning- A review" Proc. of IEEE, 67: 1092 (1979).
2. W.Parmon and H.L.Bertoni, "Ray interpretation of material signature in the acoustic microscope" Elect.Lett., 15: 685 (1979).
3. A.Atalar "Penetration depth of the scanning acoustic microscope" IEEE Trans. Son. Ultrason. 32: 164 (1985).
4. V.B.Jipson "Acoustic microscopy of interior planes" Appl.Phys.Lett. 35: 385 (1979).
5. I.R.Smith, H.K.Wickramasinghe, G.W.Farnell and C.K.Jen "Confocal surface acoustic wave microscopy" Appl.Phys.Lett. 42: 411 (1983).
6. B.Nongaillard, M.Ourak, J.M.Rouvaen, M.Houze and E.Bridoux "A new focusing method for nondestructive evaluation by acoustic surface wave" J.Appl.Phys. 55: 75 (1984).
7. C.K.Jen, P.Cielo, J.Bussiere, F.Nadeau and G.W.Farnell, Appl.Phys.Lett. 46: 241 (1985).
8. H.Koymen and A.Atalar, "Focussing surface waves using axicons" Appl.Phys.Lett. 47: 1266 (1985).
9. H.L.Bertoni and T.Tamir, "Unified theory of Rayleigh-angle phenomena for acoustic beams at liquid-solid interface" Appl.Phys. 2: 157 (1973).

10. J.Fraser, B.T.Khuri-Yakub, and A.R.Selfridge, <u>Appl.Phys.Lett.</u> 32: 698 (1978).
11. A.Atalar and H.Koymen, "Use of a conical axicon as surface acoustic wave focussing device" to be published in <u>IEEE</u> <u>Trans.</u> <u>Ultrason.</u> <u>Freq.</u> <u>Cont.</u> (1986).
12. L.M.Brekhovskikh, "Waves in layered media", 2. Ed., New York: Academic (1980).
13. F.C.Cuozzo, E.L.Cambiaggio, J-P Damiano, and E.Rivier "Influence of Elastic Properties on Rayleigh Wave Scattering by Normal Discontinuities" <u>IEEE</u> <u>Trans.</u> <u>on</u> <u>Son.</u> <u>Ultrason.</u> 24: 280 (1977).

ACOUSTICAL IMAGING TECHNIQUES--THEORETICAL AND EXPERIMENTAL RESULTS

B. Ho, L.T. Wu and R. Zapp

Biomedical Ultrasound Laboratory
Department of Electrical Engineering and Systems Science
Michigan State University
East Lansing, Michigan 48824

INTRODUCTION

Ultrasonic evaluation of materials has experienced tremendous growth in recent years. especially for composite materials in the automotive and aerospace industries. Of special interest is the ability to precisely identify small defects or faults at various depths inside the material. The range resolution is inherently limited by the transmitting pulse width and operating frequency. Improvement can be made by using large amplitude narrow pulses. However, a very narrow pulse is difficult to produce in practice, besides which its instantaneous ultrasonic intensity could cause damage to the transmitting transducer and/or the target. In addition to the range resolution limitation, we observed that the typical acoustic imaging system has some range accuracy problems related to the limited coherence of trigger time from the microprocessor controlled ultrasonic pulse transmission. This has caused a range inaccuracy of as much as one millimeter in water at an operating frequency of 2.25 MHz.

In conventional pulse-echo techniques, the imaging parameter is based on the boundary interface properties of the medium. In reality however. the return signal strength is affected by both the boundary reflection characteristics and the attenuation properties. Media without distinct boundary definition. such as early stage tumors can not be easily detected by retrieving the boundary information only. To avoid this limitation we have used a dual transducer arrangement to obtain both the boundary and the attenuation properties in order to construct target images. This paper reports various techniques recently employed in our laboratory to remove the shortcomings mentioned above.

METHODS

Most of the existing ultrasonic imaging systems, commerically available, employ detection of target echo returns. Well defined acoustic boundaries are easily identified from returned signals above a preset amplitude threshold. The range resolution of such detection schemes is heavily dependent upon the shape of the echo pulse; the narrower the transmitted pulse the higher the resolution. The location of the boundary is identified as the point where the threshold level intersects the pulse

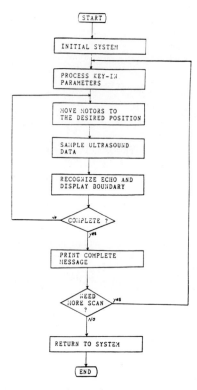

Fig. 1. Main flow chart of the imaging system.

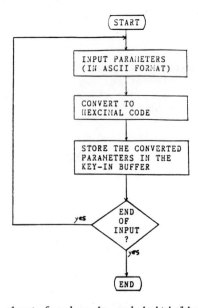

Fig. 2. Flow chart for key-in and initializing processes.

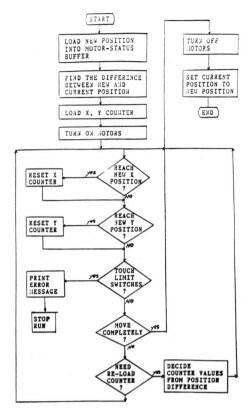

Fig. 3. Scanner program of stepping motors.

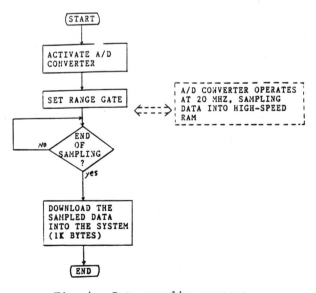

Fig. 4. Data sampling process.

envelope along the time axis. Hence, for a given echo return, the uncertainty of boundary location could be as large as the pulse width. Thus, the range uncertainty of the typical system is on the order of several wavelengths. To minimize the range inaccuracy due to amplitude processing, phase processing of the pulse r-f contents is desirable. The difficulty of retrieving the phase information from the r-f carrier lies in the high sampling rate required to satisfy the Nyquist criteria while still performing real time analog-to-digital conversion. To achieve such a strict requirement, a very high speed recording system had to be designed. This involved a very high speed sampling circuit, a memory unit to store the sampled data and the appropriate signal processing software to identify the boundaries. Figure 1 shows the over-all functional block diagram for the C scan ultrasonic imaging system. The program is initialized by inputting the desired scanning path for the transducer. Parameters such as scanning steps, limits along the x and y directions and the threshold level above which the echo signals are to be sampled are all initialized. The flow chart of a typical routine is shown in Fig. 2. Finally, the scanner motor control sequence is activated. The motor mounted transducer is programmed to follow the desired path. The sequential operation of the scanner is shown in Fig. 3.

During system operation the return signal is conditioned to a peak swing of 2 volts before it is sampled. The A/D conversion is achieved by a 20 mega sample per second circuit using a commercially available monolithic video A/D conversion chip. The converter digital output is stored in a temporary memory of 1 K bytes. Since the sampling frequency is much higher than the microprocessor clock frequency, a circuit was designed to store the output of the 15.4 MHz A/D converter. After all the sampled data is stored in temporary memory, a slower clock (100 KHz) transfers the data into the microcomputer buffer. Figure 4 shows the sampling process. After data transfer is completed, the signal processing routine identifies peak values and their relative phases. In order to ensure that the signal processed is indeed the signal from the target, a subroutine is called to screen out the unwanted artifacts and spurious noise by checking the frequency of each segment of the return data. The echo recognition and boundary display processes are depicted in Fig. 5.

In conventional pulse-echo detection the attenuation properties of the target cannot be uniquely determined due to the interaction of attenuation and boundary reflections. In order to retrieve the attenuation information, we placed two transducers on opposite sides of the object. The attenuation property of the object is obtained as follows:

1. Obtain the impulse response from both sides by using a frequency domain deconvolution technique.

2. The amplitudes of the impulse responses and the propagation times are obtained from the impulse responses.

3. The attenuation coefficients, α_i, are then obtained from the following expression:

$$\alpha_i = \frac{1}{4\tau_i} \ln[\frac{a_i b_{i+1}}{a_{i+1} b_i} (1 - r_i^2)(1 - r_{i+1}^2)]$$

where a_i, b_i are the echo amplitudes, r_i is the reflection coefficient and τ_i is the propagation time all from the ith layer.

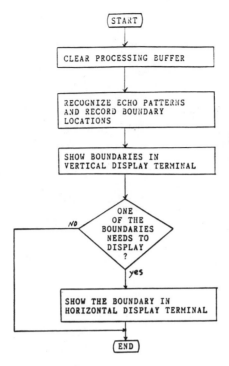

Fig. 5. Echo recognition and boundary display flow chart.

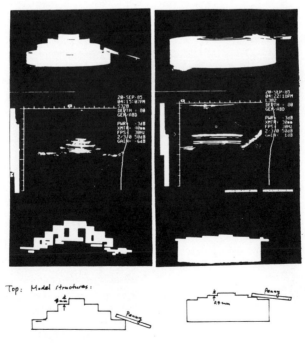

Top: Model structures:

Middle: Image from ACUSON model 128 system

Bottom::Image from our system.

Fig. 6. B scan for checking range accuracy.

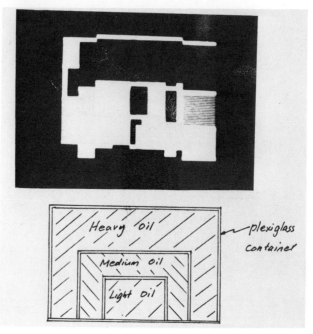

Fig. 7. Attenuation imaging.

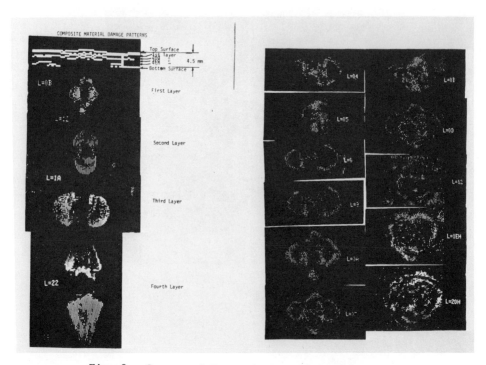

Fig. 8. C scan of layered composite material.

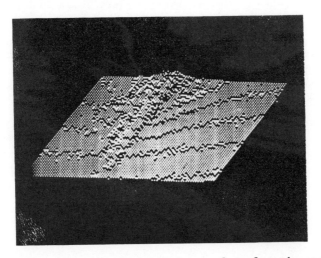

Fig. 9.   Three-dimensional image of surface damage.

RESULTS AND DISCUSSIONS

To evaluate the system range accuracy, a target model made of plexi-glass with 0.3 to 0.5 mm steps is processed by B scan ultrasonic pulses. A 2.25 MHz transducer is used in the scanning system and the returned signal is sampled at 15.4 MHz. The time interval between sampled data points is approximately 65 nanoseconds which corresponds to approximately 0.1 mm in water. Theoretically, we can distinguish target range varia-tions of 0.1 mm (65 nanoseconds). Figure 6 shows the B scan of such a model where steps of 0.3 mm are clearly shown.

The attenuation imaging of a model containing different materials with various attenuation coefficients is shown in Fig. 7. The level of attenuation in different materials is illustratd by grayscale displays. For imaging purposes, grayscale shows the relative change of attenuation, which quite often is preferred to the tedious process of obtaining the absolute value of attenuation. The image discontinuities from the model are due to the variations in propagation velocity from regions of different acoustic impedances.

C scans of layered composite materials are shown in Fig. 8. Both the 5-layered and 15-layered graphite composite samples are 4.5 mm thick. The samples were damaged by high speed projectile impact. Damage caused by the impact is mainly layer delamination and fiber fracture. Theoreti-cally, the damage patterns generally have bipolar shape (figure eight pattern). The patterns typically are shifted by 90° from layer to layer. It is important for the material scientist to know the shape and damage pattern area in order to evaluate the impact energy absorbed.

Finally, a three-dimensional scan program was recently developed in our lab for the imaging system. A 3-dimensional image of the surface damage for the sample of Fig. 8 is shown in Fig. 9. There is close correlation between surface deformation and internal structural damage. A rapid display of the 3-dimensional surface image can provide valuable information about the material structure under both static and dynamic conditions.

A FLOW IMAGING AND CW SPECTRAL

ANALYSIS SYSTEM

J.I. Mehi, R.S.C. Cobbold, K.W. Johnston, and C. Royer

Institute of Biomedical Engineering
University of Toronto
Toronto, M5S 1A4, Canada

ABSTRACT

A system for Doppler ultrasound flow imaging and CW spectral analysis of the carotid artery is described. The system uses a 24 element linear array with the long axis aligned perpendicular to the axis of the artery. Alteration of the array aperture function allows either a narrow beam to be produced for flow imaging, or a beam as wide as the artery to be produced for CW spectral analysis. For flow imaging, a narrow beam produced by an eight element crystal group is swept across the artery by sequentially shifting the group along the array. The system is designed to image flow along a line of approximately 2 cm length. A two-dimensional map of blood flow projected onto the plane of the surface of the skin is obtained by moving the array along the vessel axis using a one-dimensional position sensor. The CW spectral analysis mode of operation uses the middle twelve elements to produce a uniform 4 mm wide beam at a depth of 4 cm. Initial results with a partially tested system are described.

INTRODUCTION

Doppler ultrasound is routinely used to non-invasively assess peripheral and carotid arterial disease. The accuracy of detecting arterial stenoses can be enhanced by spectral analysis of Doppler signals. Spectral analysis provides information concerning the relative velocities of blood cells in the region of the artery which intersects the ultrasound beam, and thus yields data of a fundamental nature related to the hemodynamic phenomena. However, without the aid of imaging, the location of the insonated region is not precisely known, and in addition, with the normal variations in anatomy, proper identification of the vessels may require a certain degree of expertise for accurate and efficient patient examination. Evidently, an image will help alleviate these problems.

Imaging with B-mode, while valuable in revealing the structural characteristics of the tissue, does not always reveal arterial lesions which have an acoustic impedance similar to blood. On the other hand, a Doppler flow image is capable of providing information directly related to the time and spatial distribution of the flow velocity.

Examples of current flow imaging methods include the position sensing arm method [1,2], and real-time two-dimensional flow imaging using phased arrays [3,4,5]. In position sensing arm systems a Doppler probe, which produces a narrow beam, is connected to an articulated position sensing arm to detect the flow velocity on a point-by-point basis. This produces a two-dimensional flow map either as a projection onto the plane of the skin, or as a transverse or cross-sectional view, depending on the system design. To obtain such a flow image, the patient must lie motionless for a considerable period of time. Our previous work on the development of a real-time Doppler flow imaging system [6] made use of a special stepped linear array in conjunction with a mechanically rocked mirror. Although in-vitro images were produced with this system, some major difficulties prevented the demonstration of in-vivo carotid images. These problems will be briefly discussed later. More recently, high quality real-time carotid Doppler flow images, superimposed on the corresponding B-mode images, have been demonstrated [5] using a phased linear array system. Such systems tend to be both complex and expensive.

The system described in this paper is intended to provide flow images much more quickly than position-sensing arm systems, to be less costly than the real-time flow imaging systems, and to allow CW spectral analysis to be performed accurately.

PRINCIPLES OF OPERATION

The system uses CW Doppler for spectral analysis, and pulsed Doppler for flow imaging. Both modes of operation use the same crystal array. The flow imaging feature is intended to allow the carotid arterial system to be readily located, to see any gross vessel abnormalities, and to allow the CW beam to be quickly positioned to insonate a desired section for spectral analysis.

As shown in Fig. 1, the array is aligned perpendicular to the axis of the artery, and is tilted at an angle suitable for Doppler signal detection. In this way, the cross-section of the artery is imaged. By moving the array along the artery, different cross-sectional views can be obtained, allowing the identification of various sites within the carotid region, including the bifurcation.

The 24 elements of the linear array are multiplexed to the CW and pulsed Doppler transmitters and receivers by a network of analog switches, as illustrated in Fig. 2. By activating the array elements in a sequential manner the beam is scanned across sections of tissue for imaging.

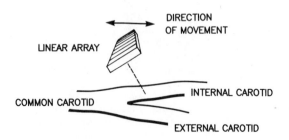

Figure 1. Alignment of the linear array with the carotid artery. The array axis is perpendicular to the artery axis, and the array is canted at an angle for Doppler signal detection.

Proper phasing and apodization enables the different beam profiles in the azimuthal plane to be optimized. The beam-forming capability of the array is important because a narrow beam is required for imaging, whereas a beam as wide as the artery is preferred for CW spectral analysis. Furthermore, certain desirable characteristics for the CW beam profile can be achieved, as will be discussed later. The field profile in the elevation plane remains the same for both modes of operation, and is determined by the geometry of the array, and an acoustic lens. A water bag is used to couple the ultrasound to the tissue.

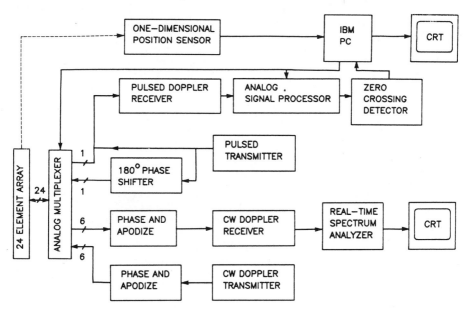

Figure 2. Block diagram of the flow imaging and CW spectral analysis system.

CW Spectral Analysis

Generally, for CW spectral analysis, the ultrasound beam should be as wide as the artery in order to include flow velocity information from the entire vessel cross-sectional area. Incomplete insonation or insonation by a non-uniform beam may cause errors in the measured Doppler spectrum [7]. Based on the knowledge that the average diameter of the internal carotid artery near the bifurcation is 4.3 mm [8], the beam was designed to have a width of about 4 mm at a distance of 4 cm from the transducer face. Furthermore, to avoid insonating adjacent vessels, the beam intensity should fall off rapidly beyond the arterial lumen [9].

Flow Imaging

Flow imaging requires a narrow ultrasound beam to be swept through various points within the tissue. To accomplish this rapidly, the network of analog switches multiplexes the pulsed Doppler transmitter and receiver to sequentially shifted sets of elements within the array. Our previous work to achieve real-time two-dimensional flow imaging made use of a stepped array and employed a rapidly scanned narrow CW beam [6]. The resulting flow image consisted of the projection of flow onto the plane of the surface of the skin. However, interference problems encountered in switching the transducer array elements, and problems in the array fabrication due to its non-planar nature, prevented the achievement of adequate Doppler sensitivity for in-vivo imaging. These difficulties led to the decision to use pulsed Doppler for imaging, and a planar array.

The range gate and transmit burst length have both been extended to ensure that the vessel always lies within the 'sample' volume. It should be noted that with multi-range gate processing, flow images at various depths could be produced. For simplicity, the prototype system does not have this capability.

An output signal approximately proportional to the mean frequency of the Doppler signal is provided by a zero-crossing detector. This signal is digitized by the IBM PC and displayed on a color monitor such that each line scanned by the array is displayed as a row of color encoded points. When the array is moved in the direction perpendicular to the scanned line, a position sensing arm records the displacement and adds another row on the display in the proper location. In this way, a two-dimensional flow map is produced.

SYSTEM DESCRIPTION

The Array

The array was designed with the aid of a computer program which simulates ultrasonic field profiles for linear arrays using the approach taken by Arenson et al. [10]. These simulations led to the selection of the element dimensions and the aperture functions used for imaging and CW spectral analysis [11].

The dimensions of the 5 MHz, 24-element array are: element width=1.0 mm, element length=10 mm, inter-element spacing=1.1 mm, array length=26.3 mm. To increase acoustic efficiency for the CW mode, the array was designed to have a narrower bandwidth than that normally used for pulse-echo imaging, and this was achieved through the use of a proprietry foam backing. Some axial resolution was thus lost, but this is not a concern since a long sample volume was desired. However, good lateral resolution is required to enable the location of the vessel boundaries for positioning the CW beam. The array was custom made (Panametrics Inc., Waltham, Mass).

In the azimuthal plane of the array the beam profile is determined by the aperture function. In the elevation plane, a convex acoustic lens, made from silicone rubber (Sylgard 170, Dow Corning) was used for focusing.

CW Transmitter and Receiver

There are six transmitting channels and six receiving channels which are phased and apodized as shown in Fig. 3. After phase shifting and apodization, the received signals are summed. The phase shifting networks and the CW preamplifier are connected to the elements through analog switches, to isolate them from the pulsed transmitter and receiver when the imaging mode is in operation. The CW receiver provides phase-quadrature outputs intended to be compatible with any real-time spectrum analyzer.

Pulsed Transmitter and Receiver

The pulsed Doppler system made use of modified circuit boards from a

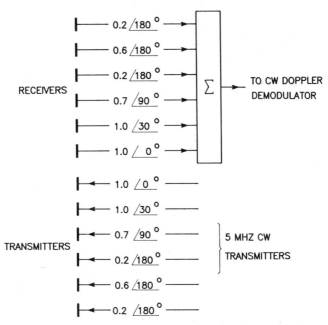

Figure 3. Phasing and apodization of the six transmitting and six receiving elements used to produce the CW ultrasound beam.

commercial pulsed Doppler system (Model CP-1, Hokanson Inc., Issaquah, Wash.). One of the modifications consisted of lengthening both the transmit burst and the range gate to 3 μs. Two transmitters producing bursts 180° out of phase are required to produce a sufficiently narrow beam. The transmit aperture function selected uses eight adjacent elements, with the elements on each end phased at 180° with respect to the six central elements. The elements are apodized equally. For the receive aperture function, the outer two elements are not used, and the remaining six are not phased or apodized. This simplifies the receiver design. The transmitters and receiver access the appropriate array elements through a network of analog switches. Only two switching paths are used, since the receive path is the same as one of the transmit paths.

Analog Processing

In switching between adjacent groups of elements large phase changes in the received signal occur. These arise from differences in the positions of the various stationary and moving interfaces as seen by each crystal group. This results in a large change in the DC offset at the demodulator output when the groups are switched. To compensate for this effect a zero-restoring circuit and a blanking circuit are used, and these are shown in Fig. 4. Immediately after a new element group is activated, the zero-restorer samples the signal at the demodulator output. This value is then held, and subtracted from the demodulator output. While the signal is being sampled, the output of the zero-restorer is blanked.

Switching Network

CMOS analog switches are used to multiplex the 24 array elements to the two pulsed Doppler channels. With eight adjacent elements transmitting, there are 17 possible locations for the pulsed aperture within the array. The switches are controlled by shift registers. A scan signal causes the parallel loading of the selected aperture activation word into the first shift registers; with each clock pulse, the aperture word is

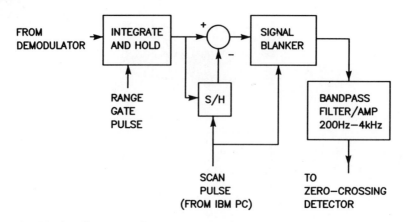

Figure 4. Block diagram of analog circuit that compensates for the large
changes in DC offset at the demodulator output when the element group
is shifted to a new location.

shifted one bit, to activate the next group of elements. At the end of
the sequence, another scan pulse reloads the aperture word into the first
registers.

System Controller

An IBM PC is used to control the operation of the system, to display
the flow data, and to store the flow data. When imaging, the assembly language controller program produces the clock and scan signals for the shift
registers in the switching network, and samples the mean flow value with
an analog to digital converter. The sampled value is then colour-coded and
displayed in the proper location. There is also a single step mode of
operation in which the narrow beam location can be advanced one step at a
time. Another function of the PC is to control the one-dimensional position tracking system, which is used to produce two-dimensional flow maps.
The prototype position sensor is based on an IBM PC 'mouse'.

PRELIMINARY RESULTS AND DISCUSSION

Field Profiles

With the water bag in place, the expected distance from the array to
the vessels is 3.5-5.0 cm. Field profiles were measured at depths within
this range. The field profile measuring system used a large water-filled
tank in which the array and a 6.3 mm diameter steel ball target were
immersed. A scanning arm under the control of a PDP-11 minicomputer moved
the target to the desired coordinates within the tank.

The CW beam aperture function produces the field profile shown in
Fig.5. The 3 dB beam width is 4.0 mm at a depth of 4.0 cm, and the side
lobe levels are 17.5 dB lower than the main lobe. Figure 6 shows the
measured field profile in the imaging mode. The 3 dB beam width at a
depth of 4.0 cm is 1.2 mm, and the side lobe levels are 11 dB lower than
the main lobe.

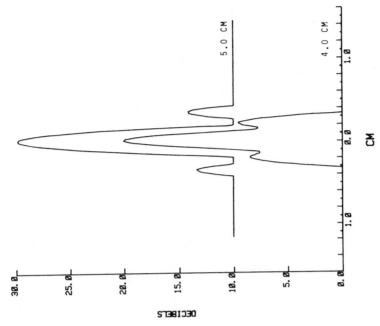

Figure 6. Imaging mode beam profile in decibels, at depths of 4.0 and 5.0 cm. There is a 10 dB offset between plots, and values more than 20 dB below the peak value are set to zero for clarity.

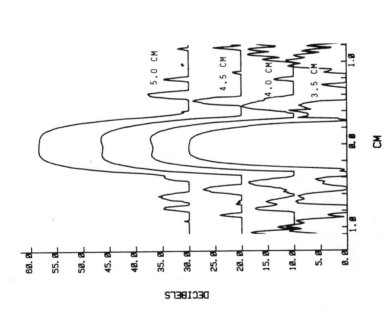

Figure 5. CW spectral analysis mode beam profile in decibels, at depths of 3.5 to 5.0 cm. There is a 10 dB offset between plots, and values more than 30 dB below the peak value are set to zero for clarity.

305

CW Spectrum

An FFT derived carotid Doppler spectrum obtained with the CW receiver is shown in Fig.7. The signal was obtained from one of the quadrature outputs of the receiver, which had a high pass filter cut-off of 300 Hz. The prototype receiver was not shielded against radio frequency interference, resulting in relatively high noise levels. Further studies will be done with the CW receiver interfaced to a commercial real-time spectrum analyzer. Spectral analysis of the pulsed Doppler output when the narrow beam is held in one position should also be possible.

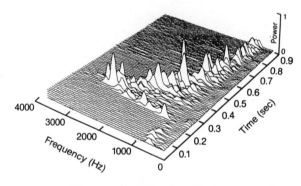

Figure 7. Frequency spectrum of CW carotid Doppler signal obtained with the array, using twelve phased and apodized elements.

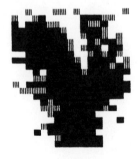 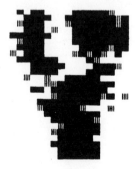

Figure 8. Examples of two preliminary flow images of the carotid bifurcation.

Flow Imaging

An initial test of the flow imaging mode of operation showed that the bifurcation can be quickly found, and the internal, external and common carotid arteries can be identified. In this test a single quadrature channel was used with a two level display (black and white). Two flow images of the bifurcation region of a presumed normal subject are shown in Fig.8. The scan time for these images was relatively long, being one second. However, the system has produced flow images with a scan time of 170 ms, i.e. 10 ms for each crystal group.

Various improvements in the system should result in images of higher quality. A combination of factors including the size and shape of the water bag and the angle of insonation resulted in the distance of the array elements from the vessel being less than required. This distance was around 2.5-3.0 cm, rather than the design distance of 4.0 cm. As a result, the 3 dB beam width at the vessel was about 4 mm. Faster imaging and better signal quality should result from improvements in the processing of the pulsed signal. Digital processing would probably be a better approach.

CONCLUSIONS

In this paper we have described a system that uses a linear array for both flow imaging and CW Doppler spectral analysis. The aperture function for flow imaging produces a beam profile with a 3 dB beam width of 1.2 mm at a depth of 4 cm. In the CW mode a different aperture function was used to ensure fairly uniform and complete vessel insonation. Very preliminary testing of the completed system has resulted in in-vivo carotid images and has shown CW spectra of reasonable quality. With further development, significant improvements in signal quality and scanning rate appear to be possible.

ACKNOWLEDGEMENTS

We are grateful to the Heart and Stroke Foundation of Ontario and the National Science and Engineering Research Council of Canada for partial financial support of this work. In addition, we wish to thank Dr Frank Ingle (Medasonics Inc.) for advice and the loan of a CW receiver.

REFERENCES

1. Reid, J.M., Spencer, M.P. and Davis, D.L., "Ultrasonic Doppler Imaging System", pp. 1127-1235 in "Ultrasound in Medicine"., D.N. White and R. Brown (Eds.), Vol. 3B, Plenum Press, New York, 1977.
2. Curry, G.R. and White, D.N., "Color Coded Ultrasonic Differential Velocity Arterial Scanner (Echoflow)," Ultrasound Med. Biol., 4:27-35, 1978.
3. Kasai, C., Namekawa, K., Koyano, A., and Omoto, R. "Real-Time Two-Dimensional Blood Flow Imaging Using an Autocorrelation Technique," IEEE Trans. Sonics Ultrason., SU-32:458-454, 1985.
4. Switzer, D.F., and Nanda, N.C., "Doppler Color Flow Mapping," Ultrasound Med. Biol., 11:403-416, 1985.
5. Powis, P.L., "Angiodynography: A New Real-Time Look at the Vascular System," Applied Radiology, 15:55-59, 1986.

6. Arenson, J.W., Cobbold, R.S.C., and Johnston, K.W., "Real-Time Two-Dimensional Blood Flow Imaging Using a Doppler Ultrasound Array", pp. 529-538 in "Acoustic Imaging", E.A. Ash and C.R. Hill (Eds.), Vol. 12, Plenum Press, New York, 1982.

7. Cobbold, R.S.C., Veltink, P.H., and Johnston, K.W., "Influence of Beam Profile and Degree of Insonation on CW Doppler Ultrasound Spectrum and Mean Velocity", IEEE Trans. Sonics Ultrason., SU-30:364-370, 1983.

8. Brown, P.M. and Johnston, K.W., "The Difficulty of Quantifying the severity of Carotid Stenoses", Surgery, 92:468-473, 1982.

9. Douville, Y., Arenson, J.W., Johnston, K.W., Cobbold, R.S.C., and Kassam, M., "Critical Evaluation of Continuous Wave Doppler Probes for Carotid Studies", J. Clin. Ultrasound, 11:83-90, 1983.

10. Arenson, J.W., Cobbold, R.S.C., and Johnston, K.W., "Computer Aided Design of Ultrasonic Imaging Arrays", Digest 8th CMBES Conf., pp.162-163, 1980.

11. Mehi, J.I. An Ultrasound Array for Arterial Doppler Flow Imaging and Spectral Analysis, MASc. Thesis, University of Toronto, 1985.

MULTIDIMENSIONAL ULTRASONIC HEART IMAGING

Jill A. Wollins, Krishnasawamy Chandrasekaran, Tom M. Kinter,
Eric A. Hoffman, and James F. Greenleaf

Biodynamics Research Unit, Department of Physiology
and Biophysics, Mayo Clinic/Foundation, Rochester, MN

ABSTRACT

Multidimensional ultrasonic imaging of the heart can provide qualitative and quantitative information describing cardiac structure and function. Two-dimensional echo fails to supply an adequate image set for assessment of specific cardiac function. By developing appropriate scanning techniques to produce compound B-scans using a conventional echo sector scanner, more objective and complete analysis can be performed. This study presents results of in vitro cardiac imaging, preliminary to application to in vivo human hearts. A motor-driven mounted transducer was incrementally rotated over 180° to obtain 50 angles of view. Two excised normal dog hearts and two pig hearts with anatomical defects were scanned with a conventional echo sector scanner. After data collection and reconstruction, three-dimensional surface displays were generated for both the endocardial and epicardial surfaces. From oblique section displays, the structural defects in the abnormal in vitro hearts were clearly visible. With further development, these techniques promise greater facility in analysis and display of three-dimensional echo images and are adaptable for in vivo cardiac imaging as well.

INTRODUCTION

Clinical evaluation of a complex moving organ, such as the heart, requires considerable training and expertise. To accurately assess cardiac structure and function, three-dimensional dynamic imaging and display of the heart is essential. As imaging technology has evolved in recent years, considerable effort has focused on development of noninvasive cardiac imaging techniques. Two-dimensional echocardiography preceded other imaging modalities to provide dynamic images of the heart. It remains one of the few techniques that is truly noninvasive. The cost of remaining noninvasive lies in the image resolution as well as inability to obtain complete dynamic 3-D data sets of the beating heart. Since the transducer must be positioned on the chest wall and the signal sent and received between the ribs, through a multi-media space, the resulting images have considerable artifactual content. To interpret echocardiograms the cardiologist typically views a videotaped image sequence in real-time, slow-motion, and stop-action modes which then provide sufficient spatial and temporal information to assist evaluation and diagnosis. Stationary two-dimensional echo images are difficult to read due to scanning artifacts.

Dynamic imaging of the heart has advanced in several imaging modalities including rapid and/or multi-source x-ray computed tomography and magnetic resonance as well as ultrasound. Fast, multi-slice x-ray CT, requiring the infusion of contrast agent into the circulation, can provide rapid acquisition of images (up to 60/sec) (Ritman et al., 1985). By rotating the x-ray source(s) around the subject, many angles of view can be obtained, with appropriate x-ray firing sequence. The limitations of this technique as with other energy modalities, including MRI, PET, and SPECT, include cost of technology and cumbersome size. Magnetic resonance imaging produces potentially high-resolution images with well-defined detail without the use of ionizing radiation but requires a long scan time with cardiac gating (Axel et al., 1983). While ultrasound has poorer image quality than some types of CT, echo scans are economical and scanners are portable.

Several investigators have attempted to reconstruct three-dimensional anatomy of the heart from two-dimensional echocardiograms from limited angles of view (Fazzalari et al., 1984, Moritz et al., 1983, Geiser et al., 1982). Most analysis of echo data to date are limited to display and computation of parameters of the left ventricle. Due to incomplete data from the epicardium as well as the difficulty identifying an accurate endocardial surface, three-dimensional analysis has not become widely utilized.

The aim of the present study is to develop scanning methodology and recently developed analysis tools (Hoffman and Ritman, 1985, Hoffman and Heffernan, 1986) to enable accurate display and interpretation of the heart in three dimensions using data obtained from conventional echo sector scanners, readily available in most medical facilities. By obtaining an appropriate data set, more complete information is available for analysis. Ultimately, quantitative cardiac parameters may be computed describing the dynamic behavior of the normal and abnormal heart.

METHODS

Data Acquisition

Scans were performed using a Diasonics Cardiovue 100 scanner with a 3.5 MHz probe (S/N 1006). The transducer was mounted on a cylindrical holder which was attached to a DC stepper motor to rotate the transducer in specific increments. This rotation was computer controlled (Perkin-Elmer 7/32) with equal steps programmed for a total rotation of 180° (3.6 degree increments for 50 angles of view). The position of the transducer was adjusted so that the acoustical beam was centered (i.e., center was unchanged with transducer rotation) in the axis of rotation prior to scanning the heart. The scanner parameters were adjusted to obtain the most visually appealing data set.

Two excised canine hearts were scanned to validate the technique. The chambers of the heart were either gelatin-filled or inflated under pressure and subsequently water filled. Similarly, two excised porcine hearts with anatomical defects were scanned. In one an atrial septal defect and in the other a ventricular septal defect was artificially created. The isolated heart was immersed in a water bath and fixed in position. The experimental set up is shown in Figure 1. The ultrasound transducer was placed in the holder, to permit motor-driven rotation. At each incremental step of the transducer rotation, the data were digitized on-line (Datacube A/D converter) and stored on disk for subsequent image reconstruction. For each single image, 256 x 256 pixel arrays containing the sector scan were sampled and stored. All image processing and reconstruction was performed on a Charles River Data System UNIVERSE 68000 microcomputer workstation.

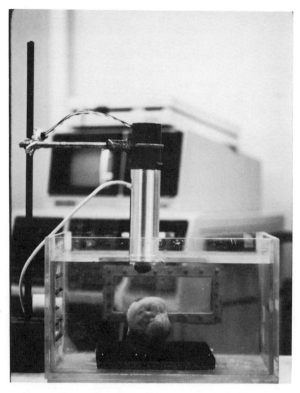

Figure 1 Experimental equipment with a motor-driven transducer immersed in a water bath containing an excised heart is shown. The transducer rotates about a fixed axis, producing sector scans incrementally over 180°.

After a complete set of data was acquired, image reconstruction proceeded off-line. The data were reduced to a 128 x 128 pixel array. The nth line of data from each sector scan was used to generate the nth level image. The corresponding lines of data were superimposed at their respective angles of rotation. Overlapping data were normalized by the number of coincident data points. Nearest neighbors were used to interpolate and fill in regions of missing data. Three x three averaging over the image replaced absent data with average values at the outer edges of the image. The volume images were then analyzed and displayed on the workstation using special-purpose software developed for three-dimensional multi-source fast CT data sets (Hoffman and Heffernan, 1986, Robb et al., 1986).

Data Analysis and Display

The data were initially examined on a three-dimensional varifocal mirror display. Existing software tools for the vibrating mirror system allowed image manipulation, generation of oblique sections, as well as visualization of the internal structures of the heart from the raw data set (Harris et al., 1986). The images were then enhanced and manipulated to generate various means of examining the data. Shaded surface displays, a three-dimensional geometric representation on a two-dimensional raster display, were created for the whole heart, showing the epicardial surface, for the atrial and/or ventricular chambers alone, displaying the endocardial surfaces as well as the myocardium (from the difference images of the whole heart minus the chambers). Prior to generating a surface display, the boundaries of the heart chambers had to be identified, either by gray level thresholding or operator-interactive tracing or editing. A binary image of the whole heart was generated; a binary image of the chambers was also created (Hoffman and Ritman, 1985). Each binary image underwent processing to identify connected borders. Ultimately, the surfaces were displayed and rotated to allow viewing from all aspects of the three-dimensional volume.

Oblique sections can also be generated for subsequent display (Harris, 1981). From this analysis module, for instance, short axis and long axis standard echocardiographic sections of the heart can be obtained. Further, to generate stereo image pairs for pseudo three-dimensional perspective, an oblique image can be computed at a 6° increment from an initial image (Greenleaf, 1982). Other analysis modules allow display of projection images, numerical biopsy (to sample regional gray levels), image manipulation and operator-interactive editing with minimal difficulty.

RESULTS

Two normal dog hearts and two pig hearts with anatomical defects were scanned. The sequential sector scans were obtained and collected as described above. The image data were reconstructed (Figure 2, left side) and interpolated (Figure 2, right side) to generate a stack of 128 images. The intensity at each pixel is represented by an 8-bit data value corresponding to gray levels between 0 and 255. Using the CRDS UNIVERSE 68000-based image analysis workstation, a variety of display modalities were investigated. For instance, oblique sections may be generated in any orientation such as long- and short-axis views (Figure 3), and used to create stereo image pairs.

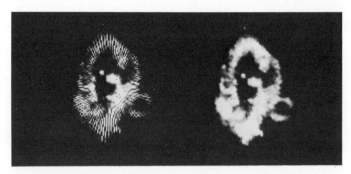

Figure 2   The reconstructed image is shown on the left prior to interpolating and filling in missing data. The resulting interpolated image is displayed on the right.

To obtain a three-dimensional representation of the endo- and epicardial surfaces of the heart, a shaded surface display was generated. For the normal dog heart, binary images of the whole heart were obtained by gray level thresholding and operator-interactive editing (Figure 4a). Binary images were created for the ventricular and/or atrial chambers alone (Figure 4b). After edge extraction, surface displays were rotated

to show the whole heart epicardium (Figure 5a) and atrial and/or ventricular endocardium (Figure 5b) from any view. The normal dog heart was
"sliced" in half to display the inside of the heart as well (Figure 5c).

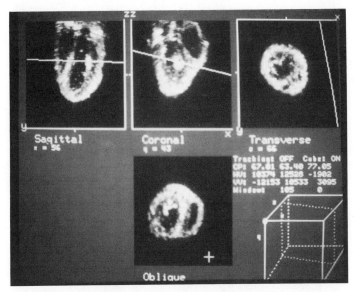

<u>Figure 3</u> The lower center image is an example of an oblique section of
a normal dog heart. Three orthogonal views with lines indicating the
orientation of the oblique views are displayed in the upper row.

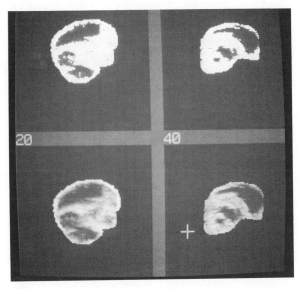

<u>Figure 4a</u> Thresholded binary images of the epicardium are shown in the
upper row and their corresponding gray level images on the lower row.

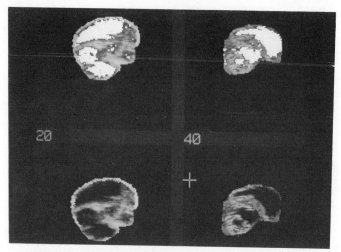

Figure 4b   Binary images are created to segment the heart chambers. Upper images show the endocardial space in white and beneath are the original gray level images.

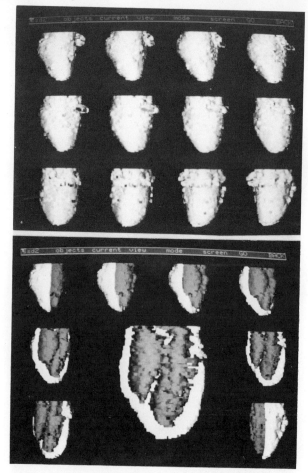

Figure 5a and b   Upper panel shows computer-generated shaded surface displays of the epicardial surfaces of a gelatin-filled normal dog heart separated by 15° increments.   Lower panel shows the same heart with half the myocardium (light gray) stripped away to show the casted surface of the ventricular chambers (dark gray). In the expanded center image, the septal division, right and left ventricular chambers, and ascending aorta are clearly visualized.

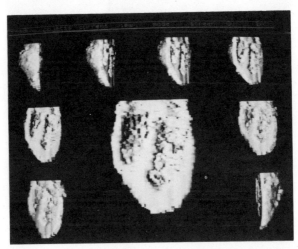

Figure 5c Shaded surfaces displayed from multiple viewing angles showing endocardial surfaces of the right and left ventricles and ascending aorta.

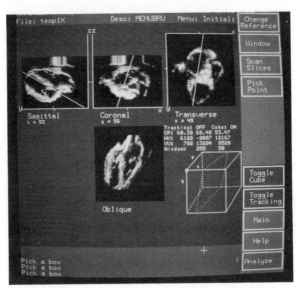

Figure 6a Oblique views of excised pig heart showing the atrial septal defect.

An alternate method for examining three-dimensional data is to move through a volume of images in any oblique orientation. By generating and displaying oblique sections, the anatomical defects in the in vitro pig heart images are visible. Figure 6a demonstrates this technique for visualizing the ventricular defect.

Thus, from a sector scanning protocol with a single transducer position, rotated to obtain scans of 50 views over 180°, adequate image

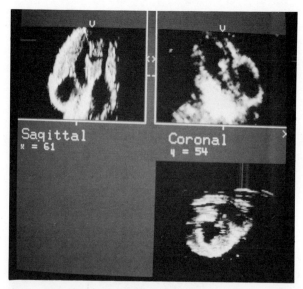

Figure 6b In vitro pig heart with ventricular septal defect is displayed here in oblique sections.

quality and sufficient data were acquired to produce three-dimensional displays of the endo- and epicardial surfaces and internal structures of the heart. Thus, without any geometrical models or assumptions, a three-dimensional reconstruction from two-dimensional echo sector scans was obtained from in vitro ultrasonic imaging of the heart.

DISCUSSION

Our preliminary findings from in vitro imaging of dog and pig hearts suggest that the techniques under development are capable of generating volume image sets which upon reconstruction produce adequate data for complete endo- and epicardial surface identification. While these results are qualitative, by obtaining more angles of view than previous work by other investigators (Sawada et al., 1983, Nixon et al., 1983, Geiser et al., 1982, Matsumoto et al., 1981), we can expect more accurate border recognition, perhaps allowing subsequent calculation of cardiac parameters. Further, incremental rotation of the transducer from a fixed position requires relatively simple subsequent image reconstruction and interpolation and lends itself to in vivo situations.

The present method does face several hurdles. The image quality of the raw data is less than desirable because of noise, extraneous reflections, and inhomogeneity of signal received over regions of heart. This creates a distinct challenge for the desired automation of image analysis. Currently, considerable operator interaction to identify noise versus signal in the images and to assist in identifying endo- and epicardial borders is required. Techniques for automated surface detection are presently under investigation.

Another limitation is the constraint on transducer positioning due to available degrees of freedom. For dynamic imaging of in vivo human hearts, this scanning system appears inadequate to scan the entire expanse of the heart. Use of an articulated arm is under consideration to assist probe placement, while allowing motor-driven transducer rotation in a fixed location.

One of the advantages of the present data acquisition method is that the transducer position can be adjusted to obtain an optimal image and view of the heart throughout the transducer rotation. Since we are not constrained to a particular scanning view (i.e., standard precordial and apical views), we can adjust transducer position to obtain the best possible data set. Other investigators have used apical long and short axis views (Sawada et al., 1983, Ghosh et al., 1982, Nixon et al., 1983), precordial views (Geiser et al., 1980, Matsumoto et al., 1981) or combinations of both (Moritz et al., 1983). The present technique, due to clear identification of transducer position, also allows reconstruction of the sector scans into tomograms using a relatively simple algorithm compared with complex computation of others (Geiser et al., 1980, Moritz et al., 1983, Stickels and Wann, 1984).

Due to the small number of views acquired in previous studies, typically 5 to 12 views (Ghosh et al., 1982, Sawada et al., 1983, Nixon et al., 1983, Geiser et al., 1980), insufficient data were available to form complete endocardial boundaries without gross interpolation or the assumption of a geometric model. Further, detection of epicardial surfaces was not even attempted in earlier work due to missing data and poor resolution. Three-dimensional displays from these previous studies were limited to wire mesh-like display of the left ventricle (Skorton et al., 1986). Although we could further improve image quality with larger numbers of views, sequential sector scans provide adequate data to not only define myocardial boundaries, but also to allow visualization of other structures within the heart as well (e.g., septal defects). Shaded surface displays also help evaluate the completeness of the volume image set.

While the present study shows preliminary results of in vitro heart scans, application to in vivo scanning appears feasible. Requisite quantitative validation of the in vitro technique is in progress. With increased angles of view available with the present technique for reconstruction, more accurate cardiac parameters, including chamber volumes, myocardial muscle mass, and wall thickness, may be achievable. Hopefully, with slight modifications, this scanning method and data analysis will be useful for three-dimensional dynamic cardiac imaging in humans. Potentially, tissue characterization and three-dimensional texture analysis will provide further information about myocardial properties. Echo sector scanning is both relatively low cost and portable. Thus, development of accurate three-dimensional imaging utilizing this modality is a promising alternative to the other available multidimensional imaging approaches.

ACKNOWLEDGMENTS

The authors wish to acknowledge the advice and technical assistance provided by Dr. Patrick Heffernan and the efforts of Ms. Elaine Quarve in manuscript preparation.

This work was supported in part by Grants HL-07111, HL-04664, and RR-02540 from the National Institutes of Health.

REFERENCES

Axel, L., Herman, G. T., Udupa, J. K., Bottomley, P. A. and Edelstein, W. A., 1983, Three-dimensional display of nuclear magnetic resonance (NMR) cardiovascular images, J. Comput. Assist. Tomogr., 7:172.

Fazzalari, N. L., Davidson, J. A., Mazumdar, J., Mahar, L. J., and DeNardi, E., 1984, Three-dimensional reconstruction of the left ventricle from four anatomically defined apical two-dimensional echocardiographic views, Acta Cardiol. (Brux), 39:409.

Geiser, E. A., Ariet, M., Conetta, D. A., Lupkiewicz, S. M., Christie, L. G., and Conti, R. C., 1982, Dynamic three-dimensional echocardiographic reconstruction of the intact human left ventricle: Technique and initial observations in patients, Am. Heart J., 103:1056.

Geiser, E. A., Lupkiewicz, S. M., Christie, L. G., Ariet, M., Conetta, D. A., and Conti, C. R., 1980, A framework for three-dimensional time-varying reconstruction of the human left ventricle: sources of error and estimation of their magnitude, Comput. Biomed. Res., 13:225.

Ghosh, A., Nanda, N. C., and Maurer, G., 1982, Three-dimensional reconstruction of echocardiographic images using the rotation method, Ultrasound Med. Biol., 8:655.

Greenleaf, J. F., 1982, Three-dimensional imaging in ultrasound, J. Med. Syst., 6(6):579.

Harris, L. D., 1981, Identification of the optimal orientation of oblique sections through multiple parallel CT images, J. Comput. Assist. Tomogr., 5:881.

Harris, L. D., Camp, J. J., Ritman, E. L., and Robb, R. A., 1986, Three-dimensional display and analysis of tomographic volume images utilizing a varifocal mirror, IEEE Trans. Med. Imag., MI-5:67.

Hoffman, E. A. and Heffernan, P. B., 1986, Investigation of the intrathoracic determinants of cardiac geometry aided by an improved interactive approach to the manipulation of surfaces. NCGA Computer Graphics '86, III:151.

Hoffman, E. A. and Ritman, E. L., 1985, Shape and dimensions of cardiac chambers via computed tomography: Role of image slice thickness and orientation, Radiol., 155:739.

Matsumoto, M., Inoue, M., Tamura, S., Tanaka, K., and Abe, H., 1981, Three-dimensional echocardiography for spatial visualization and volume calculation of cardiac structures, Ultrasound, 9:157.

Moritz, W. E., Pearlman, A. S., McCabe, D. H., Medema, D. K., Ainsworth, M. E., Boles, M. S., 1983, An ultrasonic technique for imaging the ventricle in three dimensions and calculating its volume, IEEE Trans. Biomed. Eng., BME-30:482.

Nixon, J. V., Saffer, S. I., Lipscomb, K., and Blomqvist, C. G., 1983, Three-dimensional echoventriculography, Am. Heart J., 106:435.

Ritman, E. L., Robb, R. A., and Harris, L. D., 1985, in: "Imaging Physiological Functions: Experience with the DSR," Praeger, Philadelphia, PA.

Robb, R. A., Ritman, E. L., and Harris, L. D., 1986, Digital imaging processing x-ray computed tomography: High speed volume imaging with the DSR, in: "Cardiac Imaging and Image Processing," S. M. Collins and D. J. Skorton, eds., McGraw-Hill, New York.

Sawada, H., Fugii, J., Kato, K., Onoe, M., and Kuno, Y., 1983, Three-dimensional reconstruction of the left ventricle from multiple cross sectional echocardiograms: Value for measuring left ventricular volume, Br. Heart J., 50:438.

Skorton, D. J., Collins, S. M., and Kerber, R. E., 1986, Digital image processing and analysis in echocardiography, in: "Cardiac Imaging and Image Processing," S. M. Collins and D. J. Skorton, eds., McGraw-Hill, NY.

Stickels, K. R. and Wann, L. S., 1984, An analysis of three-dimensional reconstructive echocardiography, Ultrasound Med. Biol., 10:575.

OPTIMAL INCIDENT ANGLES IN SCANNING TOMOGRAPHIC MICROSCOPY

Paul C.H. Chen and Glen Wade

Department of Electrical & Computer Engineering
University of California, Santa Barbara, CA 93106

ABSTRACT

The scanning tomographic acoustic microscope utilizes principles of digital tomography to obtain high-resolution subsurface imaging. An algorithm based on back-and-forth propagation is employed to reconstruct the tomograms. We have shown that the expected mean-squares error is a minimum and the source matrix is simply the identity matrix if the object is illuminated from certain optimal incident angles.

In usual practice, however, the object is insonified from angles separated from each other by a fixed interval thus giving a uniform angular spacing. The source matrix in this case is no longer the identity matrix as for the optimal case. This paper presents a quantitative analysis of the degradation of the image caused by using uniformly-spaced incident angles. We introduce a term we call "normalized error" and we present a theoretical analysis based on this term. We show that for a one-dimensional image the asymptote for the least upper bound of the normalized error as the number of pixels goes to infinity is $\frac{\pi}{2}-1$ or 0.5708.

1.   INTRODUCTION

The scanning tomographic acoustic microscope (STAM) utilizes principles of tomography and incorporates digital signal processing to obtain high-resolution subsurface imaging [1-5]. STAM makes use of elements from an existing ultrasonic microscope, the scanning laser acoustic microscope (SLAM), which detects the acoustic field with a scanning laser as shown in Fig. 1. In STAM, the data are acquired on a fixed receiving plane while the propagation direction of the·insonifying plane wave is varied. This is different from the case of the conventional tomographic imaging system in which the receiving plane is usually perpendicular to the direction of the propagation of the insonifying waves [6-8]. The STAM system is most suitable for imaging objects with planar structure. Because of the relatively long wavelength of ultrasound, diffraction takes place as the radiation propagates through the object being imaged. This type of ultrasonic tomography is called planar diffraction tomography.

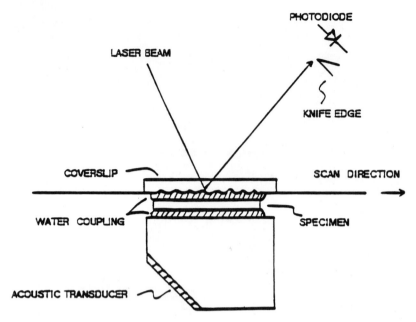

Fig. 1.   System diagram for the scanning laser acoustic
microscope (SLAM).

An algorithm called "back-and-forth propagation" has been used to reconstruct STAM tomograms [9,10]. The algorithm is most suitable for planar diffraction tomography in which the structure of interest lies in various well-defined planes. In back-and-forth propagation, the received wavefield and the source wavefield are computationally propagated back and forth respectively to a specific plane of interest. A least-squares estimate of the planar distribution within the object is then formed to obtain a tomogram of that layer.

In a previous paper an estimation that has minimum variance in the reconstruction of acoustical transmittance is treated [11]. The expected mean-squares error is determined by two factors: 1) the total number of the projections and 2) the nature of the eigenvalue distribution of the source matrix. The theoretical lower bound of the expected mean-squares error is obtained when the eigenvalues of the source matrix are all the same. The incident angles for the set of plane waves that possesses this property are called the optimal incident angles. For this optimal scheme, the source matrix is simply an identity matrix. Thus, no matrix inversion is required in computing an image. This property facilitates the computation in reconstructing images.

However, in usual practice, the object is insonified from uniformly-spaced incident angles obtained by sequentially increasing the angles through a fixed interval. We will refer to the set of angles thus obtained as the uniform incident angles. In this case, the minimum-variance solution requires computing the source matrix first and then inverting it. This computation becomes the dominant part of the data processing. In this paper, we analyze the degradation of the image caused by using this uniform scheme when we compute the image by simply assuming the source matrix as the identity matrix. We define a normalized error to give a quantitative measure of this degradation. We show that for a one-dimensional image, the asymptotic value of the least upper bound of the normalized error as the number of pixels approaches infinity is equal to $\frac{\pi}{2} - 1$ or 0.5708. This figure reveals the relative image degradation caused by using the uniform scheme rather than the optimal scheme.

In the notation observed throughout this paper lower-case letters represent scalars, a bar over a lower-case letter represents a row vector, an arrow over a lower-case letter represents a vector, a hat over a letter represents an estimation value and a capital letter represents a matrix.

2. PROBLEM FORMULATION

Assume we have an object of planar structure which is insonified by an ultrasonic wave from below as shown in Fig. 2. The object is homogeneous to the ultrasound except at plane z_2 which contains elements of different elastic composition. The wavefield at plane z_1 is $u_1(x,y)$. The acoustic waves travel through the object and the wavefield just below plane z_2 is $u_2(x,y)$. The relation between $u_1(x,y)$ and $u_2(x,y)$ can be expressed by the Rayleigh-Sommerfeld diffraction formula [12].

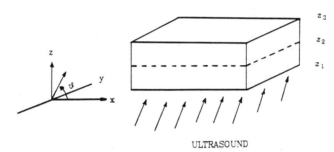

ULTRASOUND

Fig. 2. An object of planar structure insonified by ultrasound coming from below.

$$u_2(x,y) = u_1(x,y) ** w(x,y,z_1,z_2) \tag{2-1}$$

with

$$w(x,y,z_1,z_2) = \frac{|z_2-z_1|}{2\pi} \frac{1-jkr}{r^3} e^{jkr} \tag{2-2}$$

where $r = [x^2+y^2+(z_2-z_1)^2]^{\frac{1}{2}}$, $k = \frac{2\pi}{\lambda}$, λ is the wavelength, and ** denotes two-dimensional convolution. In the Fourier domain Eqs. (2-1) and (2-2) can be replaced by

$$\bar{U}_2(f_x,f_y) = \bar{U}_1(f_x,f_y)\bar{W}(f_x,f_y,z_1,z_2) \tag{2-3}$$

$$\bar{W}(f_x,f_y,z_1,z_2) = \exp[jk(z_2-z_1)(1-f_x^2\lambda^2-f_y^2\lambda^2)^{\frac{1}{2}}] \tag{2-4}$$

where $\bar{U}_1(f_x,f_y)$ is the Fourier transform of $u_1(x,y)$ and $\bar{U}_2(f_x,f_y)$ is the Fourier transform of $u_2(x,y)$. The values of the wavefield are sampled along the points of a rectangular grid of N pixels. We consider the pixels in the grid sequentially according to a certain fixed order and we can write the expression in Eq. (2-1) as

$$\bar{u}_2 = \bar{u}_1 \, W(z_1,z_2) \tag{2-5}$$

where $\bar{u}_2$ and $\bar{u}_1$ are 1xN row vectors of pixel values of the wavefields u_2 and u_1. $W(z_1,z_2)$ is an NxN Toeplitz matrix, representing forward propagation between z_1 and z_2.

At plane z_2, $u_2(x,y)$ is modified by the transmittance associated with the layer. For the general case, the wavefield transmitted through plane z_2, u_2', can be expressed as [13]

$$\bar{u}_2' = \bar{u}_2 \, T \tag{2-6}$$

where $\bar{u}_2'$ is the row vectors of the pixel values of the wavefield u_2' and T is the transmittance matrix at $z=z_2$ which characterizes the relation between the incident and transmitted wavefields. The modified wavefield u_2' then propagates to plane z_3, the receiving plane, and becomes $u_3(x,y)$ with

$$\bar{u}_3 = \bar{u}_2' \, W(z_2,z_3) \tag{2-7}$$

where $\bar{u}_3$ is the row vector of the pixel values of the wavefield u_3 and $W(z_2,z_3)$ is the forward propagation matrix between depth z_2 and z_3. Because of scattering within the object from unknown structural elements outside the z_2 plane the wavefield measured at the receiving plane, $v_3(x,y)$, is different from the calculated wavefield u_3. We can computationally back-propagate the measured wavefield $v_3(x,y)$ to z_2 by using

$$\bar{v}_2 = \bar{v}_3 \, W^{-1}(z_2,z_3) \tag{2-8}$$

where $\bar{v}_2$ and $\bar{v}_3$ are the row vectors of the pixel values of the wavefield v_2 and v_3, and $W^{-1}(z_2,z_3) = W^*(z_2,z_3)$ is the back propagation matrix between depth z_2 and z_3. W^* represents the complex congugate of W. Because of the unknown scattering outside the z_2 plane, the wavefield $v_2(x,y)$ will not be the same as $u_2'(x,y)$ and can be represented by

$$\bar{v}_2 = \bar{u}_2' + \bar{n} = \bar{u}_2 T + \bar{n} \tag{2-9}$$

where $\bar{n}$ is a 1xN row vector representing effects of the unknown scattering outside the z_2 plane. For convenience, the subscripts in Eq. (2-9) will be dropped. They should not be confused with subscripts we will need to use later in order to indicate the order of the projections. Eq. (2-9) can be written as

$$\bar{v} = \bar{u}T + \bar{n} \tag{2-10}$$

Consider M projections generated by the planar sources of insonification with M different incident angles as shown in Fig. 3. From the projections we obtain a set of equations

$$\bar{v}_m = \bar{u}_m T + \bar{n}_m, \qquad m=1,2,\ldots\ldots,M \qquad \qquad (2\text{-}11)$$

where m represents the new subscripts indicating the order of the projections. The row vectors in Eq. (2-11) can be combined into a matrix formulation as follows

$$V = UT + N \qquad \qquad (2\text{-}12)$$

where V, U, N are MxN matrices consisting of M row vectors.

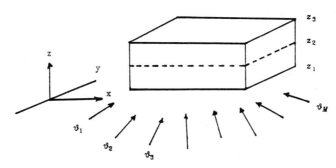

Figure 3.   Object insonification from M different incident
angles for generating M projections sequentially.

When we have no a priori information concerning the transmittance and assume the undesired signal components are uncorrelated from projection to projection, the minimum-variance estimate of T, denoted by $\hat{T}$, is given by [11]

$$\hat{T} = A_N^{-1} U^{*T}(V-N_0), \qquad \qquad (2\text{-}13)$$

where $N_0 = E(N)$ and U^{*T} represents the adjoint matrix of U. A_N is the so-called source matrix which is positive definite and given by [11]

$$A_N = [a_{pq}] = \begin{bmatrix} M & a_{12} & & & & a_{1N} \\ a_{21} & M & & & & \cdot \\ a_{31} & a_{32} & \cdot & \cdot & \cdot & \cdot & \cdot & \cdot & \cdot \\ & & \cdot & \cdot & & & \cdot \\ & & \cdot & \cdot & & & \cdot \\ & & \cdot & \cdot & & & \cdot \\ a_{N1} & a_{N2} & & & & M \end{bmatrix} \qquad (2\text{-}14)$$

with

$$a_{pq} = \sum_{m=1}^{M} \exp[j\vec{k}_m \cdot (\vec{r}_q - \vec{r}_p)] \qquad p,q = 1,2,\ldots\ldots,N \qquad (2\text{-}15)$$

where $\vec{r}_p$ and $\vec{r}_q$ are the position vectors of the p-th and q-th pixels of the rectangular grids. $\vec{k}_m$ is the wavevector of the m-th incident plane wave. From Eq. (2-15), we notice that $a_{qp} = a^*_{pq}$. For the two-dimensional case in which no variation in the y-direction is assumed, Eq. (2-15) can be expressed as

$$a_{pq} = a_{q-p} = \sum_{m=1}^{M} \exp[jk(q-p)\cos\vartheta_m \Delta x] \qquad p,q=1,2,\ldots\ldots,N \qquad (2\text{-}16)$$

where ϑ_m is the angle that the wavevector $\vec{k}_m$ makes with respect to the positive x-axis and Δx is the interval between adjacent pixels in the x-direction. In order to satisfy the Nyquist criterion we choose $\Delta x = \frac{\lambda}{2}$. Eq. (2-16) then becomes

$$a_{q-p} = \sum_{m=1}^{M} \exp[j(q-p)\pi\cos\vartheta_m] \qquad p,q=1,2,\ldots\ldots,N \qquad (2\text{-}17)$$

It has been shown that the expected mean-squares error associated with Eq. (2-13) is minimum when the angles of the incident plane waves are [11]

$$\vartheta_m = \cos^{-1}\frac{M+2-2m}{M} \qquad m = 1,2,\ldots\ldots M \qquad (2\text{-}18)$$

The set of angles given in Eq. (2-18) constitutes what may be called the "optimal incident angles." In this case, the source matrix A_N becomes identity matrix (except for a constant multiplier M) and Eq. (2-13) reduces to

$$\hat{T} = U^{*T}(V-N_0) \qquad (2\text{-}19)$$

From Eq. (2-19), we see that no matrix inversion is required in computing images. This property facilitates the computation in reconstructing images. However, as stated in the introduction, the uniform scheme which is used in practice does not possess this property. In the following section, we will analyze image degradation caused by using the uniform scheme when we compute the image from Eq. (2-19).

3. ERROR CAUSED BY USING UNIFORMLY-SPACED INCIDENT ANGLES

Consider the case of uniformly-spaced incident angles distributed between 0 and 180 degrees. If M is large, then Eq. (2-17) can be written in a integral form as

$$a_{q-p} = \frac{M}{\pi} \int_0^{\pi} \exp[j\pi(q-p)\cos\vartheta]d\vartheta$$

$$= MJ_0[(q-p)\pi] \qquad p,q = 1,2,\ldots\ldots,N \qquad (3\text{-}1)$$

where J_0 is the zero order Bessel function of the first kind. The source matrix associated with the uniform incident angles, A_N becomes

$$A_N = \begin{bmatrix} 1 & J_0(\pi) & J_0[(N-1)\pi] \\ & & \vdots \\ J_0(\pi) & 1 & \vdots \\ J_0(2\pi) & J_0(\pi) & \cdots \cdots & \vdots \\ \vdots & \vdots & & \vdots \\ J_0[(N-1)\pi] & J_0[(N-2)\pi] & & 1 \end{bmatrix} \qquad (3-2)$$

Neglecting the constant multiplier M in Eq. (3-2), we obtain from Eqs. (2-13) and (2-19)

$$\hat{T} - \hat{\hat{T}} = (A_N^{-1} - I) U^{*T} (V - N_0) \qquad (3-3)$$

where I is the identity matrix. The error associated with each column of $\hat{T} - \hat{\hat{T}}$, denoted by E_N, is given by

$$E_N = \| (A_N^{-1} - I) v' \| \qquad (3-4)$$

where v' is the corresponding column of $U^{*T}(V - N_0)$. The normalized error, e_N, is defined by

$$e_N \equiv \frac{E_N}{\| v' \|} = \frac{\| A_N^{-1} - I) v' \|}{\| v' \|} \qquad (3-5)$$

The least upper bound of e_N, denoted by sup e_N, is given by

$$\text{sup } e_N = \text{sup} \frac{\| (A_N^{-1} - I) v' \|}{\| v' \|} = \| A_N^{-1} - I \| \qquad (3-6)$$

where $\| A_N^{-1} - I \|$ is the norm of $A_N^{-1} - I$. It can be shown that [14]

$$\| A_N^{-1} - I \| = \sqrt{\lambda_{N,max}} \qquad (3-7)$$

where $\lambda_{N,max}$ is the largest eigenvalue of a matrix given by

$$Q = (A_N^{-1} - I)^{*T} (A_N^{-1} - I) \qquad (3-8)$$

Let $\lambda'_{N1}, \lambda'_{N2}, \ldots \ldots, \lambda'_{NN}$ be the eigenvalues of A_N, then the eigenvalues of Q, denoted by $\lambda_{N1}, \lambda_{N2}, \ldots \ldots, \lambda_{NN}$, are

$$\lambda_{Nn} = \left(\frac{1}{\lambda'_{Nn}}\right)^2 - \frac{2}{\lambda'_{Nn}} + 1 \qquad n = 1, 2, \ldots, N \qquad (3-9)$$

For N = 2, we have

$$A_2 = \begin{bmatrix} 1 & J_0(\pi) \\ J_0(\pi) & 1 \end{bmatrix} \qquad (3-10)$$

The eigenvalues are A_2 are given by

$$\lambda'_{21} = 1 - J_0(\pi)$$

$$\lambda'_{22} = 1 + J_0(\pi) \qquad (3-11)$$

It can be shown that

$$\sqrt{\lambda_{2,\max}} = \frac{1}{1 - J_0(\pi)} - 1$$

$$= 0.4364 \qquad (3-12)$$

For N = 3,

$$A_S = \begin{bmatrix} 1 & J_0(\pi)J_0(2\pi) \\ J_0(\pi) & 1 & J_0(\pi) \\ J_0(2\pi)J_0(\pi) & 1 \end{bmatrix} \qquad (3-13)$$

The eigenvalues of A_3 are given by

$$\lambda'_{31} = 1 + \frac{J_0(2\pi)}{2}\left[1 - \sqrt{1 + 8\left(\frac{J_0(\pi)}{J_0(2\pi)}\right)^2}\right]$$

$$\lambda'_{32} = 1 - J_0(2\pi)$$

$$\lambda'_{33} = 1 + \frac{J_0(2\pi)}{2}\left[1 + \sqrt{1 + 8\left(\frac{J_0(\pi)}{J_0(2\pi)}\right)^2}\right] \qquad (3-14)$$

and

$$\sqrt{\lambda_{3,\max}} = \frac{1}{\lambda'_{31}} - 1$$

$$= 0.5007 \tag{3-15}$$

For N = 4,

$$A_4 = \begin{bmatrix} 1 & J_0(\pi) & J_0(2\pi) & J_0(3\pi) \\ J_0(\pi) & 1 & J_0(\pi) & J_0(2\pi) \\ J_0(2\pi) & J_0(\pi) & 1 & J_0(\pi) \\ J_0(3\pi) & J_0(2\pi) & J_0(\pi) & 1 \end{bmatrix} \tag{3-16}$$

The eigenvalues of A_4 are given by

$$\lambda'_{41} = 1 - \frac{J_0(\pi)+J_0(3\pi)}{2} - \sqrt{(\frac{J_0(\pi)-J_0(3\pi)}{2})^2 + (J_0(\pi)-J_0(2\pi))^2}$$

$$\lambda'_{42} = 1 + \frac{J_0(\pi)+J_0(3\pi)}{2} - \sqrt{(\frac{J_0(\pi)-J_0(3\pi)}{2})^2 + (J_0(\pi)+J_0(2\pi))^2}$$

$$\lambda'_{43} = 1 - \frac{J_0(\pi)+J_0(3\pi)}{2} + \sqrt{(\frac{J_0(\pi)-J_0(3\pi)}{2})^2 + (J_0(\pi)-J_0(2\pi))^2}$$

$$\lambda'_{44} = 1 + \frac{J_0(\pi)+J_0(3\pi)}{2} + \sqrt{(\frac{J_0(\pi)-J_0(3\pi)}{2})^2 + (J_0(\pi)+J_0(2\pi))^2} \tag{3-17}$$

and

$$\sqrt{\lambda_{4,max}} = \frac{1}{\lambda'_{42}} - 1$$

$$= 0.5302 \tag{3-18}$$

These values of N are obviously too low to be very practical, and as N becomes large, the solutions become very complicated. In the next section, we present the asymptotic solution for N approaching infinity.

4. ASYMPTOTIC PROPERTY OF THE ERROR

We now introduce a new variable of integration s given by the equation

$$s = -\pi\cos\vartheta \tag{4-1}$$

Using this new variable, we can express Eq. (3-1) as

$$a_n = \frac{1}{\pi^2} \int_{-\pi}^{\pi} \frac{1}{\sqrt{1-(\frac{s}{\pi})^2}} e^{-jns} \, ds \qquad n = 0, \pm 1, \pm 2, \ldots \ldots, \pm N-1 \qquad (4-2)$$

We neglect the constant M in Eq. (4-2). From Eq. (4-2), we see that a_n is the Fourier coefficient of the function f(s) given by

$$f(s) = \frac{2}{\pi\sqrt{1-(\frac{s}{\pi})^2}} \qquad -\pi \leq s \leq \pi \qquad (4-3)$$

Thus, f(s) can be represented by a Fourier series

$$f(s) = \sum_{n=-\infty}^{\infty} a_n e^{jns} \qquad (4-4)$$

Consider a Hermitian function, $T_{N-1}(f)$, defined by

$$T_{N-1}(f) = \sum_{p=1}^{N} \sum_{q=1}^{N} a_{q-p} \eta_p \eta_q^* \qquad (4-5)$$

where $\eta_1, \eta_2, \ldots \ldots, \eta_N$ are N scalar variables. Substituting Eq. (4-2) into Eq. (4-5), we obtain

$$T_{N-1}(f) = \frac{1}{2\pi} \int_{-\pi}^{\pi} \left| \eta_1 e^{js} + \eta_2 e^{j2s} + \ldots \ldots + \eta_N e^{jNs} \right|^2 f(s) \, ds \qquad (4-6)$$

Equation (4-6) is the Toeplitz form of the function f(s). The eigenvalues of A_N, $\lambda'_{N1}, \lambda'_{N2}, \ldots \ldots, \lambda'_{NN}$, are defined as the roots of the characteristic equation $\det T_{N-1}(f-\lambda^N) = 0$.

The asymptotic behavior of the eigenvalues of A_N can be calculated by using the equal distributions theorem of Toeplitz forms [15]. This yields eigenvalues given by

$$\lambda_{Nn} = \frac{2}{\pi\sqrt{1-(\frac{n}{N+1})^2}} \qquad n = 1, \ldots \ldots, N, \quad N \to \infty \qquad (4-7)$$

or

$$\lambda'_\infty(s) = \frac{2}{\pi\sqrt{1-(\frac{s}{\pi})^2}} \qquad -\pi \leq s \leq \pi \qquad (4-8)$$

From Eqs. (3-9) and (4-8), we obtain

$$\lambda_\infty(s) = (\frac{1}{\lambda'_\infty(s)})^2 - \frac{2}{\lambda'_\infty(s)} + 1 \qquad (4\text{-}9)$$

Let $\lambda_{\infty,max}$ be the maximum of $\lambda_\infty(s)$. From Eqs. (4-8) and (4-9) we can show that

$$\lambda_{\infty,max} = (\frac{1}{\lambda'_\infty(0)} - 1)^2 = (\frac{\pi}{2} - 1)^2 \qquad (4\text{-}10)$$

Thus,

$$\sup e_\infty = \lim_{N \to \infty} \sup e_N = \sqrt{\lambda_{\infty,max}} = \frac{\pi}{2} - 1 \qquad (4\text{-}11)$$

or 0.5708

5. Conclusions

In this paper, we present a quantitative analysis of the image degradation caused by using uniformly-spaced incident angles and assuming that the source matrix is the identity matrix. We show that for a one-dimensional image with an infinite number of pixels, the least upper bound of normalized error associated with this degradation can be as large as 57%. When we use optimal incident angles, the source matrix is simply the identity matrix and no image degradation takes place. Therefore, the use of optimal angles can be expected to save computation time and to avoid image degradation.

6. References

1. L. W. Kessler and D. E. Yuhas, "Acoustic Microscopy - 1979", Proc. IEEE, Vol. 67, pp. 526-536, April 1979.

2. Z. C. Lin, H. Lee, G. Wade and C. F. Schueler, "Computer-Assisted Tomographic Acoustic Microscopy for Subsurface Imaging," Acoustical Imaging, Vol. 13, pp. 91-105, Eds. M. Kaveh, R. K. Mueller and J. F. Greenleaf, Plenum Press, New York, 1983.

3. Z. C. Lin, H. Lee, G. Wade, M. G. Oravecz and L. W. Kessler, "Data Acquisition in Tomographic Acoustic Microscopy," Proceedings of the 1983 IEEE Ultrasonics Symposium, pp. 627-631, Atlanta, Georgia, November 1983.

4. Z. C. Lin, H. Lee, and G. Wade, "Scanning Tomographic Acoustic Microscope," The Microelectronics Innovation and Computer Research Opportunity (MICRO) Report, University of California, pp. 138-141, 1981-1982.

5. Z. C. Lin, G. Wade and H. Lee, "Scanning Tomographic Acoustic Microscope: A Review," IEEE Trans. on Sonics and Ultrasonics and Ultrasonics, Vol. SU-32, No. 2, pp. 168-180, March 1985.

6. R. C. Brooks and G. D. Chiro, "Principles of Computer Assisted Tomography (CAT) in Radiographic and Radioisotropic Imagings," Phys. Med. Biol., Vol. 21, No. 5, pp. 689-732, 1976.

7. R. K. Mueller, M. Kaveh and G. Wade, "Reconstructive Tomography and Application to Ultrasonics," Proc. IEEE, Vol. 67, pp. 567-587, 1979.

8. S. X. Pan and A. C. Kak, "A Computational Study of Reconstruction Algorithm for Diffraction Tomography: Interpolation Versus Filtered Back-Propagation," IEEE Trans. on ASSP, Vol. ASSP-31, No. 5, pp. 1262-1275, Oct. 1983.

9. H. Lee, C. F. Schueler, G. Flesher and G. Wade, "Ultrasonic Planar Scanned Tomography," Acoustical Imaging, Vol. 11, Ed. John Powers, Plenum Press, New York, pp. 309-323, 1982.

10. Z. C. Lin, G. Wade and H. Lee, "Back-and-Forth Propagation for Diffraction Tomography," IEEE Trans. on Sonics and Ultrasonics, Vol. SU-31, No. 6, pp. 626-634, Nov. 1984.

11. P. C. H. Chen and G. Wade, "Optimal Observation Angles for Planar Tomography in STAM System," Acoustical Imaging, Vol. 14, pp. 329-342, Eds. A. J. Berkhout, J. Ridder and L. F. Van Der Wal, Plenum Press, New York, 1985.

12. J. W. Goodman, "Introduction to Fourier Optics," McGraw-Hill, New York, Chap. 3, 1968.

13. A. J. Berkhout, "Seismic Migration - Imaging of Acoustic Energy by Wave Field Extrapolation," Amsterdam/New York, Elsevier/North Holland Publ. Co., 1980.

14. D. Luenberger, "Optimization by Vector Space Method", pp. 146, John Wiley, New York, 1969.

15. U. Grenander and G. Szego, "Toeplitz Forms and Their Application," Chelsea Publishing Company, New York, 1984.

ULTRASONIC REFLECTION TOMOGRAPHY WITH

A TRANSMITTER-RECEIVER SYSTEM

D.K. Mak

Physical Metallurgy Research Laboratories
568 Booth Street
Ottawa, Canada K1A 0G1

ABSTRACT

A technique has been developed for carrying out ultrasound reflection tomography using transducers as transmitter-receiver. It has been shown that applying beam divergence angle limitation enhances the clarity of the image and also saves a lot of computer time. Convolution back projection and threshold operation can also help to improve the image.

INTRODUCTION

Modern applications of acoustical imaging take full advantage of the digital computer. Different methods of digital ultrasonic imaging have been reviewed by Schueler et al.[1]. One method, ultrasonic computed tomography, enables the reconstruction of quantitative two-dimensional mapping of various parameters in the material. It can be classified either in the transmission or reflection mode. Reflection tomography is used most effectively to determine the shapes and dimensions of cracks and voids in a material.

One particular type of reflection tomography assumes that the velocity of sound is constant in the material. Travel times along extremum paths are used for image reconstruction instead of those obtainable from diffraction theory[2,3]. A single transducer was used in the pulse-echo mode, i.e., as a transmitter/receiver. However, planar defects at an angle to the acoustic beam could escape detection. We describe here how this situation can be corrected by using separate transducers as the transmitter and the receiver. This method has the further advantage that, for n transducer scan positions, $_nC_2$ data can be collected (assuming reciprocity of a transmitter and a receiver), while only n data can be collected by a transmitter-receiver system. As using transducers as transmitter/receiver can be considered to be a particular case of using them as transmitter-receiver, the equations developed for the transmitter-receiver system also applies to the transmitter/receiver system.

METHOD

Let (x,z) be the location of a defect inside a material. The positions of the transducers can be measured and are denoted by (p_m,q_m) and (p_n,q_n) (Fig. 1). The direction of the sound beam of each transducer is given by θ', an angle described in a standard position in a Cartesian coordinate system, i.e., measured counter-clockwise from the +x-axis.

For all beams of identical transit time running from (p_m,q_m) to (p_n,q_n), the reflection points must be on an ellipse with foci (p_m,q_m) and (p_n,q_n). The centre of the ellipse will be given by $[(p_m + p_n)/2, (q_m + q_n)/2]$. Let $2f$ and $2g$ be the length of the major axis and the minor axis respectively. The properties of an ellipse show that:

$$f = \frac{\ell}{2}$$

(1)

$$g = \left[\left(\frac{\ell}{2} \right)^2 - \left(\frac{p_n - p_m}{2} \right)^2 - \left(\frac{q_n - q_m}{2} \right)^2 \right]^{1/2}$$

(2)

The equation of the ellipse in the rectangular coordinates in the x'z' reference frame (Fig. 1) is given by

$$\frac{x'^2}{f^2} + \frac{z'^2}{g^2} = 1$$

(3)

The x' axis makes an angle, β, with the positive x axis, where β is given by

$$\tan \beta = \frac{q_n - q_m}{p_n - p_m}$$

(4)

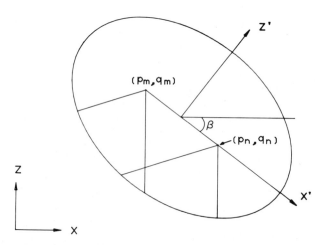

Fig. 1.   The scattered point lies on the locus of an ellipse.   The beam divergence angles of the two transducers [located at (p_m, q_m) and (p_n, q_n)] limit the location of the scattered point.   Therefore, the defect lies on the arc of the ellipse which is covered by the acoustical beams of both the transmitter and the receiver.

As a circle is a particular case of an ellipse, the algorithm has been written so that the equations reduce to those of circles when the transducers are acting as transmitter/receiver. So, if $p_m = p_n$, and $q_m = q_n$,

$$\beta \equiv \theta' + \frac{\pi}{2} \tag{5}$$

The equation of the ellipse in polar coordinates is given by

$$r'^2 = \frac{f^2 g^2}{f^2 \sin^2 \gamma + g^2 \cos^2 \gamma} \tag{6}$$

The rectangular coordinates are related to those of the polar coordinate system by

$$x' = r' \cos \gamma \tag{7}$$

$$z' = r' \sin \gamma \tag{8}$$

x, z coordinates are transformed from x', z' coordinates by translation and rotation.

$$x = x' \cos \beta - z' \sin \beta + \frac{p_m + p_n}{2} \tag{9}$$

$$z = x' \sin \beta + z' \cos \beta + \frac{q_m + q_n}{2} \tag{10}$$

Let $\eta_{h \text{ dB}}$ be the divergence angle of the transducer sound beam, where the pressure amplitude drops by h dB from that along the acoustical axis of the transducer. The direction of the sound beam at $\pm \eta_{h \text{ dB}}$ is then given by

$$\theta'_{ij} = \theta'_i + (-1)^j \eta_{h \text{ dB}} \qquad j = 1,2 \tag{11}$$

Let (p_i, q_i) be the position of a transducer. The equation of a straight line going through the point (p_i, q_i) and of gradient θ'_{ij} is given by

$$\frac{z - q_i}{x - p_i} = \tan \theta'_{ij} \tag{12}$$

Transforming Eq. (12) into the x'z' coordinate system:

$$x'L_1 = z'M_1 + N_1 \tag{13}$$

where

$$L_1 = \sin \beta - \cos \beta \tan \theta'_{ij} \tag{14}$$

$$M_1 = - (\cos \beta + \sin \beta \tan \theta'_{ij}) \tag{15}$$

$$N_1 = -\left(\frac{q_m + q_n}{2} - q_i\right) + \tan \theta'_{ij}\left(\frac{p_m + p_n}{2} - p_i\right) \qquad \text{and } i = m \text{ or } n \tag{16}$$

Substituting x' from Eq. (13) into Eq. (3) yields a quadratic equation in z'.

$$L_2 z'^2 + M_2 z' + N_2 = 0 \tag{17}$$

$$z' = \frac{-M_2 \pm [M_2^2 - 4L_2 N_2]^{1/2}}{2L_2} \tag{18}$$

where

$$L_2 = g^2 \frac{M_1^2}{L_1^2} + f^2 \tag{19}$$

$$M_2 = 2 \frac{M_1 N_1}{L_1^2} g^2 \tag{20}$$

$$N_2 = \frac{g^2 N_1^2}{L_1^2} - f^2 g^2 \tag{21}$$

Equation (18) can be substituted into Eq. (13) to find x'. As there are two solutions for Eq. (18), two solutions (x'_ℓ, z'_ℓ), $\ell = 1,2$ can be found. The solutions are transformed into the x,z coordinates using Eq. (9) and (10). θ'_ℓ are given by

$$\tan \theta'_\ell = \frac{z_\ell - q_i}{x_\ell - p_i} \qquad \ell = 1,2 \tag{22}$$

The solution (x'_ℓ, z'_ℓ) which yields $\theta'_\ell = \theta'_{ij}$ is the correct solution, the other solution is rejected since it does not lie along the path of the sound beam.

The four straight lines generated from the two transducers will intersect the ellipse at four points (Fig. 1). Their polar angles, γ_{ij} in the x'z' frame, are given by

$$\tan \gamma_{ij} = \frac{z'_{ij}}{x'_{ij}} \qquad \begin{array}{l} i = m,n \\ j = 1,2 \end{array} \tag{23}$$

The γ's are then arranged in ascending order

$$\gamma_1 \le \gamma_2 \le \gamma_3 \le \gamma_4 \tag{24}$$

Define

$$\gamma_{hk} = \frac{1}{2} (\gamma_k + \gamma_{k+1}) \qquad k = 1, 2, 3 \tag{25}$$

γ_{hk} are substituted into Eq. (6) to find r'_{hk}. Using Eq. (7) and (8), x'_{hk}, z'_{hk} can be found, and they are then transformed to the xz coordinates. θ_{hk} are calculated from:

$$\tan \theta_{hk} = \frac{z_{hk} - q_i}{x_{hk} - p_i}$$

(26)

The value of θ_{hk} that satisfies the inequalities

$$\theta'_{i1} \leq \theta_{hk} \leq \theta'_{i2} \qquad \text{for both } i = m, n$$

implies that points on the arc of the ellipse lying between γ_k and γ_{k+1} will lie inside both the beam profiles of the two transducers. The arc can be drawn in the xz coordinate frame by using Eq. (6)-(10).

The algorithm described above also applies when transducers are used as transmitter/receiver.

EXPERIMENT

A rectangular aluminum block (Fig. 2) of thickness 39.5 mm was used in the experiment. A 0.5 mm wide, 10 mm long, slot was cut at a 60° angle with a circular saw. Sixteen positions were marked on the block, five on the longer side and three on the shorter side. Transducers of 5 MHz, 6.35 mm diam were placed at these positions (Fig. 3). They were used both as transmitter/receivers and as transmitter-receivers. The times-of-flight for the first two echoes were recorded for each reading.

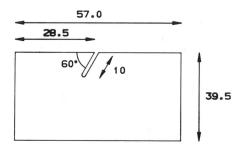

Fig. 2.   Aluminum block with crack.   All units in mm.

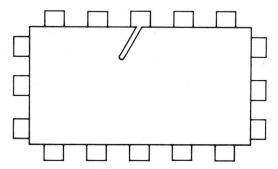

Fig. 3.   Aluminum block showing the sixteen transducer scan positions.

335

RESULTS

Figure 4 shows all the circles and ellipses that could be drawn within
the boundary of the x-y plotter. Sound beams travelling directly from a
transmitter to a receiver were eliminated by the software and were not
drawn. The picture was too unclear to show any defect. Plotting only the
arcs that lie within the beam divergence angles shows a much clearer picture
(Fig. 5). It shows a defect located in the top centre region of the block.
However, it is not very clear whether this is a point defect or a defect of
another shape. More transducer positions are required to characterize the
defect. If two transducers can move independently along the surface of the
block, specular reflections arising from the planar surface of the crack
can be detected (Fig. 6). These data, which are important in producing the
complete defect image, cannot be gathered if only a single transducer is
used as a transmitter/receiver. If these data are superimposed upon data

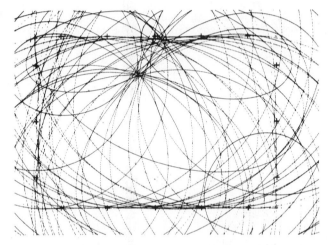

Fig. 4. Aluminum block with crack. Transducers were used as transmitter/
         receiver and transmitter-receiver. All circles and ellipses are
         drawn. + denotes transducer scan position.

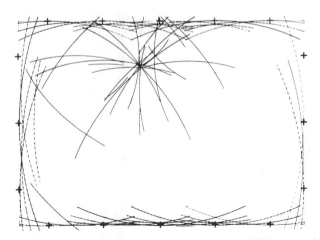

Fig. 5. Same as Fig. 4, only arcs of circles and ellipses within the beam
         divergence angle (η) are drawn. η = 25°.

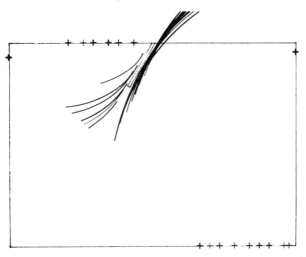

Fig. 6. Specular reflections at the plane surface of the crack. $\eta = 40°$.
The outline of the block and the crack were drawn in for reference.
+ denotes transducer scan positions.

gathered from the signals scattered from the crack tip (Fig. 7), the boundaries of the defect will show up. A window can be drawn enclosing the
defect area, and the image field can subsequently be divided into many
square picture elements. The imaging process was performed by "drawing" a
series of arcs, adding a "score" to each element transversed by the arc,
and subsequently displaying these elements with a "score" above a pre-set
threshold[4].

     An image of the flaw is displayed in Fig. 8, with a threshold level =
0. A certain amount of blurring appears as a result of simple backprojection along straight lines (as in X-ray tomography). Some blurring can be
eliminated by increasing the threshold level. Figures 9 and 10 show the
image with threshold levels of 1 and 2 respectively. Another method of

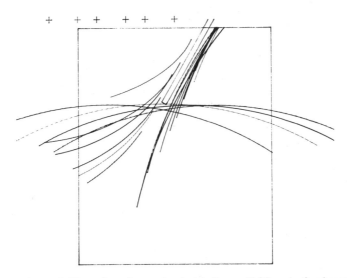

Fig. 7. A window of Fig. 6. Arcs derived from diffracted signal from
crack tip were also drawn. The outline of the crack was drawn in
for reference.

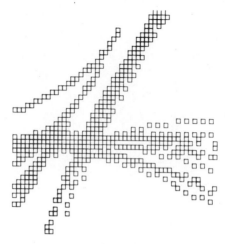

Fig. 8.   Figure 7 divided into square pixels.   Threshold level = 0.   The boundary of the crack can be seen from the image.

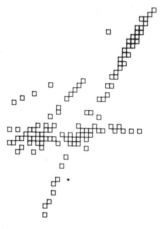

Fig. 9.   Same as Fig. 8 with threshold level = 1.   By increasing the threshold level, some of the blurring appeared in Fig. 8 was eliminated.

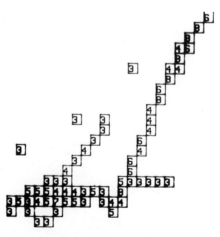

Fig. 10.   Same as Fig. 8, with threshold level = 2.   The "score" of each pixel was drawn inside the pixel.

removing blurring is to convolve the projections with a deblurring filter
and then backproject them. The deblurring filter used here for the convolution backprojection is a two-term single filter shown in Fig. 11[3].
Figure 12 shows the filtered flaw image with the threshold level set at 2.
It does show a clearer image compared with the one when no filter was used.

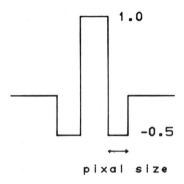

Fig. 11. The simple filter used for convolution backprojection.

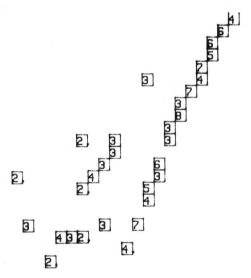

Fig. 12. Same as Fig. 10, threshold operation was applied after the
convolution backprojection. The 5's in x.5 were suppressed in
the figure.

CONCLUSIONS

An imaging technique using a transmitter-receiver system has been
described. It uses the time of flight of the echo data to construct an
image. The image can be improved when beam divergence angle limitation is
taken into account. Threshold operation and a simple deblurring filter
were tested experimentally to remove the blurring caused by simple backprojection. Edge enhancement can be improved by arranging transducer scan
positions at smaller intervals. A transmitter-receiver system has the
advantage over a transmitter/receiver system in that the former can detect
specular reflections from planar defects that can be missed by the latter.

ACKNOWLEDGEMENT

The assistance of Mr. I.R. Somerville for collecting and analyzing the data is gratefully acknowledged.

REFERENCES

1. C.F. Schueler, H. Lee, and G. Wade, Fundamentals of digital ultrasonic imaging, IEEE Sonics and Ultrasonics, SU-31:195-217 (1984).
2. M.C. Tsao and J.K. White, Reflective ultrasonic tomography, ASNT 1981 Fall Conf Proc, 491-494 (1981).
3. M. Moshfeghi and P.D. Hanstead, Ultrasound reflection tomography of cylindrical rods, Ultrasonics 23:206-214 (1985).
4. P.D. Hanstead, Fast digital ultrasonic imaging, Proc Ultrasonics Int 81 Conf, 62-66 (1981).

SPECKLE IN ULTRASOUND COMPUTERIZED REFLECTION MODE TOMOGRAPHY

Gerhard Roehrlein and Helmut Ermert

Department of Electrical Engineering
University of Erlangen-Nuremberg
Cauerstrasse 9, D-8520 Erlangen, FRG

1. INTRODUCTION

Soon after the first use of Ultrasound B-Scanners, a phenomenon was observed in the images of texture, which has been under investigation up to now: Macroscopic homogeneous texture areas are represented in the B-Scan-images not as a single homogeneous grey-level, but as very "granular" areas with characteristic "granule-size". This phenomenon is commonly called "speckle". Several different approaches were done to investigate this problem. Two of them, the analytical statistical methods of Burckhardt /3/ and Wagner et al. /4/, are extended in this paper in order to investigate speckle in ultrasound computerized reflection mode tomography (UCTR). UCTR can be explained as a numerical superposition of several B-Scans of a cross-sectional plane obtained from different aspect angles. The superposition consists of a summation and an additional inverse filtering procedure, which is equivalent to the deconvolution in X-ray-CT. UCTR has been investigated theoretically (/1/, /2/) and has also been used for clinical in-vivo imaging of female breast /5/, muscles, and thyroid gland /2/. Section 2 summarizes the theory of UCTR. Section 3 shortly reviews the results of speckle in B-Scans from Burckhardt /3/ and Wagner et al. /4/. Sections 4, 5 and 6 presents results of first and second order statistics of speckle in the summation image, and shows measurements of correlation-coefficients of two B-Scans with different aspect-angles. The statistical properties of speckle in the filtered image are included in sections 7 and 8. Chapter 9 describes a special texture phantom which was used in the measurements to verify the theory. Section 10 contains in-vivo images of testicles to demonstrate the speckle-reduction effect in UCTR images.

2. CONCEPT OF UCTR

Fig. 2-1 shows the concept of UCTR. Many B-Scans b(x,y), each of them modelled by

$$b(x,y) = \iint\limits_{-\infty}^{+\infty} a(\hat{x},\hat{y}) \cdot h_b(x-\hat{x},\ y-\hat{y})\ d\hat{x}d\hat{y} \qquad (2.1)$$

(a(x,y) = object reflectivity, $h_b(x,y)$ = point spread function (PSF) of the B-Scan) are superimposed from different aspect angles. With the relation of the fixed coordinates (x,y) and the rotated coordinates (t,u)

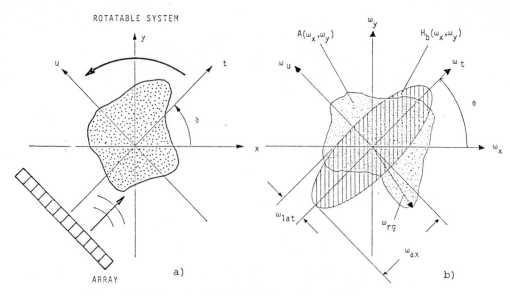

ROTATABLE SYSTEM

a)

ARRAY

b)

Fig. 2-1: Scheme of ultrasound reflection-mode CT
a) Reflection-mode imaging setup
b) Spatial frequency domain representation

$$\begin{pmatrix} t \\ u \end{pmatrix} = \begin{pmatrix} +\cos\vartheta & +\sin\vartheta \\ -\sin\vartheta & +\cos\vartheta \end{pmatrix} \begin{pmatrix} x \\ y \end{pmatrix} \qquad (2.2)$$

the summation-image $s(x,y)$ results in

$$s(x,y) = \int_0^{\vartheta_{max}} b(t,u)d\vartheta = a(x,y) ** h_s(x,y) \qquad (2.3)$$

(** denotes two-dimensional convolution)

with the summation-PSF $h_s(x,y)$

$$h_s(x,y) = \int_0^{\vartheta_{max}} h_b(x\cos\vartheta + y\sin\vartheta, -x\sin\vartheta + y\cos\vartheta)d\vartheta \qquad (2.4)$$

For both the B-Scan and the summation-image, there exist complementary
solutions in the spatial frequency domain:

$$B(\omega_x,\omega_y) = A(\omega_x,\omega_y) \cdot H_b(\omega_x,\omega_y) \qquad (2.5)$$

$$S(\omega_x,\omega_y) = A(\omega_x,\omega_y) \cdot H_S(\omega_x,\omega_y) \qquad (2.6)$$

(B = B-Scan, S = summation image, A = object reflectivity) H_b = PTF of
B-Scan, H_S = PTF of summation image; all magnitudes are in the Fourier-
domain (PTF = point transfer function))

In a second step, a two-dimensional inverse filter h_i is applied to the
summation image to increase the resolution

$$a'(x,y) = s(x,y) ** h_i(x,y) \qquad (2.7)$$

and in the Fourier-domain

342

$$A'(\omega_x, \omega_y) = S(\omega_x, \omega_y) \cdot H_i(\omega_x, \omega_y) \qquad (2.8)$$

(a'(A') = reconstructed object reflectivity,
h_i,(H_i) = PSF (PTF) of the inverse filter).

3. SPECKLE IN B-SCAN

Burckhardt /3/ and Wagner et al. /4/ have analysed the statistical behavior of the B-Scan amplitude. The following properties are of interest: "fluctuation" of the B-Scan-amplitude from a macroscopic homogeneous object. This is described by the mean <V> and variance var(V) of the B-Scan amplitude and the speckle-signal-to-noise-ratio SNR_o, which is defined as

$$SNR_o = \frac{<V>}{\sqrt{var(V)}} \qquad (3.1)$$

The SNR_o can be interpreted like a "regular" signal-to-noise-ratio. It is only a real number. If this number is large, the B-Scan of a macroscopic homogeneous object also looks homogeneous; if the number is small, the B-Scan looks very "granular". Another interesting magnitude is the mean-size of the speckles. This speckle-size can be derived from the auto-covariance function (ACVF) of the B-Scan amplitude. An analytical expression for the ACVF was found by Wagner et al. /4/. Fig. 3-1 shows the normalized ACVF of the B-Scan amplitude for the axial and lateral

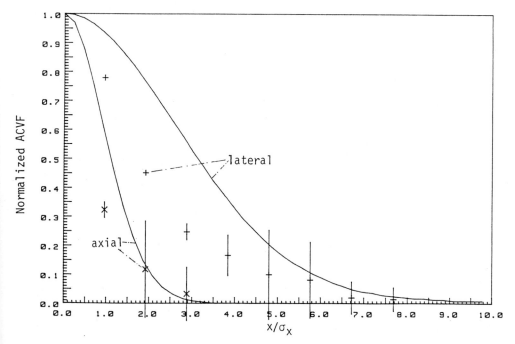

Fig. 3-1: Normalized theoretical B-scan-ACVF
(for resolution-ratio y_a/x_a =3) and experimental data obtained from a texture phantom (mean of 3 measurements $\pm$ 2 standard deviations

direction. Also measurements of the ACVF of a tissue-phantom (described in chapter 9) are included. The experimental results show a smaller ACVF than was theoretically predicted. The measurements have not been made in the center of the focal zone of the B-Scan, but in an area nearer to the transducer. That is because in the nearfield the speckle-sizes are smaller than in the focal zone, therefore the measurements are already in reasonable agreement with theory. The following result is remarkable: If the object includes many point-scatterers per resolution-cell (which is essentially the same as the point-spread-function of the B-Scan), and if the scatterers are randomly distributed, then the ACVF is only dependent on the PSF of the B-Scan. This means, that under the above conditions the speckle size is not influenced by the object.
It should be noted, that the speckle-size is defined as the infinite integral of the normalized ACVF.

The following results were obtained by the authors mentioned above:
The speckle-signal-to-noise ratio yields:

$$\text{SNR}_o = (\pi/(4-\pi)^{1/2} \approx 1,91 \tag{3.2}$$

This means, that there is a large fluctuation of the B-Scan amplitude, as opposed to a constant SNR, and this fluctuation is not influenced by the object.

The speckle-sizes are (for quadratic transducer apertures and gaussian envelope of the transmitted pulse):

$$S_{cx} = 2.43 \cdot \sigma_x \qquad \text{(axial direction)} \tag{3.3}$$

$$S_{cy} = 0,87/f_{oy} = 0,87 \cdot \lambda x_o/D \quad \text{(lateral direction)} \tag{3.4}$$

with

$$\sigma_x = 0,375/\Delta f_x$$

(Δf_x = 6 db spatial bandwidth of transmitted pulse,
λ = mean wavelength, x_o = focus of transducer,
D = width of transducer-aperture)

There are two scaling parameters σ_x, f_{oy} for speckle size in axial and in lateral direction. In order to drop one of them the resolution-ratio of the B-Scan PSF between lateral and axial direction y_a/x_a is required. Using this parameter we get:

$$\sigma_x \cdot f_{oy} = 0,3761/(y_a/x_a) \tag{3.5}$$

We now drop f_{oy}. This yields for the speckle size in lateral direction

$$S_{cy} = 2.31 \ (y_a/x_a) \cdot \sigma_x \tag{3.6}$$

This alternative type of scaling is useful for a comparison of the speckle-size between B-Scans and UCTR images.

4. SPECKLE IN THE SUMMATION IMAGE: Statistics of first order

Now we analyse the process of summation with respect to speckle. In this chapter we assume, that N B-Scans, every B-Scan rotated by the angle $\Delta\vartheta$ with respect to the previous B-Scan, are superimposed. The amplitude of the summation image is described as a stochastic variable like the B-Scan in chapter 3. As the summation amplitude V_s we get:

$$V_s = 1/N \sum_{i=1}^{N} V_i \qquad\qquad (4.1)$$

with V_i the amplitude of the i-th B-Scan.

Now the mean $<V_s>$ is simply given by

$$<V_s> = <1/N \sum_{i=1}^{N} V_i> = 1/N \sum_{i=1}^{N} <V_i> = 1/N \cdot N \cdot <V> = <V> = (\pi/2) \cdot \sigma (4.2)$$

The mean value of the summation image is the same, as the mean value $<V>$ in a single B-Scan.

To compute the variance $var(V_s)$ of the summation-image we assume, that the N superimposed B-Scans are not correlated (this assumption will be analysed in the next chapter). This yields (/6/ p. 246):

$$var(V_s) = var(V)/N = (2 - \pi/2)\sigma^2/N \qquad\qquad (4.3)$$

For correlated B-Scans, having a correlation-coefficient r, we can write:

$$var(V_s) = var(V)/N \cdot (1 + r \cdot (N - 1)) \qquad\qquad (4.4)$$

To get the speckle-signal-to-noise-ratio SNR_{Vs} of the summation image we must compute the ratio between the mean value $<V_s>$ and the square root of the variance. If the B-Scan are not correlated we get

$$SNR_{Vs} = <V_s>/\sqrt{var(V_s)} = \sqrt{(N \cdot \pi/(4-\pi))} \approx 1.91 \cdot \sqrt{N} \qquad\qquad (4.5)$$

otherwise (with eqn. 4.4)

$$SNR_{Vs} = 1.91 \cdot \sqrt{N} / \sqrt{1 + r \cdot (N - 1)} \qquad\qquad (4.6)$$

yields.

The speckle-signal-to-noise-ratio is much better in the summation-image than in a single B-Scan. Therefore, a summation image looks more "smooth" than a B-Scan-image.

5. CORRELATION OF TWO ROTATED B-SCANS

Two theories exist which describe the correlation between two linear shifted B-Scans. The first theory has been published by Burckhardt /3/ and the second by Gehlbach /7/. Burckhardt predicted for the correlation-coefficient:

$$r = \begin{cases} (1 - |d/l|)^2 & \text{for } |d| \le 1 \\ 0 & \text{otherwise} \end{cases} \qquad\qquad (5.1)$$

with d and l described in Fig.5-1. Gehlbach predicts a similar result with the same form but another exponent:

$$r = \begin{cases} (1 - |d/l|)^4 & \text{for } |d| \le 1 \\ 0 & \text{otherwise} \end{cases} \qquad\qquad (5.2)$$

To transform these linear shifts into rotational ones, we can set (see Fig. 5-1):

$$d = 2x_o \sin(\Delta\vartheta/2) \qquad\qquad (5.3)$$

with x_o the distance between focus and transducer, and $\Delta\vartheta$ the rotated angle.

We have computed the correlation coefficient r versus the rotated angle $\Delta\vartheta$ for a ratio $x_o/l = 6.6$ (Fig. 5-2) for both theories. Measurements from

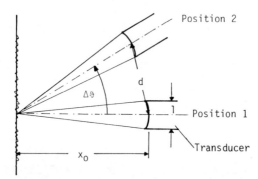

Fig. 5-1: Model (after BURCKHARDT) to evaluate the correlation-coefficient of two B-scans, rotated about the angle $\Delta\vartheta$. The object (many randomly distributed small scatterers) is in the focal-zone of the transducer.

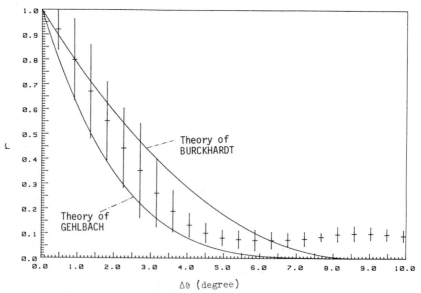

Fig. 5-2: Correlation-coefficient of two B-scans, rotated about the angle $\Delta\vartheta$ (for $x_o/l=6.6$). Theory after BURCKHARDT /3/ and GEHLBACH /7/. Experimental data were obtained from a texture phantom. The mean of 32 measurements $\pm$ 2 standard deviations is plotted.

our texture phantom show that the experimental obtained correlation-coefficients are between the results of the two theories.

6. SPECKLE IN THE SUMMATION IMAGE: Statistics of 2. order

To derive the ACVF of the amplitude of the summation-image we consider the amplitude of the summation image $V_s(x,y)$, like the B-Scan amplitude $V(t,u)$, as a statistic process. For $V_s(x,y)$ we get

$$V_s(x,y)=1/M \sum_{i=0}^{N} V_i(x \cos(i\cdot\Delta\vartheta)+y \sin(i\cdot\Delta\vartheta), -x \sin(i\cdot\Delta\vartheta)+y \cos(i\cdot\Delta\vartheta) \quad (6.1)$$

with $M = N + 1$ superimposed B-Scans. From the definition of a covariance-function we now can obtain (with 6.1) the general result for the autocovariance function of the summation image:

$$C_{Vs} = 1/M^2 \sum_{i=0}^{N} \sum_{j=0}^{N} C_{ViVj} = 1/M^2 \sum_{i=0}^{N} C_{ViVi} + 1/M^2 \sum_{\substack{i=0 \\ i\neq j}}^{N} \sum_{j=0}^{N} C_{ViVj} \quad (6.2)$$

C_{ViVi} is the ACVF of the i-th B-Scan, C_{ViVj} ($i\neq j$) the cross-covariance-function between the i-th and the j-th B-Scan.

Note, that the ACVF of the summation image consists of the sum of all ACVF s of the B-Scans and the sum of all cross-covariance-functions of all B-Scans.

Now we assume, that the B-Scans are not correlated, i.e.

$$C_{ViVj} = 0 \quad \text{for } i \neq j \quad (6.3)$$

Therefore it is obvious, with the assumption of a macroscopic homogeneous and microscopically not correlated object, that all ACVF s of the B-Scans are identical, with the exception of a rotation about the angle $i\cdot\Delta\vartheta$. This yields:

$$C_{Vs}(x,y)=1/M^2 \sum_{i=0}^{N} C_{Vi}(x \cos(i\cdot\Delta\vartheta)+y \sin(i\cdot\Delta\vartheta),-x \sin(i\cdot\Delta\vartheta)+y \cos(i\cdot\Delta\vartheta)(6.4)$$

We normalize the ACVF to get the speckle-sizes

$$k_{Vs}(x,y) = C_{Vs}(x,y)/C_{Vs}(0,0) \quad (6.5)$$

The speckle-sizes are different in different radial directions. We have therefore computed the minimum and maximum speckle sizes for different resolution-ratios, maximum aspect-angles, and numbers of superimposed B-Scans (Table 6-1). For the ACVF of a single B-Scan the result of Wagner et al. /4/ was adapted.

Table 6-1: Mean speckle-sizes of summation-image for different aspect-angle-
areas and B-scan-resolution-ratios y_a/x_a.

y_a/x_a	aspect-angle area (degree)	maximum speckle-size	minimum speckle-size.	unit
5	90	6,02	2,84	σ_x
4	90	5,61	2,83	σ_x
3	90	4,87	2,80	σ_x
5	350	4,57	4,57	σ_x
4	350	4,26	4,26	σ_x
3	350	3,85	3,85	σ_x

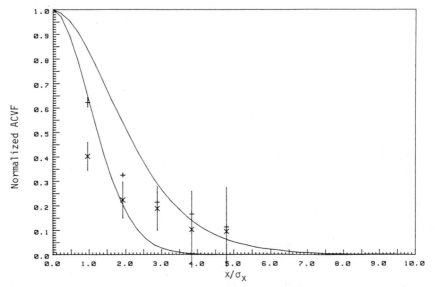

Fig. 6-2: Normalized ACVF of the summation-image (with B-scan-resolution-
ration y_a/x_a=3, aspect-angle-area = 90 degrees, 10 B-scans
superimposed). The ACVF was evaluated for the directions of
minimum and maximum speckle-size. The experimental data were
obtained from a texture phantom. The mean of 3 measurements
± 2 standard deviations is plotted.

The theoretical curves of the ACVF of the summation image and measurements of the texture phantom are shown in Fig. 6-2. The measurements do
not correspond exactly to the theory, but the same restriction applies to
the measurements as to the B-Scan.

7. SPECKLE IN THE FILTERED IMAGES: First order statistics

If we apply an inverse Filter H_i to the summation image we get the filtered images. The filtering operation describes a spatial invariant linear system. If stationary stochastic signals are applied to the input, the mean variance and ACVF can simply be evaluated from the corresponding values at the input.
For the mean $<V_i>$ in the filtered image we get:

$$<V_i> = H_i(0,0) \cdot <V_s> \qquad (7.1)$$

Because the mean in the filtered image should always be the same as in the summation image we normalize the inverse filter:

$$H_i(0,0) = 1 \qquad (7.2)$$

In this case, the means are the same in the B-Scan, in the summation-image and in the filtered image are equal.

For the variance $var(V_i)$ the following result yields:

$$var(V_i) = C_{Vi}(0,0) = 1/(4\pi^2) \int\limits_{-\infty}^{+\infty}\!\!\int T_{Vs}(\omega_x,\omega_y) \cdot |H_i(\omega_x,\omega_y)|^2 \, d\omega_x d\omega_y \qquad (7.3)$$

C_{Vi} is the ACVF of the filtered image, T_{Vs} is the power spectrum of the amplitude of the summation-image (T_{Vs} = Fourier transform of the ACVF of the summation-image). Explicit results for $var(V_i)$ can only be evaluated with special functions H_i. We have applied a filter $H_i = H_w/H_s$ with H_w an truncated bessel function as window /2/. Then the explicit results in Table 7-1 could be obtained. Obviously, the Speckle-SNR is remarkably decreased (versus the summation image), i.e. the filtered images have similar amplitude fluctuations like B-Scan-images.

Table 7-1: Theoretical variances and speckle-signal-to-noise-ratios in the filtered images for different B-scan-resolution-ratios y_a/x_a and aspect-angle-areas (N= number of summed B-scans).

y_a/x_a	aspect-angle area	N	variance	SNR
5	350°	36	$0,340 \ \sigma^2$	2,14
5	90°	10	$0,069 \ \sigma^2$	4,78
4	350°	36	$0,305 \ \sigma^2$	2,26
4	90°	10	$0,053 \ \sigma^2$	5,45
3	350°	36	$0,163 \ \sigma^2$	3,10
3	90°	10	$0,008 \ \sigma^2$	13,89

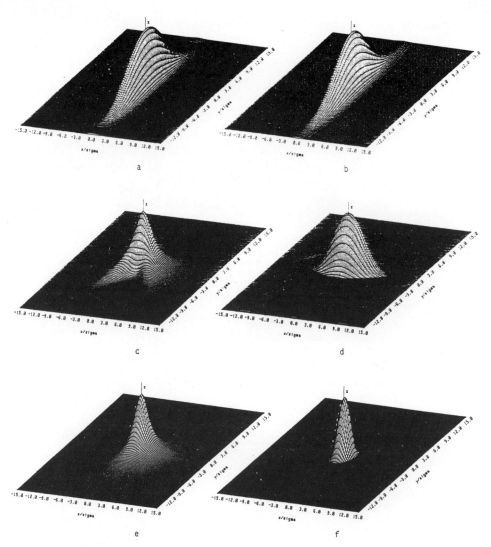

Fig. 8-3: Three-dimensional plots of auto-covariance-functions
   a) typical B-scan-point-spread-function with $y_a/x_a =4$.
   b) B-scan ACVF to a)
   c) ACVF of summation-image (aspect-angle-area 90 deg., 10 B-scans
      superimposed)
   d) ACVF of filtered image (aspect-angle-area 90 deg., 10 B-scans
      superimposed)
   e) ACVF of summation-image (aspect-angle-area 350 deg., 36 B-scans
      superimposed)
   f) ACVF of filtered image (aspect-angle-area 350 deg., 36 B-scans
      superimposed)

The ACVF C_{Vi} is the inverse fourier transformation of the fourier transform of the ACVF of the summation image T_{Vs} multiplied by the squared modulus of the inverse filter $|H_i|^2$. A computed ACVF C_{Vi} (for a specific B-Scan resolution-ratio, aspect-angle-area, and number of superimposed B-Scans) is shown in Fig. 8-1. Experimental data, obtained from our

8. SPECKLE IN THE FILTERED IMAGE: Second order statistics

In order to get speckle-sizes, we have to evaluate the ACVF of the filtered images. Because filtering is a linear and space-invariant process, this is a simple task:

$$C_{Vi}(x,y) = F^{-1} \{T_{Vs}(\omega_x,\omega_y) \; |H_i(\omega_x,\omega_y)|^2\} \qquad (8.1)$$

(F^{-1} = inverse Fourier transform)

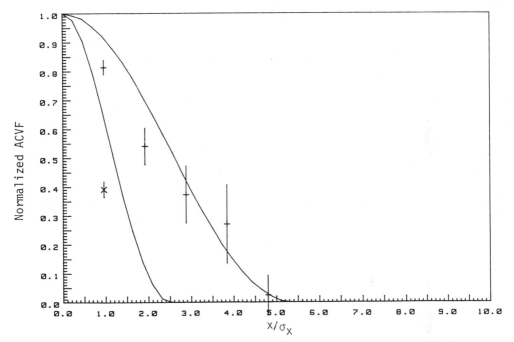

Fig. 8-1: Normalized ACVF of the filtered image (with B-scan-resolution-ratio y_a/x_a=3, aspect-angle-area = 90 degrees, 10 B-scans superimposed). The ACVF was evaluated for the directions of minimum and maximum speckle-size. The experimental data were obtained from a texture-phantom. The mean of 3 measurements $\pm$ 2 standard deviations is plotted.

y_a/x_a	aspect-angle area (degree)	maximum speckle-size	minimum speckle-size.	unit
5	90'	8,43	2,59	σ_x
4	90	9,26	2,52	σ_x
3	90	5,51	2,53	σ_x
5	350	2,78	2,78	σ_x
4	350	2,77	2,77	σ_x
3	350	2,53	2,53	σ_x

Fig. 8-2: Mean speckle-sizes in the filtered image for different aspect-angle-areas and B-scan resolution-ratios y_a/x_a.

texture phantom, are also included. The agreement between theory and experiment seems to be reasonably good.

With eqn. (8.1) speckle-sizes could be obtained also. Table 8-2 lists the calculated speckle-sizes for a number of cases.

Fig. 8-3 shows the PBF of a typical B-Scan and the corresponding ACVF s of the B-Scan, the summation-image and the filtered image (90° and 350° aspect-angle-area). From the theory and the numerical and experimental data, the following conclusion is possible: The ACVF s of the B-Scan, of the summation-image, and of the filtered image have essentially the same shape and spatial extension as the corresponding PSF s. Therefore the mean speckle sizes (in the focal-zone) are always very similar to the resolution of the corresponding images.

9. A SPECIAL TEXTURE PHANTOM

We have carried out our experiments in the previous chapters with a special texture phantom, which is commercially available from the Kretz Corp. Zipf/Austria. The phantom contains natural gelatine. Small graphite scatterers with mean-diameter of 25 μm are embedded. 50 g graphite per kg gelatine was used, which leads to an absorption of 0,5 dB/(cm MHz).

10. IN-VITRO AND IN-VIVO IMAGES

With our experimental set-up /2/ we have carried out a number of in-vitro and in-vivo-experiments.

Fig. 10-1 shows images of a sponge, which was used to simulate soft tissue. Inside the sponge are several holes with diameters from 1 mm to 10 mm. Two holes are surrounded by white circles, which are caused from rubber in the sponge. Some small white areas are air-bubbles.Fig. 10a shows a B-Scan of the object, Fig. 10b - 10f contain several summation-images with different aspect-angle areas (the term "Grad" in the head-line of the images refers to the english "degree"). Fig. 10g shows a filtered image. The speckle reduction effect with increasing aspect-angle area is obvious. The two smallest holes, which can hardly be seen in the B-Scan, are well detected in the summation image with 15° aspect-angle-area. The filtered image increases the resolution of the rubber-circles, but decreases speckle-SNR.

Fig. 10-2 to 10-4 show in-vivo images of testicles, which clearly demonstrate the speckle-reduction-effect of the summation image quite.
Fig. 10-2 shows in-vivo-images of a testicle with an unknown process on the lower left side. From the B-Scan (10-2a) it is not possible to decide, if this is a local echo within the testicle, or if it is additional tissue outside the testicles. In the summation-image (10-2b) a thin border between the normal testicle and the pathological process can be localized. The filtered image (Fig. 10-2c) also sharpens the borderlines between the testicles.
In Fig. 10-3 a special tumor (seminoma) can be seen in the upper testicle. In this case the summation image (10-3b) contains much more information about the tumor extension, than the B-Scan (10-3a). The filtered image decreases the speckle-SNR, but sharpens border-lines.
Fig. 10-4 shows a tumor within the testicle and a big hydrozele. The second testicle is invisible. In the B-Scan (10-4a) it is unclear, which extension the tumor in the testicle has. The two summation-images (10-4b, 10-4c) improve the image-quality, but the speckle-SNR s are

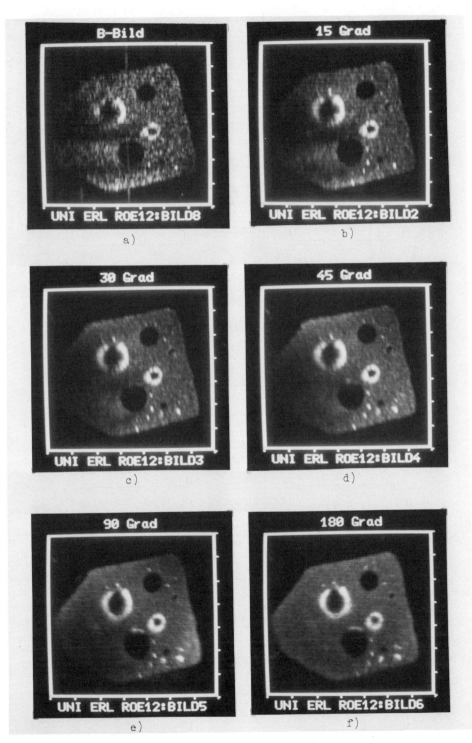

Fig. 10-1: Explanation see following side

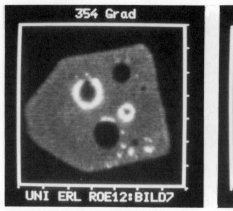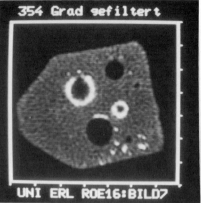

Fig. 10-1: Sponge with holes (simulation of soft tissue)
  a) B-scan
  b) - g) summation-images, aspect-angle-area is given in the head-
         lines of the images (the term "Grad" refers to "degree"),
         30 B-scans superimposed
  h) filtered image of g)

different. These differences result from distinct aspect-angle-areas and
summed B-Scans, respectively. Fig. 10-4d is the filtered version of
10-4c. Again resolution is increased, but speckle-SNR decreases.

11. CONCLUSION

     Ultrasound reflection mode computerized tomography is a special kind
of cross-sectional imaging. Conventional B-Scans of a single plane
obtained from different angles are used for a numerical image reconstruction. First the B-Scans are summed taking into account their angular position, in a second step the summation image is filtered by two dimensional inverse filtering to increase resolution. We have developed a theory
to explain the speckle-characteristics in the summation-image and filtered image. Therefore we have adapted the theory of Burckhardt /3/ and
Wagner et al. /4/ for B-Scan speckle. The results of the extension of the
theory to UCTR can be summarized:
     1. The mean speckle size in the B-Scan, summation-image and filte-
red image is very similar to the resolution of these images.
     2. The speckle-signal-to-noise-ratio is increased by a factor of $\sqrt{N}$
        in the summation image (compared to a single B-Scan) if the N
        summed B-Scans are not correlated.
     3. Because of the high-pass-character of the filter the speckle-
        signal-to-noise-ratio in the filtered image is significantly de-
        creased as compared to the corresponding summation-image.
Measurements of a texture phantom are in reasonable agreement with
theory, and in-vivo-images of testicles clearly show the predicted
speckle characteristics.

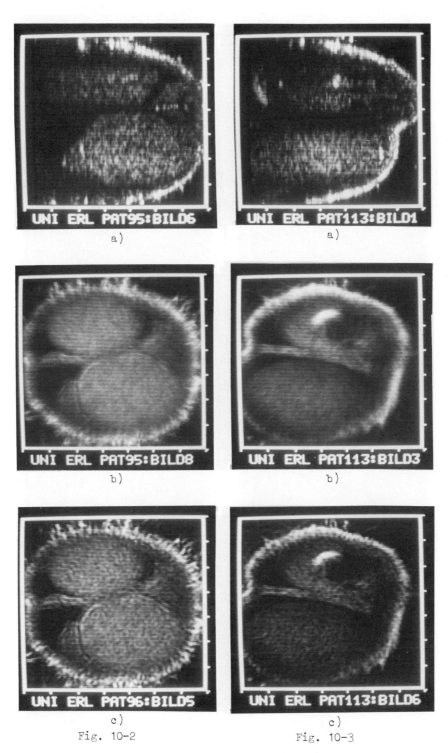

a)

a)

UNI ERL PAT95:BILD6

UNI ERL PAT113:BILD1

b)

b)

UNI ERL PAT95:BILD8

UNI ERL PAT113:BILD3

c)

c)

UNI ERL PAT96:BILD5

UNI ERL PAT113:BILD6

Fig. 10-2

Fig. 10-3

Explanation see following side

Fig. 10-2: Testicle with unknown pathological process
     a) B-scan
     b) summation-image, aspect-angle-area=354 deg, 30 B-scans summed
     c) filtered image of b)

Fig. 10-3: Testicle with seminoma
     a) B-scan
     b) summation-image, aspect-angle-area=180 deg., 30 B-scans summed
     c) filtered image of b)

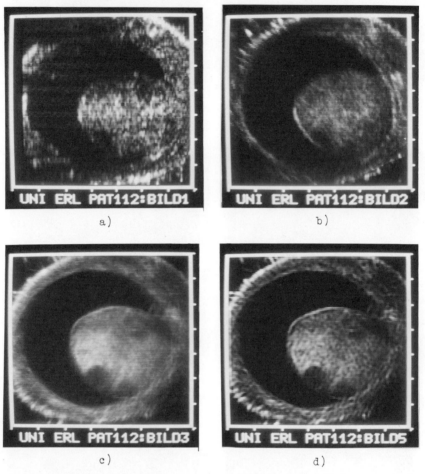

a)   b)

c)   d)

Fig. 10-4: Testicle with tumor and hydrozele
     a) B-scan
     b) summation-image,aspect-angle-area=50 deg., 5 B-scans summed
     c) summation-image,aspect-angle-area=180 deg., 30 B-scans summed
     d) filtered image of c)

12. ACKNOWLEDGEMENTS

These investigations were supported by research grant no. BMFT 01 ZS 172 5 from Bundesministerium für Forschung und Technologie, Fed. Rep. of Germany.
This work was carried out within the framework of the Concerted Action Program on Ultrasonic Tissue Characterization of the European Community.

13. REFERENCES

/1/ HILLER D., ERMERT H.: System analysis of reflection mode computerized
    tomography. IEEE Trans. Sonics and Ultrasonics, Vol. SU-31, No. 4,
    Juli 1984, pp. 240 - 250
/2/ ROEHRLEIN G, ERMERT H.: Limited angle reflection mode computerized
    tomography. Acoustical Imaging, Vol. 14, Plenum Press 1985, New York
    and London, edts. A.J. Berkhout et al.
/3/ BURCKHARDT D.B.: Speckle in ultrasound B-mode scans. IEEE Trans. on
    Sonics and Ultrasonics, Vol. SU-25, No. 1, January 1978, pp. 1-6
/4/ WAGNER R.F., SMITH S.W., SANDRIK J.M., LOPEZ H.: Statistics of
    speckle in ultrasound B-scans. IEEE Trans. on Sonics and Ultrasonics,
    Vol. SU-30, No. 3, May 1983, pp. 156-163
/5/ HASSLER D.A., TRAUTENBERG E.A., FRIEDRICH M., SPARRENBERG A.:
    Breast-scanner for clinical evaluation of ultrasonic computed
    tomography in reflection mode. Proc. of WFUMB 85, Sydney, 14-19 July
    1985, Pergamon Press, pp. 360-361
/6/ PAPOULIS A.: Probability, Random Variables and Stochastic Processes.
    McGraw-Hill, Hamburg, 1965
/7/ GEHLBACH S.M.: Quantitative analysis of acoustic speckle.
    Ultrasonic Imaging, Vol. 5, No. 2, 1983, p. 190

ANALYSIS OF INVERSE SCATTERING SOLUTIONS FROM SINGLE FREQUENCY,
COMBINED TRANSMISSION AND REFLECTION DATA FOR THE HELMHOLTZ
AND RICCATI EXACT WAVE EQUATIONS

W. W. Kim[1], S. A. Johnson[1,2,3], M. J. Berggren[2], F. Stenger[4], and
C. H. Wilcox[4]

[1] Department of Electrical Engineering
[2] Department of Bioengineering
[3] Department of Radiology and
[4] Department of Mathematics

University of Utah, Salt Lake City, Utah 84112

ABSTRACT

Various numerical methods to solve the exact inverse scattering problem are presented here. These methods consist of the following steps: first, modeling the scattering of acoustic waves by an accurate wave equation; second, discretizing this equation; and third, numerically solving the discretized equations. The fixed-point method and the nonlinear Newton-Raphson method are applied to both the Helmholtz and Riccati exact wave equations after discretizations by the moment method or by the discrete Fourier transform methods. Validity of the proposed methods is verified by computer simulation, using exact scattering data from the analytical solution for scattering from right circular cylindrical objects. (*Acoustical Imaging 15*, Halifax, Nova Scotia, July, 1986)

INTRODUCTION

Ultrasound imaging is one of the most promising areas of research for looking into the human body noninvasively, because the weak scattering interactions of ultrasound reveal small details of soft tissue structures which may be invisible to other energy sources. Furthermore, ultrasound is known to be one of the few medical imaging modalities that uses nonhazardous energy. The present ultrasound B-scan image is limited in its use, and is not adequate for some sophisticated diagnostic tests, because it is not quantitative and does not reach its potential spatial resolving power. These limitations arise because diffraction effects are not adequately taken into account. The most commonly advocated model equations for sound waves which will overcome these shortcomings of B-scan imaging are the Helmholtz and Riccati wave equations. To our knowledge, no complete numerically demonstrable inversion of these wave equations has been reported for objects with dimensions and refractive indices as large as those we have studied. In this paper, we suggest and investigate various numerical methods which converge to the exact inverse scattering inversion of these wave equations. We also give some simulation results which validate our approaches.

The Helmholtz and Riccati wave equations are, respectively, given by [1,2,3]

$$\nabla^2 f(\mathbf{r}) + k_o^2 f(\mathbf{r}) = k_o^2 \gamma(\mathbf{r}) f(\mathbf{r}) \tag{1}$$

and

$$\nabla^2 w(\mathbf{r}) + \nabla w(\mathbf{r}) \cdot \nabla w(\mathbf{r}) + 2 \nabla \ln f^{(in)}(\mathbf{r}) \cdot \nabla w(\mathbf{r}) - k_o^2 \gamma(\mathbf{r}) = 0. \tag{2}$$

Eq. (2) is obtained by substituting $f(\mathbf{r}) = f^{(in)}(\mathbf{r}) e^{w(\mathbf{r})}$ in Eq. (1), where $w(\mathbf{r})$ is called the complex scattered phase or scattered eikonal. Here, $f(\mathbf{r})$ and $f^{(in)}(\mathbf{r})$ are the transformed field and the transformed incident field (or simply the field and the incident field), and are given, respectively, by $f(\mathbf{r}) = p(\mathbf{r})\rho^{-1/2}(\mathbf{r})$ and $f^{(in)}(\mathbf{r}) = p^{(in)}(\mathbf{r})/\rho^{-1/2}(\mathbf{r})$, where $p(\mathbf{r})$ is the acoustic pressure, $p^{(in)}(\mathbf{r})$ is the incident acoustic pressure, and $\rho(\mathbf{r})$ is the density distribution in the object and the surrounding medium. Here, $\gamma(\mathbf{r})$ is called the scattering potential, and is given by [1]

$$\gamma(\mathbf{r}) = 1 - [c_o^2/ c^2(\mathbf{r})] + [c_o^2/ \omega^2] [\rho^{1/2}(\mathbf{r})\nabla^2\rho^{-1/2}(\mathbf{r})] - j\, 2\{c_o^2/ [\omega c(\mathbf{r})]\}\alpha(\mathbf{r}), \tag{3}$$

where $c(\mathbf{r})$ represents the speed-of-sound distribution, c_o is the speed of sound in the homogeneous coupling medium, ω is the temporal angular frequency of the sound wave, and $\alpha(\mathbf{r})$ is the pressure modulus absorption coefficient. A more intuitive equation [4] can be derived from Eq. (2), after some mathematical arrangements; this is given by

$$\nabla^2[f^{(in)}(\mathbf{r})\, w(\mathbf{r})]+k_o^2[f^{(in)}(\mathbf{r})\, w(\mathbf{r})] = -f^{(in)}(\mathbf{r})\{-k_o^2\, \gamma(\mathbf{r})+\nabla w(\mathbf{r}) \cdot \nabla w(\mathbf{r})\}. \tag{4}$$

In Eq. (4), the right-hand side represents the scattering departure from the homogeneous wave equation given by the left-hand side. Exact inversion methods to solve Eqs. (1) and (4) for γ follow.

A FIXED-POINT METHOD FOR SOLVING THE RICCATI EXACT WAVE EQUATION

The fixed-point method is an approach to solve the equation $f(x)=0$ by changing the equation into the form $x=g(x)$ [5]. In order to approximate the fixed point of a function g, we choose an initial approximation $p^{(0)}$ and generate the sequence $\{p^{(n)}\}$ by letting $p^{(n)}= g(p^{(n-1)})$ for each n greater than or equal to 1. Here the superscript in parenthesis means a trial value, and not an exponent. If the sequence converges to p and g is continuous, then a solution to $x=g(x)$, i.e., $f(x)=0$ is obtained. We have proposed and verified the fixed-point iterative technique to find an exact solution to the Riccati wave equation, Eq. (4), for plane incident waves [6]. In this method, the fixed-point algorithm is alternately applied to solve two equations derived from Eq. (4): the detector equation and the field equation. These two equations are more clearly seen in their respective rotated-coordinate spatial-frequency domain representations, and a more complete derivation is given by [6]

$$FT[w^{(sc)}(x=d,y)-\{FT^{-1}[G(\Lambda+k_o)FT\{\nabla w^{(m-1)}(\mathbf{r})\cdot\nabla w^{(m-1)}(\mathbf{r})\}\circ(\Lambda)]\}|_{(x=d,y)}]$$

$$= j\, O^{(m)}(k_x,\, -k_o+[k_o^2 - k_x^2]^{1/2})[4(k_o^2 - k_x^2)]^{-1/2} \exp\{j\, [k_o^2 - k_x^2]^{1/2}\, d\} \tag{5}$$

and

$$W^{(n)}(\Lambda) = G(\Lambda+k_o)\, [O(\Lambda) + FT\, [\nabla w^{(n-1)}(\mathbf{r}) \cdot \nabla w^{(n-1)}(\mathbf{r})]\circ(\Lambda)], \tag{6}$$

where $w^{(sc)}$ is the scattered phase measured at the detector, $W^{(n)}(\Lambda)$ and G are the Fourier transform of $w^{(n)}$ and the Green's function, respectively, and $O(\Lambda)$ is the Fourier transform of the object function $o(\mathbf{r}) = -k_o^2\gamma(\mathbf{r})$. The symbol $\circ$ means "is a function of." Here, $\Lambda = (k_x, k_y)$ represents the Fourier domain coordinates, and FT and FT^{-1} represent the forward and inverse Fourier transforms, respectively. Here, d designates the detector position, and m and n are the iteration indices. It is further assumed that Eqs. (5) and (6) are discretized by using the discrete Fourier transform (DFT), and that the number of incident plane-waves exceeds k_oD, where D is the diameter of the object, and they are equally spaced around 2π radians [6,7].

The procedure of the fixed-point method is summarized in the following [6].

(1) Guess an initial value for $\nabla w \cdot \nabla w$.

(2) Solve Eq. (5) for $O^{(m)}(\Lambda)$ [7].

(3) Iterate on index n in Eq. (6) until the internal eikonal field $W^{(n)}(\Lambda)$ converges.
(4) Test for overall convergence by testing the residual.
(5) Stop if the convergence is satisfied; else go to step (2) again.

We have previously shown that the above fixed-point method converges for cylindrical objects only when the diameter is less than a certain maximum value for a given maximum value of γ [6]. This limitation is removed for a larger class of objects by the methods presented next.

MOMENT METHOD DISCRETIZATION OF THE HELMHOLTZ EXACT WAVE EQUATION

Suppose we have multiple single-frequency plane-wave sources placed outside of the object grid. We designate the direction of such a plane-wave source by a source angle ϕ, which is measured by the angle between the wave-number vector $\mathbf{k}$ generated by that source at the origin and the positive x-axis. Then all the fields and scattered phases in Eqs. (1) and (4) will depend on the source angle ϕ. It should be pointed out that the multiple views are neccesary so that, at least in the simplest case where the Born approximation holds, the rotation of the Ewald circle will cover the entire spatial-frequency object plane [7]. Two separate systems of equations are obtained by solving Eq. (1) for the field at the detector and at the object grid. These are designated as the detector equation and the field equation, respectively, and are given by

$$f_\phi^{(sc)}(\mathbf{r}) = -k_o^2 \int g(\mathbf{r}-\mathbf{r}')\,\gamma(\mathbf{r}')\,f_\phi(\mathbf{r}')\,d\mathbf{r}' \qquad (7)$$

and

$$f_\phi(\mathbf{r}) - f_\phi^{(in)}(\mathbf{r}) = -k_o^2 \int g(\mathbf{r}-\mathbf{r}')\,\gamma(\mathbf{r}')\,f_\phi(\mathbf{r}')\,d\mathbf{r}'. \qquad (8)$$

The subscript ϕ represents the ϕ-dependence of the field, and $f_\phi^{(sc)}$ represents the scattered field. The detector equation is solved for γ using the scattered field $f_\phi^{(sc)}$ measured at the detector and the field f_ϕ calculated by the field equation, Eq. (8). On the other hand, the field equation is solved for f_ϕ using given the incident field $f_\phi^{(in)}$ and the scattering potential γ calculated from the detector equation, Eq. (7). For digital computer implementation, the analytic equations (7) and (8) must somehow be discretized. This has been done by a sinc-basis moment method [1]. The discretized versions of Eqs. (7) and (8), respectively, are given by [1]

$$f_{\phi m}^{(sc)} = \sum_{j=1}^{N} D_{mj}\, \gamma_j\, f_{\phi j} \qquad \begin{array}{l} m = 1, \ldots, M \\ j = 1, \ldots, N \\ \phi = 1, \ldots, \Phi \end{array} \qquad (9)$$

and

$$f_{\phi l} = f_{\phi l}^{(in)} + \sum_{j=1}^{N} C_{lj}\, \gamma_j\, f_{\phi j} \qquad \begin{array}{l} l = 1, \ldots, N \\ j = 1, \ldots, N \\ \phi = 1, \ldots, \Phi \end{array} \qquad (10)$$

Here, the subscript m implies the functional values at a discretized detector position m, and the subscripts l and j represent the discretized pixel points l and j of the object grid. Here, the coefficients D_{mj} and C_{lj} are, respectively, given by [1]

$$D_{mj} = - k_o^2 \int \psi(\mathbf{r}'-\mathbf{r}_j')\, g(\mathbf{r}_m-\mathbf{r}')\, d\mathbf{r}' \qquad (11)$$

and

$$C_{lj} = - k_o^2 \int \psi(\mathbf{r}'-\mathbf{r}_j')\, g(\mathbf{r}_l-\mathbf{r}')\, d\mathbf{r}', \qquad (12)$$

where $\psi\,(\mathbf{r}\text{-}\mathbf{r}_j)$ is the sinc-basis function given for the Q-dimensional problem, with uniform grid point spacing h, by [1]

$$\psi\,(\mathbf{r}-\mathbf{r}_j) = \prod_{q=1}^{Q} \sin\left[\,(\pi/h)\,(r_q - n_{qj}\,h)\,\right] / \left[\,(\pi/h)\,(r_q - n_{qj}\,h)\,\right]. \qquad (13)$$

It is, in fact, the above coefficients D_{mj} and C_{lj} that set up the relations between the source and response, i.e., the detector point m and the pixel point j, and the two pixel points j and l, respectively. These discrete coefficients may be obtained by taking the inverse DFT of the sampled version of a particular analytic expression corresponding to the Fourier transform of the supported Green's function [6].

The above equations (9) and (10) are generally well-posed algebraic equations, and can therefore be solved by any standard linear-system solution algorithm. Here, the conjugate gradient algorithm is used for fast convergence. Also note that Eqs. (9) and (10) are general and hold for sources other than plane waves.

NEWTON-RAPHSON METHOD FOR SOLVING THE HELMHOLTZ EXACT WAVE EQUATION

The Newton-Raphson method is one of the most powerful and well-known numerical methods for finding a root of f(x)=0 where f is a scalar function of a single independent variable x. It is known to have generally better performance than most other fixed-point schemes close to the solution [5]. Starting with a given initial approximation $x^{(0)}$, a sequence $x^{(1)}, x^{(2)}, x^{(3)}, \ldots$ is computed, where $x^{(n)}$ is determined by the following iteration formula:

$$x^{(n+1)} = x^{(n)} + \delta x^{(n)} \quad \text{and} \quad \delta x^{(n)} = - [df(x^{(n)})/dx]^{-1} f(x^{(n)}) .$$

The iterations can be stopped when $| \delta x^{(n)} |$ has become less than the largest error one is willing to permit in the root. Note that $x^{(n)} + \delta x^{(n)}$ can be associated with $g(x^{(n)})$ so that $x^{(n+1)} = g(x^{(n)})$; thus Newton-Raphson is a special fixed-point method. The Newton-Raphson method can be generalized to be applicable to systems of non-linear equations, and has been suggested [6] as a means for solving the inverse scattering problems. In this section, we apply the Newton-Raphson method, first to the Helmholtz exact wave equation and finally, in the next section to the Riccati exact wave equation. We also derive the respective formulas for computer implementation. Some of simulation results will be shown.

Let $R_\phi^{(sc)}(\mathbf{r})$ be the residual of the detector equation, Eq. (7) and let $R_\phi^{(fld)}(\mathbf{r})$ be the residual of the field equation, Eq. (8). They are given from Eqs. (7) and (8), respectively, by

$$R_\phi^{(sc)}(\mathbf{r}) = f_\phi^{(sc)}(\mathbf{r}) + k_o^2 \int g(\mathbf{r}-\mathbf{r}') \, \gamma \, (\mathbf{r}') \, f_\phi(\mathbf{r}') \, d\mathbf{r}' \tag{14}$$

and

$$R_\phi^{(fld)}(\mathbf{r}) = f_\phi^{(in)}(\mathbf{r}) - f_\phi(\mathbf{r}) - k_o^2 \int g(\mathbf{r}-\mathbf{r}') \, \gamma \, (\mathbf{r}') \, f_\phi(\mathbf{r}') \, d\mathbf{r}'. \tag{15}$$

Let the column vector $\mathbf{R} \equiv [R_\phi^{(sc)}, R_\phi^{(fld)}]^T$, where T means transpose, represent the accumulation of all residuals from all equations. Let $\mathbf{v} \equiv [\gamma, f_\phi]^T$ be a column vector of sampled values of γ and f_ϕ at each pixel for each discrete plane-wave source and incident-field direction ϕ. Similarly, let $R_\phi^{(sc)}$ and $R_\phi^{(fld)}$ be discretized to represent the residuals at each pixel and each detector for each incident-field direction. Then the solution to the inverse scattering problem is the solution to the equation

$$\mathbf{R} \, (\mathbf{v}) = 0, \tag{16}$$

and may be found by Newton-Raphson iteration:

$$\mathbf{v}^{(k+1)} = \mathbf{v}^{(k)} + \delta \mathbf{v}^{(k)} . \tag{17}$$

Here, $\delta \mathbf{v}^{(k)} \equiv [\delta\gamma^{(k)}, \delta f_\phi^{(k)}]^T$ is a column vector that is the solution to the following system of linear equations:

$$[(\partial \mathbf{R}/ \partial \mathbf{v})|_{\mathbf{v}=\mathbf{v}(k)}] \, \delta \mathbf{v}^{(k)} = - \mathbf{R} \, (\mathbf{v}^{(k)}) . \tag{18}$$

The matrix $[\partial \mathbf{R}/ \partial \mathbf{v}]$ is known as the Jacobian, and is also written in the intuitive notation $[\partial (R_\phi^{(sc)}, R_\phi^{(fld)})/ \partial (\gamma, f_\phi)]$, which demonstrates that it is composed of four submatrices $[\partial R_\phi^{(sc)}/ \partial\gamma]$, $[\partial R_\phi^{(sc)}/ \partial f_\phi]$, $[\partial R_\phi^{(fld)}/ \partial\gamma]$, and $[\partial R_\phi^{(fld)}/ \partial f_\phi]$. Using this notation, Eq. (18) can be written as

$$\begin{bmatrix} -\partial R_\phi^{(sc)}/\partial\gamma & \partial R_\phi^{(sc)}/\partial f_\phi \\ \partial R_\phi^{(fld)}/\partial\gamma & \partial R_\phi^{(fld)}/\partial f_\phi \end{bmatrix} \begin{bmatrix} \delta\gamma \\ \delta f_\phi \end{bmatrix} = - \begin{bmatrix} R_\phi^{(sc)} \\ R_\phi^{(fld)} \end{bmatrix} \tag{19}$$

The product of the Jacobian matrix elements and the differential displacements $\delta\gamma$ and δf_ϕ may be found by means of the Frechet derivatives or by means of the calculus of variations or other methods. One way of doing this is by using the following identity:

$$\{[\partial R_\phi^{(sc)}(\gamma + \varepsilon\,\delta\gamma,\, f_\phi)/\,\partial\varepsilon]\}|_{\varepsilon=0}$$

$$= \{[\partial R_\phi^{(sc)}(\gamma + \varepsilon\,\delta\gamma,\, f_\phi)\,/\,\partial(\gamma + \varepsilon\,\delta\gamma)]\,[\partial(\gamma + \varepsilon\,\delta\gamma)/\,\partial\varepsilon]\}|_{\varepsilon=0}$$

$$= [\partial R_\phi^{(sc)}(\gamma,\, f_\phi)/\,\partial\gamma]\,\delta\gamma\,. \tag{20}$$

The partial derivative on the far left of Eq. (20) can be calculated directly from Eq. (14), and similar arguments are used for obtaining the elements of the other submatrices. These matrix elements are then given, respectively, by the discretized versions of the following equations:

$$[\partial R_\phi^{(sc)}/\,\partial\gamma]\,\delta\gamma\,(\mathbf{r}) \;=\; k_0^2\int g\,(\mathbf{r-r'})\,f_\phi(\mathbf{r'})\,\delta\gamma\,(\mathbf{r'})\,d\mathbf{r'} \tag{21}$$

$$[\partial R_\phi^{(sc)}/\,\partial f_\phi]\,\delta f_\phi\,(\mathbf{r}) \;=\; k_0^2\int g\,(\mathbf{r-r'})\,\gamma\,(\mathbf{r'})\,\delta f_\phi(\mathbf{r'})\,d\mathbf{r'} \tag{22}$$

$$[\partial R_\phi^{(fld)}/\,\partial\gamma]\,\delta\gamma\,(\mathbf{r}) \;=\; -\,k_0^2\int g\,(\mathbf{r-r'})\,f_\phi(\mathbf{r'})\,\delta\gamma\,(\mathbf{r'})\,d\mathbf{r'} \tag{23}$$

$$[\partial R_\phi^{(fld)}/\,\partial f_\phi]\,\delta f_\phi\,(\mathbf{r}) \;=\; -\,\delta f_\phi(\mathbf{r}) - k_0^2\int g\,(\mathbf{r-r'})\,\gamma\,(\mathbf{r'})\,\delta f_\phi(\mathbf{r'})\,d\mathbf{r'}\,. \tag{24}$$

To discretize Eqs. (21) through (24), and, thus, to obtain the matrix elements of Eq. (19), the previously mentioned sinc-basis moment method may be used. After discretization, the following linear system of equations, with the size of each submatrix indicated, is obtained:

$$\begin{array}{cccc} & N & \Phi N & 1 & 1 \end{array}$$

$$\begin{array}{c} \Phi M \\ \Phi N \end{array} \begin{bmatrix} -D_{mj}\,f_{\phi j} & -D_{mj}\,\gamma_j \\ C_{1j}\,f_{\phi j} & -\delta_{1j} + C_{1j}\,\gamma_j \end{bmatrix} \begin{bmatrix} \delta\gamma_j \\ \delta f_{\phi j} \end{bmatrix}\begin{array}{c} N \\ \Phi N \end{array} = \begin{bmatrix} -R_{\phi m}^{(sc)} \\ -R_{\phi l}^{(fld)} \end{bmatrix}\begin{array}{c} \Phi M \\ \Phi N \end{array} \tag{25}$$

We can make Eq. (25) overdetermined by taking $\Phi M > N$. The solutions δv from Eq. (25) are used to update Eq. (17). The new value $v^{(k+1)}$ from Eq. (17) is then inserted in Eq. (25) to find a new $\delta v^{(k)}$. This process is repeated until convergence is satisfactory. The solutions of the linear system in Eq. (25) may be found by Kaczmarz, Gauss-Siedel, or other iteration methods. In our present simulation work, the conjugate gradient algorithm is used for fast convergence.

NEWTON-RAPHSON METHOD FOR SOLVING THE RICCATI EXACT WAVE EQUATION

The Newton-Raphson method is also applicable to the Riccati wave equation. The residual equations similar to Eqs. (14) and (15) are obtained by solving Eq. (4) as described in [4]. Including the ϕ dependence, we have

$$R_\phi^{(sc)}(r) = f_\phi^{(in)}(r) w_\phi^{(sc)}(r)$$

$$- \int g(r-r') f_\phi^{(in)}(r') [- k_o^2 \gamma(r') + (\nabla w \cdot \nabla w) \circ (r')] dr' \qquad (26)$$

and

$$R_\phi^{(fld)}(r) = f_\phi^{(in)}(r) w_\phi(r)$$

$$- \int g(r-r') f_\phi^{(in)}(r') [- k_o^2 \gamma(r') + (\nabla w \cdot \nabla w) \circ (r')] dr'. \qquad (27)$$

In this problem, the known value is the scattered phase $w_\phi^{(sc)}$ measured at the detector, and the unknown variables are the scattering potential γ and the scattered phase w_ϕ inside the object grid. The solution procedure is very similar to that for the Helmholtz exact wave equation. Here, however, $v \equiv [\gamma, w_\phi]^T$ and $\delta v^{(k)} \equiv [\delta\gamma^{(k)}, \delta w_\phi^{(k)}]^T$. The matrix product of the Jacobian matrix elements and $\delta\gamma$ and δw can also be found using the same argument as that for the Helmholtz equation in the previous section. The four equations similar to Eqs. (21) through (24) are given by

$$[\partial R_\phi^{(sc)}/ \partial\gamma] \delta\gamma(r) = k_o^2 \int g(r-r') f_\phi^{(in)}(r') \delta\gamma(r') dr' \qquad (28)$$

$$[\partial R_\phi^{(sc)}/ \partial w] \delta w(r) = 2 \int \{\nabla \cdot [g(r-r') f_\phi^{(in)}(r') \nabla w(r')]\} \delta w(r') dr' \qquad (29)$$

$$[\partial R_\phi^{(fld)}/ \partial\gamma] \delta\gamma(r) = k_o^2 \int g(r-r') f_\phi^{(in)}(r') \delta\gamma(r') dr' \qquad (30)$$

$$[\partial R_\phi^{(fld)}/ \partial w] \delta w(r) = f_\phi^{(in)}(r) \delta w(r)$$

$$+ 2 \int \{\nabla \cdot [g(r-r') f_\phi^{(in)}(r') \nabla w(r')]\} \delta w(r') dr'. \qquad (31)$$

Eq. (31) is obtained by integration by parts as follows;

$$[\partial R_\phi^{(fld)}/ \partial w] \delta w(r)$$

$$= f_\phi^{(in)}(r) \delta w(r) - \int g(r-r') f_\phi^{(in)}(r') \{[2\nabla w \cdot \nabla(\delta w)] \circ (r')\} dr'$$

$$= f_\phi^{(in)}(r) \delta w(r) + 2 \int \{\nabla \cdot [g(r-r') f_\phi^{(in)}(r') \nabla w(r')]\} \delta w(r') dr. \qquad (32)$$

Eq. (29) is obtained in a similar manner. Discretization and computer implementation of Eqs. (28) through (31) are more involved because of the $\nabla w \cdot \nabla w$ term in the original equation. These steps are now under development.

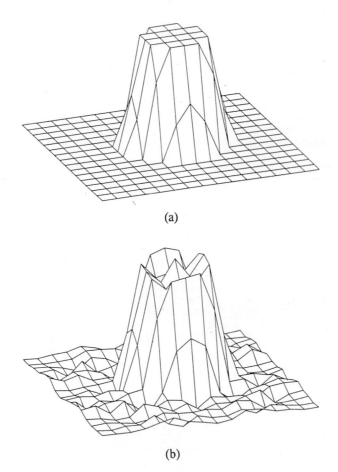

(a)

(b)

Fig. 1   Simulation results by isometric plots: (a) original cylinder, and
(b) reconstruction after 4 linearizations.

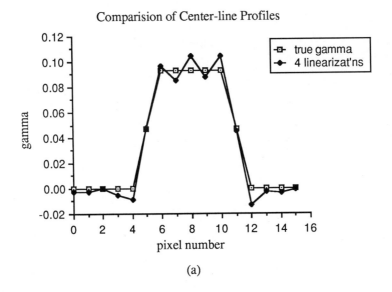

(a)

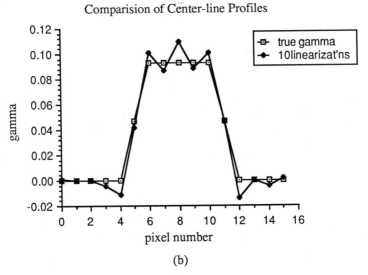

(b)

Fig. 2　Comparison of the center-line profiles of reconstructed images of test object shown in Fig. 1(a): (a) after 4 linearizations, and (b) after 10 linearizations.

SIMULATION EXAMPLES

Examples of the direct scattering and inverse scattering problems of a right circular cylindrical object using the fixed-point iteration method on the Riccati wave equation were shown in [6]. In [6], the region of convergency of the direct scattering problem was also shown. Another example of reconstruction of a right circular cylinder using the single-frequency moment method on the Helmholtz wave equation was shown in [8]. In those papers, we verified the validity of the proposed methods by using an alternating variable fixed-point method; the system of equations to be solved at each step was linear. Here, however, we present a simulation resulting from reconstructing a right circular cylindrical object using the nonlinear Newton-Raphson method on the Helmholtz equation, as described by Eqs. (14) through (25). Fig. 1(a) shows the original cylinder, while Fig. 1(b) shows the reconstructed cylinder. The center-line profiles are compared in Fig. 2. Fig. 2(a) shows the result obtained after 4 linearizations, and Fig. 2(b) shows the result after 10 linearizations. The detector data were generated by a program which uses the exact analytic formula for scattering from such a cylinder [9]. We used an object grid of $N=256$ pixels (16x16) with a spacing between adjacent pixels of $\lambda/4$. The object was a cylinder of radius 0.75λ with a speed of sound of 1.575×10^5 cm/sec. The speed of sound in the medium was 1.5×10^5 cm/sec. This means that the real part of γ was 0.093. The imaginary part of γ was set equal to zero. The perimeter of the object grid was sampled uniformly at 60 detector locations. A satisfactory convergence (Fig. 1(b) or Fig. 2(a)) was obtained after 4 linearizations and associated linear inversions. This joint process took a c.p.u. time of 39.8 minutes using a Gould 9080 computer. A 10 linearization process took a c.p.u. time of 99.4 minutes on the same computer. We observed that $\| \gamma - \gamma_{true} \|_2 / \| \gamma_{true} \|_2$ for the center-line profiles in Fig. 2 had values of 0.105 and 0.114 after 4 and 10 linearizations, respectively. However, $\| R \|_2$ had values of 0.045 and 0.013 after 4 and 10 linearizations, respectively, for all sources and detectors. This is consistent with the notion that an object not spatially bandlimited cannot be reconstructed perfectly from undersampled data, even though the resulting equations may have a minimum square-norm solution.

CONCLUSION AND SUGGESTED FURTHER RESEARCH

Mathematical derivation and computer implementation for some exact solution methods to the Helmholtz and Riccati wave equations are presented. Validity of these methods is also verified by computer simulation giving the reconstruction of right circular cylindrical objects from the scattered field at the detectors. An example of application of the nonlinear Newton-Raphson method to imaging is provided by a numerical inversion of the Helmholtz exact wave equation.

The implementation of the nonlinear Newton-Raphson method on the Riccati equation is under development with the results expected soon. More complete comparison of those various methods on the accuracy, region of convergence, rate of convergence, c.p.u. time, robustness, etc. as functions of size of object, contrast range in scattering potential, number of detectors, number of sources, etc. should be done to predict optimum practical application. The best combination of the number of linearizations and the number of iterations for linear inversion at each linearization step, given a fixed c.p.u. time, is also being investigated.

ACKNOWLEDGEMENTS

Use of a closed-form formula of the Fourier integral transform of the supported Green's function developed by Mr. David Borup, department of Electrical Engineering, University of Utah, for rapid computation of the D_{mj} and C_{1j} coefficients, is greatly appreciated. This work was supported by PHS Grant No. 2 R01 CA29728-04 from NCI and PHS Grant No. 1 HL34995-01 from NHLBI.

REFERENCES

1. S. A. Johnson and M. L. Tracy, "Inverse Scattering Solutions by a Sinc Basis, Multiple Source, Moment Method -- Part I: Theory," *Ultrasonic Imaging 5*, pp. 361-375, 1983.
2. S. A. Johnson, Y. Zhou, M. L. Tracy, M. J. Berggren, and F. Stenger, "Inverse Scattering Solutions by a Sinc Basis, Multiple Source, Moment Method -- Part III: Fast Algorithms," *Ultrasonic Imaging 6*, pp. 103-116, 1984.
3. S. A. Johnson, F. Stenger, C. Wilcox, J. Ball, and M. Berggren, "Wave Equations and Inverse Solutions for Soft Tissue," *Acoustical Imaging 11*, pp. 409-424, 1982.
4. M. Slaney, A. C. Kak, and L. E. Larson,"Limitations of Imaging with First Order Diffraction Tomography," *IEEE Transactions on Microwave Theory and Techniques*, Vol. MTT-32, No. 8, pp. 860-873, 1984.
5. R. L. Burden, J. D. Faires, and A. C. Reynolds, *Numerical Analysis*, 2nd ed., Prindle, Weber & Schmidt, Boston, Massachusetts, 1981.
6. W. W. Kim, M. J. Berggren, S. A. Johnson, F. Stenger, and C. H. Wilcox, "Inverse Scattering Solutions to the Exact Riccati Wave Equations by Iterative Rytov Approximations and Internal Field Calculations," *IEEE Sonics and Ultrasonics Symposium Proceedings*, pp. 878-882, 1985.
7. R. K. Mueller, M. Kaveh, and G. Wade, "Reconstructive Tomography and Applications to Ultrasonics," *Proceedings of IEEE*, Vol. 67, No. 4, pp. 567-587, 1979.
8. M. J. Berggren, S. A. Johnson, B. L. Curruth, W. W. Kim, F. Stenger, and P. K. Kuhn, "Ultrasound Inverse Scattering Solutions from Transmission and/or Reflection Data," *Proceedings of International Workshop on Physics and Engineering of Computerized Multidimensional Imaging and Processing*, 1986. (Submitted to SPIE Vol. 671)
9. P. M. Morse and K. U. Ingard, *Theoretical Acoustics*, McGraw-Hill Book Co., New York, 1968.

ATTEMPT TO INCLUDE REFRACTION IN AN ULTRASONIC TOMOGRAPHY ALGORITHM

F. Denis, G. Gimenez and F. Peyrin

Laboratoire de Traitement du Signal et Ultrasons, INSA 502

69621 Villeurbanne Cedex, France

ABSTRACT

This paper is concerned with reconstruction of ultrasonic tomography from time-of-flight projections. The use of conventional CT methods, assuming straight line propagation, generally yields to insufficient quality images. In order to improve the reconstruction, the refraction phenomenon has to be taken into account. Some ray tracing and reconstruction methods are compared then implemented and tested on simulated objects. Finally, reconstructed images are displayed.

INTRODUCTION

Image reconstruction from projections has had a large success in the last few years, especially due to good results obtained in X-ray computerized tomography [1-2]. The application of these methods to ultrasonic tomography is particularly interesting in medical imaging because of the harmlessness of this technique. Images of various acoustic parameters of biological tissues may be reconstructed.[3-5]. However the direct transposition of X-ray reconstruction methods to the ultrasonic case, assuming implicitly rectilinear propagation, has been proved to result in insufficiently precise images [4, 6]. In order to improve the quality of the reconstructions, studies have been carried out trying to take into account the curvature of rays due to refraction [7-14]. Let us note that the knowledge of the ray path is necessary to reconstruct the values of the acoustic parameter in the medium, and that conversely, the knowledge of the medium is necessary for ray-tracing. Consequently it is interesting to use an iterative method which at each step corrects the image according to the rays computed from the image of the previous step.

In this paper we present the results of a comparison between different types of iterative ultrasonic tomographic reconstruction methods of time-of-flight images. In this case the experimental data are the propagation times of pulses through the studied medium.This time-of-flight is expressed as the integral along the ray of the inverse of the ultrasonic celerity (or equivalently the acoustic refractive index) which is the reconstructed parameter.

Usually, the ultrasonic rays are not confined in a plane. Then, taking into account the refraction phenomenon, leads to a three dimensional approach. However, at the present stage, the study is performed in 2D assuming a cylindrical symmetry of the medium. This is done in order to choose the most appropriate method for a further three-dimensional reconstruction.

The general reconstruction process we have used begins by a complete reconstruction assuming straight rays (this is rapid and gives a good first approximation of the image).

Then, a reconstruction with curved rays is performed which includes two steps :

. computation of the rays and of their times-of-flight from the reconstructed image ;

. distribution along the rays of the difference between computed and measured times-of-flight with the Algebraïc Reconstruction Technique (ART) [2].

We shall only describe here these two steps, since tomography in the case of rectilinear propagation has already been widely discussed in the relevant literature.

RAY TRACING

Ray-tracing methods are based on integration of differential equations. These equations are generally derived from the eikonal equation that describes propagation in an inhomogeneous medium [7,9].

$$\nabla S \cdot \nabla S = (\frac{C_0}{C(r)})^2 = n(r)^2 \qquad (1)$$

where the surfaces $S(r) = cte$ represent wave surfaces, C_0 is the reference for acoustic speeds, $C(r)$ is the local acoustic speed, $n(r) = C_0/C(r)$ is the local refractive index, and vector r with (x,y,z) coordinates characterizes the point position.
As for geometrical optics, rays can be defined as the orthogonal trajectories to the wave surfaces.

To trace the rays, Schomberg [8,10,11] proposes to solve the equation :

$$\frac{\partial^2 r}{\partial \sigma^2} = 4 n \nabla n \qquad (2)$$

where σ is the curve parameter. This last equation may be converted into a first order differential system that can be numerically integrated by Runge-Kutta's method for example.

However a commonly used differential equation is :

$$\frac{d}{ds} (n \frac{dr}{ds}) = \nabla n \qquad (3)$$

where s represents the curvilinear coordinate along the ray.

Johnson et al. [12], Andersen and Kak [9] have studied different means of integrating this equation. One of them consists of computing the vector r from its second order development in a Taylor series :

$$r(s+\Delta s) = r(s) + \frac{dr}{ds} \Delta s + \frac{1}{2} \frac{d^2 r}{ds^2} \Delta s^2 \qquad (4)$$

Equation (3) gives an evaluation of d^2r/ds^2 :

$$n \frac{d^2r}{ds^2} + (\nabla n \cdot \frac{dr}{ds}) \frac{dr}{ds} = \nabla n \qquad (5)$$

Then, equations (4) and (5) lead to :

$$r(s+\Delta s)=r(s) + \frac{dr}{ds} \Delta s + \frac{1}{2n} \left[\nabla n -(n. \frac{dr}{ds}) \frac{dr}{ds} \right] s^2 \qquad (6)$$

Here, the main difficulty is to estimate dr/ds. Johnson et al. [12] proposed to approximate dr/ds by :

$$\frac{1}{s} \left[r(s)-r(s-\Delta s) \right] \qquad (7)$$

However this evaluation is not precise enough and the computed ray rapidly diverges from its theoretical trajectory, unless a very small step size s is used . For our ray tracing, we use an auxiliary computation of the tangent to the ray. The angular displacement form, described by Andersen and Kak [9] is a good means to obtain this evaluation. Using the Snell Descartes law, the following holds :

$$\frac{d\theta}{ds} = \frac{1}{n} (\cos \theta \frac{dn}{dy_1} - \sin \theta \frac{dn}{dx_1}) \qquad (8)$$

where θ is given by $\begin{cases} \cos \theta = dx_1/ds \\ \sin \theta = dy_1/ds \end{cases} \qquad (9)$

(x_1,y_1) are the coordinates in the plane defined by the tangent to the ray, the gradient vector n and the point determined by $r(s)$. In case of cylindrical symmetry, only two dimensions have to be considered and this plane is the (x,y) plane. Then dr/ds results from :

$$\begin{cases} \frac{dx_1}{ds} = \cos (\theta + d\theta) \\ \\ \frac{dy_1}{ds} = \sin (\theta + d\theta) \end{cases} \qquad (10)$$

We have implemented both the method proposed by Schomberg (equation (2)) and the one given by equations (6) (8) (9). Using the latter, the evaluation of dr/ds is quite correct and the ray tracing provides good results. Furthermore, computation times are about three times shorter than those required for the fourth order Runge- Kutta integration of Schomberg's equation (2) for a similar precision.

Another problem that arises in ray tracing is interpolation. Indeed, because of sampling, the refractive index value $n(r)$ is only known on a grid of points. As the rays do not necessarily run through these points, we need, to improve tracing a good knowledge of n and n at all points. The traditional pixel representation, for which n is constant on a square surface centered on each point, gives bad results. So, it is better to look for a continuous representation of n. For this purpose, the simplest way to insure function continuity is to use a bilinear interpolation, where the function value at any point depends on the values at its four nearest sampling points. This is simple and rapid but the continuity of the function derivatives on the sampling grid lines is not insured.

To satisfy this further condition, we hence use a two dimensional cubic spline interpolation which has been implemented by Lytle and Dynes [11]. In view to determine the interpolated function, we impose the condition that the function and its first partial derivatives are continuous for the four nearest grid points. The derivatives with respect to x, y and xy being defined with the four nearest grid points again, the interpolated function at a point depends therefore on the sixteen neighboring points of the sampling grid.
Figure 1 shows an example of ray tracing with this last type of interpolation.

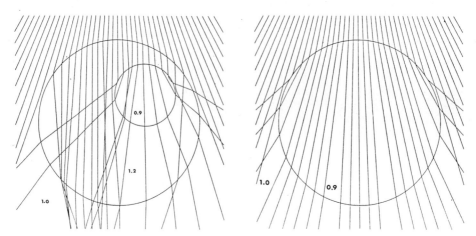

Fig.1. :   Ray tracing with cubic spline interpolation an second order algorithm. Left : medium of refractive index values 0.9 and 1.2 embedded in a medium of refractive index 1.0. Right : medium of refractive index value 0.9 embedded in a medium of index 1.

For the present work, we only consider bidimensional ray tracing. Though, let us note that computation of rays in a three dimensional space would be exactly the same for equation (2) integration. It seems not so direct for equation (6) when dr/ds estimation is done with the angular displacement method. For interpolation, complication comes from the number of coefficients to be computed, 8 instead of 4 for bilinear interpolation, and 64 instead of 16 for spline interpolation.

RECONSTRUCTION

The line integral of the refractive index n along a ray gives the value of the time-of-flight :

$$T = \frac{1}{Co} \int_\gamma n \, ds \tag{11}$$

where γ is the ray trajectory. To use this equation, we must find a discrete representation for n, such as :

$$n = \sum_1^N n_i \, b_i \tag{12}$$

where n_i is the value of function n at point i of the sampling grid and b_i is a basis function verifying :

$$\begin{cases} b_i = 1 & \text{at point } i \\ b_i = 0 & \text{at all other points of the lattice.} \end{cases}$$

Andersen and Kak have shown [14] that equation (11), for a ray j along a trajectory γ_j, may be written :

$$\text{CoT}_j = \int_{\gamma_j} \sum_{i=1}^{N} n_i \, b_i \, ds = \sum_{i=1}^{N} n_i \int_{\gamma_j} b_i \, ds$$

or :

$$\text{CoT}_j = \sum_{i=1}^{N} a_{ij} \, n_i$$

$$\tag{13}$$

$$a_{ij} = \int_{\gamma_j} b_i \, ds$$

The a_{ij} coefficients represent the line integrals along the ray path γ_j of the basis functions b_i.

Data acquisition of Tj for many ray paths γ_j, provides a system of equations of type (13). A common method to solve this system is A.R.T. which is an application of the Kaczmarz method [2, 15, 16]. It is an iterative algorithm whose form is :

$$k = 0, 1, \ldots$$
$$j = k \bmod LM + 1$$
$$i = 1, \ldots N$$

$$n_i^{(k+1)} = n_i^{(k)} + \omega^{(k)} \cdot a_{ij} \frac{\text{CoT}_j - \sum\limits_{l=1}^{N} a_{1j} n_1^{(k)}}{\sum\limits_{l=1}^{N} (a_{1j})^2} \tag{14}$$

where (k+1) denotes the (k+1)[th] iteration, L is the number of rays per projection and M is the total number of projections. $\omega^{(k)}$ is a relaxation parameter which must be carefully chosen in order to ensure convergence and to reduce noise in the reconstructed images. In the present work, we have considered the resolution problem with $\omega^{(k)} = 1$ for all k, but it seems that some artefacts in the images could be reduced with a more appropriate choice of $\omega^{(k)}$.

To implement the reconstruction method it is necessary to compute the a_{ij} coefficients. As n must be expressed as a linear combination of N basis functions b_i (see (12)) different methods are then available depending on the choice made for b_i functions. Among all possible choices, we have picked out and compared the four following examples.
In the following we denote "d" the size of the square lattice.

"Cubic" basis

The first function b_i is the simplest one, i.e a function of constant value 1 at all points of a square of side d around point i (Fig.2a). The a_{ij} coefficients are then equivalent to the length of the ray intersecting the square.

"Cosine" function

The second basis function b_i is defined on a square area of side 2d around point i, as :

$$b_i(x,y) = \frac{1}{4} (1 - \cos \pi (\frac{x-x_i}{d} - 1)) (1 - \cos \pi(\frac{y-y_i}{d})) \qquad (15)$$

With this basis, the representation of function n is continuous, opposite to the first one, and its variations are smoother. The a_{ij} coefficients are computed by a discrete integration of b_i along the ray.

"Pyramidal" pixels

This basis and the next one correspond to the two types of inter-polation previously described in the ray tracing section. The present one is for bilinear interpolation and has been used and explained by Andersen and Kak [14]. We describe it briefly.

Consider a point P(x,y), and its four nearest neighbours i_1, i_2, i_3, i_4 (Fig.3). We call (x_o, y_o) the coordinates of one of these four points, for example i_1. Under these assumptions the interpolated value of n at point P is :

$$n(x,y)=n_{i_1}(1-X-Y+XY)+n_{i_2}(X-XY)+n_{i_3}(Y-XY)+n_{i_4} XY$$
with :

$$X = \frac{x - x_o}{d} \qquad\qquad Y = \frac{y - y_o}{d} \qquad (16)$$

Fig.3. :   Point positions for
            bilinear interpolation

This interpolation is equivalent to a representation of the image with "pyramid-shaped" basis function, as called by Andersen and Kak. These functions are defined on a square surface of side 2d (Fig.2c). The coefficients of n_i terms in eq. (16) directly give the value of the basis function b_i at point P. The discrete integration of b_i along the ray is then immediate and gives the coefficients a_{ij}.

Spline functions

The last type of basis function that we shall mention is related to cubic spline interpolation. In this case, the value n(x,y) at point P is calculated with its sixteen neighbours i_1 to i_{16}.

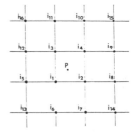

Fig.4 .:   Point positions for cubic
            spline interpolation

(x_o, y_o) denotes i_1 coordinates again, and X and Y have the same signi-fication as in (16).

376

a)

b)

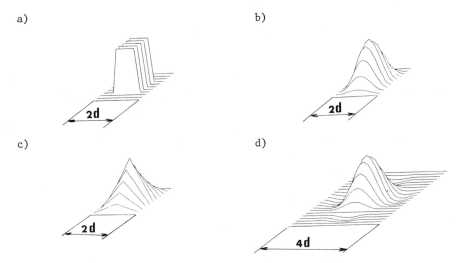

c)

d)

Fig. 2. : Different basis functions.
           a) "cubic" basis.   b) "cosine" function.
           c) "pyramidal" function. d) "Spline" function.

a)

b)

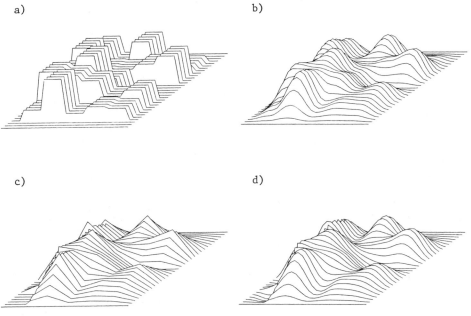

c)

d)

Fig. 5. : Example of representation of a small image with different
           basis functions.
           a) "cubic" basis.   b) "cosine" function.
           c) "pyramidal" basis.   d) "Spline" function.

It can be shown that $n(x,y)$ is given by :

$$n(x,y) = n_{i_1}\left[(2-5X^2+3X^3)(2-5Y^2+3Y^3)-2(X^2-X^3)(Y^2-Y^3)\right]/4$$

$$+ n_{i_2}\left[(X+4X^2-3X^3)(2-5Y^2+3Y^3)-2(X-2X^2+X^3)(Y^2-Y^3)\right]/4$$

$$+ n_{i_3}\left[(2-5X+3X^3)(Y+4Y^2-3Y^3)-2(X^2-X^3)(Y-2Y^2+Y^3)\right]/4$$

$$+ n_{i_4}\left[(X+4X^2-3X^3)(Y+4Y^2-3Y^3)-2(X-2X^2+X^3)(Y-2Y^2+Y^3)\right]/4$$

$$+ n_{i_5}\left[-(X-2X^2+X^3)(2-7Y^2+5Y^3)\right]/4+n_{i_6}\left[-(2-7X^2+5X^3)(Y-2Y^2+Y^3)\right]/4$$

$$+ n_{i_7}\left[(X-8X^2+5X^3)(Y-2Y^2+Y^3)\right]/4+n_{i_8}\left[-(X^2-X^3)(2-7Y^2+5Y^3)\right]/4$$

$$+ n_{i_9}\left[(X^2-X^3)(Y-8Y^2+5Y^3)\right]/4+n_{i_{10}}\left[(X-8X^2+5X^3)(Y^2-Y^3)\right]/4$$

$$+ n_{i_{11}}\left[-(2-7X^2+5X^3)(Y^2-Y^3)\right]/4+n_{i_{12}}\left[(X-2X^2+X^3)(Y-8Y^2+5Y^3)\right]/4$$

$$+ n_{i_{13}}\left[-(X-2X^2+X^3)(Y-2Y^2+Y^3)\right]/4 +n_{i_{14}}\left[-(X^2-X^3)(Y-2Y^2+Y^3)\right]/4$$

$$+ n_{i_{15}}\left[-(X^2-X^3)(Y^2-Y^3)\right]/4 + n_{i_{16}}\left[-(X-2X^2+X^3)(Y^2-Y^3)\right]/4 \qquad (17)$$

The corresponding basis function is defined on a square of side 4d, (Fig.2d) and the a_{ij} terms are again computed by discrete integration along the ray of the factors of n_i terms. For example, Fig.5 shows the different representations of an image using these four different basis functions.

RESULTS

Reconstructed images are presented in Fig.6. The simulated acqui-sition geometry is of fan-beam type. At the present stage, reconstructed images are limited to 31 x 31 pixels in view to keep the computation time at a resonable value. Initial data are simulated assuming a cylindrical object of constant refractive index value $n = 0.9$ surrounded with a medium of refractive index $n = 1.0$ (Fig.6a). Reconstruction is carried out with 43 projections of 33 rays, and the two first iterations are done assuming straight rays (Fig.6b). Then curved rays are calculated, the images being corrected after each ray computation. Figures 6c and 6d represent reconstructions of the images after two iterations for respec-tively cubic and cosine basis functions. To improve the image quality, a filtering procedure has been performed after each iteration. The results for the same basis functions are displayed on Fig.6e and 6f.

To estimate the precision of the reconstruction methods, we have drawn curves giving the arrival point on the detector line, of a ray traced in the reconstructed images. Here the variable is the starting incidence angle of the ray. These curves are compared with the theo-retical ones and presented on Fig.7. According to these curves and the reconstructed images the method using the cosine function basis seems better than the reconstruction with the cubic function basis. This is not surprising because of the similitude between the spline function used for ray tracing and the cosine function used in the reconstruction step (see Fig. 2 and 5). The reconstruction with a spline function, although interesting is much more time consuming for similar results.

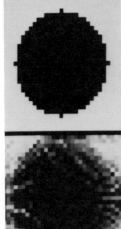

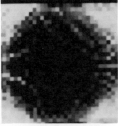

Fig. 6. : Reconstructed
          images.

a) Theoretical result.

b) Reconstructed image after
   two straight line iterations.

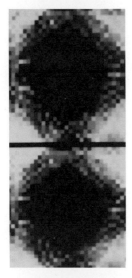

Reconstructions after two
iterations with curved rays :

c) using cubic pixels.

d) using cosine basis.

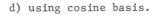

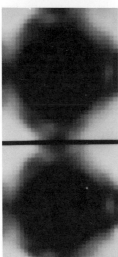

Reconstructions after two
iterations with curved rays
and with filtering procedure :

e) using cubic pixels.

f) using cosine pixels.

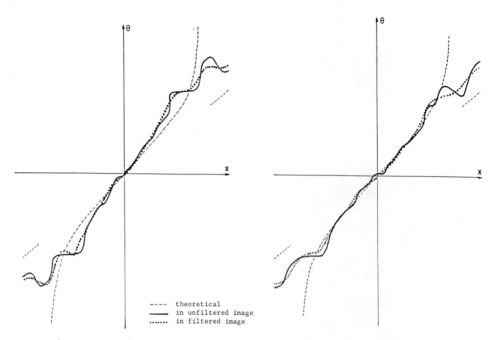

Fig. 7 : Arrival point on the line detector versus ray
angle at point source. Left : cubic pixel
reconstruction. Right : cosine basis reconstruction

CONCLUSION

We have presented some ray tracing and reconstruction methods
developed for ultrasonic computerized tomography. It appears that the
best reconstruction results are obtained with an iterative method using a
decomposition of the image on a cosine function basis. The decomposition
of the image on a spline basis function is quite time consuming and then
seems not to be a good choice for an actual three dimensional reconstruction.

REFERENCES

1 . A.C. Kak, Computerized tomography with X-ray, emission, and
    ultrasound sources, Proceedings of the IEEE, vol. 67, n°9, sept.
    1979, pp.1245-1272.
2 . R. Gordon and G.T. Hermann, Three-dimensional reconstruction from
    projections : a review of algorithms, International Review of
    Citology, G.H. Bourne and J.R. Danielli eds, vol.38, Acad. Press,
    New-York, 1973.
3 . C.V. Jakowatz and A.C. Kak, Computerized Tomographic imaging using
    X-Rays and ultrasound, School of Electrical Engineering, Purdue
    univ., west Lafayette, Indiana, Technical Report TR EE, 76-26,
    1976.
4 . J.F. Greenleaf, S.A. Johnson, and A.H. Lent, Measurement of spatial
    distribution of refractive index in tissues by ultrasonic computer
    assisted tomography, Ultrasound in Med & Biol., Vol.3, pp.327-339,
    Pergamon Press, 1978 (Great Britain).
5 . J.F. Greenleaf, Computerized tomography with ultrasound, Proceedings
    of the IEEE, vol. 71, N°3, March 1983, pp.330-337.

6 . F. Peyrin, C. Odet, P. Fleischmann, and M. Perdrix, Mapping of internal material temperature with ultrasonic computed Tomography, Ultrason. Imag., July 1983, Halifax, conference proceedings, pp.31-36.

7 . J.F. Greenleaf, Computerized transmission tomography, in : Methods of experimental physics, vol.19, Ultrasonics, P.D. Edmonds ED, Academic Press, New-York, 1981, pp.563-589.

8 . M. Schomberg, Non linear image reconstruction from projection of ultrasonic travel times and electric current densities, Mathematical aspects of computerized tomography, G.T. Herman, F. Natterer ed., New-York, Springer, 1981.

9 . A.H. Andersen and A.C. Kak, Digital ray tracing in two dimensional refractive fields, J. Acoust. Soc. Am., 75(5), Nov. 1982, pp.1593-1606.

10 . H. Schomberg, Non linear image reconstruction from ultrasonic time of flight projections, Acoustical imaging, P. Alais, A.F. Metherell ed., New-York, Plenum Press, 1982, pp.381-396.

11 . H. Schomberg, An improved approach to reconstructive ultrasound tomography, J. Phys. D : Appl. Phys., Vol.11, 1978, L.181.

12 . S.A. Johnson, J.F. Greenleaf, W.A. Samayoa, F.A. Duck, and J. Sjostrand, Reconstruction of three dimensional velocity fields and other parameters by acoustic ray tracing, Ultrasonics symposium proceedings, IEEE, cat 75, CHO 994, 4SU, 1975.

13 . R.J. Lytle and K.A. Dynes, Iterative ray tracing between boreholes for underground image reconstruction, IEEE TRANS; Geosci. Remote Sensing, GE-18, 234-240 (1980).

14 . A.H. Andersen and A.C. Kak, Simultaneous algebraïc reconstruction technique (SART) : a superior implementation of the ART algorithm, Ultrason. Imag. (1984), 6, N°1, pp.1-12.

15 . K. Tanabe, Projection method for solving a singular system of linear equations and its applications, Numer. Math. 17, 203-214, 1971.

16 . R. Gordon, A tutorial on ART, IEEE Trans. on Nuclear Science, Juin 1974, NS-21, pp.78-93.

BACK-PROJECTION ALGORITHMS FOR A COMPUTER-CONTROLLED SCANNING LASER

ACOUSTIC MICROSCOPE

R. K. Mueller*, W. P. Robbins*, E. Rudd*, and Z. Q. Zhou†

* University of Minnesota   † Wuhan Institute of Physics
  Department of Electrical Engineering   Academia Sinica
  Minneapolis, MN 55455   Wuhan Hubar
                                      The People's Republic of
                                      China

I. Introduction and Summary

In this paper we evaluate the capability of a scanning laser acoustic microscope (SLAM) to produce images of buried flaws or artifacts in objects which support both shear and compressional waves. First we describe a method of imaging near-surface flaws or artifacts by surface wave insonification, and give some experimental results. We then show that a conventional SLAM does not acquire sufficient data for the back-projection imaging in solids. However appropriate spatial filtering of the acquired data can produce acceptable quasi-back-projected images of deeply buried flaws. This is shown analytically and demonstrated with some images obtained with a computer-controlled SLAM developed in our laboratory.

II. The Instrument

The images described in this paper are obtained with a SLAM which is computer controlled and equipped with digital data acquisition. A detailed description of the instrument is given by Rudd, et al. [1].

In principle a SLAM is a scanning laser optical microscope which samples an optically reflecting and acoustically excited surface. The acoustic surface excursion causes the reflected laser beam to become phase modulated. A modulation converter transforms the phase modulation into amplitude modulation, which is subsequently converted into electrical signals by a photodetector. The electrical signals contain both the phase and amplitude of the acoustic surface excursion, which are retrieved by quadrature detection. A schematic of the acousto-optic subsystem is shown in Fig. 1. The acoustic frequency used is 100 MHz. The scanning laser beam diameter is 10 μm. Our system offers the choice of two modulation converters, the "time-delay interferometer" and the "knife-edge demodulator". The performance characteristics of these two demodulators are described and compared by Mueller and Rylander [2]. A block diagram of the total microscope system is shown in Fig. 2. The analog signal processor provides three independent data channels: an optical channel which carries the information on the optical reflectivity of the scanned surface, and two acoustic channels which give the real and imaginary part of the "complex amplitude" of the acoustic surface excursion. An IBM Systems 9000 computer is used to supervise the data

acquisition, A/D conversion, data handling and storage. The image
reconstruction and data processing is done by the S9000 in conjunction
with a vector processor from Sky Computers, Inc.

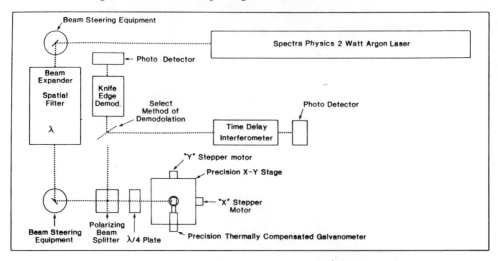

Fig. 1 Acousto-optical subsystem.

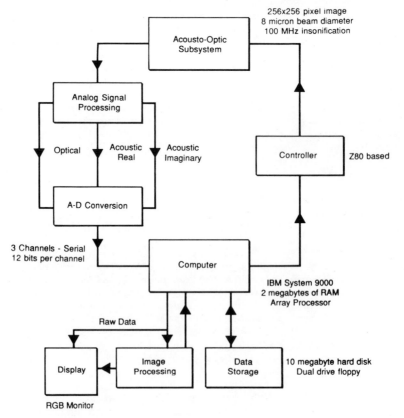

Fig. 2 Block diagram of microscope system.

III. Modes of Operation

The objective of acoustic microscopy is to image, on a microscopic
scale, artifacts or flaws in optically opaque but acoustically transparent

objects. Such flaws or artifacts can be described generally as local inhomogeneities in an otherwise homogeneous elastic medium. We have mentioned above that the data from which such images must be reconstructed is the observed surface excursion of an acoustically excited and optically reflecting interface. In the most simple case this interface is the polished surface of the test object itself. However, a large class of objects cannot be polished, as for example biological specimens on the one hand, and objects with sensitive surface structures such as integrated circuits on the other. For the study of these objects a cover plate is used.

A cover plate is an optically transparent plastic block with a flat and optically-reflecting surface. This cover plate is placed on the object with the reflecting surface touching the "rough" object surface. An acoustic coupling medium connects the cover plate to the object. The observed surface excursion depends linearly, but in a rather complex fashion, on the elastic shear and compressional waves which impinge upon and interact with this interface. It is therefore to be expected that the appropriate image reconstruction algorithm depends to a large measure on the nature of this interface. We assume a Cartesian coordinate system x,y,z and let the interface be the x,y plane $z=0$. Medium 1 is the medium below the interface, i.e. occupying the half space $z<0$. The inhomogeneities to be imaged are in this half space. Medium 2 represents the cover plate material, or air or vacuum if the specimen itself provides the optically reflecting (polished) surface.

With our limitation to isotropic media transparent to elastic waves, we are left with essentially two classes of media: those which support propagating shear waves and those which do not. For the purpose of the following discussion we shall loosely call the first class solids, the second fluids. Since one of the media must support a flat optically reflecting surface we are left with only three kinds of interfaces useful for a SLAM. They are given in Table 1.

Table 1

Interface	Medium 1	Medium 2
a	Fluid	Solid
b	Solid	Solid
c	Solid	Fluid (Vacuum)

Besides the nature of the interface, it is the mode of insonification which determines the appropriate reconstruction algorithm. We consider here two modes of insonification: nominally plane bulk waves insonifying the objects of interest from below the interface, and surface waves supported by the interface and generated outside the scanned surface area. The different imaging modes which are possible with these two insonification schemes are schematically shown in Fig. 3. The most straightforward imaging mode is proximity or shadow-projection imaging, schematically shown in Fig. 3a. Here surface or near-surface artifacts are insonified from underneath, and acceptable images are produced by displaying the amplitude of the observed surface excursion. Some improvement in resolution is attainable by appropriate filtering [3,4]. We shall not further discuss this imaging mode which can be employed with all three interface categories.

Another imaging mode suited for imaging surface or subsurface artifacts is to use a surface wave insonification shown in Fig. 3b. We shall discuss this imaging mode in the following section. Finally the imaging of artifacts which are buried deep below the observation surface

require back-projection methods for image reconstruction which will be
discussed in section V.

IV.   Surface-Wave Imaging

    Surface-wave imaging can be used with solid-fluid interfaces (cases
"a" and "c" of Table 1). These interfaces always support surface waves,
in contrast to solid interfaces which support them only for special
material combinations (Stonely waves).

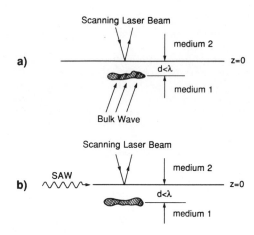

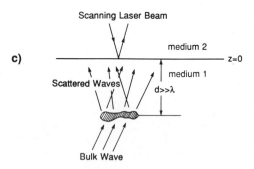

Fig. 3   Insonification schemes.

    The setup for surface-wave imaging is shown schematically in Fig.
3b. A surface acoustic wave (SAW), generated outside the area of
interest, passes over flaws located underneath the surface. We then
observe the phasor field corresponding to the normal component a_z of the
surface excursion. With no flaw present the surface excursion satisfies
a two-dimensional Helmholtz equation:

$$\left(\frac{\partial^2}{\partial x^2} + \frac{\partial^2}{\partial y^2} + {}^o k_s^2\right) a_z = 0 \ , \tag{1}$$

where ${}^o k_s$ is the propagation constant of the surface wave. At the flaw the impinging surface wave is partially scattered and partially converted into bulk waves.

The bulk waves carry energy into the material away from the interface and therefore give only minor contribution to the surface excursion outside the immediate disturbed area. We can therefore describe the observed surface excursion approximately as resulting from surface waves generated by a local inhomogeneity $\Delta(x,y)$ of the propagation constant $k_s = {}^o k_s + \Delta$:

$$(\nabla^2 + {}^o k_s^2) a_z = -2 \Delta {}^o k_s a_z \ . \tag{2}$$

Energy loss due to bulkwave conversion is reflected in a possibly complex value of Δ. Since we observe a_z over the total area including the locus of the inhomogeneities there is no need to resort to the usual Born or Rytov approximations [4] to solve for Δ. One can reconstruct Δ by simply applying the differential operator $\nabla^2 + {}^o k_s^2$ to the observed normal surface excursion a_z and divide the result by a_z. In our system this is most effectively done by Fourier transformations. Letting $\tilde{a}_z$ be the two dimensional Fourier transform of the observed surface excursion a_z one obtains for Δ:

$$\Delta = \frac{FT^{-1}\{(\Lambda^2 - {}^o k_s^2)\tilde{a}_z\}}{2 {}^o k_s a_z} \ , \tag{3}$$

where Λ is the norm

$$\Lambda = \sqrt{\xi^2 + \eta^2} \tag{4}$$

of the radius vector $\vec{\Lambda} = \{\xi, \eta\}$ in spatial frequency space ξ, η.

In Fig. 4 we show the actual reconstruction of a 5000-Å tungsten finger evaporated on a lithium niobate substrate, which was subsequently coated with 1000 Å of aluminum. The tungsten finger represents a 2% change in surface wave velocity due to mass loading. Fig. 5 is a cross-section through the image of Fig. 4 showing the good quantitative agreement obtained with our simple algorithm.

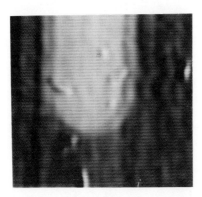

Fig. 4   Surface wave image of tungsten finger.

V. Back-Projection Imaging

Back-projection imaging is indicated if flaws deeply buried inside a test sample have to be imaged. This situation is shown schematically in Fig. 3c. A plane elastic wave impinges upon and is scattered by a deep-lying flaw. The scattered wave impinges on and intracts with the optically reflecting interface where it generates a surface excursion which is sensed by the scanning laser beam. The observed normal component of this surface excursion represents the data base for image reconstruction.

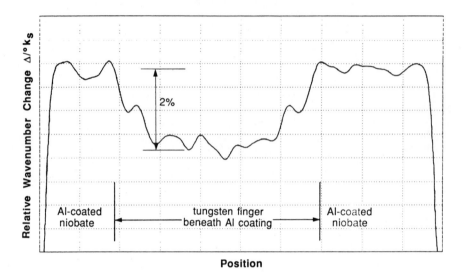

Fig. 5 Computer printout of one line through image of Fig. 4.

The image reconstruction must proceed in two stages. First the impinging wavefront must be derived from the observed surface excursion. The reconstructed wavefront is then "back-projected" to the object plane, yielding the source distribution of the scattered wave; that is, the acoustic image of the flaw or inhomogeneity. Only in the fluid-solid configuration (case "a" of Table 1) does one have sufficient information to carry out the image reconstruction procedure outlined above.

The fluid medium which contains the artifact of interest supports only compressional waves. These waves are described by a scalar potential φ, which satisfies the Helmholtz equation:

$$(\nabla^2 + k_{1c}^2) \varphi = 0 .$$ (5)

We have shown elsewhere [2,3] that in this case the boundary conditions at the interface together with equation (5) yield a simple relation between the potential φ^I of the impinging wave at the interface z=0 and the observed normal component a_z of the surface excursion:

$$\varphi^I = q * a_z .$$ (6)

The star indicates convolution. Fourier transformation of equation (6) yields

$$\tilde{\varphi}^I = \tilde{q} \cdot \tilde{a}_z ,$$ (7)

where $\tilde{x}$ indicates the Fourier transform of x. The quantity $\tilde{q}$ is a function of the elastic constants of the two media and of the spatial frequencies ς and η

$$\tilde{q} = \frac{1}{2\sqrt{k_{1c}^2 - \Lambda^2}} + \frac{\mu_2(k_{2s}^2 - 2\Lambda^2)^2}{2\mu_1 k_{2s}^4 \sqrt{k_{2c}^2 - \Lambda^2}} + \frac{2\mu_2\Lambda_2\sqrt{k_{2s}^2 - \Lambda_2}}{\mu_1 k_{1s}^4} , \qquad (8)$$

where ρ_1, ρ_2 are the densities in media 1 and 2, $k_{i\alpha}$ are the wavenumbers of compressional ($\alpha=c$) and shear ($\alpha=s$) waves in the two media (i=1,2).

Since only propagating waves reach the interface from a deep-lying flaw, the surface excursion is spatially band limited to $\Lambda < k_{1c}$ where k_{1c} is the propagation constant of the compressional waves in medium 1.

The filter function $\tilde{q}$ which restores the impinging wavefront φ at z=0 from the observed surface excursion is singular for $\Lambda=k_{2c}$, and $\Lambda=k_{2s}$ where k_{2c} and k_{2s} are the wave numbers of the compressional and shear waves in the cover plate material (medium 2). The singularities are due to the fact that a_z vanishes for the critical frequencies $\Lambda_{crit}=k_{2c}, k_{2s}$. If one or both of the critical frequencies lie within the band of interest: $\Lambda<k_{1c}$ the spectrum $\tilde{\Phi}(\xi,\eta)$ of the impinging wave in the neighborhood of the critical frequencies cannot be determined from equation (7), but since $\varphi(\xi,\eta)$ is regular it can be recovered by interpolation.

If one limits the bandwidth of the observed surface excursion to $\Lambda<k_{2c}$ (the smaller of the two critical frequencies) one can avoid the singularities in $\tilde{q}$ and obtain (although with some reduction in resolution) the approximation

$$\tilde{\varphi} \simeq \tilde{a}_z . \qquad (9)$$

In other words, the observed surface excursion a_z itself can be used as an approximation for the impinging wavefront. With $\varphi(x,y)$ restored, one obtains the desired image by back-projection. An example of this imaging mode is given by Mueller and Li [4].

The situation is less straightforward if the artifacts of interest are imbedded in a solid matrix as in cases "b" and "c" of Table 1. The scattered wave (which carries the image information) consists in this case of both shear and compressional waves. We have shown elsewhere [2,3] that one must therefore acquire all three linearly independent components a_x, a_y and a_z of the surface impinging shear and compressional wavefronts individually. A conventional SLAM which acquires only the normal component a_z of the surface excursion vector a thus does not give a sufficient data base to reconstruct the impinging wavefronts. The best one can do is to express the observed normal surface excursion in terms of the normal surface excursions a_{zs} and a_{zc} caused by the impinging shear and compressional waves

$$a_z(x,y) = Q_1 * a_{zs} + Q_2 * a_{zc} , \quad z = 0 ; \qquad (10)$$

or in Fourier transform space,

$$\tilde{a}_z = \tilde{Q}_1 * a_{zs} + \tilde{Q}_2 * a_{zc} , \qquad (11)$$

where the $\tilde{Q}_1$ and $\tilde{Q}_2$ are derived by Mueller and Soumekh [3], and given for the case of vacuum as medium 2 by:

$$\tilde{Q}_1 = \frac{2k_{1s}^2 \sqrt{k_{1s}^2 - \Lambda^2} \sqrt{k_{1c}^2 - \Lambda^2}}{\rho_1 [(k_{1s}^2 - 2\Lambda^2)^2 + 4\Lambda^2 \sqrt{k_{1s}^2 - \Lambda^2} \sqrt{k_{1c}^2 - \Lambda^2}]}$$

$$\tilde{Q}_2 = \frac{(k_{1s}^2 - 2\Lambda^2)}{\rho_1 k_{1s}^2 [(k_{1s}^2 - 2\Lambda^2)^2 + 4\Lambda^2 \sqrt{k_{1s}^2 - \Lambda^2} \sqrt{k_{1c}^2 - \Lambda^2}]} .$$

The a_{zs} and a_{zc} have the same back-propagation characteristics as the impinging wave potentials, that is a_{zs} can be back-propagated with the propagation constant k_{1s}, and a_{zc} with k_{1c}. If one therefore back-propagates the observed surface excursion a_z as if it were caused by a shear wave one obtains in the image plane a distorted (convolved with Q_1) image of the sources of the scattered shearwave, superimposed by a distorted and out-of-focus image of the sources of the compressional wave, and vice versa if one back-propagates assuming a_z is caused by a compressional wave. One obtains an improved image by back-projecting either

$$\frac{\tilde{a}_z}{\tilde{Q}_1} = \tilde{a}_{zs} + \frac{\tilde{Q}_2}{\tilde{Q}_1} \tilde{a}_{zc} , \quad \Lambda < k_{1s} \tag{13}$$

as a shear wave, or

$$\frac{\tilde{a}_z}{\tilde{Q}_2} = \frac{\tilde{Q}_1}{\tilde{Q}_2} \tilde{a}_{zs} + \tilde{a}_{zc} , \quad \Lambda < k_{1c} \tag{14}$$

as a compressional wave. This gives an undistorted image of the sources of the shear wave, or the sources of the compressional waves, superimposed by a distorted and out of focus image of the sources of the other wave components. Since the wavenumber k_{1c} of the compressional wave is smaller than the wavenumber k_{1s} of the compressional wave one obtains in general a better image by back-projecting the filtered surface excursion as a compressional wave, than by back-projecting as a shear wave. The reason is that any filter which reduces the bandwidth of the observed data rejects relatively more of the shear wave contributions than of the compressional wave distribution.

To demonstrate these features we have imaged a microscope locator grid which was fastened to the underside of a 1-cm-thick glass plate. The top surface of the glass block was coated with a thin film of aluminum which served as the optically reflecting reference surface. The insonification geometry is shown in Fig. 6. Fig. 7 shows the obtained images. Fig. 7a is the amplitude of the unprocessed surface excursion. Fig. 7b shows the amplitude of the filtered and back-projected surface excursion using compressional wave back-projection. Fig. 7c finally shows the shear wave back-projection. As expected, the locator grid is recognizable but the image is much noisier than the compressional wave image.

390

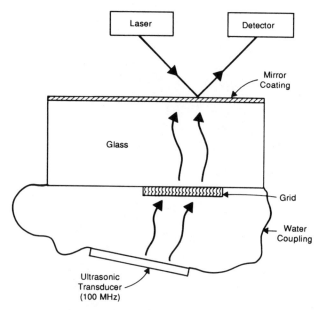

Fig. 6   Insonification geometry.

a)   Unprocessed amplitude image.

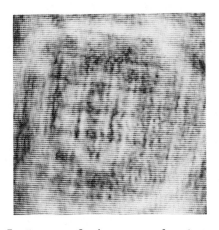

Fig. 7   Images of microscope locator grid.
(continued)

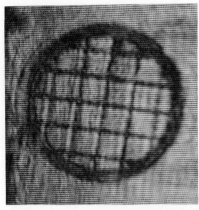

b) Compressional wave back-projection image.

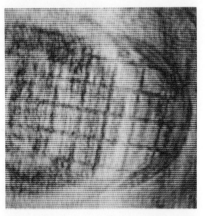

c) Shear wave back-projection image.

VI. References

1. "A Scanning Laser Acoustic Microscope with Digital Data Acquisition",
    E. P. Rudd, et al., to be published Rev. of Sci. Instr.
2. "New Demodulation Scheme for Laser Scanned Acoustic Imaging Systems",
    R. K. Mueller, R. L. Rylander, J. Opt. Soc. Am. 69, 407-412 (1979).
3. Theory of Image Reconstruction for Scanned Laser Acoustic
    Microscopy, R. K. Mueller, B. Soumekh, Proc. Ultrasonics Symposium
    (IEEE, San Francisco, 1985) 720-724.
4. Acoustic Microscopy with Shear and Compressional Waves, R. K.
    Mueller, X. D. Li, to be published this volume.

DIRECTIONAL ACOUSTIC MICROSCOPE WITH ELECTRICAL REFERENCE SIGNALS

Toshio Sannomiya and Noriyoshi Chubachi

Department of Electrical Engineering,
Faculty of Engineering, Tohoku University
Sendai 980, Japan

INTRODUCTION

The acoustic microscopes have been expected to be widely used in the fields of biological science, material characterization, nondestructive evaluation and others[1-2]. For the quantitative measurements, several types of scanning acoustic interference microscope (SAIM) have been developed so far, to measure the velocity distributions in thin materials and/or topological profiles on the solid surfaces[3-8]. In most imaging systems including SAIMs, a point-focus-beam has been employed for high resolution. On the other hand, with the nonscanning reflection acoustic microscope, a line-focus-beam has been introduced for the quantitative measurement of acoustic properties including anisotropy on various solid surfaces[9]. A measurement system for the anisotropic materials have been successfully established with high accuracy[10]. However, the line-focus-beam usually has a line width wider than 1mm, so that the results obtained by the system show the mean values over the line width. A directional scanning acoustic microscope has been already proposed, which reveals elastic anisotropy with high spatial resolution[11]. In that acoustic microscope, however, directly reflected waves from the sample is necessary to interfere with re-radiated leaky surface waves on the sample for the V(z) curve establishment. If only the leaky surface waves can be excited and detected with perfect elimination of the directly reflected waves from the sample[12], the shapes of V(z) curves can be preferentially controlled by mixing the received signals with the electrical reference signal. Recently, "Ultrasonic Micro-Spectroscopy (UMS)" has been expected for the development of a new field in material science and technology[13].

In this paper, a new directional point-focus-beam acoustic microscope with a variable phase shifter is demonstrated for the UMS system with which both quantitative measurement of surface wave velocity and two-dimensional imaging can be made including the angular dependence on a small area of the samples. The construction of the system and some experiments on the imaging and V(z) curve measurement are described. Anisotropic measurements of leaky SAW velocity for a Y-cut $LiNbO_3$ wafer and images obtained for Mn-Zn ferrite ceramics are demonstrated in the frequency range between 60 and 200MHz.

CONSTRUCTION OF THE SYSTEM

Figure 1 shows a block diagram of the directional acoustic inter-ference microscope system for two-dimensional imaging and V(z) curve measurement. In this system, the focused acoustic pulse signal radiated by a transducer(transmitter) is reflected at the sample surface and received by another transducer(receiver). The received signal is mixed with the electrical reference signal through the variable phase shifter and the variable attenuator so that acoustic image contrast can be desirably controlled. This system can be said to be a modified system of the scanning acoustic interference microscope (SAIM) for the reflection mode[8]. The cross-correlation signal[14] between the received and the reference signal is obtained as the V(z) signal so that both the amplitude and the phase information can be detected.

Acoustical images can be displayed on the CRT by the conventional electronic techniques, as the acoustic beam is scanned in the X and Y directions synchronously with the raster scan of the CRT. In the V(z) curve measurements, the received output signals are observed as a function of moving distance z when the sample is moved along Z axis toward the acoustic transducers by a Z-stage controller. In this system, with the digitally controlled variable phase shifter newly introduced in the reference signal line, the phase difference between the received and the reference signal can be varied in association with the variation of dis-tance between the acoustic transducer and the sample. The correlation output signals are taken into a computer through the A/D converter, and are recorded on the X-Y recorder. The dip interval Δz of V(z) curve is determined by the FFT analysis[9] and then the leaky SAW velocity v_{lsaw} of sample is calculated. For the directional measurements, the sample stage can be rotated around Z axis.

In this system, the phase variation $\delta\phi_r$ of reference signal is con-trolled to be proportional to the variation δz of distance z between the transducer and the sample. The relation between $\delta\phi_r$ and δz is expressed as,

$$\delta\phi_r = 2k_r \delta z \tag{1}$$

where the proportional constant k_r is the equivalent wave number. The phase velocity v_{lsaw} of leaky SAW can be determined from the dip interval Δz of V(z) curve by the similar manner as the conventional V(z) measurement. Using the equivalent wave number k_r, the dip interval Δz is given approximately by the following equation,

$$\Delta z = v_l/2f(k_r/k_l - \cos\theta_{lsaw}) \tag{2}$$

where $\theta_{lsaw} = \sin^{-1}(v_l/v_{lsaw})$ is the critical angle of leaky SAW, v_l and k_l is the longitudinal velocity and the wave number of coupling liquid respectively, f is the acoustic frequency. Equation (1) can be repre-sented also in terms of v_{lsaw} as

$$v_{lsaw} = v_l/[1-(R_k - v_l/2f\Delta z)^2]^{1/2} \tag{3}$$

where $R_k = k_r/k_l$ is the equivalent wave number ratio. Equation (2) shows that in case of $R_k > \cos\theta_{lsaw}$, the changing rate of Δz against v_{lsaw} is increased as R_k is decreased, while in case of $R_k < \cos\theta_{lsaw}$, the changing rate of Δz against v_{lsaw} is decreased with reversed sign as R_k is decreased.

Figure 2 shows the normalized dip interval $f\Delta z$ as a function of v_{lsaw} where a parameter is R_k. The curve of $R_k=0$ corresponds to the case of

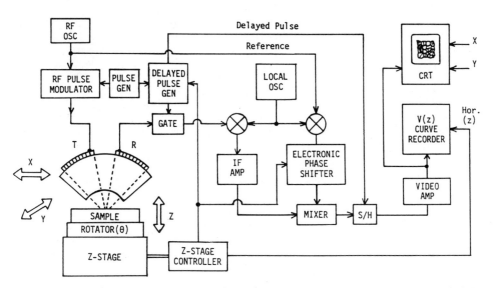

Fig.1 Block diagram of the directional SAIM system for imaging and V(z) curve measurement.

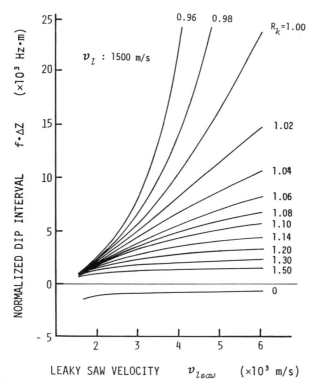

Fig. 2 Normalized dip interval f·Δz of V(z) curve as a function of v_{lsaw} where the parameter is R_k.

which the phase of reference signal is fixed, while the curve of $R_k=1$ corresponds to the case of the conventional $V(z)$ curve measurement. In this system, it is desirable to set R_k either small or large depending on the cases, $R_k < \cos\theta_{lsaw}$ or $R_k > \cos\theta_{lsaw}$. For the materials with extraordinarily large values of v_{lsaw}, movable distance of the lens along the Z-axis will be limited due to the large opening angle and Δz. On the other hand, it will be hard to observe the dip pattern for the materials with high attenuation. Even in such cases, it will be possible to measure Δz by using a suitable value of R_k which is determined by changing the phase of reference signal.

EXPERIMENTS

Transducers

In these experiments, a couple of directional point focusing elements, DFE-80 and DFE-200, have been employed. The configuration of the focusing element is shown in Fig.3. A pair of concave transducers are fabricated on a convex surface of concentric spherical glass shells with a concave radiation surface as shown in the figure.

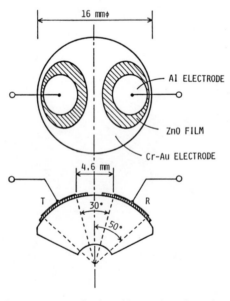

Fig.3 Configuration of the directional point focusing element.

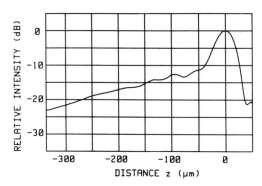

Fig.4 V(z) curve observed at 80 MHz with a sample of SiO$_2$
without reference signal for mixing.

For the DFE-80, the convex-concave glass shells were formed with
radii, 9mm and 2.5mm, respectively.   The transducers are ZnO
piezoelectric films of 5.4mm in diameter.   The center frequency of the
transducers is about 80MHz.   A pair of point focus beams with the opening
angles of 35° are focused confocally in a minute area of the coupling liquid medium by these concave transducers.   Half width of the beam is expected to be about 16µm at 80MHz.   The sound field distribution has been
measured at 80MHz, and the sound intensity on the Z-axis at a position
more than 100µm apart from the focal point was suppressed below −25dB as
compared with that at the focal point.   To study the response of the
transducers, the V(z) curve measured at a frequency of 80MHz with a sample
of fused quartz of 2mm in thickness is shown in Fig.4 without the
reference signal for mixing.   The result shows that the direct reflected
wave component has been almost eliminated.

Another directional point-focusing transducer of DFE-200 has been
fabricated by the convex-concave glass shells with radii of curvature, 9mm
and 1.25mm, respectively, for the imaging at frequency of 200MHz.

V(z) curve measurements

To confirm the capability of the present system, the experiments of
V(z) curve measurement have been made at a frequency of 60MHz which is a
center frequency of electronic phase shifter, with a sample of the fused
quartz plate of 2mm in thickness.   The V(z) curves have been observed
with a water as a coupling liquid medium at various equivalent wave number
ratios R_k.   The V(z) curves obtained at R_k of 1.625 and 1.219 are shown
in Fig.5 (a) and (b), respectively, as examples.   Using the Eq.(3), the
leaky SAW velocities have been calculated from the dip intervals determined by the FFT analysis.   The measured values of v_{lsaw} are shown in
table 1.   Larger errors are seen for large R_k of 1.625 ($R_k > \cos\theta_{lsaw}$) or
$R_k=0$ ($R_k < \cos\theta_{lsaw}$).

Experiments have been further performed at a frequency of 80MHz to investigate the dependence of leaky SAW velocity with respect to the propagation direction. Angular dependence of the leaky SAW velocities measured on the sample of Y-cut $LiNbO_3$ wafer is shown Fig.6 (R_k=0). It can be said that the results should be satisfied at the present stage, although there are some discrepancies between the values obtained with the present system(circle) and those obtained with the line-focus-beam acoustic microscope(dashed line)[15].

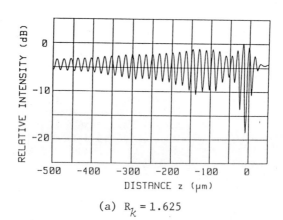

(a) $R_k = 1.625$

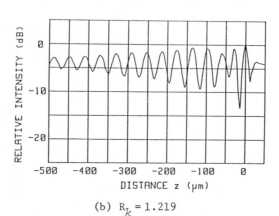

(b) $R_k = 1.219$

Fig.5 V(z) curves obtained on a SiO2 sample for different value of R_k.

Table 1. Measured v_{lsaw} for a SiO_2 sample

Equivalent Wavenumber Ratio R_k	Dip Interval ΔZ (μm)	v_{lsaw} (m/s)		Difference ε (%)
		Calculated	Measured	
1.625	17.08		3347.1	-2.42
1.393	25.14		3378.4	-1.50
1.219	38.96	3430	3406.8	-0.68
1.083	67.53		3406.6	-0.68
0	13.92		3378.4	-1.50

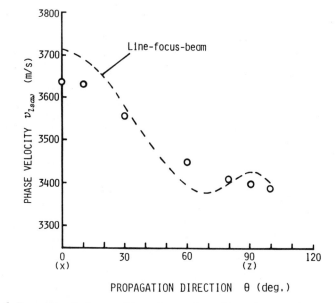

Fig.6 Experimental results of angular dependence of leaky SAW
velocity on a sample of Y-cut $LiNbO_3$ plate (R_k=0).

Image observations

    To obtain the directional images, only the sample has been rotated by
90°.   Figure 7 shows the acoustic images of the optically polished surface of Mn-Zn ferrite plate observed at a frequency of 80MHz.   These
images have been taken at the same defocus length of -60um. As expected,
different contrasts are imaged in the same area on the surface due to the
anisotropy of grain faces, although the resolution is insufficient.

Figure 8 shows the acoustic images obtained for the same ferrite sample at a frequency of 200MHz. The defocus length is -40μm. The grain boundaries are displayed clearly as compared with the Fig.7.

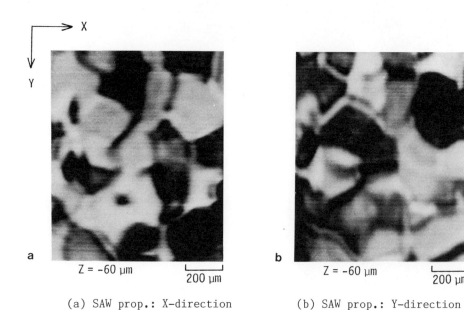

(a) SAW prop.: X-direction   (b) SAW prop.: Y-direction

Fig.7   Acoustic images of the surface of Mn-Zn ferrite plate
         observed at 80MHz.   The sample was rotated by 90° at
         the same defocus length of z=-60μm.

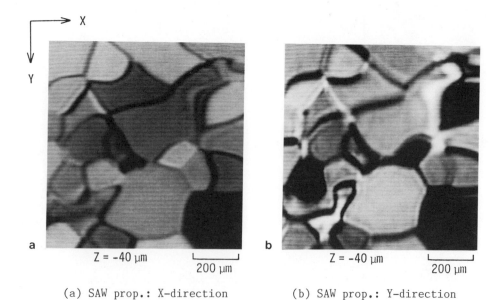

(a) SAW prop.: X-direction   (b) SAW prop.: Y-direction

Fig.8   Acoustic images of the surface of Mn-Zn ferrite plate
         observed at 200MHz.   The sample was rotated by 90° at
         the same defocus length of z=-40μm.

CLOSING REMARKS

In this paper, a new directional acoustic interference microscope system with a variable phase shifter has been described. The acoustic anisotropy measurements for a Y-cut $LiNbO_3$ crystal and the imaging for a Mn-Zn ferrite have been demonstrated in the frequency range between 60 and 200 MHz. The system is expected to be developed for the use in higher frequency regions above 200MHz to cultivate the ultrasonic micro-spectroscopy.

ACKNOWLEDGMENTS

The authors are grateful to Prof. H. Shimizu, Dr. J. Kushibiki, and Mr. Y. Matsumoto for their useful discussions on this work. We would like to thank Honda Electron Co. which provided us the electronic phase shifter. This work was supported in part by the Research Grant-in-Aids from Japan Ministry of Education, Science & Culture, and also the Toray Science and Technology Grants, Japan.

REFERENCES

1. C.F.Quate, A.Atalar, and H.K.Wickramasinghe, Acoustic microscope with mechanical scanning - A review, Proc. IEEE 67 :1092(1979).
2. H.K.Wickramasinghe, Acoustic microscopy:present and future, Proc. IEE 131,a-4 :282(1984).
3. N.Chubachi, Mechanically scanned acoustic microscope composed of plane and concave transducers for transmission mode, "Scanned Image Microscopy", E.A.Ash Ed., Academic Press, London, :119(1980).
4. N.Chubachi, T.Sannomiya, J.Kushibiki, H.Horii, H.Maehara and H.Okazaki, Scanning acoustic microscope with transducer swing along beam axis,IEEE Ultrasonics symp. Proc., :629(1982).
5. N.Chubachi and T.Sannomiya, Scanning acoustic microscope in interference mode using frequency modulation method, IEEE Ultrasonics Symp. Proc. :611(1983).
6. N.Chubachi and H.Okazaki, Scanning acoustic interference micro-scope with wedge delay line, Electron. Lett, 20:113(1984).
7. N.Chubachi. T.Jindo and R.Suganuma, Acoustic interference micro-scope with electronic delay line, Report of spring meeting of Acoustical soc. Japan :625(1984).
8. N.Chubachi and T.Sannomiya, Acoustic interference microscope with electrical mixing method for reflection mode, IEEE Ultrasonic Symp. Proc. :604(1984).
9. J.Kushibiki, A.Ohkubo, and N.Chubachi, Linearly focused acoustic beams for acoustic microscopy, Electron. Lett. 17 :520(1981).
10. J.Kushibiki and N.Chubachi, Material characterization by line-focus-beam acoustic microscope, IEEE Trans. SU-32 :189(1985).
11. J.A.Hildebrand and L.K.Lam, Directional acoustic microscopy for observation of elastic anisotropy, Appl. Phys. Lett. 42(5):413(1983).
12. I.R.Smith and H.K.Wickramasinghe, SAW attenuation measurement in the acoustic microscope, Electron. Lett. 18(22):955(1982).
13. N.Chubachi, Ultrasonic micro-spectroscopy via Rayleigh wave, Proc. Rayleigh wave centenary Symp. :291(Springer Verlag, 1985).
14. N.Chubachi, T.Sannomiya, and K.Imano, Reflection ultrasonic microspectrometer for a small quantity of liquid using correlation method, Electron. Lett. 22(1):44(1986).
15. J.Kushibiki, A.Ohkubo, and N.Chubachi, Propagation characteristics of leaky SAWs on water/$LiNbO_3$ boundary measured by acoustic microscope with line-focus beam, Electron. Lett. 18:6(1982).

FOCAL PLANE DETECTION IN ACOUSTICAL IMAGING

L. Germain and J.D.N. Cheeke

Département de physique, Université de Sherbrooke

Sherbrooke, Québec, Canada   J1K 2R1

ABSTRACT

We present a new configuration for the transmission acoustic micro-scope using a piezoelectric transducer at the focal plane as the receiver. This configuration appears to be easier to use than the standard two-lens system. Examples of images taken in water and liquid nitrogen with this method are presented. The potential of this configuration for non-linear imaging is also discussed.

INTRODUCTION

The transmission mode acoustic microscope using two lenses aligned in a confocal pattern is well known (R.A. Lemons and C.F. Quate, 1979). This configuration is however not very practical due to the critical lens alignment that it necessitates. In this paper, we report a new config-uration for transmission microscopy which is much simpler to use. The method makes use of a piezoelectric transducer placed at the focal plane as the receiving element. This configuration has been employed primarily for the characterization of transducer vibration modes (L. Germain and J.D.N. Cheeke, 1985a) and also for the development of ultrasonic point detectors (L. Germain and J.D.N. Cheeke, 1985b). Here we are concerned with the potential of this method for transmission acoustic imaging. Typical images obtained in water and liquid nitrogen will be presented. Results on nonlinear imaging using this configuration will also be discussed.

LINEAR TRANSMISSION IMAGING

The experimental set up for the transmission scanning acoustic micro-scope with focal plane detection is presented in fig. 1. The set up is essentially similar to a standard reflection microscope except that the signal directed to the receiver comes from the transducer at the focal plane rather than back from the lens. Here we used a Matec 6600 system for emission and reception of the pulsed high frequency signal. The received signal is sampled by a boxcar integrator, digitized by an A/D converter and sent to a microcomputer. The image is then displayed on a high resolution monitor or saved on a disk for later use. The lens used

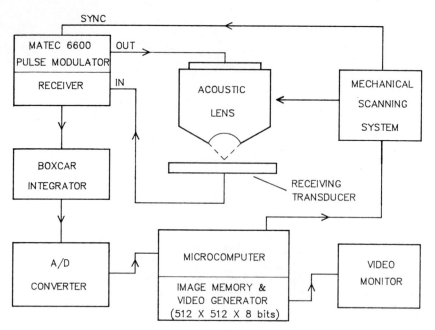

Fig. 1. Experimental set up for the transmission acoustic microscope with focal plane detection.

here is a small quartz rod with a hemispherical cavity of 1,6 mm in diameter at one end and a piezoelectric transducer at the other end. Both transducers (on the lens and at focus) are longitudinal 30° Y-cut LiNbO$_3$ plates resonant at 30 MHz. The receiving transducer in this case has been glued on a backing substrate to attenuate the vibration patterns observed on free transducers (L. Germain and J.D.N. Cheeke, 1985a). The scanning mechanism is made of two small electromagnets similar to those used at Stanford (J. Heiserman et al., 1980), fixed on a semi-rigid coaxial cable at the top of which is placed the lens. The lens is scanned in the habitual raster pattern over the receiving transducer. This microscope can be used either at room temperature or in cryogenic baths. Frequencies between 10 and 300 MHz could be used.

Figures 2 and 3 give a comparison of reflection and transmission images of a microscope test grid obtained in water at 270 MHz. On the reflection image we get very good contrast which is mainly due to the well known signature (or V(z)) phenomenon (A. Atalar, 1979). Scattering of acoustic energy out of the lens from inclined surfaces of the object will also contribute to the structure of this image. The transmission image does not present as much contrast as the reflection one but still gives a very good idea of the structure of the grid. The contrast in this case will now be due to the acoustic attenuation of the material and to the transmission coefficient at the liquid-specimen interface, hence giving a complementary set of information on the studied object. One small inconvenience of this imaging configuration are the dim fringes that can be observed on the image in the free areas around the object. These fringes are thought to be residual standing surface wave patterns on the receiving transducer and no method has been found yet to suppress them totally.

Figures 4 to 7 show results obtained in liquid nitrogen for a similar grid at many frequencies. For these images, the scanning system was

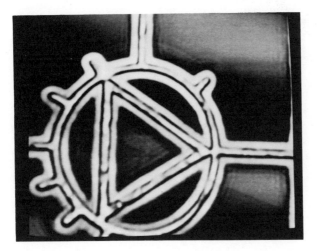

50 μ

Fig. 2. Reflection image of a microscope test grid obtained in water
(25°C) at a frequency of 270 MHz.

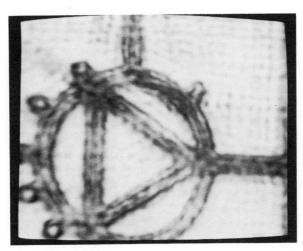

Fig. 3. Transmission image of the same grid as in figure 1, obtained with
the focal plane detection configuration (in water, at 270 MHz).

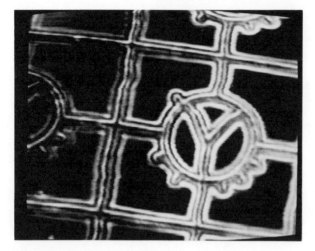

100 μ

Fig. 4. Reflection image of the grid taken in liquid nitrogen (77 K) at a frequency of 90 MHz.

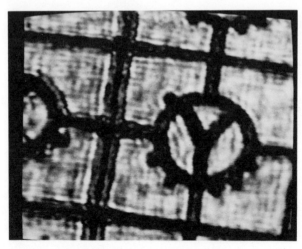

Fig. 5. Transmission image of the grid obtained in the same conditions as in figure 4 (liquid nitrogen, 90 MHz) with the focal plane detection configuration.

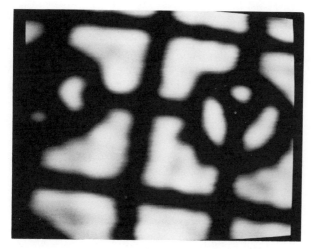

100 μ

Fig. 6.   Transmission image in liquid nitrogen of the same grid as in
figure 5, but obtained at a frequency of 30 MHz.

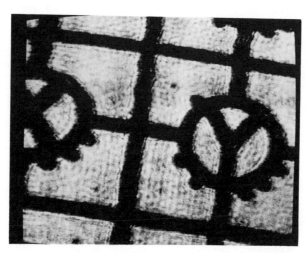

Fig. 7.   Transmission image in liquid nitrogen of the same grid as in
figure 5, but obtained at a frequency of 270 MHz.

immersed in a cryostat filled with liquid nitrogen and supported by three large springs for protection from pumps and floor vibrations. Figures 4 and 6 show the differences between reflection and transmission images at 90 MHz. The reflection image is again clearer than the transmission one but one can still obtain good information from the latter. Fig. 5 to 7 are other examples of transmission images obtained at different frequencies, showing very well the increase in resolution with the frequency used.

We have seen, in this first part, that the focal plane detection configuration can be a very practical way to obtain transmission images since there is no complicated lenses alignment to do. Images produced with this configuration are probably a little bit less clear due to the remaining fringes on the free surface of the transducer but interesting information on the attenuation in the specimen and on the transmission coefficient at the liquid-object interface can nevertheless be obtained from them.

NONLINEAR TRANSMISSION IMAGING

Nonlinear imaging has been studied for some time both in reflection mode (D. Rugar, 1984) and in transmission mode using the two-lens configuration (R. Kompfner and R.A. Lemons, 1976; H.K. Wickramasinghe and Celia Yeack, 1977). The nonlinear behavior of the acoustic wave in the microscope is due to the sharp focussing of the sound beam by the lens, yielding to very high acoustic intensity near the focal point. This high intensity produces a deformation of the sound wave which generates acoustic signal at harmonics of the emitted frequency.

When doing nonlinear imaging, one is interested in receiving the signal generated at the harmonic frequencies by the coupling liquid and by the imaged object. The receiving lens is then tuned to the frequency of the harmonic signal. We know however that the harmonic content of the transmitted beam is rapidly depleted due to the greater attenuation of higher frequencies in liquids and also to the down-conversion phenomenon observed in the diverging part of the beam (D. Rugar, 1984). This depletion usually limits the nonlinear imaging at the second harmonic.

The transmission configuration presented here is particularily well suited for nonlinear imaging because the reception is done directly at the focal point where the harmonic content of the beam is the most important. Indeed, this configuration has been used sucessfully to study the dependence of the power transfered in the harmonics at the focus of a lens in some liquids, as a function of the emitted power. Dependence of up to the tenth harmonic could be observed in some cases (L. Germain and J.D.N. Cheeke, 1986).

In the following, nonlinear imaging capability of the focal plane detection configuration will be demonstrated. The set up used here is similar to the one showed in figure 1 except that now, two separate Matec systems are used to permit emission and reception at different frequencies. The emitting transducer has also been changed to one resonating at 15 MHz, hence avoiding the possibility of reception of direct signal at the fundamental frequency and still permitting the reception of the 2nd, 6th and 10th harmonics (remember that $LiNbO_3$ transducer can emit or receive only at odd harmonics of the fundamental frequency).

Figure 8 shows a typical nonlinear image obtained in water with this configuration. Here the emission frequency was fixed at 45 MHz while the receiver was tuned at the second harmonic, i.e. at 90 MHz. This image shows a good signal to noise ratio, demonstrating the sensitivity of the

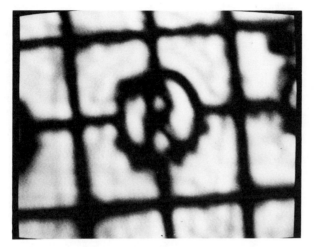

100 μ

Fig. 8. Nonlinear transmission image of a microscope grid obtained in water (25°C) for an emission frequency of 45 MHz and a reception frequency of 90 MHz (second harmonic).

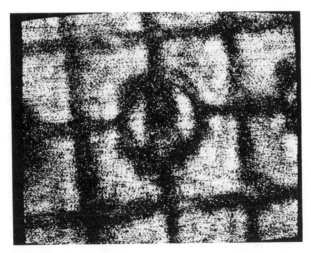

Fig. 9. Nonlinear transmission image of the same grid as in figure 8 but for emission at 15 MHz and reception at 90 MHz (sixth harmonic).

set up to the second harmonic.

Figure 9 shows an other example of nonlinear imaging, this time for the sixth harmonic obtained in water at an emission frequency of 15 MHz and reception at 90 MHz. This image shows a really good resolution if we compare it to a linear image at 15 MHz where we would not detect the grid at all. We see in fact that the resolution is almost as good as that on figure 8. The image is however quite noisy since the sixth harmonic in water was very weak for the emission power used here. In fact, this signal was so weak that it could never have been detected with the standard two lens configuration. This shows again the great potential of the focal plane detection configuration for nonlinear acoustical imaging. Imaging of nonlinear specimen other than liquid has not been tried yet but the use of this configuration should also certainly lead to very interesting results.

CONCLUSION

A new configuration for transmission acoustical imaging using focal plane detection has been reported. This method appears to be much easier to use than the standard two lens configuration since there is no difficult lens alignment to do. Image quality is however not as good as in reflection mode, due to the presence of the dim fringes in the free parts of the receiving transducer.

On the other hand, this configuration seems very interesting for nonlinear imaging since the detection is made near the focal point, where the harmonic content in the acoustic beam is the greatest. Examples of nonlinear images using up to the sixth harmonic were presented to demonstrate the potential of this configuration for nonlinear imaging.

ACKNOWLEDGEMENTS

We would like to thank André Beauséjour for technical assistance with the microscope imaging. This project was supported by a strategic grant from the Natural Sciences and Engineering Research Council of Canada.

REFERENCES

Atalar, A., 1979, J. Appl. Phys., 50:8237.
Germain, L. and Cheeke, J.D.N., 1985a, Acoust. Lett., 9:75.
Germain, L. and Cheeke, J.D.N., 1985b, Journal de Physique, suppl. no 12,
    46:C10-759.
Germain, L. and Cheeke, J.D.N., 1986, to be published.
Heiserman, J., Rugar, D. and Quate, C.F., 1980, J. Acoust. Soc. Am.,
    67:1629.
Kompfner, R. and Lemons, R.A., 1976, Appl. Phys. Lett., 28:295.
Lemons, R.A. and Quate, C.F., 1979, in: "Physical Acoustics", vol. XIV,
    W.P. Mason and R.N. Thurston, ed., Academic Press, New York.
Rugar, D., 1984, J. Appl. Phys., 56:1338.
Wickramasinghe, H.K. and Yeack, Celia, 1977, J. Appl. Phys., 48:4951.

PROGRESS TOWARD A PRACTICAL 100 MHZ SCANNING LASER

TOMOGRAPHIC ACOUSTIC MICROSCOPE[*]

Michael Oravecz and Lawrence Gibbons

Sonoscan, Inc.
530 East Green Street
Bensenville, IL 60106

ABSTRACT- This paper presents the results of research into the development
of a Scanning Laser Acoustic Microscope (SLAM) which produces diffraction
corrected tomographs from a series of shadowgraphic micrographs. This
demonstration is based on the following work. By modifying an in-house 100
Mhz SLAM, we acquired data containing both the amplitude and phase
information needed for diffraction tomography algorithms. The principle
modification was a new general purpose single sideband synchronous
demodulation receiver based on phase coherent quadrature detection with
selectable output of either the upper or lower sideband. The images produced
by the system were digitized in real-time into a 256 x 240 grid of 6-bit
pixels. An analysis of the principle characteristics of the system transfer
function was performed to allow modification of the acquired data so that a
better representation of the detected sound field could be used in
reconstruction algorithms. We demonstrated extraction of the amplitude and
phase information by digitally reconstructing both amplitude and phase images
of a series of phantoms. The phantoms were constructed to produce
understandable images of a series of amplitude and phase variations, fine
spatial detail, and known diffraction from a circular aperture. Some
phantoms were used to obtain two dimensional diffraction-corrected
holographic reconstructions by back propagation in Fourier space. (See the
companion paper "Subsurface Imaging in Acoustic Microscopy" by Z-C. Lin, H.
Lee and G. Wade.) The tomographic acoustic microscope could produce
unambiguous images needed in materials characterization, detailed inspection
of micro-electronic components, nondestructive evaluation of solid-state
materials and non-invasive imaging of biological samples.

I. INTRODUCTION

Scanning Laser Acoustic Microscopy (SLAM) is a method of imaging high
frequency, 10 Mhz to 500 Mhz, ultrasound. With ultrasonic energy, the
surface and internal mechanical (elastic) structure of specimens is
studied. Since most materials support ultrasonic propagation, SLAM
technology can be used to study specimens ranging from hard structural
ceramics to soft biological tissues[1,2,3].

---

[*]Supported by Nat'l Science Foundation's SBIR Contract ECS-8460665.

In the SLAM, a specimen is insonified with plane acoustic waves. As the sound passes through the specimen, it is scattered and absorbed according to the internal elastic microstructure. An optically reflective surface placed in the sound field directly behind the specimen will become distorted in proportion to the localized pressure. A focused scanning laser beam is reflected off this surface and is first angularly (spatially) modulated by these distortions. A knife-edge detector is used to change the spatial modulation into intensity modulation for pickup by a photodiode. The electronic signal processing includes down-conversion, amplification, band-pass filtering, synchronous detection and a fixed black-clamp relative to blanking. Scanning laser technology allows real-time imaging, that is, conventional video rates of 30 frames per second.

The SLAM's qualitative, grey-scale display of spatial attenuation variations has been accepted as a nondestructive testing tool[4]. This is due to the high visual impact of regions of high attenuation caused by air gaps and discontinuities associated with internal cracks, delaminations, voids, inclusions, etc.

However, practical application of SLAM technology has also revealed two fundamental limitations to the technique. First, the micrographs are two-dimensional shadowgraphic views of three-dimensional objects, analogous to x-ray skiagraphs. To obtain an unambiguous image without a confusing overlapping of internal structure, the specimens must have little or no structural variation in the depth direction. A partial solution that has proven practical for certain applications uses a double-view stereo-optic technique in which the depth information is extracted manually. In general this technique is limited to samples that are structurally simple; the technique does not approach theoretical limitations of depth resolution.

Second, many potential applications involve imaging structures which are comparable in size to the acoustic wavelength used. The images of such small structures are actually far-field diffraction patterns. These patterns are easily recognizable with minimal training, and thus identification is routine. However, without a detailed knowledge of the sample, little more than the most basic characterization of the structure is possible. Using frequencies high enough to solve this problem is generally impractical due to the resulting increase in the ultrasonic attenuation in the sample and the difficulty of obtaining any useful signal.

The overall objective of this research is to develop techniques to overcome the problems associated with overlapping features in the images of internally complex objects and with diffraction effects common to acoustic imaging. The proposed solution is to develop a scanning laser acoustic microscope which produces diffraction-corrected tomographic micrographs. Such an instrument could produce the unambiguous images necessary to open up new horizons in materials characterization, detailed inspection of micro-electronic commponents, non-destructive evaluation of solid-state materials, process control and non-invasive imaging of biological samples.

Critical to the development of a tomographic acoustic microscope is the availability of an appropriate diffraction tomography algorithm. As discussed by Robinson and Greenleaf[5], there has recently been a high level of theoretical activity in ultrasonic diffraction tomography as well as some experimental results using relatively simple biological objects and phantoms. Currently, then, there are a number of very promising algorithms whose capabilities are being expanded and studied. There has been comparatively little experimental verification of the assumptions involved in each algorithm. Also, the algorithms have not yet been developed for general experimental conditions involving solid samples which support

412

multiple types of waves and in which there is considerable refraction at interfaces.

An important part of this project is to develop an experimental test-bed for research into and verification of a practical diffraction tomographic algorithm. The basic insonification conditions used in the current SLAM technology parallel assumptions under which a number of algorithms have been developed -- plane wave insonification and transmission methods. The interest in applications covering a wide range of materials, however, means that algorithms based on the first Born and Rytov approximations may not be sufficiently general for the long term.

II. DEVICE

A standard SLAM was modified so that the data necessary for input into diffraction holography and tomography algorithms could be obtained using 100 MHz ultrasound. As yet, not all decisive modifications have been accomplished. The modifications implemented were those that allowed the acquisition of data suitable, but not yet optimized, for holographic and tomographic image processing.

There are several features in the detection process that are critical to proper signal processing. In standard SLAM's, the detected signal is proportional to the normal component of the acoustic pressure. If an external reflective coverplate is used it alters the signal only when sound is incident onto the coverplate from the coupling medium at the critical angle, Rayleigh angle, etc. of this interface. The knife-edge detection process contributes significantly to the final signal, and this contribution is a strong function of the laser spot size at the detection plane. This was originally described by Korpel and Kessler[6] and more recently in greater detail by Rylander[7]. During the scanned detection, the speed of the laser is sufficient (57.1 m/sec) to Doppler shift the frequency of the waves in proportion to their velocity component parallel to the laser velocity. In particular, sound incident with a component of velocity along the laser scan is down-shifted; sound incident with a component opposite the laser scan is up-shifted. The band-pass filter in a standard SLAM is designed to pass only one of these shifted sidebands. The standard SLAM obtains its phase sensitive interferogram mode by simply adding in a reference signal prior to the synchronous detector (Figure 1). Although the resulting video image appears similar to the sinusoidally modulated output of one channel of a quadrature detector, analysis such as that done by Lin et al[8] shows it to be much more complex (Figure 2).

The development and breadboarding of a receiver based on a phase coherent quadrature detector (Figure 3) provided the basic improvement required for acquistion of holographic data. This receiver eliminates the complications arising from the standard SLAM's synchronous detector and the SLAM interferogram. The two sinusoidally varying, 90-degree out-of-phase outputs of a quadrature detector are easily combined to give the required amplitude and phase information. The newly developed quadrature receiver provides both the up-shifted and down-shifted side bands for processing. The two sidebands are separately processed. As a practical consequence, the receiver has four outputs. Thus, four separate video images constitute the data for a single, complex amplitude image. This separation greatly simplifies the correction due to the knife-edge response and minimizes the requirements on the Fourier transform routines. Special consideration was given to the filters used for the quadrature receiver. Surface Acoustic Wave filters with excellent phase characteristics were chosen.

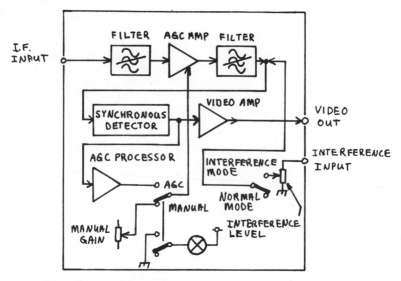

Figure 1- Schematic of standard SLAM receiver.

The back-to-back filters employed in the quadrature receiver (Figure 4) dictated a change in I.F. frequency from the standard SLAM's 36.4 MHz to 40.25 Mhz. Such a change in I.F. frequency requires modifications of the ultrasonic driver and the preamp to accommodate this new frequency. Standard SLAM modules were modified as required while trying to maintain bandwidth and gain.

In order to use most fully the limited resolution provided by the 6-bit video digitizer employed in this work, control of the video signal's reference black level and reference white level were required.

Prior to this work, Lin et al.[9] had already published a description of an algorithm which could, in principle, calculate diffraction-corrected tomographic images from SLAM data. The published results also included the successful application of the algorithm on simulated SLAM data.

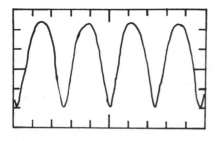

STANDARD SLAM INTERFEROGRAM

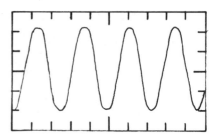

NEW SLAM QUADRATURE OUTPUT

Figure 2- An oscilloscope display representation showing a portion of a horizontal line of the video output of the two receivers. The standard SLAM fringes are equivalent to the beat envelope resulting from adding two slightly different frequencies, the detected and reference signals. Zero signal occurs at the fringe troughs. The quadrature fringes arise from the sinusoidal modulation of the amplitude information. Zero signal occurs in the middle of the wave with the amplitude oscillating both positive and negative.

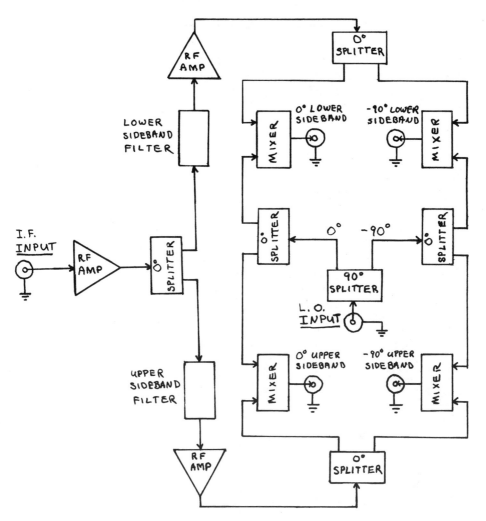

Figure 3- Schematic of quadrature receiver designed and built for this work.

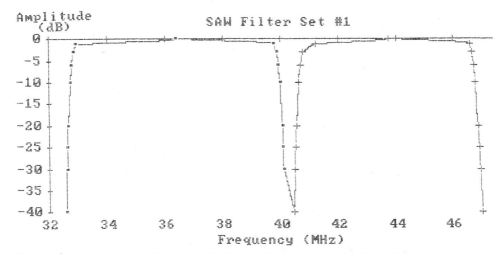

Figure 4- Graphical display of the bandpass, back-to-back filters used in
the quadrature receiver.

SPATIAL FREQ. (Megacycles/m)

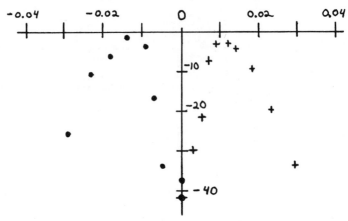

RELATIVE SIGNAL (dB)

Figure 5- Measured system response as a function of spatial frequency at the coverslip for the quadrature SLAM.

SPATIAL FREQ. (Megacycles/m)

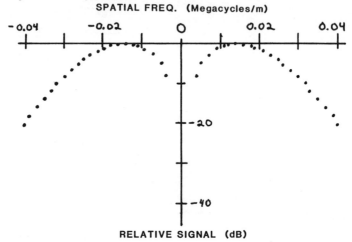

RELATIVE SIGNAL (dB)

Figure 6- Ideal system response based on a knife-edge transfer function with a 20 micron laser spot size.

As originally designed, the back-and-forth propagation algorithm required an equal spatial density of pixels along the two image axes. To accomodate this, the field of view was changed from 3.0 mm x 2.25 mm to 3.0 mm x 2.81 mm. This provided a 240 x 240 block of pixels measuring 2.81 mm on each side. As a side effect, some of the images appear compressed in the vertical direction.

The overall effects of the quadrature SLAM detection process on the signal to be measured were lumped together as a single transfer function. This function was measured experimentally, and the raw data are shown in Figure 5. This function plots relative signal in decibels versus the spatial frequency being detected. The zero decibel point was defined as the highest signal. The baseband video frequency associated with the plotted spatial frequencies can be calculated directly in MHz by multiplying the axis value by the laser velocity (57.14 m/sec). Thus the spatial frequency value 0.035 megacycles/m corresponds to 2 MHz. The data were obtained by rotating a transducer through ± 25 degrees using a goniometer whose center of rotation was about at the detection plane.

Since the images were to be digitized into 256 pixels horizontally, a design goal for the frequency bandwidth for each sideband was 2 to 2.5 MHz as dictated by the 256 pixels per horizontal line. Unfortunately, the measured transfer function fell short of this goal. Examination of the modified electronic modules - preamp, receiver, and video display - showed that the bandwidth specification was applied to each module separately so that each contributed roughly 3 dB loss at 2-2.5 MHz. This accounts for roughly 6 to 10 dB of the high frequency droop. Correction of the data due to measurement of only the normal component of the incident wave adds only 2 more dB. All of this fails to account for the measured lack of high frequency response.

If the electronics are designed for flat response and the data are corrected for the normal component of the wave, the best possible frequency response is limited by the knife-edge response. Figure 6 shows a calculation based on a 20 micron spot size for a Gaussian beam. This expected response is based on measurements of the laser spot using a USAF 1951 Resolution Test Target. For detection of 100 MHz sound, the SLAM optical resolution is about 50 line pairs/mm which corresponds to 20 microns per line pair. A comparison of our measured transfer function with calculations for 10, 20 and 40 micron spots indicate that the measured transfer function is more characteristic of a laser spot size of about 30 microns. Such a spot size could result from incorrect interpretation of the test target measurements, or from taking the transfer function measurments without fully optimizing focus. More direct measurements of spot size are planned.

II. METHOD

The following is a brief description of the typical procedure used for acquiring data on a test sample.

The insonification geometry was typically set to optimize the signal-to-noise ratio of the experimental SLAM. Thus the transducer was set to a 10 degree angle relative to the laser-scanned detection plane. The test samples were oriented flat with respect to the detection plane and so were insonified at a 10 degree angle. The transducer was operated at 101.8 - 101.9 MHz, and distilled water was used as a couplant. The electrical power into an efficient air-backed transducer was limited to about one half watt. Higher power has a tendency to cause nonlinear propagation in the water so a safe level was chosen. The video signal carrying the image data was connected to the real-time video frame grabber inside the computer and to an oscilloscope. The frame grabber was first operated in pass-through mode so that the image could be monitored during set-up. In preparation for digitization, the video's reference black level and the signal's topmost white level were adjusted to carefully match the voltage range of the digitizer using the oscilloscope. This was fine-tuned using the frame grabber in an analysis mode. Preliminary data was digitized (one video field takes 1/60 sec)., and the actual pixel values were examined to ensure that the voltage range of the digitizer was not exceeded.

After adjustments were complete, an image from each of the four receiver outputs in turn was digitized and stored on floppy disk. Often slides were taken to document the images during this process.

IV. RESULTS

The most significant results of our work are embodied in the amplitude and phase images we calculated from our data and in the one- and two-dimensional holographic reconstructions calculated by Lin et al. from our data. The results are given in a logical fashion moving from simple to more complex.

There are a number of images related to the quadrature receiver SLAM data so that a brief description of each is needed. The real-time video images produced by the system can be any one of the four outputs: lower sideband, 0 degrees; lower sideband , 90 degrees; upper sideband, 0 degrees; upper sideband 90 degrees. The lower sideband data result from sound propagating with a velocity component along the direction of the laser scan; the upper sideband data result from sound propagating with a velocity component opposite the laser scan direction. The 0-degree outputs are obtained by mixing the detected signal with the reference signal; the 90-degree outputs are obtained by mixing the detected signal with the reference signal after it has been shifted by -90 degrees. The first type of image is simply an image of one of these outputs, characterized by the amplitude of the sound at the coverslip being sinusoidally modulated. This modulation produces the alternating bright and dark vertical bands seen in these images.

From the quadrature data we directly calculated images which separately display the amplitude and phase of the sound field at the detection plane as detected. These are thus referred to simply as the amplitude and the phase images. The amplitude images are presently calculated by taking the square root of the sum of the squares of the quadrature outputs of the principal sideband for a given image. The phase images are calculated by first dividing the 90-degree data by the 0-degree data and then taking the inverse tangent of the result. All of these calculations are done pixel-by-pixel. The amplitude image is essentially equivalent to the amplitude image obtained with a standard SLAM. Standard SLAM amplitude photos are presented for comparison to the quadrature receiver SLAM photos.

Also, one- and two-dimensional holographic amplitude images were calculated by Lin et al. from quadrature data we obtained. These images were obtained by combining the dominant quadrature sideband outputs of the modified SLAM and backpropagating the detected wavefield in the spatial frequency domain. The backpropagated wavefield is divided by an assumed incident plane wavefield yielding the transmission profile. The holographic amplitude images show the amplitude associated with this transmission profile.

The first series of images (Figure 7) show amplitude and phase images calculated from data acquired on the modified SLAM. This data is based on continuous 100 MHz plane waves incident upon a detection plane at 10 degrees. In the bottom half of these images we see a thin homogeneous plastic sheet with a moderate amount of insertion loss and phase change on the transmitted wave. This is compared to a simple water field, sound which has travelled only through water, in the top half of the images. The right corner of the images is dominated by an air bubble, adjacent to the detection plane, which illustrates the results when no signal is present. The lower transmission in the plastic region is mainly due to reflection losses since the 0.004 inch thick material is only about 5 wavelengths thick. The phase change due to the plastic as compared to water is seen as a horizontal shift of the entire field of vertical fringes in the region of the plastic sheet. A standard SLAM amplitude image, which has been digitized, is shown for comparison to the amplitude image calculated from quadrature SLAM data.

As expected the amplitude image compares well with the standard SLAM amplitude image. However, a pattern of vertical lines is apparent in the quadrature amplitude image. These small modulations occur at twice the frequency at which the quadrature images are sinusoidally modulated. This is consistent with the assumption that the 0- and 90-degree data used to calculate the amplitude image are not truly separated by 90 degrees. The magnitude of this modulation indicates that there may be a roughly 5 degree error. When the reference signal is shifted by 90 degrees, there should be less than 1 degree error. Most likely there is a drift in the system during the time interval between acquiring the 0-degree data and the 90-degree data. These data were not acquired simultaneously. Also at the current pixel density there are only about 7.1 pixels per 360 degree phase change.

The phantom imaged in Figure 8 was chosen as a test of resolution for the quadrature SLAM system. The phantom, a finder grid used in electron microscopy, is shown at a similar magnification with a standard optical microscope, the standard SLAM, and the quadrature SLAM. The grid dimensions are nominally as follows: the open areas between parallel sides of the hexagons are 210 microns across and the thin bars making up the sides of the hexagons are 25 microns across.

To allow reconstruction from a well known case of diffraction, a circular aperture phantom was designed. The sample was constructed of three layers bonded together, each layer being between 0.5 and 1.0 thousandths of an inch thick. The top two layers were apertures whose nominal diameter was 400 microns. Measurements indicate a diameter of about 370 microns. The center layer was simply a ring to provide an air gap between the top layers. This three-layer construction was necessary since the single layer of copper around the aperture attenuated the sound by only about 10 dB.

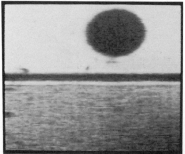

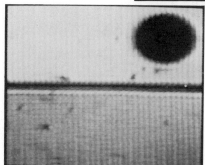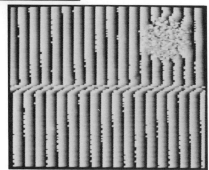

Figure 7- Images showing amplitude (bottom left) and phase (bottom right) images calculated from data acquired on the quadrature SLAM. The images compare a water field (top half of image), a thin homogeneous plastic sheet (bottom half) and a void (air bubble adjacent to the detection plane). The plastic sheet induces a moderate reduction in transmission and a phase change. The void produces a no signal condition. A standard SLAM amplitude image (digitized) is shown at top.

Reassurance of our basic capability to obtain holographic reconstructions with SLAM technology is found by studying a circular aperture in one dimension (Figure 9) and a honeycomb finder grid in two dimensions (Figure 10). The reconstructions were obtained by Dr. Lin using our data.

Figures 9a and 9b show the two, 256-pixel lines of quadrature data used in the one-dimensional aperture reconstruction. Since most of the information was contained in one sideband, the other sideband was neglected at this time. Figure 9c shows the one-dimensional amplitude image calculated from the quadrature data. This should resemble the Bessel function, J_1. The second ring is so low in amplitude that it is lost in the high frequency noise of this image. Figure 9d shows the holographically reconstructed image in which the data was backpropagated 4 mm. This reconstruction was performed using a single, unaveraged set of data.

Note the improved definition of the reconstructed image compared to the diffracted image of the aperture. A set of vertical lines marks the optically measured diameter of the aperture. Also note that the image has moved toward the center of the field-of-view where the aperture itself was located. Given a 10 degree angle of propagation and a depth of 4 mm, one expects the reconstructed image to be 0.7 mm (60 pixels) to the left of the detected position. In Fig. 9c the signal is centered at pixel 182. In Fig. 9d the signal is centered at pixel 124. This gives a measured movement of 58 pixels in excellent agreement with expectations.

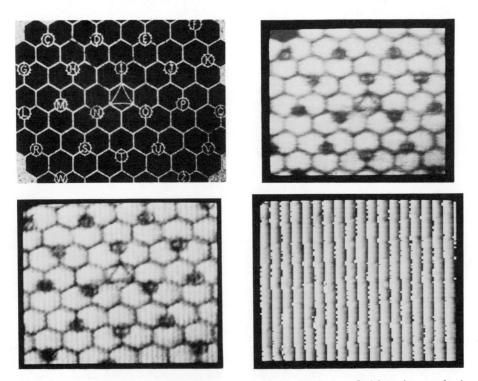

Figure 8— A honeycomb finder grid is used to test resolution in quadrature SLAM images. The nominal grid dimensions are: open areas between parallel sides of the hexagon are 210 microns wide and the thin bars making the hexagon sides are 25 microns wide. The grid is 15 to 25 microns thick. The grid is shown with an optical microscope (top left), with the standard SLAM (top right), and with the amplitude (bottom left) and phase (bottom right) images calculated from quadrature SLAM data.

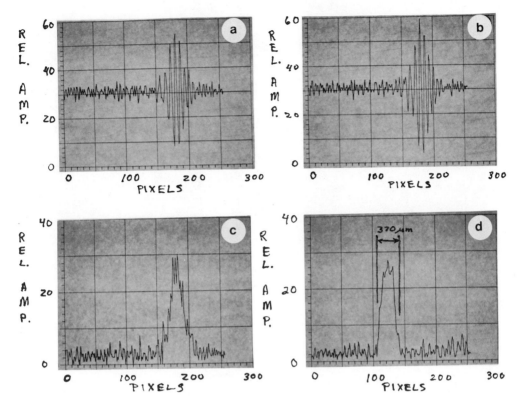

Figure 9- A one-dimensional holographic reconstruction and the input data. Shown in (a) and (b) are the two, 256-pixel lines of quadrature data. The one-dimensional amplitude image calculated from the quadrature data is shown in (c). The holographically reconstructed image appears in (d). The data were backpropagated 4 mm to obtain this reconstruction. The aperture diameter was measured at 370 microns.

To demonstrate the ability we have developed to obtain and manipulate data with ultrasonically limited accuracy, a holographic reconstruction of a honeycomb finder grid was performed. Figure 10a shows a diffraction distorted image of the grid obtained by raising the coverslip off the grid.

Our first holographic reconstruction of the grid is shown in Figure 10b. This reconstruction was at a backpropagation distance of about 0.6 mm. This was the optimum reconstruction found using 0.1 mm steps. Because the grid is so close to the resolution limit of the microscope, we were not expecting to obtain a very detailed reconstruction. Our results for 0.6 mm are very remarkable. The detail in the reconstructed image actually rivals the detail in the direct contact images from the standard SLAM and the quadrature SLAM.

To correct for the transfer function of the knife edge detector, the reconstruction routine was modified and performed again. The corrected holographic reconstruction of the diffracted grid appears in Figure 10c. The high frequency background artifact of the previous image has been eliminated and there is better edge definition in the corrected image.

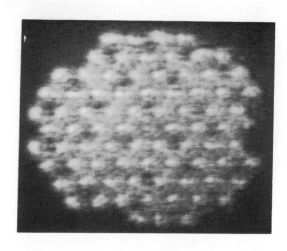
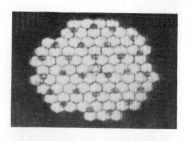
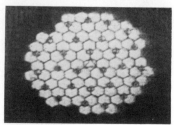

Figure 10- A two-dimensional holographic reconstruction shows detail rivalling direct contact images. The data were backpropagated 0.6 mm. The left image is a standard SLAM image of the diffracted grid. The top right image is a standard reconstruction. The bottom right image results from considering the knife-edge response in the reconstruction. This gives the best results.

REFERENCES

1 L.W. Kessler and D.E. Yuhas, "Acoustic Microscopy - 1979," Proc. IEEE, Invited Manuscript, Vol. 67, No. 4, April 1979, pp. 526-536.
2 L.W. Kessler and D.E. Yuhas, "Principles and Analytical Capabilities of the Scanning Laser Acoustic Microscopy (SLAM)," SEM/1978, Vol. 1, pp.555.
3 L.W. Kessler, "Imaging with Dynamic-Ripple Diffraction," Acoustical Imaging, Chap. 10, pp. 229-239, Ed. G. Wade, Plenum Press, New York, 1976.
4 S.K. Prasad,"S.L.A.M. Study of Die attach Integrity," Proc. of ISTFA 1985.

   J.A. Michael and W.W. Fultz, "Nondestructive evaluation by Acoustic Microscopy as Applied to the Failure Analysis of Microelectronics," Proc. of ISTFA 1985.
5 B.S. Robinson and J.F. Greenleaf, "Results of Diffraction Tomography of Complex Objects," Symposium on Computers in Ultrasound, Vol. 2, Drexel Univ., Philadelphia, PA, Sept. 1985.
6 A. Korpel and L. Kessler, Comparison of methods of Acoustic Microscopy," Acoustic Holography, ed. A.F. Metherell, Vol. 3, Chap. 3, Plenum Press, 1971.
7 R.L. Rylander, Appendix to "A Laser-Scanned Ultrasonic Microscope Incorporating Time-Delay Interferometric Detection," Ph.D. dissertation, U. of Minnesota, Mineapolis, MN, Dec. 1982.
8 Z.-C. Lin, H. Lee, G. Wade, M.G. Oravecz, L. W. Kessler, "Data Acquisition in Tomographic Acoustic Microscopy," Proc. IEEE 1983 Ultrasonics Symp., pp. 627-631, Nov. 1983.
9 Z.-C. Lin, H. Lee and G. Wade, "Back-and-Forth Propagation for Diffraction Tomography," IEEE Trans. Sonics & Ultrasonics, Vol. SU-31, No. 6, Nov. 1984, pp. 626-634.

THERMOACOUSTIC IMAGING USING A LASER PROBE

Bernard Cretin, and Daniel Hauden

Laboratoire de Physique et Métrologie des Oscillateurs
du Centre National de la Recherche Scientifique
associé à l'Université de Franche-Comté-Besançon
32, avenue de l'Observatoire - 25000 Besançon - France

ABSTRACT

In transmission thermoacoustic scanning microscopy, the thermally
induced bulk waves are detected on the opposite surface of the sample by a
piezoelectric transducer or a laser probe. The use of a compact heterodyne
interferometric laser probe enables high resolution and wide frequency
range imaging. Such a microscope is described in this paper. Results obtained for inhomogeneous or layered samples are presented and discussed,
showing potential applications.

INTRODUCTION

When a modulated laser or electron beam hits an absorbing material,
photon's or electron's energy is converted into heat by a non radiative
deexcitation process. Since the generated thermal waves are exponentially
dumped as they propagate from the source, they are difficult to detect
directly. Therefore, various indirect ways for probing the thermal response
of the material have been developed [1,6] In solids, elastic waves propagate
with relatively low attenuation. Then, the detection of thermally generated
elastic waves is a convenient solution for obtaining thermal and elastic
properties of materials. As the sample is translated relatively to the beam
focused point, the magnitude and phase of the acoustical signal gives information on the sample properties. This technique is known as scanning
thermoacoustic microscopy (STAM).

In this paper, a STAM system operating in the 1 kHz - 250 kHz frequency range is reported. Some images of subsurface structure of metal and
layered material are presented, showing potential applications of this
instrument in non-destructive testing.

SCANNING TRANSMISSION THERMOACOUSTIC MICROSCOPE

The principle of the microscope was previously presented.[7] An adjus-
table-power NdYag laser beam is intensity modulated and focalized on the
material under test. Displacements associated to the thermally generated
bulk elastic waves are colinearly detected on the opposite surface of the

sample by a laser probe. The sample scanning is operated by means of two stepping motor translators. Amplitude and phase information are separated by a lock-in amplifier. Then, they are digitized and stored in a computer that synchronizes scanning and acquisition. Corresponding images are displayed on a video screen or plotted under the form of cross-section line.

The operating range of this STAM was previously limited by the heterodyne laser probe noise.[8] Therefore, a more compact laser probe was achieved, providing sufficient resolution.

Heterodyne interferometric laser probe

The heterodyne interferometer is a very sensitive tool for probing surface displacement.[9] Its wide dynamic range ($\sim 10^{-4}$ Å to 100 Å) and large bandwidth (typically 1 kHz - 0.5 GHz) enables the detection in STAM. Nevertheless, a classical heterodyne interferometer exhibits large low frequency noise due to mechanical vibrations, spurious beams and thermal disturbances. In STAM, the resolution of such an interferometer is not always sufficient for detecting the small displacements of the sample surface at frequencies above 10 kHz ($\delta \sim 0.01$ to 0.1 Å at 10 kHz for 0.1 W effective excitation power).

Following recent work from D. Royer and al.,[10] a compact asymmetrical heterodyne probe was developed for probing displacements in transmission STAM. The probe diagram is shown on Figure 1. The HeNe laser beam is horizontally polarized. One half of the power is split by cube 1 ; the reference beam is reflected inside the Dove prism and is directed towards the p.i.n. photodetector. The signal beam is upshifted ($f_L + f_B$) by a colinear input-output Bragg cell, and after passing through the quarter-wave plate is reflected and phase modulated by the sample surface. After the second passing through the quarter-wave plate, the signal beam is vertically polarized. It is reflected by the polarizing beamsplitter (cube 2) and directed onto the photodetector. The polarizer is oriented at $\pi/4$ relatively to the polarizations of the two beams interfering on the photodetector. When operating, the photocurrent spectrum contains a carrier at frequency f_B and sidebands those amplitude and number depends on the sample surface displacements.

The use of this probe allowed to increase the S/N ratio in the microscope frequency range (increasing by a factor $\simeq 20$ at 10 kHz). In noisy environments, due to NdYag laser cooler and ventilation, the probe exhibits a resolution $\simeq 3.10^{-4}$ Å/√Hz at 10 kHz and shows several improvements.

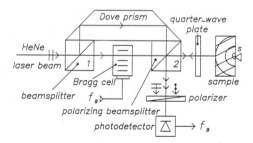

Fig. 1. Asymmetrical probe diagram

Because the optical path lengths are shortened, the beams alignment and the planeity of the sample surface are less critical (in a classical probe, a misalignment of about 0.1 mrad cancels the signal). The alignment planeity tolerance increases by one order of magnitude compared with a classical probe. The high resolution enables noncontact, wide bandwidth, transmission thermoacoustic imaging.

A specific chain (Fig. 2), including AGC and PLL, reduces low frequency noise (under 1 kHz) and immediatly calibrates the probe

$$v_p = \frac{4\pi s}{\lambda_L} \delta$$

where v_p is the probe output voltage in the linear range, δ the surface displacement, λ_L the laser wavelength and s the PLL phase detector slope ($V.rad^{-1}$) in the operating conditions.

Microscope improvement

Probing the surface displacement with this new heterodyne interferometer allows wide bandwidth operating in STAM. As in a classical interferometer, mechanical resonances of the different supports prevent the bulk waves detection at low frequencies. A P.L.L. was then used with a 700 Hz cut-off frequency. The lock-in amplifier sets the high operating frequency at 250 kHz. Nevertheless, operating above 1 MHz is possible by using a frequency mixing.

Acquisition time improvement is the main interest in using this new probe. Previously a lock-in amplifier time constant of 1 s was required at a few kilohertz for sufficient S/N ratio. This time has been reduced under 0.1 s. Thus, image acquisition time is now limited by the stepping motor's speed.

In the 1 kHz - 250 kHz frequency range, the acoustical wavelength is typically 5 m - 2 cm. Therefore, acoustical inhomogeneities are not detectable and the probe beam may be unfocused. The STAM images contain information about optical absorption, thermal expansion and, principally, thermal properties. The thermal resolution ($\sim \mu = \sqrt{2\beta/\omega}$ where β is the thermal diffusivity and ω the excitation pulsation) is typically in the range 5 μm - 100 μm depending on the materials.

The image size is software limited at 64 × 64 pixels and 16 gray levels or false colors.

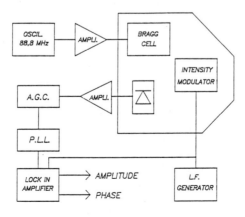

Fig. 2. Microscope electronics

RESULTS AND DISCUSSION

Nonhomogeneous sample

Figure 3 shows amplitude and phase images of simulated defects in a plate. The sample is a 4 mm thick metallic disc in AU4G duralumin. The probe side is optically polished for the displacement detection. Two square sectional slots of 300 μm size were machined on the excitation face, allowing the sample positioning. Two 1 mm diameter drillings simulate volume defects. They are respectively 150 and 350 μm under the excitation surface. The sample was excited by a 1 W power focused beam at a modulation frequency of 2.7 kHz. The holes were horizontally positioned.

The surface slots are clearly visible on the images. The amplitude image is optically affected by the displacement out of the focal plane but the two images also show the thermal discontinuity on the slots edges. Under the slots crossing, only one of the holes outline appears near the slots crossing due to the thermal diffusion length at the operating frequency ($\mu \simeq 100$ μm). The images contain 64 × 64 pixels corresponding to a 6 400 × 6400 μm scan size. These results follow previous theory and results obtained with other thermal wave microscopes.[11],[12]

Metal layered sample

The sample is a 4 mm thick stainless steel plate. Letters were engraved and the corresponding holes were filled in with glue. After that, the sample surface was planed and covered by a 20 μm thick Aℓ layer. Then the letters were optically invisible.

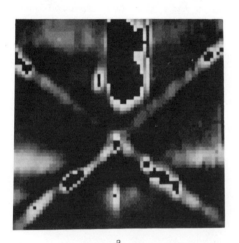
a

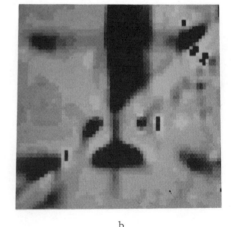
b

Fig. 3. Duralumin sample : (a) amplitude image ; (b) phase image ;
(c) sample

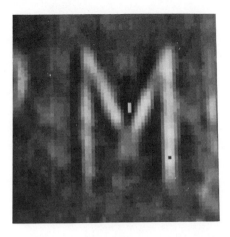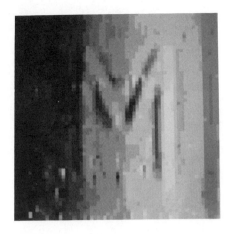

Fig. 4. Amplitude and phase images of an engraved overlayered letter

Figure 4 shows amplitude and phase images (size : 64 × 64 pixels) of an overlayered letter. Each 75 µm scan step is obvious on the pictures. The 15 kHz excitation frequency enables the crossing of the Aℓ layer ($\mu \simeq$ 40 µm) by thermal waves. The different reflexion coefficients at the interfaces Aℓ - stainless steel and Aℓ - glue give a good contrast on the amplitude image. (For a plane wave, the reflexion coefficient is expressed :

$$r = \frac{Z_2 - Z_1}{Z_2 + Z_1} \text{ with } Z_i = \frac{1 - j}{\sqrt{2}} \left(\frac{1}{\omega K_i \rho_i C_i} \right)^{1/2}$$

where K_i is the thermal conductivity, ρ_i the volume density and C_i the specific heat). The letter edges are visible on the phase image (phase rotation $\simeq 15°$) as in the previous example.

Limitations in the case of insulated semiconductor

We attempted studies about implanted areas in semiconductors such as silicon and GaAs (implantation depth 0.5 µm).

At the excitation beam wavelength (1.06 µm) the optical depth penetration is ~ 100 µm in semiconductors.[13] Thus an absorption overlayer is necessary for the detection of thin insulated layers. Then, a 800 Å Aℓ layer was deposited on a ion implanted GaAs sample. We have noted that electron microscopes yield a pattern image without Aℓ only. The Aℓ overlayer inhibits such an observation.

No significative results have been obtained in the 150-200 kHz frequency range with our STAM. Previous results have shown the difficulty for obtaining an accurate observation at such low frequencies[14,15] ($\mu \simeq$ 10 µm), pointing out the great influence of the absorption coefficient in these images. Other experiments will be done with visible light to verify this point.

CONCLUSION

These results show the interest of STAM using an high resolution laser probe. This method permits wide bandwidth operating, now limited by electronics at 250 kHz. Electronics improvement may increase the cut-off frequency into the MHz range, and thus enable a resolution into the sub-micron range. The modulation frequencies are low enough so that no imaging can be performed by the acoustic waves themselves. Therefore the thermal features provide the dominant contribution to images in the case of an optically uniform sample.

We are working on several microscope improvements : increasing of the image size up to 128 × 128 pixels, higher operating frequency by mixing, reduction of the global acquisition time and studies on depth profiling.

Micromechanics defects detection, multilayered sample analysis and insulated semiconductors observations are some potential applications for this STAM.

ACKNOWLEDGMENTS

The authors would like to acknowledge R.D. Weglein who provided us GaAs and Si implanted samples and C. Tellier for electron micrographs of samples.

REFERENCES

1. A. Rosencwaig, R.M. White, Imaging of dopant regions in silicon with thermal-wave electron microscopy, Appl. Phys. Lett., 38(3), 165-167 (1981).

2. Y. Martin, E.A. Ash, Photodisplacement microscopy using a semiconductor laser, Electron. Lett., vol. 18, n ° 18, 763-764 (1982).

3. T. Baumann, F. Dacol, R.L. Melcher, Transmission thermal wave microscopy with pyroelectric detection, Appl. Phys. Lett., 43(1), 71-73 (1983).

4. I.J. Cox, C.J.R. Sheppard, Imaging in scanning photoacoustic microscope, J. Acoust. Soc. Am., 76(2), 513-515 (1984).

5. F. Lepoutre, D. Fournier, A.C. Boccara, Non destructive control of weldings using the mirage detection, J. Appl. Phys., 57(4), 1009-1015 (1985).

6. C.C. Williams, High resolution photothermal laser probe, Appl. Phys. Lett., 44(12), 1115-1117 (1984).

7. B. Cretin, D. Hauden, Thermoacoustic scanning microscope using a laser probe, IEEE Ultrasonics Symposium Proceedings, 656-659 (1984).

8. B. Cretin, D. Hauden, Transmission thermoacoustic imaging without contact, "Acoustical Imaging", vol. 14 (A.J. Berkhout, J. Ridder and L.F. Van der Wal, Ed.), Plenum Press, 653-655 (1985).

9. H.K. Wickramasinghe, Y. Martin, D.A.H. Spear and E.A. Ash, Optical hete-rodyne techniques for photoacoustic and photothermal detection, J. Phys. C6, vol. 44, 191-196 (1983).

10 D. Royer, E. Dieulesaint, Y. Martin, Improved version of a polarized beam heterodyne interferometer, IEEE Ultr. Symp. Proc., 432-435 (1985).

11 G. Busse, A. Rosencwaig, Sursurface imaging with photoacoustics, Appl. Phys. Lett., 36(10), 815-816 (1980).

12 E.A. Ash, Y. Martin, S. Sheard, "Acoustic and thermal wave microscopy", Acoustical Imaging, vol. 14 (A.J. Berkhout, J. Ridder and L.F. Van der Wal, Ed.), Plenum Press, 343-360 (1985).

13 J.R. Meyer, M.R. Druer, F.J. Bartoli, Optical heating in semiconductors : laser damage in Ge, Si, InSb and GaAs, J. Appl. Phys., 51(10), 5513-5522 (1980).

14 A. Rosencwaig, G. Busse, High-resolution photoacoustic thermal-wave microscopy, Appl. Phys. Lett., 36(9), 725-727 (1980).

15 A. Rosencwaig, Thermal-wave imaging, Science, vol. 218, 223-228 (1982).

A HIGH PERFORMANCE ACOUSTIC MICROSCOPE - TECHNICAL ASPECTS

AND SELECTED APPLICATIONS

Abdullah Atalar[+] and Martin Hoppe[*]

[+]Electrical and Electronics Engineering Department
Middle East Technical University
06531 Ankara, Turkey

[*]Ernst Leitz Wetzlar GmbH
P.Box 2020
D-6330 Wetzlar, FRG

ABSTRACT

Technical aspects of a scanning acoustic microscope
with broad frequency coverage (50...2000 MHz) are described.
Images demonstrating the capabilities of the microscope are
shown.

INTRODUCTION

The scanning acoustic microscope is finding applications
as a powerful scientific instrument for imaging and
characterization of materials (Ash, 1980; IEEE Trans. Sonics
Ultrasonics SU-32, 1985). A few commercial instruments have
 shown up recently at the marketplace. In this paper, we
decribe the scanning acoustic microscope (ELSAM)* developed
at Ernst Leitz Wetzlar GmbH, West Germany (Hoppe et al., 1983;
Hoppe et al., 1985) following the guidelines of Stanford
microscope (Lemons, 1974; Quate et al., 1979; Jipson et al.,
1978).

ELSAM is an acoustic microscope combined with an optical
microscope capable of generating visual or hard-copy acoustic
images. Use of microprocessors released the user from routine
adjustments of the complicated system, and also the hardware
and wiring is simplified to result in a reliable system. In
this paper, we also present some selected acoustic images
obtained with ELSAM which show the capabilities of the
scanning acoustic microscope.

---

*TM

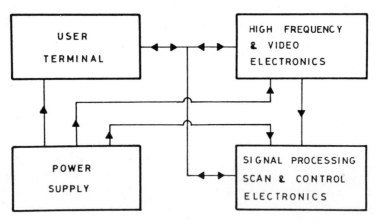

Fig. 1. The main sections of the acoustic
microscope

GENERAL DESIGN FEATURES

The wavelength of the acoustic waves used in imaging is determined by the frequency of operation. To serve both high resolution and high penetration depth applications, an acoustic microscope with broad frequency coverage is necessary. The 50 - 2000 MHz frequency band is selected to be the operation range. For ease of operation and for compatibility with many objects the coupling liquid is selected to be water. To get both optical and acoustical information from the same area of the object, a reflected-light microscope is combined with the acoustic microscope. The mechanical accuracy of conversion between the two micorscopes is such that the obtained images are centered to within a few micrometers of each other.

The main sections of the acoustic microscope are its mechanical parts, its electrical parts and its acoustic part as depicted in Fig. 1 in block diagram form. The critical mechanical parts include the X-Y scan mechanism, the Z adjustment mechanics, the object leveling apparatus. The X-Y scan mechanism is able to generate a 1 mm by 0.8 mm raster scan with less than 0.3 micrometer deviation in the Z direction. It is a electromechanical scan utilizing electromagnets and long leaf springs. Z adjustment can be done either manually or remotely by an electrical motor. The object leveling apparatus is coupled to the object stage to adjust the object surface parallel to the X-Y scan plane.

The user terminal is a small terminal designed around an 8-bit microprocessor to take commands from the user and send it to the other parts of the microscope for the selected operating mode to act as a controller for the acoustic microscope system. It is also used to inform the user on the modes of the microscope. The terminal has a dedicated keyboard and a joy-stick through which all the commands and adjustments are easily entered, and a 40 x 2 character plasma display on which all the relevant information is shown. Through the keyboard the user can select the various display and signal processing modes, change the magnification or the operation frequency.

HIGH FREQUENCY ELECTRONICS

The high frequency electronics operates in the pulse-echo mode. It receives commands from the user terminal and sets its operating point accordingly. The 50 - 2000 MHz frequency band is divided between two units. A block diagram of the high frequency electronics operating at 0.8 GHz to 2.0 GHz is shown in Fig. 2. It is basically composed of transmitter oscillators, pulse generating circuits and a superheterodyne receiver. The transmitted signal is generated by varactor tuned oscillators whose frequency can be controlled by a voltage applied from a D/A converter driven by a computer. This signal is pulsed by a solidstate switch to generate 10 nsec pulses. The switch is driven by a pulse drive electronics again controlled by the computer. The pulsed rf signal is amplified to a level of 1 W. The signal is fed to one of the arms of a double throw switch. The

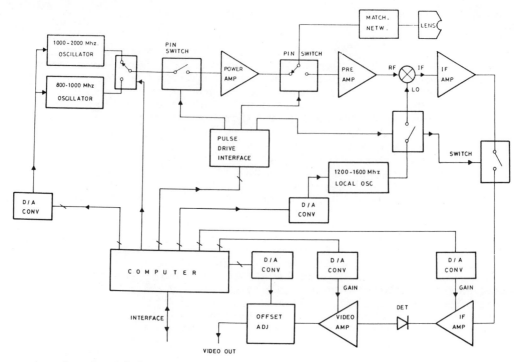

Fig. 2. The high frequency electronics for the 800 - 2000 MHz range

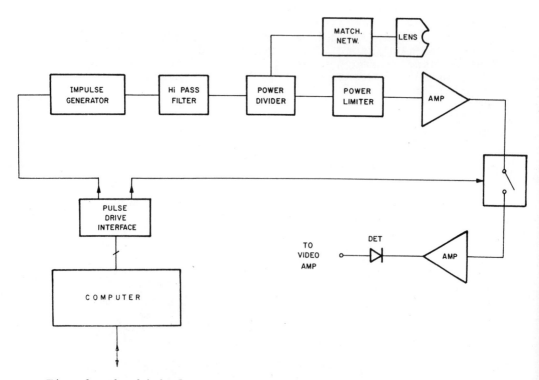

Fig. 3. The high frequency electronics for the 50 - 800 MHz range

common arm of the switch is connected to the acoustic lens
element. The second arm of the switch goes to a wide-band
preamplifier. The pulse drive interface driving this switch
is adjusted such that the first arm is connected to the common
arm only when the first switch is on and the second arm is
connected to common arm at a time slightly after the transmitter pulse is applied to the lens element. The output of the
preamplifier is fed to a wide band mixer. The local oscillator
is also pulsed to keep the IF amplifiers away from the
saturation caused by the spurious reflections. The local
oscillator is turned on only during the time the object pulse
may appear. The necessary pulse is created by the pulse drive
electronics using computer controlled digital delay techniques.
The frequency of the local oscillator is corrected by the
microprocessor to maximize the output voltage each time a
new frequency is selected. The two intermediate frequency
(IF)amplifiers in cascade provide the necessary gain. There
is another switch between the two IF amplifiers to further
reduce the undesired pulses. The gain of the IF amplifier is
adjustable by the computer to the desired level. Finally, the
output of the IF amplifier is detected by a detector diode to
generate the video signal which is proportional to the
amplitude of the received acoustic signal. The computer
responsible for the whole high frequency electronics is built
around an 8-bit single-chip microprocessor.

A block diagram of the high frequency electronics suitable for the 50 - 800 MHz range is depicted in Fig. 3.
A 1 nanosecond duration base-band pulse is used to excite the
transducer. This pulse is fed to the transducer through a
power divider. The output of the power divider is connected
to a limiter to protect the input of the receiver amplifier.
After amplification a mixer is used as a switch to gate out
the unwanted parts of the incoming pulse train. After the
time-gating operation further amplification is performed.
High pass filters are placed in the receiving chain to get
rid of switching spikes caused by the time gating operation.
The amplitude detection of the amplifier output provides the
necessary video signal for further processing.

The basic functions of video electronics are to shift
the DC level of the video signal and to change the video gain.
Those variables can be adjusted by the user with the joy-stick
on the user terminal. The signal processing electronics is
responsible to make some simple signal processing functions
like inverting the video signal to get reverse video images,
or differentiating it to get emphasized edges in the images.
The video gain can be adjusted either automatically or
manually. The circuitry is controlled by the third computer
of the acoustic microscope system. The output of this section
is fed to either a high persistence cathode-ray-tube (CRT)
for display or to a high resolution CRT for photographing
purposes.

SCAN AND CONTROL ELECTRONICS

The scan electronics takes care of various display
modes by generating the appropriate scan drive signals for
mechanical scan parts. It is possible to change the magnification just by changing the drive amplitude for X and Y scans.

A complete raster scan may contain 64, 128, 512 or 1024 horizontal lines and will be completed within a time interval which varies between 1 to 17 seconds depending on the scan magnitude and on the number of lines selected. If desired, the Y scan can be stopped to investigate just a single scan line. The video signal can be applied to Z input of CRT or to the Y input or a combination of both to get three-dimensional-like display forms. All the functions of the scan electronics are directed by the third computer and they are selected by the user at the user terminal.

The control electronics performs the miscellaneous functions like controlling the temperature of liquid medium, changing the object to lens distance all under computer command and under user instructions.

ACOUSTIC OBJECTIVE

The heart of the acoustic microscope system is its acoustic objective. It converts the electrical signals fed to it into ultrasonic signals, focusses them to a diffraction limited spot and converts the reflected acoustic signals back to the electrical form. The lenses are manufactured from single-crystal sapphire material. A spherical lens cavity is ground on one side of the sapphire with mechanical means. A ZnO thin film tranducer is deposited on the flat side of the crystal. The transducer generates planar acoustic wavefronts when used as transmitter, and as a receiver it is sensitive to the shape of the wavefronts impinging on it. The lens cavity is coated with a quarter-wavelength thick glass anti-reflection layer to reduce the reflection loss. The two-way conversion loss of tranducers is typically 10 dB. The lens units are housed in small metallic tubes with the high frequency connector on one end and the lens on the other. Matching networks are included within the lens housing.

Due to bandwidth limitations the whole frequency range can not be taken care of with a single acoustic objective. Instead, the 0.8 to 2.0 GHz range is divided between two objectives: One centered at 1 GHz and the other at 1.7 GHz. The lower frequency 50 to 800 MHz range is covered by objectives operating at the following center frequencies: 100 MHz, 200 MHz and 400 MHz. A 50 MHz objective is in preparation. All the objectives have the associated matching networks to give the necessary bandwidth. The acoustic objectives differ not only in frequency but also in radius of lens cavity. At high frequencies the loss in the liquid medium is very high. In this case lenses with a cavity radius of 40 micrometers are used. On the other hand, at low frequencies the liquid losses drop very rapidly making large radius lenses feasible. At the low frequency end, 2000 micrometer radius lenses are used to increase the working distance and to make higher imaging depth possible. Working with large radius lenses is easy both from mechanical and from electrical points of view. Mechanically there is a big playroom and electrically the various internal reflection pulses are well separated from each other. On the other hand, for a 40 micrometer radius lens there is only 60 nsec separation between the first internal reflection pulse and the object pulse. Additionally the size of the object pulse is

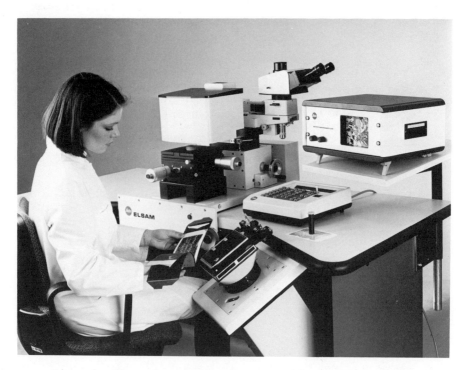

Fig. 4. The microscope in acoustic imaging mode

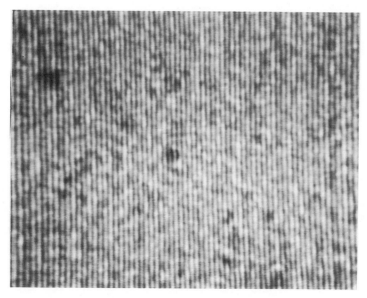

Fig. 5. Acoustic image of a resolution test grating with a
period of 0.83 μm, taken at f = 1,5 GHz (corresponding wavelength in water ∿ 1 μm).

60 dB below the spurious pulse. Any reflection in electronics or in cables will manifest itself as interference of object pulse with a reference. The high frequency electronics described above is capable of separating the small object pulse from its large and close neighboring spurious pulses to generate interference free images.

The objectives of varying lens radii have varying time delays. The object pulse will not appear at the same place for the different objectives. Hence, the delays of time gating pulses as generated by the pulse drive circuitry should be different. This time delay adjustment is made automatically for every acoustic objective by the microprocessors.

IMAGES

Fig. 4 depicts the ELSAM in its acoustic imaging mode. Referring to the figure, the housing close to the center contains the scanning mechanism for x-y movement of the acoustic objective and the stage with micrometer spindles. The acoustic objective cannot be seen in this picture. The light microscope, here out of its operating position, is on the right side of the scanner housing. At the rear right is a long-persistence CRT screen for real-time display of the acoustic slow scan image. On the table below is the user terminal with joystick and function display. A photomicrographic unit with a high-resolution CRT screen is located in front of the user terminal.

Figs. 5 - 7 demonstrate the high resolution and depth penetration ability of the acoustic microscope. All images were obtained from ELSAM high resolution CRT screen with a 35-mm camera attached to it. Brighter pixels represent higher levels of received signal from the corresponding object point. Darker pixels do not necessarily indicate that the acoustic energy at the object is absorbed; the reduction of the signal may be as a result of a cancellation at the phase sensitive transducer (Quate et al., 1979.)

OUTLOOK

The scanning acoustic microscope is a microscope capable of subsurface imaging with a resolution equalling a good optical microscope. Optically opaque materials or layers, which are unsuitable for the optical microscope, become the objects of the acoustic microscope. The acoustic microscope can be used with almost all objects and nondestructively. It is sensitive to a change in density or stiffness of the material. Voids within the body of the materials or delaminations in thin film structures are easily detected due to very high acoustic impedance change at the interface. The scanning acoustic microscope has found applications in such diverse fields as materials science, thin film technology, geology, biology and new fields are emerging as the application research continues.

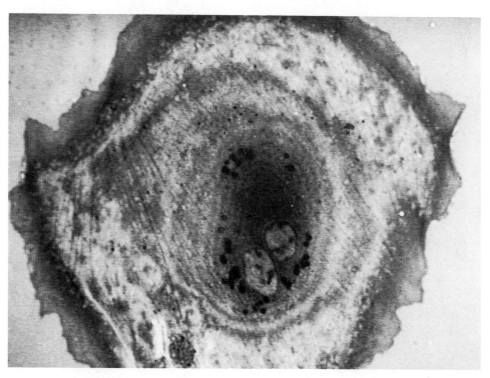

Fig. 6. Single-frame acoustic image of a fixed frog heart cell.
Frequency 1.6 GHz, picture width 200 µm. The image
shows fringes due to cell topography. Structural
details in the 1 µm-range are visible (stress fibers).

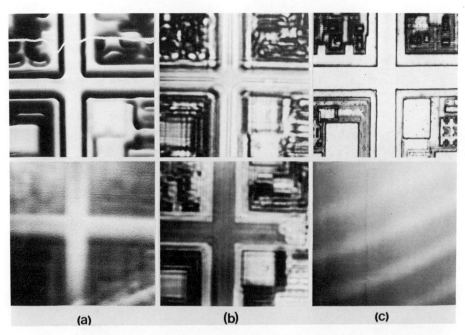

(a)   (b)   (c)

Fig. 7. Depth penetration ability of the acoustic microscope
at different frequencies: (a) 100 MHz, (b) 200 MHz,
(c) 400 MHz; width of images 0.8 mm.

Upper row shows surface images of an integrated
circuit (IC).

Bottom row shows pictures of the same area, but
imaged through a 250 µm thick sheet of mica
(water - coupled to the IC surface). At 400 MHz, the
mica is not penetrated (c).

Enhanced resolution vs. higher frequencies is clearly
visible, too.

REFERENCES

Ash, E.A., 1980, "Scanned Image Microscopy", Academic, London.

IEEE Trans. Sonics Ultrasonics, 1985, SU-32.

Hoppe, M., Atalar, A., Patzelt, W.J. and Thaer, A., 1983, "LEITZ-Akustomikroskop ELSAM: Anwendungen in der Materialuntersuchung - erste Ergebnisse", Leitz - Mitt. Wiss. u. Techn., VIII: 125

Hoppe, M. and Bereiter-Hahn, J., "Applications of Scanning Acoustic Microscopy - Survey and New Aspects", 1985, IEEE Trans. Son.Ultrason., 32: 289.

Lemons, R. and Quate, C.F., 1974, Appl. Phys. Lett.,24: 163.

Quate, C.F., Atalar, A. and Wickramasinghe, K.K., 1979, Proc. IEEE 67: 1092.

Jipson, V. and Quate, C.F., 1978, Appl. Phys. Lett.,32: 789.

SUBSURFACE IMAGING IN ACOUSTIC MICROSCOPY

Zse-Cherng Lin*, Glen Wade,
Hua Lee†, and Michael G. Oravecz**

Department of Electrical and Computer Engineering
University of California, Santa Barbara, CA 93106

ABSTRACT

Acoustic microscopy is capable of producing micrographs with a high degree of resolution. When an acoustic microscope operates in the transmission mode, the micrograph is simply a shadowgraph of all the structure encountered by the paths of acoustic rays passing through the objects. Because of diffraction and overlapping, the resultant images are difficult to comprehend in the case of specimens of substantial thickness and structural complexity. The principles of diffraction tomography and acoustic holography can be used to overcome this problem. In this paper, we present experimental results of subsurface imaging using holographic image reconstruction with a modified scanning laser acoustic microscope (SLAM). We describe how to model the imaging process as a two-dimensional linear system. The compensation for the nonuniform frequency response of the wavefield detection and the computation of wave propagation are discussed. We show a series of images to demonstrate that high-quality, high-resolution subsurface images can be obtained from holographic data with image processing.

INTRODUCTION

Acoustic microscopy [1-3], which employs ultrasound in the range of hundreds and thousands of megahertz, represents an outstanding example of acoustic imaging. It is capable of producing micrographs with a high degree of resolution. In contrast with the conventional optical microscopy, ultrasound can image the internal structure of opaque specimens. Such microscope can be used to study solid-state surfaces, the layers beneath the surface, and the interior structure of microscopic life.

This research is supported by the National Science Foundation under Grants ECS-8406511 and ECS-8460665.
*Zse-Cherng Lin is now with SRI International, 333 Ravenswood Ave., Menlo Park, CA 94025.
†Hua Lee is with the Department of Electrical and Computer Engineering, University of Illinois, Urbana, IL 61801.
**Michael G. Oravecz is with Sonoscan, Inc., 530 E. Green St., Bensenville, IL 60106.

The scanning laser acoustic microscope (SLAM) is a typical example of an acoustic microscope that operates in the transmission mode. Its principles of operation have been presented and discussed extensively in the literature [4,5]. Micrographs obtained with SLAM are simply shadowgraphs of all the structure encountered by the paths of the acoustic rays passing through the objects. Because of diffraction and overlapping, the resultant images are difficult to comprehend in the case of specimens of substantial thickness and structural complexity. With the technique of digital signal processing, the ideas of acoustical holography and diffraction tomography can be used to overcome this difficulty [6].

Although the principle of acoustical holography has existed for a long period of time, the images reconstructed were usually very noisy and the resolution was far from satisfactory because of the difficulties encountered in the actual data acquisition, signal processing and image reconstruction. Recently, we have been successful in obtaining high-resolution subsurface images with a properly modified SLAM by applying these principles.

The modification of conventional SLAM to acquire proper data for the holographic image reconstruction is presented in a companion paper "Progress toward a practical 100 MHz scanning laser tomographic acoustic microscope" by M. Oravecz and L. Gibbons. In this paper, we describe how to model the subsurface imaging process as a two-dimensional linear system. A series of images reconstructed using the data collected from a suitably modified SLAM are presented to show the first high-quality high-resolution microscopic subsurface images obtained by digital acoustical holography.

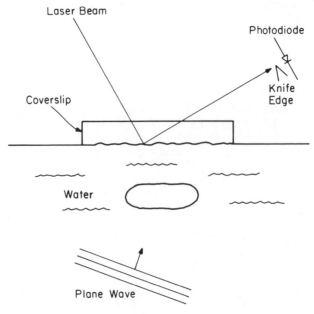

Figure 1.   Schematic diagram of SLAM.

SUBSURFACE IMAGING WITH SLAM

As shown in Fig. 1, plane-wave ultrasound is used as the insonification source. The planar wavefield is modulated by the object distribution and propagates to the receiving plane of the data acquisition. The image data are read out by means of a scanning laser beam reflected from the coverslip (mirror surface) [5]. A knife-edge and photodiode combination is used to detect the acoustical signal [4]. The detected signal represents the ultrasound wavefield scattered or shadowed by the object distribution. The problem of image reconstruction becomes first compensating for the nonuniform frequency response of the wavefield detection that involves the knife-edge demodulation. The object distribution can then be recovered by computing the back-propagation of the ultrasound wavefield to correct for the diffraction experienced in the forward propagation.

The object being imaged is a thin planar test pattern submerged in water. This setup simulates the imaging of a particular internal planar distribution of inhomogeneities within a homogeneous material. Under the circumstances, the imaging process can be modeled as a linear system as shown in Fig. 2. The input to this system is the wavefield distribution at the plane where the test pattern is located. The system contains two two-dimensional linear filters. One is a dispersive phase filter which governs the wave propagation through the homogeneous medium. The transfer function of this filter can be expressed as follows [7]

$$H_1(f_x,f_y) = \begin{cases} \exp\left[j\,2\pi z\,(\frac{1}{\lambda^2} - f_x^2 - f_y^2)^{\frac{1}{2}}\right], & f_x^2 + f_y^2 \leq \frac{1}{\lambda^2} \\ 0, & \text{otherwise}, \end{cases} \tag{1}$$

where we have neglected the evanescent waves, λ is the wavelength of the ultrasound within the water and z is the distance between the plane of the object and the receiving plane.

The other filter is the one which characterizes the response of the knife-edge demodulation. Its transfer function has been derived as [8]

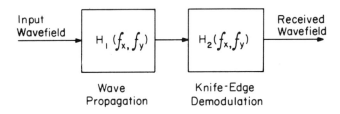

Input Wavefield → $H_1(f_x, f_y)$ → $H_2(f_x, f_y)$ → Received Wavefield

Wave Propagation   Knife-Edge Demodulation

Figure 2.   A linear-system model of the imaging process. $H_1(f_x,f_y)$ is a linear filter representing the wave propagation. $H_2(f_x,f_y)$ is a linear filter representing the knife-edge demodulation.

$$H_2(f_x, f_y) = j \, \text{erf}\left[\frac{\pi r_o f_x}{\sqrt{2}}\right] \exp\left[-\frac{\pi^2 r_o^2}{2}(f_x^2 + f_y^2)\right]$$

$$= j\left\{\text{erf}\left[\frac{\pi r_o f_x}{\sqrt{2}}\right] \exp\left[-\frac{\pi^2 r_o^2 f_x^2}{2}\right]\right\} \cdot \left\{\exp\left[-\frac{\pi^2 r_o^2 f_y^2}{2}\right]\right\}$$

$$= j H_x(r_o f_x) \cdot H_y(r_o f_y). \tag{2}$$

in which we have assumed that a laser beam of Gaussian intensity profile is used and its effective beam radius is r_o. The notation erf represents the error function. The laser beam is assumed to scan in the direction of x. Fig. 3 shows the two separable functions $H_x(r_o f_x)$ and $H_y(r_o f_y)$ composing the transfer function.

Since the detected wavefield is the output of the linear system, the holographic image reconstruction becomes designing the inverse filters to estimate the object distribution. The block diagram of the image reconstruction is shown in Fig. 4. We first compensate for the imperfect frequency response of the knife-edge detection.

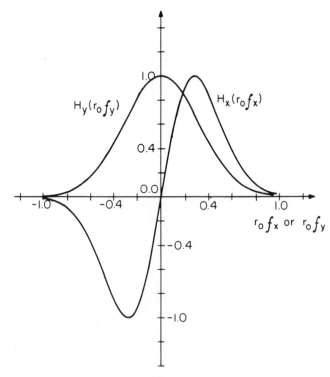

Figure 3. Transfer function of the knife-edge detector oriented perpendicular to the scan direction of the laser beam which is assumed to have a Gaussian intensity profile. The plots are normalized to their maximum responses. The function can be separated into two functions. $H_x(r_o f_x)$ is the response function in the scan direction. $H_y(r_o f_y)$ is the response function perpendicular to the scan direction.

As can be deduced from Fig. 1, both the low and high frequency components in the x direction will have a very small signal to noise ratio. In the y direction, high-frequency components will have a small signal to noise ratio. Inverse filtering may therefore amplify the noise and degrade the reconstructed image. To minimize this, we must choose a threshold for the transfer function. Only those frequency components for which the transfer function has values greater than the threshold will be compensated. The inverse filter for $H_2(f_x, f_y)$ is designed as follows:

$$
\hat{H}_2(f_x, f_y) = \begin{cases} \dfrac{H_{max} \exp\left[\dfrac{\pi^2 r_o^2}{2}(f_x^2 + f_y^2)\right]}{\left[j\, \mathrm{erf}(\dfrac{\pi r_o f_x}{\sqrt{2}})\right]} & \text{if } |H_2(f_x, f_y)| \geqslant H_s \\[6pt] 1 & \text{otherwise .} \end{cases}
\tag{3}
$$

where H_s is the threshold chosen in such a way that after inverse filtering the main spectrum of the signal is recovered and the noise amplification does not degrade the image reconstruction. H_{max} is the amplitude of the maximum response for $H_2(f_x, f_y)$.

The diffraction experienced by wavefield propagation can be corrected by computing the corresponding backward propagation. The corresponding inverse filter to accomplish this is

$$
\hat{H}_1(f_x, f_y) = \begin{cases} \exp\left[-j2\pi z(\dfrac{1}{\lambda^2} - f_x^2 - f_y^2)^{1/2}\right] & f_x^2 + f_y^2 \leqslant \dfrac{1}{\lambda^2} \\[6pt] 0 & \text{otherwise .} \end{cases}
\tag{4}
$$

As before, we neglect the evanescent waves because they will not be detected.

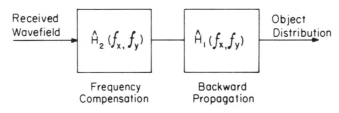

Figure 4.   Model corresponding to image reconstruction by inverse filtering.

EXPERIMENTAL RESULTS

A conventional SLAM was modified to acquire data for reconstructing an image. The ultrasound source for the system operated at 101.8 MHz. Proper electronic filters and quadrature detectors were designed and built to collect the data for holographic reconstruction. Several phantoms were fabricated as the test object. To simplify the experiment, the phantoms were made of thin material and supported in water which served as the surrounding homogeneous material. The wavelength of the ultrasound in the water was approximately 15 microns. The thickness of the phantoms was about 15 to 25 microns. The field of view was 3.0 mm by 2.81 mm. For each phantom, data corresponding to four images from the modified instrument and one image from a conventional SLAM were taken and digitized. There were 256 by 240 samples in each image and each sample had 6 bits of intensity information.

The test specimens were placed in a plane parallel to but some distance away from the detection plane (coverslip). The angle of incidence of the ultrasound onto the specimens was 10 degrees. This gave a maximum signal to noise ratio. In the modified SLAM, a set of data contains four images. Two images represent the real and imaginary parts of the positive spatial-frequency band of the wavefield. The other two images represent the real and imaginary parts of the negative spatial-frequency band. However, with this angle of incidence, the signal spectrum was largely confined to the positive spatial-frequency band. Hence, only the two images corresponding to positive spatial-frequency band were used for the image reconstruction. We discovered a small relative phase error between the two images. This error could be due to the fact that the two images were not acquired simultaneously or to the possibility that the two reference signals did not have an exact 90 degree phase difference as required in the quadrature detector.

Figs. 5, 6 and 7 show the result of image reconstructions for three different test patterns. In the figure, (a) and (b) are the two image data used for the holographic reconstruction. (c) is the image obtained from a conventional SLAM. (d) is the reconstructed image for the subsurface where the test pattern is located. The test pattern in Fig. (5) represents a small aperture in the center of the field of view. The distance between the coverslip and the test pattern is 3 mm. From Fig. 5(c), we can see that the aperture is shifted to the right-hand side and blurred because of the wave propagation and diffraction. The subsurface image shown in Fig. 5(d) is well defined and the aperture is located in the center.

Fig. 6 shows the result of a test pattern which contains three vertical bars. The distance between the pattern and the coverslip is 0.6 mm. Since the dimension of the bar is big compared to the wavelength of the ultrasound and the distance is small, diffraction is not very significant. Nevertheless, the vertical bars shown in the conventional SLAM image in Fig. 6(c) are still blurred. Fig. 6(d) shows a reconstructed image which has better resolution and sharper edges.

In Fig. 7, the test pattern is a honeycomb finder grid. The center-to-center spacing between parallel faces of the hexagons is 225 microns, the circle diameters are 100 microns, and the thin bars making up sides of the hexagons are about 15 microns across. The honeycomb finder grid was placed 0.6 mm below the coverslip when the data were acquired. The conventional SLAM image for this situation as shown in Fig. 7(c) is so blurred that the honeycomb pattern is not discernable. Only dark and bright spots can be seen in the picture. The two uncompensated images from the real and imaginary parts of the complex amplitude of the wavefield are shown in Figs. 7 (a) and (b). These images are difficult to comprehend. Fig. 7 (d) shows a well focused image with the honeycomb pattern easily identified. The pattern is well defined and has excellent resolution.

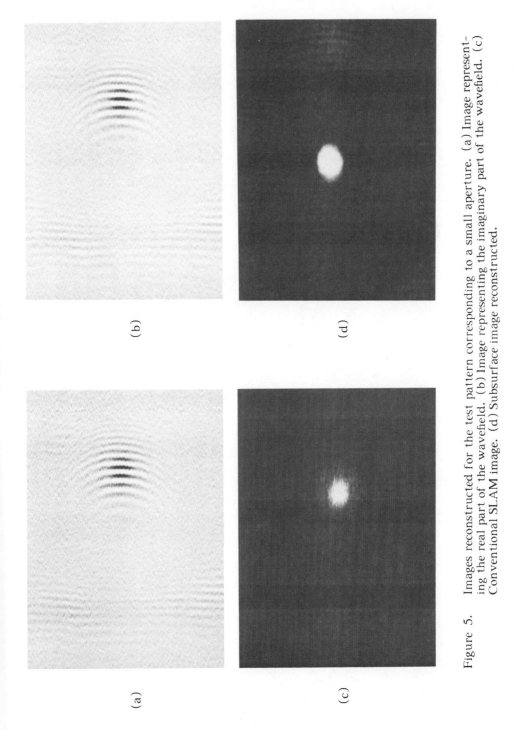

(a)

(b)

(c)

(d)

Figure 5.   Images reconstructed for the test pattern corresponding to a small aperture. (a) Image representing the real part of the wavefield. (b) Image representing the imaginary part of the wavefield. (c)
Conventional SLAM image. (d) Subsurface image reconstructed.

449

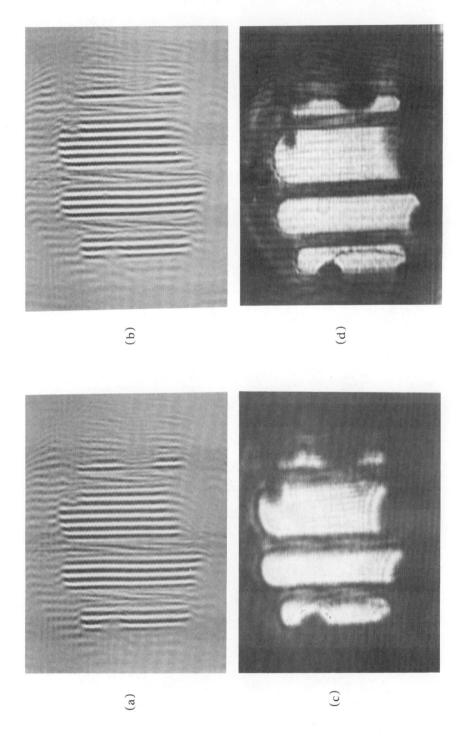

(a)

(b)

(c)

(d)

Figure 6. Images reconstructed for the test pattern containing three vertical bars. (a) Image representing the real part of the wavefield. (b) Image representing the imaginary part of the wavefield. (c) Conventional SLAM image. (d) Subsurface image reconstructed.

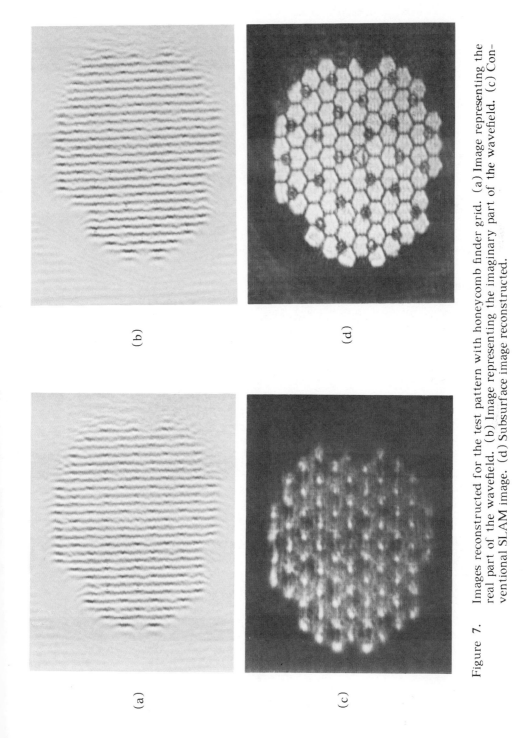

Figure 7.   Images reconstructed for the test pattern with honeycomb finder grid. (a) Image representing the real part of the wavefield. (b) Image representing the imaginary part of the wavefield. (c) Conventional SLAM image reconstructed. (d) Subsurface image reconstructed.

451

CONCLUSION

We have discussed how to model the subsurface imaging in acoustic microscopy as a two-dimensional linear system. The two transfer functions representing the wave propagation and the ultrasonic wavefield detection are described. The inverse filtering technique for the holographic image reconstruction is presented. The inverse filter compensates for SLAM's nonideal transfer function and the computed back-propagation takes into account diffraction and produces a focused image of any particular plane of interest.

Several experiments were performed to collect data by using phantoms as the test samples. Both conventional SLAM images and the holographic images were reconstructed. The results demonstrate that SLAM, modified appropriately, can acquire the data needed for successful holographic image reconstruction. The reconstructed images show that high-quality, high-resolution subsurface images can be obtained in scanning laser acoustic microscopy.

ACKNOWLEDGEMENT

The authors would like to acknowledge Lawrence K. Gibbons of Sonoscan, Inc. for his extremely valuable efforts in performing the experiment and taking the data.

REFERENCES

[1] L.W. Kessler and D.E. Yuhas, "Acoustic microscopy - 1979," *Proc. IEEE*, vol. 67, pp. 526-536, Apr. 1979.

[2] C.F. Quate, A. Atalar, and H.K. Wickramasinghe, "Acoustic microscopy with mechanical scanning - A Review," *Proc. IEEE*, vol. 67, pp. 1092-1114, Aug. 1979.

[3] L.W. Kessler, "Acoustic microscopy commentary: SLAM and SAM," *IEEE Trans. Sonics Ultrason.* vol. SU-32, no. 2, pp. 136-137, March 1985.

[4] R.L. Whitman and A. Korpel, "Probing of acoustic surface perturbations by coherent light," *Applied Optics*, vol. 8, no. 8, pp. 1567-1576, Aug. 1969.

[5] L.W. Kessler, "Imaging with dynamic-ripple diffraction," in *Acoustic Imaging*, G. Wade, Ed. New York: Plenum, 1976, chap. 10, pp. 229-239.

[6] Z.C. Lin, H. Lee and G. Wade, "Scanning tomographic acoustic microscope: A Review," *IEEE Trans. Sonics Ultrason.*, vol. SU-32, no. 2, pp. 168-180, Mar. 1985.

[7] J.W. Goodman, *Introduction to Fourier Optics*. New York: McGraw-Hill, 1968, pp. 54.

[8] R.K. Mueller and R.L. Rylander, "New demodulation scheme for laser scanned-acoustic imaging systems," *J. Opt. Soc. Am.*, vol. 69, no. 3, pp. 407-412, March 1979.

RELATION BETWEEN SPATIAL FREQUENCY SAMPLING WINDOW AND LATERAL

RESOLUTION IN BACKWARD PROPAGATION ACOUSTICAL IMAGING

Xianhua Xia and Dejun Zhang

Wuhan Institute of Physics
Academia Sinica
Wuhan , Hubei
People's Republic of China

ABSTRACT

An acoustical imaging could be numerically reconstructed by several methods, one of which is Backward Propagation method. This method has many advantages;especially it could be used in nearer distance where it is no longer in the region of Fresnel diffraction. Using traditional backward propagation method, the lateral resolution of the imaging system would be constrained by spatial sampling interval when the imaging distance is very short. This problem is discussed and the solution worked out using the method of data augmenting in spatial frequency domain. The details of the method and the results of computer simulant experiments are given in the paper.

INTRODUCTION

With the advance in arithmetic technology, the various numerical methods of processing and reconstructing images are more and more extensively used in the field of acoustical imaging. There exist two common kinds of image reconstructing methods, one of which is Fourier-Fresnel transform method, the other is Backward Propagation method (BP method) which is to be considered in this paper. For the sake of the following discussion we first introduce the principle of BP method briefly.

Let $u_s(x, y)$ and $u(x, y)$ represent the complex amplitude distribution functions of the wavefields on the object plane ($z=-z_s$) and receiving plane ($z=0$) respectively. Assuming

$$A(f_x, f_y) = F \{ u(x,y) \}$$

$$A_s(f_x, f_y) = F \{u_s(x,y) \}$$

$$H(f_x, f_y, z_s) = F \{ h(x,y,z_s) \}$$

Where

$$h(x,y,z_s) = \exp\{j2\pi(x^2 + y^2 + z_s^2)^{1/2}/\lambda\}$$

λ is the wavelenth used by the system. F and F^{-1} are defined as the operators of two-dimensional Fourier transform and its inverse transform respectively. We have

$$A(f_x, f_v) = A_s(f_x, f_v)H(f_x, f_v, z_s) \tag{1}$$

Then

$$u_s(x_i, y_i) = F^{-1}\{A(f_x, f_v)H^{-1}(f_x, f_v, z_s)\} \tag{2}$$

It seems that from the distribution of the wavefield on the receiving plane one could know the exact distribution of the wavefield on the object plane. But it is impossible in reality. As all the receiving apertures are of limited sizes, the spectrum of the signal one could get on the receiving aperture is

$$A_1(f_x, f_v) = A(f_x, f_v) * F\{\sigma(x, y)\} \tag{3}$$

$\sigma(x, y)$ is the aperture function whose value equals one within the aperture and zero otherwise. Asterisk "*" is a convenient symbol indicating that the two functions are to be convolved. From the above equations the complex amplitude function of the image could be deduced

$$u_i(x_i, y_i) = \{[u_s(x_i, y_i) * h(x_i, y_i, z_s)]\sigma(x_i, y_i)\} * h^{-1}(x_i, y_i, z_s) \tag{4}$$

Eq.4 shows that the image is no longer the perfect replica of the object and the image obtained is a smoothed version of the object [1],[2]. The lateral resolution of the system is $\lambda z_s/L$ (Rayleigh criterion), where L is the dimension of the aperture. When the distribution of the wavefield on the aperture $\sigma(x, y)$ is sampled discretely it is sure that the repetition of the original object's image occurs. Only when the condition that the dimension of the object which is to be imaged is smaller than the that of the field of view (i.e. $\lambda z_s/D$, where D is the equal sampling interval) is satisfied, the spatial positions of a set of images could be separated from each other. The relation of the object and the images could be written

$$u_i(x_i, y_i) = \{[u_s(x_i, y_i) * h(x_i, y_i, z_s)]\sigma(x_i, y_i)\text{comb}(x_i/D)_m$$

$$\text{comb}(y_i/D)_n\} * h^{-1}(x_i, y_i, z_s) \tag{5}$$

Where $\quad \text{comb}(x)_m = \sum_{m=-\infty}^{\infty} \delta(x-m)$

METHOD OF DATA AUGMENTING IN FREQUENCY DOMAIN

Usually the steps of the image reconstruction using BP method are taken as follows:

First sample the wavefield on the receiving aperture to get the sampling data $u(mD, nD)$ (m, n = $-(N-1)/2$, $-(N-1)/2+1$, ..., $(N-1)/2$, where the total number of the sampling is N^2) and figure out its discrete Fourier transform

$$A_2(k\Omega, l\Omega) = \sum_{m,n=-\frac{N-1}{2}}^{\frac{N-1}{2}} u(mD, nD) \exp\{-j2\pi(mk+nl)\}$$

$$= F\{u(mD, nD)\}_{N \times N} \tag{6}$$

$$k, l = -(N-1)/2, \quad 1-(N-1)/2, \quad ..., \quad (N-1)/2 \qquad \Omega = 1/N/D$$

symbol $F(\ )_{N \times N}$ stands for the NXN points two-dimensional discrete Fourier transform of the function.

Second multiply $A(k\Omega,l\Omega)$ by the filtering function and then take the inverse transforming of it. The complex amplitude distribution of the image is found out

$$u_{1,2}(mD,nD)=F^{-1}\{A_2(k\Omega,l\Omega)H^{-1}(k\Omega,l\Omega,z_{\ast})\}_{N\times N} \tag{7}$$

From the above-mentioned process we could see that the sampling interval on the image plane equals to that on the receiving aperture and the area of the imaging region equals to that of the receiving aperture because we have to adopt FFT algorithm in the procedure of calculation. Difficulties arise out of the affair.

When the imaging distance is very large $(\lambda z_{\ast}/D > L)$, the field of view of the system would be reduced to L, it is no longer $\lambda z_{\ast}/L$. For further discussion of this aspect see Ref. [3],[4].

When the imaging distance is short $(\lambda z_{\ast}/D < L)$, the lateral resolution of the system would be restricted. It is not the one determined by aperture diffraction but the sampling spacing D .

The trouble is caused by the cutoff of the two windows in BP method. One is the cutoff of the window of the holographic operation which determines the information content obtained by the system so that the lateral resolution the system may have is determined as $\lambda z_{\ast}/L$. The other is the cutoff by the window in the spatial frequency domain for the need of the adoption of the FFT algorithm. If the window function in the spatial frequency domain is given by

$$G(f_x,f_y)=rect(f_x/N/\Omega)rect(f_y/N/\Omega)$$

then the point spread function of the system can be written

$$v_{1,2}(mD,nD)= \sum_{k,l=-\infty}^{\infty}\sum \{[Sin(\pi NLx/z_{\ast}\lambda)Sin(\pi NLy/z_{\ast}\lambda)]$$
$$/[Sin(\pi Lx/z_{\ast}\lambda)\ Sin(\pi Ly/z_{\ast}\lambda)]\}$$
$$* \{Sinc[(x-kND)/D]\ Sinc[(y-lND)/D]\}_{x=mD,y=nD} \tag{8}$$

Our attention is focused here on the zero-order image (the influence of the higher order images will be discussed in the other paper) and we have the distribution of the zero-order image's amplitude of the system

$$v_{1,\ast}(mD,nD)=Sinc(m)\ Sinc(n) \tag{9}$$

$$m\ ,\ n = -(N-1)/2,\ 1-(N-1)/2,\ \ldots,\ (N-1)/2$$

It is obvious that the lateral resolution of the system becomes D.

Above constraint is disadvantageous for BP method to be used in the short distance imaging process. It does not make the best of the lateral resolution the system has. To conquer the drawback one could employ the method of decreasing sampling interval D . But it means that to reach the inherent resolution of the system the number of receiving elements must be increased so as not to reduce the aperture dimension. In many cases this is not flexible and economical.

There is another way to reach the same purpose that is what we called "Data augmenting in spatial frequency domain". Through the analysis we get to know that what we need to do is to expand the function of the sampling window in spatial frequency domain . We may seek the form of it as

$$G(f_x, f_y) = \text{rect}[f_x/(N+\varDelta)/\Omega] \; \text{rect}[f_y/(N+\varDelta)/\Omega] \qquad (10)$$

where $\varDelta$ is a minimal integer which simultaneously satisfies inequality

$$\varDelta \geq -N(1-LD/z_s/\lambda)$$

and

$$\varDelta + N = 2^k \qquad\qquad \text{(k is a positive integer)}$$

the last equality is only for the need of base-2 FFT algorithm. Such expansion of the window function will eliminate the influence of the window cutoff in the spatial frequency domain on the lateral resolution of the system.

It is noteworthy that the spectrum components calculated from Eq.(6) do not include the following parts

$$D^{-1} < [\; 1f_x1 \; , \quad 1f_y1 \;] < (N + \varDelta)\Omega$$

due to $(N + \varDelta) > D^{-1}$. They must be determined. But those parts are not independent. Having the aid of the property of FFT and analysing Eq.(6) we could write

$$A_2(k\Omega, 1\Omega) = (-1)^{1+J} A_2(k\Omega + IN\Omega, 1\Omega + JN\Omega) \qquad (11)$$

where I,J are arbitrary integers. One possible result from the expansion would be the reconstruction of some higher order images. In this paper we leave it out of consideration.

To sum up the above discussion we may turn out the steps of the method as follows

1. Add zero value points to u(mD, nD) which are the N X N points complex data series of the samples of the wavefield, so it becomes a M X M points complex data series

$$u_2(mD,nD) = \begin{cases} u(mD,nD) & \text{when } [1m1,1n1] \leq (N-1)/2 \\ \emptyset & \text{when } (M-1)/2 \geq [1m1,1n1] \geq (N-1)/2 \end{cases} \qquad (12)$$

$$m, \; n = -(M-1)/2, \; 1-(M-1)/2, \; \ldots, \; (M-1)/2$$

considering the location of the imaged object is paraxial, the value of M could be chosen to be an integer which is greater than 2N and equals to 2^k (where k is an arbitrary integer)

2. Process $u_2(mD, nD)$ using M X M points FFT algorithm to obtain one part of spatial frequency distribution on the receiving aperture

$$A_2(k\Omega, 1\Omega) = \sum_{m,n=-\frac{M-1}{2}}^{\frac{M-1}{2}} u_2(mD,nD) \exp\{ -j2\pi(mk+nl)/M \} \qquad (13)$$

$$k, \; 1 = -(M-1)/2, \; 1-(M-1)/2, \; \ldots, \; (M-1)/2$$

3. Using the result of the Eq.(13) we get the spectrum function

$$A_3(k'\Omega, 1'\Omega) = \sum_{I,J=1-n_0}^{n_0-1} (-1)^{(1+J)} A_2[(k'-IM)\Omega, (1'-JM)\Omega]$$
$$\text{rect}[(k'-IM)/(M-1)] \; \text{rect}[(1'-JM)/(M-1)] \qquad (14)$$

where

$$k', \quad l' = -(M+\Delta-1)/2, 1-(M+\Delta-1)/2, \quad \ldots, \quad (M+\Delta-1)/2$$

Δ is a minimum integer satisfying

$$\Delta \geq -M(1-LD/z_s/\lambda)$$

and

$$\Delta + M = 2^k \qquad (k \text{ is a positive integer })$$

n_s is a minimum integer satisfying the inequality

$$n_s \geq [1+(\Delta-1)/M]$$

4. After multiplying $A_3(k'\Omega, l'\Omega)$ with the filtering function we get the distribution function of the image field by turning out the inverse Fourier transform with FFT algorithm

$$u_{1,2}(m'D', n'D') = F^{-1}\{A_3(k'\Omega, l'\Omega) \ H^{-1}(k'\Omega, l'\Omega, z_s)\}_{M' \times M'} \qquad (15)$$

where

$$m', \ n' = -(M+\Delta-1)/2, \ 1-(M+\Delta-1)/2, \quad \ldots, \quad (M+\Delta-1)/2$$

$$D' = DM/(M+\Delta)$$

$$M' = M+\Delta$$

RESULTS OF SIMULANT EXPERIMENT

We have made a simulant experiment to examine the above analysis using a computer. Fig.1 shows its results. What we simulated was a $N=16$ one dimensional holographic receiving array. It does not lose the generality . Its sampling function in spatial domain was

$$\text{rect}(x/L) \ \text{comb}(x/D)_n$$

where $L=ND$. The object distribution function on the object plane was

$$u_s(x) = \delta(x+D/2)$$

In reconstructing process we let $M=64$ (i.e.,imaging region was $-L$ by $+L$). In order to make the sampling points in the image field sufficient close so as to observe it easily we added some extra zero value points to the spectrum data series in the experiment. Symbol "." in Fig.1 represents the experimental value and the continuous curve is the intensity distribution of the point spread function determined by the limited aperture diffraction. They are both the unitized values.

In Fig.1-a, because of using the traditional BP method and $\lambda z_s/L = D/2$ the lateral resolution of the system is not $\lambda z_s/L$ but D ; While in Fig.1-b all the conditions are the same except the use of the method of data augmenting in the spatial frequency domain, it is clear that the resolution is $\lambda z_s/L$. From the figure we could also see that there exist two first-order images which are defocussing and located about $\pm(\lambda z_s/D)$. The intensity of zero-order image is far greater than that of the two higher order images

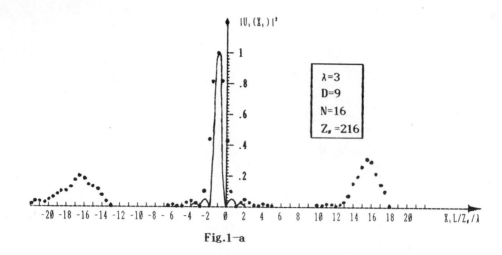

Fig.1-a

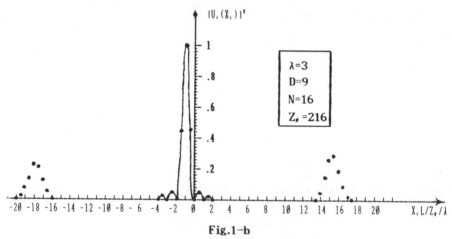

Fig.1-b

Fig.1 The intensity distribution of the point spread function
"●" experiment sampling points

SUMMARY

As one kind of method to reconstruct image numerically BP method has
its own advantages. Short-distance imaging is a very important aspect of
its applications. Fresnel approximation is not a good one under such
circumstances. Adopting the method suggested in the paper will make the
applications of BP method in various fields more flexible and more
extensive.

ACKNOWLEDGMENT

The authors would like to acknowledge Professor J.P.N. Wei for his
encouragement and his assistance in preparing the manuscript.

458

REFERENCES

[1] J. W. Goodman,1968, "Introduction to Fourier Optics," Mc Graw Hill, New York

[2] E. Lalor, Inverse Wave Propagation, J. Math. Phys., 9(1968), 2001

[3] J. P. Power, Computer Simulation of Linear Acoustic Diffraction, Acoustical Holography , Vol.7, Plenum Press, New York, (1976), 193

[4] C. Schueler, et al, Spatial Replication in Back-Propagated Acoustic Holograms, Proc. IEEE , 69(1981), No.12, 1580

APPLICATIONS OF DIGITAL IMAGE ENHANCEMENT TECHNIQUES

TO THE ULTRASONIC NDE OF COMPOSITE MATERIALS

Brian G. Frock and Richard W. Martin

University of Dayton
Research Institute
Dayton, Ohio 45469

ABSTRACT

Results of the applications of local and global digital image enhancement techniques to ultrasonic C-scan images of damaged graphite/epoxy composites are presented. The original unenhanced images were generated by using focused ultrasonic transducers with center frequencies between 3.5 and 25 MHz. Small defects were often difficult to detect in the unenhanced images because the relatively small signal amplitude changes resulting from the defects were obscured by the larger signal amplitude changes caused by variations in: (1) surface roughness, (2) material attenuation, and (3) material morphology. Results given in this paper indicate that those enhancement techniques which emphasize the higher spatial frequencies at the expense of the lower spatial frequencies and those techniques which operate on local pixel regions can often remove enough of the undesirable variations to make small defects visible in the enhanced images.

INTRODUCTION

Conventional analog ultrasonic C-scan images such as are often generated in industrial NDE fail to display all of the information which has been acquired. There are at least two reasons for this. First, the display mode is often binary, and the breakpoint between the two levels must be set before the scan is made. Second, variations in material attenuation, thickness, surface roughness, etc., cause the edge information to occur at considerably different amplitudes. Thus, the entire edge definition information for a feature may fall entirely within one or the other of the two levels, resulting in invisible edges. Even in those cases where multi-level analog C-scans can be made there are still considerable drawbacks, since the threshold levels are set prior to scanning, and the number of levels is fixed.

Digitizing and storing the C-scan signals overcomes these problems because the number of grey levels and their threshold settings are selected after the scanning is completed. The image can be redisplayed as often as desired and with an almost unlimited number of different choices of grey level threshold values. With these capabilities, a far greater percentage of the total information content in the data can be displayed to the viewer than is the case for the non-digitized C-scan.

The advantages to the user do not end at this point. Once the data have been digitized and stored, many of the digital image enhancement techniques which have been so well developed in other disciplines[1,2,3] are available to those working in the field of ultrasonic NDE. In particular, noisy images can be linearly or nonlinearly smoothed[4], global histogram stretching (histogram equalization) can be used, and local histogram stretching techniques such as variable gain filtering[5-8] can be applied to improve the visibility of features which are suppressed by low spatial frequency variations in image intensity. Also, directional edge enhancement techniques[9-13] can be used to improve the visual definitions of feature outlines, and images can be added to or subtracted from each other to produce composite images which are better than either image taken by itself.

In this paper we will demonstrate how some of the more common digital image enhancement techniques can be applied to the ultrasonic NDE of graphite/epoxy composites to improve the visualization and spatial resolution of image features of interest. In particular, we will illustrate the use of histogram equalization, variable gain filtering, edge enhancing, image smoothing, and image summing techniques.

SCANNING SYSTEM

A high-precision, automated scanning system was developed for the acquisition, storage, enhancement, and display of ultrasonic images of up to 512 x 512 points in size. The system can perform both B-scans and C-scans. Control of the system is accomplished by an LSI-11/23 microcomputer operating under the RT-11 operating system through a high speed IEEE-488 DMA interface to a data acquisition module and a stepper motor controller.

The data acquisition module utilizes a 6809 microcomputer to control the operation of a 12-bit 40,000 sample-per-second digitizer and stores an entire C-scan line in a 42 KByte memory during collection. The transducer is in continuous movement and data are collected at operator selected points as the transducer moves. The 6809 microcomputer reads the transducer's position through an interface to linear optical encoders mounted on the scanning axes. Positional resolution is 0.0005 inch (0.0125 mm). When a line of data is collected it is transferred to the LSI-11/23 and stored on a 30 MByte Winchester disk.

The stepper motor controller receives commands from the LSI-11/23 and controls the position of the scanning system to a minimum step size of 0.001 inch (0.025 mm) during a scan. The image is displayed on a color video monitor and a hardcopy can be obtained by directing output to either an 8 color ink jet printer or to a grey-scale laser printer. Other equipment includes a pulser/receiver, a boxcar integrator used to detect and gate the signal to the digitizer, and an oscilloscope for simultaneous viewing of the RF waveform, detected signal and time gate position. A schematic diagram and additional information are available in prior publications[14-15].

DISPLAY CAPABILITIES

The video display system is capable of displaying from 1 to 16 colors or levels of grey-scale representing the signal amplitude. The image display software initially sets the breakpoint amplitude levels such that the entire amplitude range of the data is divided into 16 equally spaced intervals. This technique improves the contrast of the video image because all 16 colors will be displayed on each image regardless of the amplitude range of the actual scan data.

Other standard features allow the user to display the image in an equalized histogram format and to specify both the number of breakpoints and the threshold values of the breakpoints. A zoom feature is utilized to expand the size of selected parts of an image and multiple images may be displayed on the screen for comparisons. The grey-scale can be inverted and amplitude plots of selected video lines can also be displayed.

DIGITAL IMAGE ENHANCEMENT TECHNIQUES

With the exception of histogram equalization, all of the image enhancement techniques presented in this paper were implemented through the use of a moving 3 pixel by 3 pixel mask. The numbering system for the individual elements in the mask is illustrated in Fig. 1a.

Mean Value Filter

The simplest of the techniques is the mean value filter[6] in which the amplitude of the central pixel in the mask is replaced by the mean value of the amplitudes of the nine pixel elements within the mask. This type of filter is used mostly for noise removal in cases where the noise severely interferes with visual interpretation of image features. It is also used as a preprocessing step to remove low level noise in images which will be subjected to high frequency enhancements for improved edge detection and visualization. Unfortunately, while the mean value filter suppresses noise, it also blurs edges in the image, thus somewhat degrading the quality.

Variable Gain Filter[6,7,8]

The equation for the variable gain filter implemented in this paper is:

$$\hat{A}_1 = (KM_G/\sigma_L)(A_1 - M_L) + BM_L + C \tag{1}$$

where,

A_1 = original amplitude of pixel 1 in the 3 x 3 mask

$\hat{A}_1$ = amplitude of pixel 1 in the 3 x 3 mask of the transformed image

K = user chosen constant to control the filter gain

M_G = global mean amplitude for all pixels in the original image

M_L = local mean amplitude for the 9 pixels in the 3 x 3 mask in the original image

σ_L = local standard deviation of pixel amplitudes for the 9 pixels in the 3 x 3 mask in the original image

B = user supplied constant

C = user supplied constant

The gain factor, "KM_G/σ_L", in Eq. 1 is controlled on a local basis by "σ_L", since both "K" and "M_G" are constant for the entire image. In regions where the variation in pixel amplitudes within the local 3 x 3 mask is high, "σ_L" will be large, and the gain factor will be correspondingly small. In regions where the variation in pixel amplitudes within the mask is small, "σ_L" will be small, and the resulting gain will be large. The effect of this variable gain filtering is to amplify or enhance features in regions where the overall variation in amplitudes is small and to suppress (in a relative sense, at least) features in regions where the overall variation in pixel amplitudes is high. This technique is sometimes referred to as local area histogram equalization or stretching[8].

Fig. 1. Enhancement masks: (a) numbering system; (b) vertical edge enhancement; (c) horizontal edge enhancement; (d) sum of "b" and "c".

Vertical Edge Enhancement

There are a large number of directional edge enhancement techniques described in the literature[2,3,9-13]. Most of the techniques use an approximation to the first derivative in which the amplitude of the central pixel in the original image is replaced by the sum of first differences of pixel amplitudes within the mask. The mask[3] which is presented in this paper is given in Fig. 1b. In equation form the transformed pixel amplitude becomes:

$$\hat{A}_1 = A_4 - A_2 + 2(A_5 - A_9) + A_6 - A_8 \tag{2}$$

In Eq. 2 the "A's" are the amplitudes of the pixel elements represented by the subscripts. Thus, if the difference across the vertical region enclosed by the mask is large and positive, the value of the corresponding central pixel in the transformed image will be large and positive. If the difference is large and negative, the value of the corresponding central pixel in the transformed image is large and negative. Not only are vertical edges enhanced or sharpened, but they are also directionally "shaded", thus creating a three-dimensional effect.

Horizontal Edge Enhancement

As with vertical edge enhancements, this technique uses an approximation to the first derivative, but, in this case the derivative is taken across the horizontal direction in the image. The mask[3] used in this paper is given in Fig. 1c. In equation form the transformed pixel value is:

$$\hat{A}_1 = A_8 - A_2 + 2(A_7 - A_3) + A_6 - A_4 \tag{3}$$

Edges in the resultant image are both sharpened and shaded.

Sum of Vertical and Horizontal Edge Enhancements

Images which are both visually pleasing and very useful for feature identification can be created by adding the vertical edge enhanced image to the horizontal edge enhanced image. The resultant image has sharpened edges and directionally dependent shading which creates a three-dimensional effect. The mask for this transformation is given in Fig. 1d. The equation for the transformation is:

$$\hat{A}_1 = 2(A_6 - A_2) + 2(A_7 - A_9) + 2(A_5 - A_3) \tag{4}$$

It can be seen from the mask in Fig. 1d that this transformation is just an approximation to a first derivative across a 45 degree diagonal in the image.

464

Histogram Equalization

This technique[2] sets the grey level thresholds for image display such that each grey level has approximately the same number of pixel elements. In the conventional percent of range thresholding, the grey level thresholds are uniformly spaced across the range of amplitudes which occur in the image. Unfortunately, in many images most of the information content is contained in a relatively small portion of the total range of values. Thus, many of the edges which delineate features in images may not be visible because the amplitudes of the pixels on both sides of the edge are within the same grey level. Histogram equalization partially overcomes this problem by placing most of the grey level thresholds in regions of the image histogram where most of the pixel amplitudes occur. This greatly increases the probability that amplitudes of pixels on different sides of an edge will be placed in different grey levels, making the edge visible.

SAMPLES

Two samples, both with defects, were used for this study. The first sample is an 8 ply thick graphite/epoxy sample with a $[0_2/90_2]_s$ fiber orientation. The physical dimensions of this sample are 7 inches (177.8 mm) by 2 inches (50.8 mm) by 0.045 inch (1.14 mm). The dye enhanced x-ray radiograph of this sample (Fig. 2a) reveals that it has numerous matrix cracks in the vertical direction as well as delaminations of large extent between the 0 degree plies and the 90 degree plies.

The second sample is a 16 ply graphite/epoxy specimen with a $[90_4/0_4]_s$ fiber orientation. Its physical dimensions are 2.5 inches (63.5 mm) long by 1 inch (25.4 mm) wide by 0.1 inch (2.54 mm) thick. As is evident from the dye-enhanced x-ray radiograph in Fig. 2b, this sample contains matrix cracks in both the 90 degree plies and in the 0 degree plies.

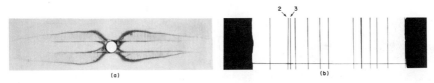

Fig. 2. X-ray radiographs: (a) delaminated sample; (b) cure crack sample.

DATA COLLECTION

All data were collected using ultrasonic immersion C-scanning techniques with focused transducers aligned so that the ultrasonic waves entered the sample along the normal to the sample surface. The transducers were focused on the back surfaces of the samples by maximizing the amplitudes of the echoes from the back surfaces of the samples. The RF echoes were amplified by a pre-amplification stage, and then further amplified, rectified and low-pass filtered (5MHz cutoff) with a MATEC Broadband Receiver. A sampling gate was centered over the rectified and filtered back surface echo and the averaged value of the signal in the gate was digitized and stored during scanning. The step sizes for scans on the 8 ply thick delaminated sample were 0.015 inch (0.381 mm) by 0.015 inch (0.381 mm). For the 16 ply thick sample with cure cracks, the step sizes for all scans were 0.005 inch (0.127 mm) by 0.005 inch (0.127 mm).

465

Low noise images were produced by using very low attenuation in the pre-amplifier stage and low gain in the Broadband Receiver stage. A high noise image was generated by using larger amounts of attenuation in the pre-amplifier stage which resulted in very low signal strength (and a much lower signal-to-noise ratio) at the Broadband Receiver stage. Subsequent amplification in the Broadband Receiver resulted in a noisy signal at the digitization stage and a correspondingly noisy image.

IMAGES

Delaminated Sample

Binary images of the delaminated 8 ply sample (corresponding to typical industrial C-scan images) are shown in Fig. 3. The data for these images were collected with a 25 MHZ, 1 inch (25.4 mm) focal length, 0.25 inch (6.35 mm) diameter transducer. The delamination and several of the matrix cracks are visible in the images. However, the matrix cracks are not visible in some parts of the sample due to high echo amplitudes in some regions and lower echo amplitudes in others. Since the crack information is super-imposed on the larger echo amplitude variations due to changes in attenu-ation, sample warping, etc., only some of the cracks can be displayed in this binary image. Changes in the threshold level bring out the matrix cracks in different regions of the sample as can be seen in Figs. 3a and 3b. A considerable improvement over the simple binary presentation is attained by making use of the 16 grey-level imaging capabilities of our system. Two 16 grey-level images using the same data as that for Figs. 3a and 3b are shown in Figs. 3c and 3d. Figure 3c is displayed in an equal percent of range thresholding format, while Fig. 3d is displayed in an equalized his-togram thresholding format. In the cases illustrated in Figs. 3c and 3d the delamination and matrix cracks are visible everywhere in the images. More detail is visible in the equalized histogram display format than is the case for the equal percent of range format. Despite the improvements in image quality, there are still light and dark areas in the image which partially obscure features of interest.

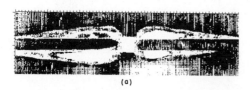
(a)

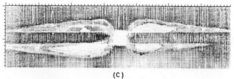
(c)

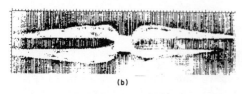
(b)

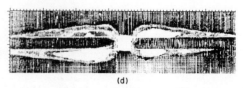
(d)

Fig. 3. Images of delaminated sample using 25 MHz transducer: (a) binary images with threshold at 30% of range; (b) binary image with threshold at 40% of range; (c) sixteen grey-level image with equal percent of range thresholding; (d) sixteen grey-level image with equalized histogram thresholding.

Since these areas represent very spatially slow changes in amplitude, a variable gain filter can be used to suppress the spatially slow variations while amplifying the local variations due to the matrix cracks. The results of applying the variable gain filter (with K = 0.1, B = 0.1, and C = 0.0) to the original data are presented in Fig. 4a. It is obvious that the spatially slow variations in intensity have been almost entirely suppressed, while the local matrix crack features have been emphasized. The image formed from the sum of the vertically and horizontally edge enhanced versions of the original image (Fig. 3) are shown in Fig. 4b. The delamination and matrix cracks are clearly visible everywhere in the image, and the directional "shading" has produced a three-dimensional effect in the image.

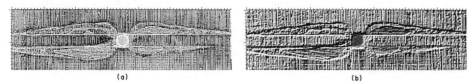

Fig. 4. Enhanced images of delaminated sample using 16 grey levels with equalized histogram thresholds: (a) variable gain filtering (K=0.1, B=0.1, C=0.0) of original images; (b) sum of vertically and horizontally edge enhanced versions of original image.

The corresponding lower ultrasonic frequency images for the delaminated sample are shown in Fig. 5. Data for these images were acquired with a 3.5 MHz, 2 inch (50.8 mm) focal length, 0.50 inch (12.7 mm) diameter transducer. Note that even in the equalized histogram version of the image (Fig. 5b), the details are blurred and suppressed due to both variations in material attenuation and to the larger spot size of the lower frequency transducer. Even with this blurring, the equalized histogram thresholding is clearly superior to the equal percent of range thresholding (Fig. 5a) for visualizing features in the image. The image formed by summing the vertically and horizontally edge enhanced versions of the original lower frequency image is shown in Fig. 5c.

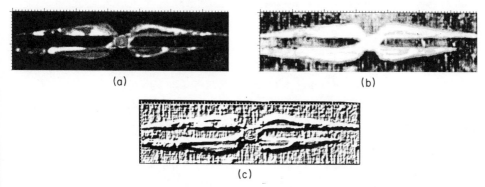

Fig. 5. Low frequency (3.5 MHz) images of delaminated sample: (a) sixteen grey levels with equal percent of range thresholding; (b) sixteen grey levels with equalized histogram thresholding; (c) sum of vertically and horizontally edge enhanced versions of the original data.

Cure Cracked Sample

A noise-free equalized histogram image of the sample with cure cracks is given in Fig. 6a. Data for this image were acquired with a 10 MHz, 3 inch (76.2 mm) focal length, 0.50 inch (12.7 mm) diameter transducer. The transducer was focused on the back surface of the sample and the gate was placed over the echo from the back surface. The two cracks labeled 2 and 3 in the X-ray radiograph of Fig. 2b can not be resolved using the "unenhanced" image produced from data taken with the 10 MHz transducer. However, these two cracks are visually resolvable in the image shown in Fig. 6b. This image was created by summing the vertically and horizontally edge enhanced versions of the original data as displayed in Fig. 6a. The image in Fig. 6b is displayed using equalized histogram thresholding.

Finally, we present the results of enhancing a "noisy" image. These data were acquired using the same transducer, focusing, and gating as that used to acquire the data for Fig. 6a. The noisy image is shown in Fig. 6c. The noise was reduced by two successive applications of the mean value filter to the original data. This technique suppressed the noise, but also blurred the image. Details of the cracks were brought out again by summing the vertically and horizontally edge enhanced versions of the noise suppressed data. Cracks 2 and 3 are now visually resolvable in the "enhanced" image of Fig. 6d.

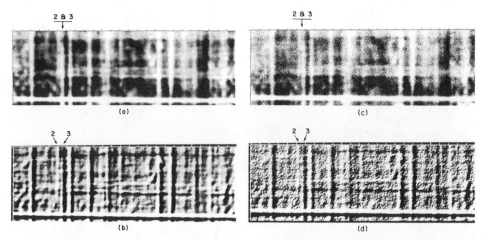

Fig. 6. Images of cure crack sample using 10 MHz transducer: (a) noiseless image; (b) sum of vertically and horizontally edge enhanced versions of noiseless image; (c) noisy image; (d) image created by smoothing the noisy data and then summing the vertically and horizontally edge enhanced versions of the smoothed data.

SUMMARY

In this paper we have demonstrated some of the advantages to be gained by applying digital image enhancement techniques to the ultrasonic NDE of graphite/epoxy composites. We have shown that the visualization of important features can be improved by using multiple grey levels rather than just two levels and by using global histogram modification techniques. Further improvements are often possible with variable gain filtering (local histogram modification) and by edge enhancement and image summing techniques which were also illustrated in this paper. As was discussed earlier, features which are unresolvable in the original image are resolvable in some of the enhanced images. Finally, we have shown that noise can be removed from image data, and that the data with the noise removed can be processed to produce an image with improved feature resolution.

ACKNOWLEDGMENTS

This research was sponsored by the AFWAL Materials Laboratory under contract Number F33615-83-C-5036. The authors acknowledge Dr. Thomas J. Moran and Mr. Robert J. Andrews for their support and encouragement in the area of image enhancements. The authors also thank Mr. Mark Ruddell for his data collection efforts.

REFERENCES

1. K. R. Castleman, "Digital Image Processing," Prentice-Hall Inc., Englewood Cliffs, New Jersey, (1979).
2. R. C. Gonzalez and P. Wintz, "Digital Image Processing," Addison-Wesley Publishing Company, Reading Massachusetts, (1977).
3. H. C. Andrews and B.R. Hunt, "Digital Image Restoration," Prentice-Hall Inc., Englewood Cliffs, New Jersey, (1977).
4. A. N. Venetsanopoulos and V. Cappellini, "Real-Time Image Processing," S. G. Tzafestas, Ed., Marcel Dekker, Inc., New York, NY, (1986).
5. V. T. Tom, Adaptive Filter Techniques for Digital Image Enhancement, SPIE, Digital Image Processing: Critical Review of Technology, Vol. 528, (1985).
6. J. Lee, Digital Image Enhancement and Noise Filtering by Use of Local Statistics, IEEE Transactions on Pattern Analysis and Machine Intelligence, Vol. PAMI-2, No. 2, (1980), pp. 165-168.
7. P. M. Narendra and R. C Fitch, Real-Time Adaptive Contrast Enhancement, IEEE Transactions on Pattern Analysis and Machine Intelligence, Vol. PAMI-3, No. 6, (1981), pp. 655-661.
8. D. J. Ketcham, Real-Time Image Enhancement Techniques, SPIE/OSA Image Processing, Vol. 74, (1976), pp. 120-125.
9. L. S. Davis, A Survey of Edge Detection Techniques, Computer Graphics and Image Processing, 4, (1975), pp. 248-270.
10. W. Frei and C. Chen, Fast Boundary Detection: A Generalization and a New Algorithm, IEEE Transactions on Computers, Vol. C-26, No. 10, (1977), pp. 988-998.
11. A. Rosenfeld and M. Thurston, Edge and Curve Detection for Visual Scene Analysis, IEEE Transactions on Computers, (May 1971), pp. 183-190.
12. J. E. Hall and J. D. Awtrey, Real-Time Image Enhancement Using 3 x 3 Pixel Neighborhood Operator Functions, Optical Engineering, Vol. 19, No. 3, (1980), pp. 421-424.
13. E. L. Hall, R. P. Kruger, S. J. Dwyer, D. L. Hall, R. W. McLaren and G. S. Lodwick, A Survey of Preprocessing and Feature Extraction Techniques for Radiographic Images, IEEE Transactions on Computers, Vol. C-20, No. 9, (1971), pp. 1032-1044.
14. T. J. Moran, R. L. Crane and R. J. Andrews, High Resolution Imaging of Microcracks in Composites, Materials Evaluation, Vol. 43, No. 5, (April 1985), pp. 536-540.
15. R. W. Martin and R. J. Andrews, Backscatter B-Scan Images of Defects in Composites, in: "Review of Progress in Quantitative Nondestructive Evaluation," Vol. 5, Plenum Press, New York, NY, (1986), pp. 1189-1198.

SOME PROBLEMS AND EXPERIMENTAL RESULTS

OF SEISMIC SHALLOW PROSPECTING

J.C. Tricot, B. Dellanoy, B. Piwakowski*, and P. Pernod

Laboratoire de Physique de Vibrations et d'Acoustique
(C.N.R.S. U.A. 832 Valenciennes)
Institut Industriel du Nord, B.P. 48

INTRODUCTION

In spite of the relatively small depth, the detection of underground empty spaces by means of seismic reflections methods creates a
problem not resolved fundamentally, up to now. The difficulties result
from the impossibility of the resolution of ground roll signals and the
refractions on the one hand, and the reflections from detected object, on
the other. The problems increase, when decreasing the depth of the object
(only depths of several meters make a limit at which the detection becomes
easier[1]). Few references show that, in spite of the universal principles
of the proceeding, the method and the way of detection must be carefully
chosen according to the geological conditions and the detected object
parameters.

The paper concerns the problems of the detection of the underground
empty spaces appearing in the north of France, which are the remains of
old chalk-pits, now unexploited. These spaces[2] form a network of
underground tunnels situated at depths of 8–12 m, and their positions are
partially unknown. To develop the method of mapping these underground
tunnels which represent a serious danger to building activities, is the
author's task. In the paper the system applied to the acquisition of
seismic signals, first measurements results and conclusions are presented.

INSTRUMENTATION

The schematic diagram of the instrumentation destined and applied
to shallow reflection surveys is shown in fig. 1.

Seismic pulses are generated by the shotgun charged with typical
hunting cartridges without the bullet. Such a source of limited power was
chosen with regard to available larger spectral characteristics, essential

---

* Permanent Affiliation : Institute of Telecommunication Technical
University of Gdansk, Poland.

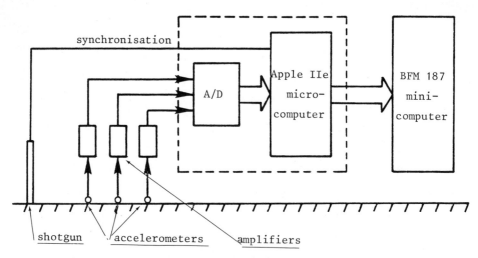

Fig. 1.   Functional block diagram of shallow reflection
acquisition and processing system.

for obtaining better survey resolution[3]. Seismic signals are detected by
3, B & K, type 4368 accelerometers and next amplified in B & K, type 2635
charge amplifiers. Choice of accelerometers results from their spectral
characteristic which have high-pass response of 6dB/octave with respect
to the response of velocity geophone, commonly used in seismic measurements.
Application of such low-cut filters emphasises the high frequency components
of signal and aims to improve the relation of the suspected high frequency
reflections to the low frequency ground roll disturbances[4]. The recording
system, made on the base of Apple IIe microcomputer, records simultaneously
the 3-Channel input signal via a 12-bit analog/digital converter (sampling
rate = 0.2 ms).

The solution as above is an approach to high resolution seismic reflection acquisition system. Its disadvantage is the relatively small
number of channels which involves the prolongation of time needed for
measurements, and insignificantly worsens the complex section record
quality due to source signal's repetitivity.

The recorded signals are then recopied in the laboratory on the BFM
187 microcomputer where they are processed. Processing possibilities contain static corrections, gain trace equalisation, filtering, deconvolution,
automatic gain control and graphic exposition.

GEOLOGICAL AND ACOUSTIC CONDITIONS

Typical geological structure of the area with appearance of underground tunnels, is as follows : the area is covered by a clay layer of

Table 1. Geophysical data obtained from borehole
measurements[5] in the region nearby of
experiments, and acoustic velocities
of the layers situated above the tunnels.

depth [m]	thick-ness [m]	type of layer		acoustic velocity [m.s^{-1}]	
				P	S
0					
2.3	2.3	clay		320	120
3	0,7	clay + chalk		560	200
		white chalk		1 250	440
	15	zone of tunnels			
18					
28	10	silicate chalk			
59	31	marl			

thickness 1-3 m, below which lies the chalk layer of thickness 25-31 m,
followed by the 30 m layer of marl. Between the chalk and clay occurs
the 70 cm mixed layer, which is the mixture of chalk and clay. In the
chalk two sublayers could be distinguished : white chalk of the thickness
~ 11-15 m and ~ 10 m silicate chalk. The tunnels occurs typically at depth
below surface of 8-12 m; their height is 1,5 - 3,5 m and width 2-4 m.

Geophysical section[5] which results in borehole measurement performed
nearby the place of the experiments is shown in table 1. In the same table
the acoustic velocities of the layers occuring above the tunnels are displayed. The velocities were obtained by means of classic measurements as
well as refraction methods.

FIELD MEASUREMENTS AND INTERPRETATION

The first records preceding those presented below were conducted in the
places positioned vertically over the known tunnel, and then in the areas
where there are none of it. The obtained data (not presented) showed the
impossibility of distinguishing any credible difference between the two
cases.

The following measurements were performed along the specially chosen
profile AA', the position of which is displayed in the Fig. 2. The selection of such conditions with the sharp tunnel boundary assure the possibility of comparing the seismic signals recorded over and apart from it,
in nearly the same geological conditions.

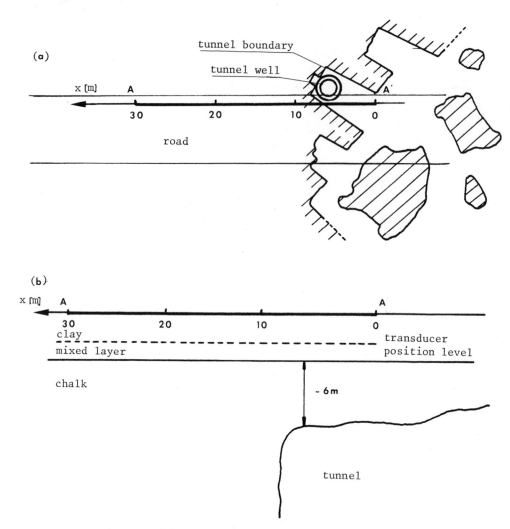

Fig. 2.   (a) Locality plan of chosen seismic
profile AA' with regard to the tunnel
position ; (b) geological cross section
of the profile.

Walkaway Test

      During the measurements, the transducers and the source were placed
at the beginning of mixed layer, in the specially prepared holes. Such a
solution aimed to improve the conditions of reflection detection by means
of avoiding the double passage of signals by a strongly attenuating clay
layer. To evaluate the general seismic properties the walkaway test[3] was
performed for two source positions : x=0 and x=26.6 m, with the trace
spacing of 0,33. The obtained seismic data, after static correction and
gain trace equalisation are presented in the Fig. 3. The first arrival
lines are the refractions : lines A and B corresponding to the velocities
of 1075 and 1250 ms-1 are the refractions on chalk. Line C, with the velocity 580 ms-1, must be refraction on mixed layer. Lines D are the air-
coupled wave arrivals.

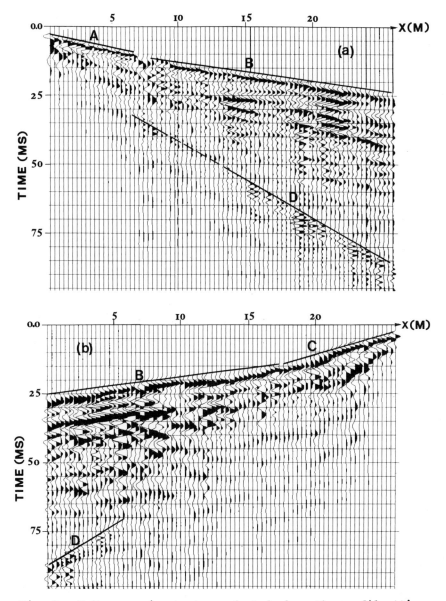

Fig. 3. Walkaway noise tests conducted along the profile AA'
(see Fig. 2), for two source positions. Trace spacing
is 0.33 m ; (a) source position x = 0 ; (b) x = 26.6 m.

475

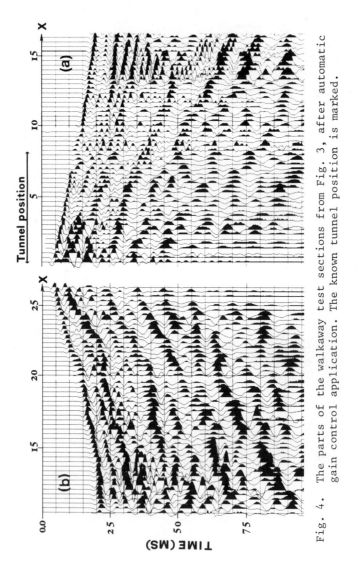

Fig. 4. The parts of the walkaway test sections from Fig. 3, after automatic gain control application. The known tunnel position is marked.

It is seen that to further analyse, gain control corrections must be applied. Because the time dependant amplitude of signals varies strongly as a function of offset, time-programmed gain correction is not useful. Therefore the automatic gain control was applied. The more interesting parts of the processed sections are presented in the Fig. 4. The comparison of these sections (corresponding to the different source positions, above and apart from the tunnel) should enable the common features to be found, which could be interpreted as seismic characteristic of the area, and the differences to be found which could be assumed as the tunnel presence indicates.To facilite the comparison, the sections are presented by the sides. Note that for the section Fig. 4 (b), the tunnel position is outside the drawing.

The line drawing interpretation of Fig. 4 is presented in Fig. 5. Except for the arrivals A, B, C, D mentioned before, the following signals assumed as recognized seismic events are displayed : multiple refraction B1, ground rolls E, E1, E2, E3 corresponding to the velocity of clay of 320 ms-1 (note the nearly same slope as of D line of 340 ms-1), several reflections G, H, I, J, K, the direct arrival in mixed layer M and primary surface reflection L. To evaluate correctly the time of suspected tunnel reflections, the run times between the tunnel vault and the vertically over placed transducer were measured, for the waves type P and S. The obtained average velocities were used to determine the hyperboles of suspected reflections type P-P, S-S and P-S, which are displayed in Fig. 5 in dotted lines.

The analysis of the figures 4 and 5 enables us to state that the following events can be assumed as the differences possibly proving the presence of the tunnel :

1. appearance of the event X1, replacing E2, which can be assumed as reflection P-S (but also as multiple refraction A),

2. absence of reflections G, H, I perhaps because of masking action of the tunnel,

3. presence of the event X2 which can be reflection S-S (as well as the part of ground-roll E),

4. relatively more complicated signal distribution in area of the circle X3.

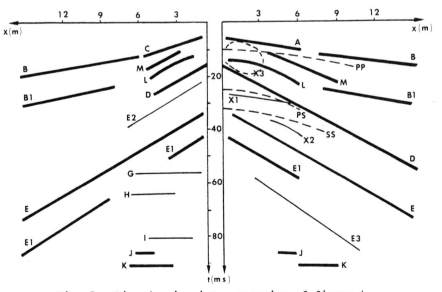

Fig. 5. Line drawing interpretation of figure 4

477

Possibility of tunnel reflections

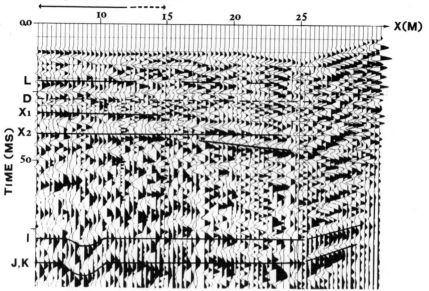

Fig. 6. The common offset section of the profile AA' with the
seismic events found – X1, X2, D, L, J, K (the last
part of the section is the common receiver gather).

Common offset survey

To verify the hypothesis 1, 2, 3, common offset measurements, with
the offset 6 m, were conducted. The last part of the section was continued
as common receiver gather, with the accelerometer at the constant position :
x = 26.6 m. The comparison of Figs. 4, 5 and 6 enables events X1, X2, D, L,
J, K, to be found. It is clearly visible that the events X2, J, K are not
the reflections but the ground rolls (note the slope of these lines in
common receiver gather area of the section). The absence of the regular
events G, H with regard to known position of the tunnel shows that these
signals are not linked to its presence. Meanwhile the appearance of the
signal X1 is well correlated with the tunnel position.

CONCLUSIONS

- the presented data analysis shows that the walkaway test performance is
  indispensable for interpretation of shallow seismic data,

- the P-P type tunnel reflections are relatively too small to distinguish
  them from the background of ground rolls,

- in the presented geological conditions ground roll signals appear as
  the numerous multiple modes. They should be filtered with 500 Hz cut-off
  high-pass filter. To take advantage of the dynamics characteristic of
  A/D converter[3], filtering should be applied before conversion,

- further research of P-P type reflections requires the additional mea-
  sures of air-coupled wave attenuation application.

478

- it can be supposed that the signal X1, assumed as P-S type reflection, can be used for tunnel detection. To confirm this, the additional common offset survey should be performed. The optimum[6] offset value should be 2-3 m,

- in the conditions of measurements presented, the reflections from the silicate chalk and from the marl were not observed. Therefore the masking action of the tunnel[7] is not confirmed as a way of its detection.

ACKNOWLEDGMENTS

The authors wish to express their great appreciation to Z. Kielczewski, who had participated in the first measurements sessions and had prepared the signal processing software, but left the laboratory before the application of his work.

We thank the employees of Bureau de Recherches Geologique et Minières and of Service d'Inspection des Carrières Souterraines of North Department of France for their help, advice and valuable discussions. We wish also to thank M. Quayle for the language corrections and F. Vyncke for her work in preparing the manuscript.

REFERENCES

1. J. Peragallo, Méthodes sismiques de subsurface : contribution à la détection des cavités souterraines, Thèse de doctorat, Université de Bordeaux I, 1976.

2. Y. Leplat, les cavités souterraines de la craie dans le nord de la France, Bull. Liaison Labo P. et Ch. 63, janv. - fév. 1983.

3. R.W. Knapp, Don. W. Steeples, High resolution common-depth - point reflection profiling : Field acquisition parameter design, Geophysics 51, 2, 1986.

4. R.W. Knapp, Don. W. Steeples, High resolution common-depth - point seismic reflection profiling : Instrumentation, Geophysics, 51, 2, 1986.

5. Data from the geological map, made by Bureau de Recherches Geologique et Minières, Borehole nr. 7.229.

6. Y.A. Hunter, S.E. Pullan, R.A. Burns, R.M. Gagne and R.L. Good, Shallow seismic reflection mapping of the overburden-bedrock interface with the engineering seismograph - some simple techniques, Geophysic-, 49, 8, 1984.

7. J.H. Cook, Seismic mapping of underground cavities using reflection amplitudes, Geophysics, XXX, 4, 1965.

A MODIFIED SUM FOCUSSING APPROACH TO ULTRASONIC

SPECKLE REDUCTION

Satpal Singh, S.N. Tandon and H.M. Gupta*

Centre for Biomedical Engineering,
Indian Institute of Technology Delhi-16, India

*Electrical Engineering Department,
Indian Institute of Technology Delhi-16, India

ABSTRACT

Ultrasonic speckle is inherrent in coherent imaging systems and is modelled as an interference. It occurs due to random inhomogeneties within the specimen under observation. This interference leads to a detection of randomly varying signal which manifests as a random variation of the gray level in the B scan. The resulting textural appearance in the image masks the details of specimen structure. The random variation due to speckle can be reduced by a factor of $1/\sqrt{N}$ by averaging N B-scans obtained by suitably displacing the transducer in space. Alternatively an N element array can be used to produce N images. However, the conventional use of an array for beam steering and focusing does not lead to a reduction in speckle. A technique is proposed which utilises sequential activation of the array elements. The signal received is first quadrature demodulated and multiplied by a depth dependent factor. The signals from all the elements are then delayed and summed. This technique leads to the reduction in speckle by a factor of $1/\sqrt{N}$ and yet maintains the high resolution.

INTRODUCTION

The B scan images of human tissues exhibit a granular texture[1,2]. This texture is different from the tissue structure and it limits the low contrast resolution in the image[3]. This degradation is termed as speckle and is modelled as an interference of the backscattered waves. The backscattering arises from a large number of acoustical inhomogeneties present within the specimen. The presence of speckle masks the details of the specimen and hence its reduction is desired. The various reduction methods reported, can be broadly classified as filtering or compounding techniques. The filtering methods employ a low pass filter to suppress the high frequency speckle noise[4]. However, this leads to a loss in the resolution. The compounding techniques work on the principle that when N images with uncorrelated speckle are averaged, there is a reduction in the speckle by a factor of $1/\sqrt{N}$. The compounding techniques operate either in the spatial domain[1,2,5,6] or in the frequency domain[6,7]. The reduction in speckle by frequency compounding has been reported in the range of 1.3 to 1.84[7] and by spatial compounding by a factor of 1 to 2[5]. It has been shown[1] that when a transducer is displaced by a distance equal to its width then the A mode speckle obtained in the two positions are uncorrelated. Therefore, if the echoes received individually by N elements of an array are averaged, there should be reduction in speckle by $1/\sqrt{N}$. However, the conventional use of a linear array[8,9] is primarily limited to beam steering and focussing and does not lead to speckle reduction. A modified focussing approach for speckle reduction is given below.

MODIFIED FOCUSSING

In the proposed scheme, the elements of a linear array are activated sequentially. Let the k th element in the array transmit a burst of ultrasound which impinges the specimen under observation. The received echo $g_k (t)$ can be written as,

$$g_k (t) = a_o . h (t - k.L - d_{k,o}) + \sum_{n\neq o} a_n . h(t-k.L-d_{k,n}) \quad (1)$$

Where L = time interval between the activation of successive elements of the array, h(t) = transmitted pulse, a_n = amplitude of backscattered wave from the n th random backscatterer, $d_{k,n}$= time delay for the echo to be received by the k th element from the n th scatterer. Let the backscatter for n=o be of interest, then the second term in Eq.(1) is the undesired interference. This is the time delayed summation with a random value and is used to explain the appearance speckle[10,11]. Let the signal received by the k th element be delayed by an amount τ_k given as,

$$\tau_k = d - k.L - d_{k,o} \quad (2)$$

Where d is some constant, then the delayed signal can be written from Eq(1) for a sinusoidal burst of excitation as,

$$g_k (t - \tau_k) = a_o . Cos (wt - wd) . U_T (t - d)$$
$$+ \sum_{n\neq o} a_n . Cos (w (t-d_{k,n}+d_{k,o}-d)) . U_T(t-d_{k,n}+d_{k,o}-d) \quad (3)$$

Where
$$U_T (t) = 1, o \leq t \leq T$$
$$= o \text{ otherwise} \quad (4)$$

The summation term on the R.H.S. of Eq (3) is a random variable[10,11] to which a mean m and a variance v can be assigned. The ratio of the desired signal (corresponding to the o th scatterer) to the square root of variance denotes the SNR and is,

$$SNR = a_o/\sqrt{v} \quad (5)$$

If the delayed echoes in Eq(3) are summed up for all elements k, then

$$g\,(t) = \sum_{k=1}^{N} g_k\,(t - \tau_k) \qquad\qquad (6a)$$

$$= N \cdot a_o \cdot \cos\,(wt-wd)\,\cdot\,U_T\,(t-d)$$

$$+ \sum_{k=1}^{N} f_k\,(t) \qquad\qquad (6b)$$

Where $f_k\,(t)$ represents the 2nd term in the R.H.S. of Eq(3). Since $f_k(t)$ is a random variable with variance v, then g(t) in Eq (6) is also a random variable but with variance N.v. The first term on the R.H.S. of Eq(6) shows that due to the suitable choice of delays τ_k (Eq.(2)), the echoes received at all array elements k from the o th scatterer, add up in phase. Thus the choice of τ_k according to Eq.(2), results in focus at the location of the o th scatterer. The SNR for g(t) in Eq.(6) can be written as,

$$SNR = \frac{N \cdot a_o}{\sqrt{N \cdot v}} = \frac{a_o}{\sqrt{v}/\sqrt{N}} \qquad\qquad (7)$$

Comparison of Eq.(5) and Eq.(7) reveals an improvement in SNR by a factor of $\sqrt{N}$, or a reduction in speckle by a factor of $1/\sqrt{N}$. This reduction has been possible because $f_k(t)$ in Eq(6) (or the summation term in Eq.(3)) is assumed to be uncorrelated for all values of k. This can be achieved if the inter-element spacing is at least equal to the width of an individual element[1].

The reduction for a sequential scanning and focussed system, described above, is not achievable in conventional array systems. In these systems, all the elements of the array are activated in overlapping time periods and as a result any point in the medium is insonified by more than one array element. The signal received by an element k in Eq.(1) is now modified as, as,

$$g_k\,(t) = \sum_{i=1}^{N} \sum_{n} a_n \cdot h\,(t-d_{n,i} - b_{n,k}) \qquad\qquad (8)$$

Where h(t) = transmitted pulse, $d_{n,i}$ = time required by the wave to travel from the transmitter element i to the n th scatterer, $b_{n,k}$ = time required for travel from n th scatterer to the kth element. The above equation denotes a random summation to which all elements of the array are associated. Due to this cross coupling between any two elements i and k of the array, there is only a single speckle pattern associated with the entire array. Therefore due to speckle, the degradation in the signal received by any element k will be highly correlated to that received by other elements of the array. Hence, the summation of delayed signals (Eq.6a) will not lead to speckle reduction in the conventional focussed array systems.

The scheme shown in Fig.1 requires additional hardware burden as in each channel there are large delays(k.L) and very small delays required for focussing.For the proper phase addition required for focussing (Eq.6), the delays should be precisely calculated according to Eq.(2). For a tapped delay line which introduces a quantization error Q, the focusing is degraded as the side lobes are found to increase[12,13]. For the side lobes to remain small, it is desired that the delay steps Q be much smaller than one time period of the RF sound. Therefore the task of designing a large delay, k.L, in Fig.2 with a very small fraction of error (Q/(k.L)) is difficult. To overcome this difficulty a processing scheme is suggested which does not require the fine focussing delays. This is achieved by a quadrature demodulation scheme which has same effect of introducing the delays τ_k in Eq.(2).

Let the array be focused at the position of n=o scatterer and for simplicity, it is assumed that there are no other scatterers. If the output of each channel k be mixed in quadrature with a local oscillator, then its low pass filtered outputs, as shown in Fig.2, can be derived from Eq.(1) for a sinusoidal burst as,

$$h = a_o . \text{Cos} (\theta_k) . U_T(t-d_{k,o}) \qquad (9a)$$

$$h_q = a_o . \text{Cos} (\pi/2 + \theta_k) . U_T (t-d_{k,o}) \qquad (9b)$$

Where $d_{k,o}$ is defined with respect to Eq.(1), the delay factor k.L has been dropped for simplicity and θ_k is,

$$\theta_k = w.d_{k,o} = 2\pi r_k/\lambda \qquad (10)$$

Where λ = wavelength of excitation and r_k = distance of the o th scatterer from the k th element. On multiplying the signals h and h_q with $\text{Cos} \emptyset_k$ and $\sin \emptyset_k$ respectively and summing, the output is,

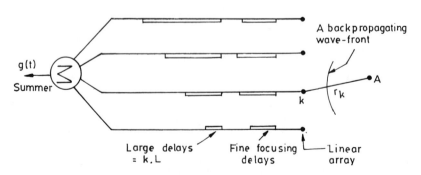

FIG.1. A modified focusing system with sequential activation of the array elements

$$g'_k (t) = h.\cos \emptyset_k + h_q . \sin \emptyset_k$$

$$= a_o. \cos (\Theta_k - \emptyset_k) . U_T(t - d_{k,o}) \tag{11}$$

If $\emptyset_k$ is made depth dependent and equal to Θ_k in Eq.(10), then the phase factor $\cos (\Theta_k - \emptyset_k)$ in Eq.(11) vanishes. Subjecting the signal in the k th channel to an envelope delay $\mathcal{T}'_k$,

$$\mathcal{T}'_k = d - d_{k,o} \tag{12}$$

Where d is some constant, and summing up the signals from all the channels, a focussed signal g'(t) is obtained as,

$$g'(t) = \sum_{k=1}^{N} a_o . U_T(t - d) \tag{13}$$

The above equation shows an inphase addition to generate a strong signal for the focal point at the location of o th scatterer. For an off-focal point, Θ_k will be different from the compensation $\emptyset_k$ and the summation in Eq.(13) will be out of phase leading to a loss of signal. Thus the desired inter-ference due to which focussing is achieved, is retained in the modified focussing approach.

CONCLUSIONS

A scanned focussing approach using a linear array has been suggested for reduction of ultrasonic speckle. This is a modi-fication of the conventional array systems. The scheme propo-sed, involves quadrature modulators followed by multiplication by depth dependent factors. This factor is chosen to nullify the phase shift effect due to propogation from the focal point. The proposed scheme does not require fine precision delays as required in conventional focussing using tapped delay lines. Therefore it can tolerate larger errors in the delay lines as the delays are required only for introducing delays in the envelope. The proposed technique needs to be validated by either experimental or computer simulation work.

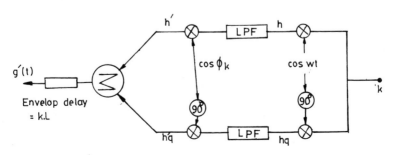

FIG 2 THE QUADRATURE DEMODULATION SCHEME

REFERENCES

1. C.B.Burckhardt, Speckle in Ultrasound B-mode scans, IEEE Trans. Son. Ult., Vol SU-25, No.1 : 1 (1978).

2. J.G. Abott and F.L. Thurstone, A-coustic Speckle: Theory and Experimental Analysis, Ultrasonic Imaging, 1; 303(1979)

3. S.W.Smith, R.F. Wagner, J.M. Sandrik and H. Lopez, Low contrast detectability and contrast/Detail analysis in Medical Ultrasound, IEEE Trans. Son. Ult., Vol.30, No. 3:164(1983).

4. D.L. Parker and T.A. Pryor, Analysis of B Scan speckle reduction by resolution limited filtering, Ultrasonic Imaging 4: 108 (1982).

5. D.P. Shattuck and O.T.V. Ramm, Compound scanning with a phased array, ultrasonic Imaging, 4 : 93(1982)

6. P.M. Shanker and V.L. Newhouse, Speckle reduction with improved resolution in ultrasound Images, IEEE Trans. Son. Ult., Vol. SU-32, No.4:(1985).

7. P.A. Magnin, O.T.V. Ramm and F.L. Thurstone, Frequency Compounding for speckle contrast reduction in phased array images, Ultrasonic Imaging, 4: 267 (1982).

8. A. Macovski, "Medical Imaging System," Prent. Hall Inc., Englewood Cliffs, New Jersey, 1983.

9. O.T.V. Ramm and S.W. Smith, Beam Steering with linear Arrays, IEEE Trans. Biomed. Engg., BME 30, No.8:438(1983)

10. S.W. Flax, G.H. Glover and N.J. Pelc, Textural Variations in B mode Ultrasonography : A stochastic Model, Ultrasonic Imaging, 3: 235 (1981).

11. D.R. Foster, M. Arditi, F.S. Foster, M.S. Patterson and J.W. Hundt, Computer simulations of speckle in B scan images, Ultrasonic Imaging, 5: 308 (1983)

12. W.L. Beaver, Phase error effects in phased Array Beam Steering, IEEE Ultrasonic Symp. Proc. 1977; 264 (1977).

13. P.A. Magnin, F.L. Thurstone and O.T.V. Ramm, Anomalous Quentization error lobes in phased array images, in "Acoustical Imaging", Vol.II, J.P. Powers, ed., Plenum Press, N.York, London: 491 (1982).

DEREVERBERATION TECHNIQUES

Juval Mantel

Dr. Mantel & Partners GmbH
Inninger Str. 7a
8000 Muenchen 70, West Germany

Several methods for dereverberation were applied in the past. Two application methods should be represented here.

1. Discrete Dereverberation

Loudspeaksers usually transmit sound from the membrane and due to the reverberation of the loudspeaker itself /2/. There is a reverberation of air-borne sound in the enclosure and dereverberation time due to the body-borne sound of the housing itself.

Whenever one needs a short acoustic burst with sharp shut-off, one has to dereverberate the sound of the loud-speaker. The dereverberation can be done for example by transmitting a short time later (b) after the original transmitted burst another damped burst. Such weak new bursts with alternating polarity might be necessary so that the series of compensating bursts should compensate for the reverberation according to formula 1:

$$
\begin{aligned}
F_1 &= F_0 + aF_0(t-b)\ (-1) \\
F_2 &= F_1 + a^2F_0(t-2b)(+1) \\
F_3 &= F_2 + a^3F_0(t-3b)(-1)
\end{aligned}
\qquad (1)
$$

$$
\vdots \qquad \vdots
$$

$$
F_n = F_{(n-1)} + a^n F_0(t-n\cdot b)(-1)^n
$$

The above form of dereverberation can be done for every discrete echo, whenever the amplitude of the reflected sound and its time delay are known.

It had been shown /1/ (see figure 1) that the periodical transmitting of such signals enables to compress the duration of such bursts and square waves can be transmitted.

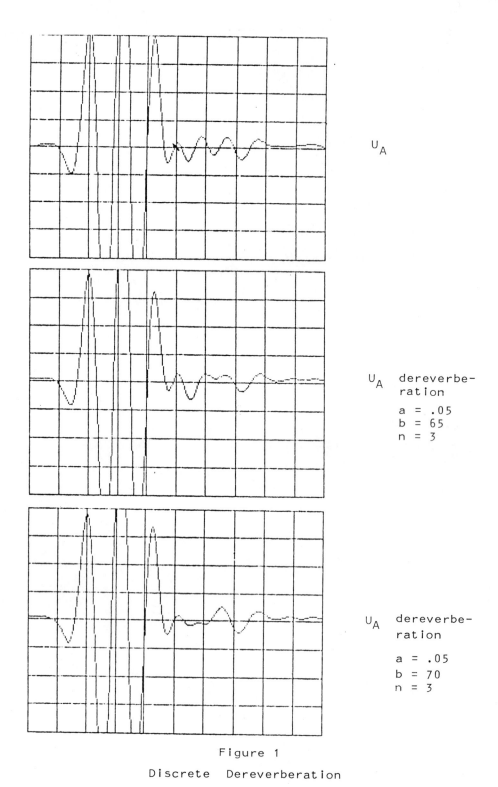

U_A

U_A dereverbe-
ration

a = .05
b = 65
n = 3

U_A dereverbe-
ration

a = .05
b = 70
n = 3

Figure 1

Discrete   Dereverberation

2. General Dereverberation

The purpose of dereverberation which had been shown over-
leaf can be generalized without knowledge of time – delay and
strength of reflexion of sounds. This can be done due to the
fact that a flutter echo shows in the time domain periodicity which in a fourier transformation represents a line
spectrum.

For the purpose of transmitting a clean acoustical burst,
one can use a programmable generator in which the signal
which will be transmitted had to be corregated, according to
formula 2:

$$U_{EK} = \frac{U_{E0}^2}{U_{A0}} \qquad (2)$$

In this formula U_{EK} is the corregated output voltage of the
generator, which feeds to an amplifier and the loudspeaker.
E0 is the initial signal, which is a result of the multiplication of a Gauss-pulse and a carrier frequency. U_{A0} is the
acoustically transmitted signal of U_{E0}.

This form of dereverberation according to formula 2 is
also a compensation for the time limitation of the signal.
The transmissibility H is:

$$H = \frac{U_{A0}}{U_{E0}} \qquad (3)$$

So is:

$$U_{EK} = \frac{U_{E0}}{H} \qquad (4)$$

It is obvious that with the aid of the general reverberation better time compressed pulses can be realized. The
criterium we used for quantifying this is

$$Q = \frac{U_{MAX} \ (t > t_p)}{U_{MAX} \ (t < t_p)} \qquad (5)$$

The advantage of the discrete dereverberation can be combined with those of the general dereverberation, as can be
seen in figure 3.

In the upper part one can see the acoustical signal in
the time domain with general dereverberation but without
the discrete dereverberation. In the lower part of this
picture there is shown the combination of both dereverberation methods. In this case the general dereverberation had
been carried out first, the discrete dereverberation afterwards /3/. In time compressing of signals and in measurements these techniques can be applied.

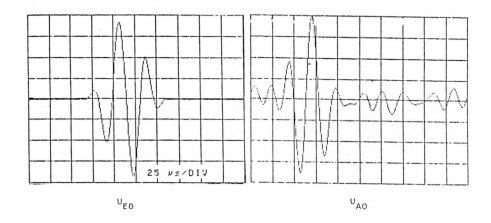

U_{EO} U_{AO}

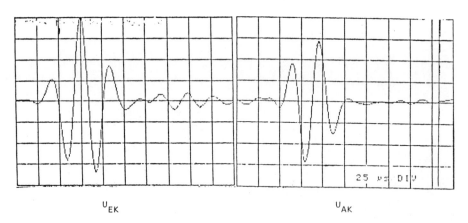

U_{EK} U_{AK}

Figure 2

General   Dereverberation

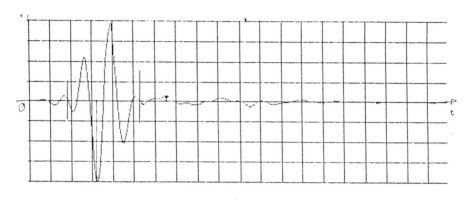

25 μs/DIV

Without discrete dereverberation

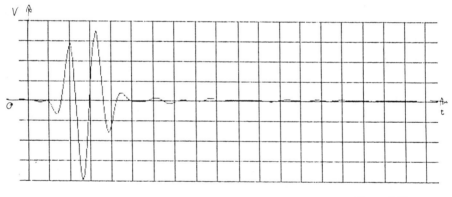

25 μs/DIV

With discrete dereverberation

Figure 3

REFERENCES

/1/ Mantel, J. (1986): "Studienvertrag T/R 325/E0017/E2313"
      report No. 84130/III of Messrs. Dr. Mantel & Part-
      ners GmbH, Munich, of 1986 January 30

/2/ Mantel, J. (1982): "Nachhallzeiten von Lautsprechern,
      ein Effekt und dessen Veränderung (Dereverberation
      times of loudspeakers, an effect and its change)"
      Hörrundfunk, Mannheim, 1982 November 23-25

/3/ Mantel, J. (1986): "Enthallungstechniken für Lautspre-
      cherimpulse (Dereverberation techniques for loud-
      speaker pulses)"
      DAGA '86, Oldenburg, 1986 March 11-13

POLARITY-SENSITIVE DETECTION OF PULSED ULTRASOUND SIGNALS

Ron J. Geluk and Marcel R. de la Fonteijne

OLDELFT Research Laboratory

P.O. Box 72, 2600 MD
Delft, The Netherlands

1   INTRODUCTION

The signal-processing methods to be described, permit the extraction of more information from the H.F.-echo signal than the traditionally used envelope detector does. The latter detector ignores for instance the polarity of the reflection, which is obviously a part of the information as polarity represents the "most significant bit" of a signal. [1]

Several methods have been suggested to preserve more of the information contained in the high frequency (receiver) signal. Such methods are:
- a complex fourier-transform of the H.F.-signal to generate both amplitude and phase spectra.[2]
- determination of the central frequency of HF-pulses based on measurement of the time-intervals between the zero crossings of the H.F.-signal.[3]
- determination of the frequency-dependancy of the attenuation-coefficient of tissue.[4,5]
- mixing of the H.F.-signal with two reference signals with 90° phase shift. The two quadrature output signals provide information on particle velocities. [6,7]

All these methods have draw-backs of either a fundamental or a practical nature.

The fourier-transform, for instance, requires some kind of time-gating in order to separate the spectra of individual pulses.
In addition, with presently available hardware, the operation requires too much time to be executed in real time.
The measurement of the signal zero-crossings does give a value of the average frequency and its change with depth but the phase information on individual echo-pulses remains unknown.
The mixing-method with quadrature signals generates essentially velocity information and provides no extra signal on stationary objects.
The detection methods to be described here, permit instantaneous detection of H.F. echo pulses, while preserving the polarity of the reflection. Moreover, one of the methods to be described provides quantative values of the phase of individual H.F. impulse signals.

Once the phase angles of pulses are available, different ways of displaying the extra information is imaginable. Such further elaborations, however, are beyond the scope of this article.

2   A PRIORI FILTERING

An ultrasound imager with an ideal transducer, (meant is a flat amplitude and phase response), would not require a signal rectifier or "detector" at all, as every reflection could be displayed as a "δ-impulse", the polarity of which represents the type of each reflection. Unfortunately practical transducers have a limited bandwidth centered around the central frequency. Consequently, echo-impulses from even an ideal reflector have an oscillating shape which lasts over several periods. What comes to mind first, as a counter measure against such an oscillating pulse shape is the excitation of the transducer with an electrical signal such, that after reflection, a δ-pulse is the approximate result.

Fig. 1. Shows how such an inverse filtering can be realized in practice. Firstly an echo impulse (f) is measured and digitized.
From this measured signal the inverse function (g) is (approximately) calculated according to[8]:

$$\widetilde{F}(g) = \frac{1}{\widetilde{F}(f)} \tag{1}$$

Where: $\widetilde{F}$ denotes Fourier transformation.

This excitation function g is loaded into an arbitrary waveform generator which is connected to the transducer. As a result "δ-impulses" are received. (fig. 2)
    This pre-filtering technique looks very effective, as the received pulse-shape could be displayed directly, giving a good indication of signal-polarity (which is the polarity of the reflection). However, such stringent filtering reduces the maximum signal level drastically, as the transducer is forced to operate mainly at frequencies where its efficiency is very low, and consequently the depth-range of a practical scanner would be reduced. Moreover, the D.C.-content of the reflection will not be restored.
    We must conclude that prefiltering provides any pulse shape we desire, but strong amplitude filtering has to be avoided, if we want to maintain practical signal levels.

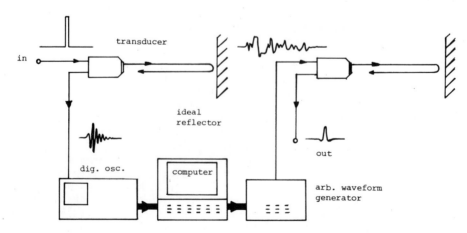

Fig. 1. Configuration for a-priori filtering.

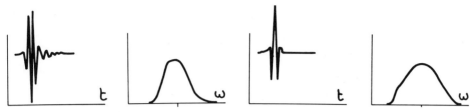

Fig. 2. Impulse shape and spectrum for a 10 MHz echo signal without
filtering (left) and prefiltered (right).

3   DETECTION BY INVOLUTION

The prefiltering technique alone is clearly not sufficient to
produce polarity-preserving detection. However, a moderate amplitude
filtering and stringent phase filtering can be applied to obtain, for
instance, symmetrical H.F.-pulses with a relative spectral bandwidth
between 0.4 and 0.6. Although, in such signals no D.C.-component is
available, we can try to exploit the difference between positive and
negative peak values of such symmetrical signals.

It will be clear that, presuming a flat phase spectrum, the
difference between the positive and the negative peak value increases
with the relative bandwidth of the signal.

To this end we distort the H.F.-signal in such a way that higher
peak values are amplified with a larger value than smaller peak values.
The effect of this distortion must be equally effective over the full
dynamic range of the H.F.-signal. In addition, this operation must be
identical for positive and negative signal values. Involution of
signals can meet these conditions, if we preserve the polarity of the
signal. Here we will limit ourselves to involution to the power of two.
Negative signal values are reversed in polarity, after squaring and in
this way the polarity of the H.F.-signal is maintained.

Fig. 3 shows the calculated effect of "polarity preserving
squaring" on a H.F.-pulse with a relative bandwidth (RBW) of 0.7.

The DC-component as introduced is small as compared to the peak
signal value at the central frequency, and insignificantly small at a
realistic RBW of 0.4.

From fig. 4 we conclude, that for a reasonable DC-contribution, an
RBW larger than 0.4 is required.

Another aspect of the described method is the quadratic
relationship of the output signal amplitude and the original signal.

Fig. 5 shows a "non-linear processor" which has a linear
relationship between input- and output-signal amplitudes and yet uses
the involution technique to introduce a DC-component.
Note that the filtering is done before the square root operation is
introduced.

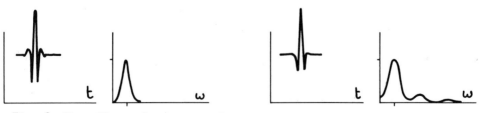

Fig. 3. The effect of squaring of a symmetrical H.F.-impulse with a RBW
of 0.7 and Gaussian envelope. (right = squared)

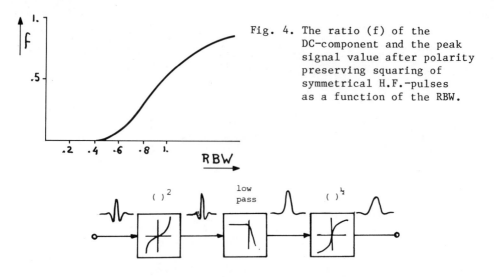

Fig. 4. The ratio (f) of the
DC-component and the peak
signal value after polarity
preserving squaring of
symmetrical H.F.-pulses
as a function of the RBW.

Fig. 5. non-linear filter operation using polarity-preserving squaring
of a H.F.-pulse with a RBW of 1.

4   DETECTION BY DIVISION

The method of § 3 looks useful if the echo pulse has a relative
bandwidth larger than 0.5, but even then the obtained DC-component is
relatively small. A better detection method will now be explained with
the help of fig. 6.
We start with an anti-symmetrical echo pulse with Gaussian envelope.
Prior to any nonlinear processing, the echo signal is delayed over a
half period and added to the input signal.
Over a half period in the centre of the H.F.-pulse almost zero response
is introduced. This signal is now rectified. If we divide the original
echo by signal "N", a half period is selectively amplified. The delay
determines which "half period".
We can even execute this operation for a number of half periods
simultaneously by operating more dividers in parallel.

This detection process, by division, produces an output signal, of
which the amplitude is independent of the input amplitude.
If we want a linear relationship, a "quadratic" circuit according to
the one described in the previous paragraph can be connected in the
denominator signal circuit.

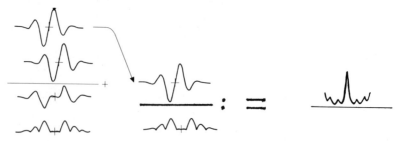

Fig. 6. Nonlinear filter operation using signal division.
Note, that the detected impulse is as short as only half a period,
independent of the length of the original H.F.-pulse.

496

5   DETECTION BY MULTIPLICATION

The detection by division gives an excellent response. However, for
H.F.-pulses with a longer response time (more oscillations in one
pulse), it requires more divider circuits operating simultaneously, if
we want to extract signal from the whole length of the H.F.-signal.

Fig. 7 explains an other detection method, which is effective for
longer echo pulses. Again an anti-symmetrical pulse with a gaussian
envelope is presumed.

Like in the previous §, the input signal is delayed over a half
period and added to itself, which results in a pulse with a half period
of practically zero response.

After rectification, this signal is again delayed over half a
period and now subtracted from the signal before delay. The resulting
reference signal oscillates over two full periods, and does not change
with the polarity of the input pulse. Finally, detection is done by
multiplication of this reference signal with the input signal.
(Here the output amplitude is the square of the input amplitude)

For other pulse shapes, the amplitude ratio of the first addition
has to be adjusted to obtain signal cancellation over a half period.

For odd (anti-symmetric) shapes this ratio is always 1,
independent of the relative bandwidth of the signal spectrum. For even
functions this ratio depends on the RBW, and approximates 1 as the RBW
decreases.

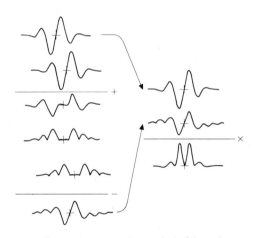

Fig. 7. Detection by multiplication.

6   PHASE MEASUREMENT

As stated in §5, the detection method by multiplication can be
adjusted to even or odd pulse-shapes. (0° resp. 90° phase angle)

Other pulse shapes (with the same envelope), can be regarded
as a linear combination of an odd and an even pulse.

Let us now have two detectors according to fig. 7, of which one is
tuned for maximum output for even functions and the other for maximum
output for odd functions.

Then we define the phase of the input pulse as the ratio of
output voltages of the two detectors according to:

$$tg\,\varphi = \frac{\text{output even detector}}{\text{output odd detector}} \qquad (2)$$

Equation 2 was tested with a computer simulation as follows:

An input signal "h" was used according to:

$$h = f(t)\cos\theta + f_{Hi}(t)\sin\theta \qquad (3)$$

where f is an even function and f_{Hi} is the Hilbert transform of f.

In this special case $\varphi = \theta$ is constant for all frequencies and can be regarded as a real angle.
The calculated DC-component of the output of the even detector as a function of the phase angle φ of function h was calculated.
    The shape was compared with a true sine-function, and no deviation larger than 1 % was found. A similar result was found for the odd detector.
From this we conclude, that it is correct to measure the phase angle of pulse signals according to eq. 2.

7   NOISE

    In order to get an idea of the behaviour of the detector with noise, we simulated additive white noise on odd functions.
We define the signal to noise ratio S/N as:

$$S/N = \frac{S}{\sigma} \qquad (4)$$

Where S is the peak value of the H.F.-pulse and σ the standard

deviation of the noise on the signal.
The result depends on both the RBW and the S-to-N ratio of the input signal (Fig. 8.).
We conclude, that for a practical RBW = 0.4 the S to N ratio decreases about 10 dB due to the phase-sensitive detection process.

    To understand this loss of S/N ratio, we must take into consideration the first signal addition in the detector according to fig. 7.
    Essentially, we convolve with two δ-pulses with a half period delay. The spectrum of this convolution has a dip at the centre-frequency of the H.F.-signal and consequently the remaining spectrum has a reduced S-to-N ratio, of which the effect is transmitted through the further stages of the detector. (fig.9)
    It will be clear, that the influence of this spectral weighing becomes worse as the RBW of the H.F.-signal decreases.

498

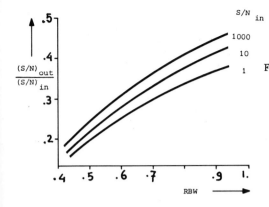

Fig. 8. Reduction factor of S/N for
detection by multiplication
as a function of the
relative bandwidth.
Parameter: S/N of input
signal.

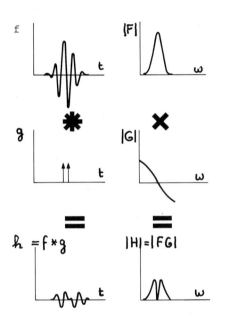

Fig. 9. The effect of addition and
a time delay over half a
period. The dip in the
frequency spectrum causes
the reduction of S/N-ratio.

8   EXPERIMENTS

The detector of fig. 7 was built and tested with continuous
signals in real time.
Fig. 11 shows the response on computer generated pulses that were
generated by an arbitrary waveform generator at a centre-frequency of
10 MHz. The phase angle increases with steps of 45°.
To show the DC-component as a function of the input phase, the
signal was integrated after detection.
Next, echo pulses from a mechanical sector scanner were supplied
to the detector. The central frequency was again 10 MHz, but the pulse
shape was kept unfiltered.
We see, that the detector is also effective on unfiltered
echo-signals (fig. 11 a).
The detected signal was also integrated and used to control
the intensity of a brightness display (fig. 11 b).
Clearly, we can now image homogeneous materials rather than just
the transients.

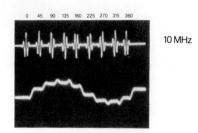

10 MHz

Fig. 10. Response on phase of the detector according to fig. 7 after detection and integration

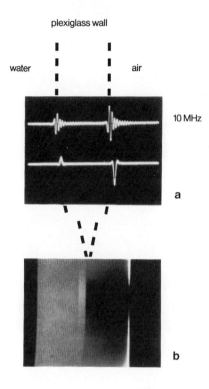

plexiglass wall

water   air

10 MHz

a

b

Fig. 11. (a) Response on unfiltered echo-signals from plexiglass wall of watertank
(b) brightness display of 11 a after integration

9   CONCLUSION

Three real time detection-methods have been described that preserve the polarity information of ultrasound echo pulses.
All methods are based on some kind of "time selective amplification" of the H.F.-signal, with a signal derived from the same H.F.-signal. Consequently, the polarity and/or phase signal is a function of the pulse-shape only, rather than the time of flight.
Detection by involution requires H.F.-pulses with a very wide spectrum, which in turn requires heavy pre-filtering. Pre-filtering, however, causes loss of signal level and should be applied with care.
Detection by division produces very short responses, but requires considerable instrumentation, if we want to exploit all information contained in the signal.
Detection by multiplication produces reasonably good responses on practical echo pulses with a moderate amount of instrumentation. The method is suitable for continuous phase detection on pulses with a relative bandwidth of 0.4. The detector has also been demonstrated on a mechanical sector scanner. No pre-filtering was required and short response-pulses were obtained.

10 ACKNOWLEDGEMENT

The following students contributed significantly to the computer simulation and performance testing of the proposed methods: Marcel Struis, Albert J. Everts, Maurice R.J. Faatz and Alex J. Schooneveld.

11 REFERENCES

1 Miyashita T., Schwettick H. and Kessel W.: "Recovery of ultrasonic impulse response by spectral extrapolation". Acoustical Imaging 14 p. 247; (1985)
2 Hottier F. and Bernatets J.L.: "Estimation of ultrasonic attenuation in biological tissues". Acta Electronica 26 p 33-58; (1985)
3 Seggie D.A. et al.: "Ultrasonic imaging using the instantaneous frequency of pulse-echo signals". Acoustical Imaging Vol 14 p. 487; (1985)
4 Cloosterman M.J. Verhoef W.A. and thijssen J.M.: "Generalized description and tracking estimation of the frequency dependent attenuation of ultrasound in biological tissues", Ultrasonic Imaging 7 p. 133-141 (1985).
5 Gehlback S.M., Sommer F.G. and Stern R.A.: "Scatter induced frequency variations in reflected acoustic pulses: implications for tissue characterization". Ultrasonic imaging 7. p. 172-178 (1985)
6 Matsumoto Kenzo: European Patent application 0139242
7 Rader Charles M.: "A simple Method for sampling In-phase and Quadrature Components". IEEE transactions on Aerospace and electronic systems. Vol. AES-20 No. 6 November 1985
8 Kim J.H. Etal: "Prior Inverse filtering for the improvement of axial resolution". Ultrasonic Imaging 7. p. 179-190 (1985)

ULTRASONIC DEFECT VISUALIZATION IN A METAL BLOCK

D.K. Mak, M. Macecek* and A. Kovacs*

CANMET Physical Metallurgy Research Laboratories
Ottawa, Ontario K1A 0G1

*Techno Scientific Inc.
205 Champagne Dr. #1
Downsview, Ontario M3J 2C6

ABSTRACT

A technique has been developed to produce a three-dimensional image
of internal defects in a metal block. In the experiment, a rectangular
block (approximately 9cm X 7cm X 7cm) with a hole drilled through it
diagonally was inspected. The block was scanned with narrow beam,
focused transducers and the time of flight (TOF) to the defect was
measured.

The initial transducer position and scanning parameters were taken as
input, and the TOF data were processed. The software used the position
and orientation of the transducer to determine which surfaces of the
block had been penetrated by the beam. The program assumed that the
scanned block was rectangular. Knowing the surface of penetration
allowed the angle of incidence to be found, and Snell's Law was used to
calculate the angle of refraction. If the flaw was located inside the
block it was stored in a data file, otherwise it was considered to be
noise and was eliminated.

The shape of the defect was mathematically reconstructed from the
data file of the defect points and displayed on a 3-D colour graphics
system.

INTRODUCTION

There are a number of techniques for the ultrasonic imaging of
internal defects. The majority are very complex and require extensive
hardware and software to produce an image of the defect (for example:
acoustical holography (1), synthetic aperture imaging system (2,3), and
computerized ultrasonic tomography (4)). Most imaging methods do not take
into account refraction at the surface inspected, as a normal beam is
generally assumed. We describe a method where an angled beam was used,
and a refracted ray in three dimensional space was tested. Only TOF data
and transfer position and orientation are required to reconstruct the
image of the defect. Objects to be imaged usually have regular external
boundaries, e.g. cube, prism. If the surface through which the ultrasonic
beam enters is known, the refracted ray can be determined and path of the
beam within the body established.

503

Snell's Law defines the relationship between the sine of the angles of incidence and refraction, and the acoustical velocity in both media. It is expressed mathematically as (5):

$$SIN (\theta) / V1 = SIN (\phi) / V2 \qquad [1]$$

where θ is the angle of incidence in material 1, ϕ is the angle of refraction in material 2, and V1 and V2 are the respective velocities in the two materials.

Equation [1] holds true only if $SIN(\theta) * V2 / V1 \leq 1$.

Software developed for this experiment processes a file of amplitude time of flight ultrasonic data and generates a new file of data points in the Cartesian coordinate system.

The software assumes that the object being scanned is a rectangular block, with edges running parallel with those of the scanning tank.

METHOD

An aluminum block, 9cm X 7 cm X 7cm with a 1.2 cm hole drilled through its diagonal was manufactured (Figure 1). The outside surface was polished until smooth while the inside (the surface of the hole) was left rough.

Selection of Transducers

Five focused transducers were tested for their sensitivity in detecting the defect. The frequencies of the tested transducers were 1 MHz, 3.75 MHz, 5 MHz, 7.5 MHz and 10 MHz.

The 1 MHz transducer was unable to detect the defect while the signal from the hole was barely visible with the 3.75 MHz transducer. The 5 MHz transducer was more sensitive and the signal was slightly above the noise level. The 10 MHz yielded the best result with a signal to noise ratio of four to one and was used for all scans. The peak amplitude of the 10 MHz transducer's radio frequency waveform from the flaw was 0.48 Volts after a 40 dB gain. After the signal was passed through the video amplifier, the amplitude was lowered to 0.03 V.

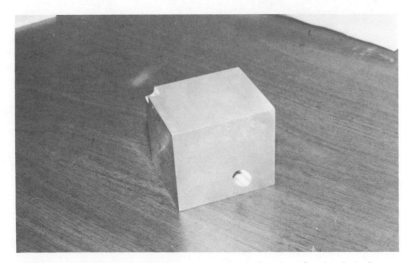

Fig. 1. Aluminum rectangular block with a diagonal hole

The 10 MHz transducer had the smallest beam spread: 4° in water. Although divergence was small in water, the beam spread was greatly increased in aluminum due to refraction.

Calculations show that with an incident angle of 12° the beam would be refracted to 60.6° inside the test block. With a 4° beam spread the angle of incidence would vary from 8° to 16°. An incident angle of 8° would refract to 35.7°. A 16° incident angle is beyond the critical point for a water-aluminum boundary. The 10 MHz was the least divergent and the 1 MHz the most (15°).

Testing was performed in a conventional immersion tank with a scanning transducer mast. The system had resolution and repeatability of better than .001". The slave computer controlled the motion in the scanning tank while the master computer handled the data acquisition, processing and display (Figures 2a and 2b). The heart of the system was an A/D board sampling data at 40 to 160 MHz with eight bit resolution. The signal from the transducer was amplified by 40 dB and then run through a video filter. The video filter lowered the background noise level to 25% of the defect signal. The computer digitized each A-Scan in real time to extract the amplitude and the time of flight data from the signal. The data was stored in the master computer's hard disk for further processing.

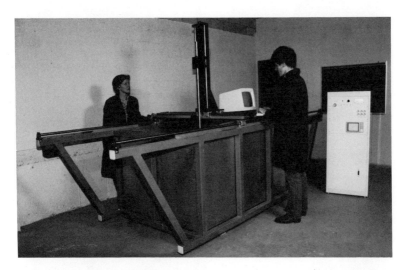

Fig. 2a. Overall view of the immersion scanning system

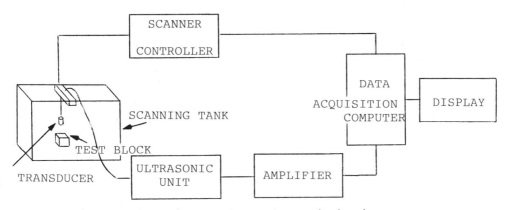

Fig. 2b. Block diagram of the ultrasonic imaging system.

The block was first scanned using a conventional C-Scan (Figure 3) to determine which transducer was best, as well as the angle of inspection. It was found that an angle of 12° yielded the best results. The first critical angle was approximately 14°. A video filter was added to the system to reduce the noise (Figure 4).

For the experiment the block was scanned in a 30 x 30 point matrix. The program SNELL.FTN was used to translate amplitude and time of flight data to the Cartesian coordinate system. The program required the user to input the initial conditions of the scan, and data points were analyzed. The program found the beam path for each data point and determined which, if any of the block's surfaces might have been penetrated. The angle of incidence was determined and Snell's Law taken into account at the surface of penetration to determine the angle of refraction. From the angle of refraction and the TOF, the location of the defect was calculated. If the location of the defect was inside the cube then the data point was stored, otherwise it was rejected.

The Cartesian data file generated above was displayed using three-dimensional imaging software.

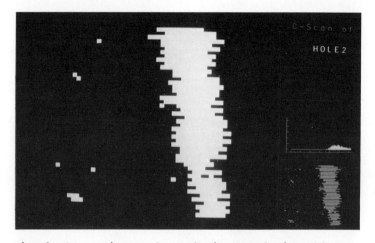

Fig. 3. C-scan image of a hole in the aluminum block.

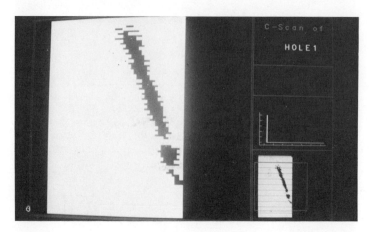

Fig. 4. C-scan image of the aluminum cube with video
filtering applied.

Software: SNELL.FTN

The software's analysis of the amplitude time of flight data can be divided into 10 steps.

1) A sample from the Amplitude-TOF data file is read.
2) The position and orientation of the transducer at the time of sampling is calculated.
3) The program determines which of the block's walls could not have been penetrated by the beam from the transducer's position.
4) The program further determines which of the walls could not have been penetrated from the transducer's orientation.
5) The time required for an ultrasonic beam to travel from the transducer to the planes of each of the remaining walls is calculated. If the calculated time is greater than the recorded time of flight for the data point, the wall is eliminated.
6) The point of intersection of the plane of the wall with the beam is found. If it is found to be part of the surface of the block, the wall of penetration has been found, otherwise the wall is eliminated.
7) If no wall of penetration is found the program returns to step one to analyze the next point; otherwise Snell's Law is applied to find the angle of refraction inside the cube.
8) The TOF from the transducer to the surface of the cube is subtracted from the total time of flight of the data points. The remaining TOF is multiplied by the velocity of sound in aluminum to find the distance to the defect. Using the point of penetration and the angle of refraction the precise location of the defect is found.
9) The location of the defect is compared with the limits of the cube. If the point is found to be inside the cube it is stored in another data file.
10) The program returns to step one to analyze the next point.

Display Software

The data files generated by SNELL.FTN are displayed on a high resolution graphics screen. Figure 5 shows the data produced by the program being plotted in three dimensions. The PLOT software is capable of joining groups of data points which are in close proximity, and representing these groups as a geometric shape. This was first reported for imaging surfaces of objects immersed in water (6). Figure 6 shows the data after it had been grouped together using PLOT.

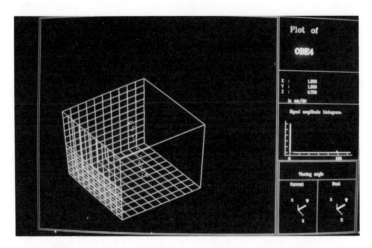

Fig. 5. Three-dimensional plot of raw data

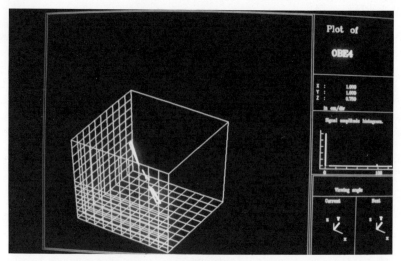

Fig. 6. Three-dimensional plot of ultrasonic data after
grouping points together via PLOT routines.

DISCUSSION

The block was scanned in a 30 by 30 point matrix, taking roughly 6
seconds per scan line, i.e. 4 minutes to complete a scan. Calculations
show a small (4°) beam spread in water becomes extremely large (25°) in an
aluminum test piece. The greater the beam spread the lower the signal
amplitude. This sugests that beam spread, not frequency, is the most
important factor in transducer sensitivity.

Figure 3 illustrates a gap in the data. Several scans were run, but
in each the gap remained present. A visual inspection of the cube's
exterior revealed no flaws on the surface. It was difficult to visually
inspect the surface of the hole. A possible cause for the signal gap
would be a short length of the hole's surface being relatively smooth. In
this case the beam would reflect similarly to one off of a mirrored
surface.

Accurate measurement of the angle of the transducer is critical when
an ultrasonic beam transmits from an acoustically slow material to a
faster one (7). Calculations show that the angle of refraction in aluminum
was 60.6°. If the measurement of the angle of incidence was in error by
the calculated angle of refraction would be in error by 7°.

CONCLUSIONS

An immersion method for the imaging of internal defects in solids was
developed that takes into account the effects of surface refraction. The
technique requires the exterior surface of the object being inspected to
be known a priori.

The choice of transducer and divergence of its ultrasonic beam is
critical. Accurate measurement of initial scanning conditions are
essential, especially the angle of incidence of the imaging transducer.

Decision logic, computational and imaging software have been written
and successfuly tested on objects with simple surface topology.

508

ACKNOWLEDGEMENTS

The authors wish to thank CANMET (Canada Centre for Mineral and Energy Technology) for support of this project.

REFERENCES

1. B. P. Hildebrand, "Acoustic Holography", Methods of Experimental Physics; Vol 19, Ultrasonics, Academic Press, 1981; pp 533-562.
2. V. Schmitz, P. Holler, "Reconstruction of Defects by Ultrasonic Synthetic Aperture Procedures", Review of Progress in Quantitative Nondestructive Evaluation; V 4A Plenum Press 1985; pp 297-307.
3. D. R. Hamlin, J. L. Jackson, T.A. Mueller, "Program for field Validation of the Synthetic Aperture Focussing Technique for Ultrasonic Testing (SAFT UT), Quarterly Progress Report, Nov. 1980 - Jan. 1981, NUREG/CR-1885, Vol. 2; Southwest Research Institute, San Antonio, TX.
4. J. F. Greenleaf, "Computerized Transmission Tomography", Methods of Experimental Physics; Vol 19, Ultrasonics, Academic Press, 1981; pp 563-589.
5. ASM Handbook Committee, Nondestructive Testing and Quality Control, ASM Committee on Ultrasonic Inspection, American Society for Metals, Metals Park, Ohio 44073, pp 161-198.
6. D. K. Mak, M. Macecek, K. Luscott and J. Wells, "Three-Dimensional Imaging of Defects", Proceedings of the IEEE Ultrasonics Symposium, Dallas, TX; November 14-16, 1984, pp 856-859.
7. Raymond Powis and Wendy Powis, A Thinker's Guide to Ultrasonic Imaging, Urban and Schwarzenberg, Baltimore-Munich 1984, pp 153-162

GENERALIZED HOLOGRAPHY AS AN IMPROVED VERSION OF CONVENTIONAL ACOUSTICAL HOLOGRAPHY

W.S. Gan

Acoustical Services PTE ltd.
29 Telok Ayer Street
Singapore 0104

INTRODUCTION

Generalized Holography (GENHOL) as an imaging tool provides more information than conventional acoustical holography which is restricted by using experimental techniques borrowed over from optical holography. GENHOL exploits all informations given by the basic principles of holography.

DERIVATION OF EXPRESSIONS OF GENHOL

The Bojarski[1] exact inverse scattering theory is the basis of GENHOL. The theory is derived in the form leading to an integral equation which can be solved numerically.

Consider a source $\rho(x)$ in a domain D bounded by a surface S. Then the time harmonic field, $\phi(\underline{x})$, due to $\rho(\underline{x})$, is the solution to the inhomogeneous wave equation

$$\nabla^2 \phi(\underline{x}) + k^2 \phi(\underline{x}) = -\rho(\underline{x}), \quad \underline{x} \in D$$

where $k = 2\pi/\lambda$ (1)

The inverse scattering problem is one in which $\phi(\underline{x})$ is known, and $\rho(\underline{x})$ is sought. For the inverse source problem, $\phi(\underline{x})$ is measured over some surface, and the object is to determine $\rho(\underline{x})$. Acoustical holography is a type of inverse source problem.

In general, $\rho(x) = \rho_m(x) + \rho_s(x)$, where ρ_m is due to interaction with the medium and ρ_s is due to actual sources. If $n(\underline{x})$ is the complex refractive index of the medium, then

$$\rho_m(x) = k^2 \left[n^2(\underline{x}) - 1 \right] \phi(\underline{x})$$ (2)

In most remote sensing problem, $\rho_s(x)$ is known and $\rho_m(x)$ is sought to yield $n(x)$. This is termed the inverse medium problem.

In this paper only the inverse source problem will be considered.

For acoustical waves, equation (1) can be reduced to

$$\nabla^2 \phi(\underline{x}, \omega) + k_m^2 \; \phi(\underline{x}, \omega) = 0 \tag{1a}$$

where $k_m = \omega/v_m$ $(\underline{x} \; \omega)$ where

v_m is the velocity of the medium,
ω is the angular frequency. Equation (2) can be written as

$$\rho(\underline{x}, \omega) = \left[(\omega^2/c^2) - (\omega^2/v_m^2) \right] \phi(\underline{x}, \omega) \tag{2a}$$

where c is the homogeneous medium propagation velocity.

Substitution of equation (2a) into equation (1a) yields equation (1).

Let the field $\phi_H(x)$ be defined as:

$$\phi_H(\underline{x}) = \oint \left[g^* \, (\underline{x} - \underline{x}') \; \nabla \phi(\underline{x}') - \phi(\underline{x}') \; \nabla g^* (\underline{x} - \underline{x}) \right] d\underline{S}' \tag{3}$$

where $g(\underline{x})$ is the free space (Green's function and the asterisk denotes complex conjugation. g satisfies Eqn 1 with $\rho(\underline{x}) = \delta(\underline{x})$. ϕ_H is in the form of the Kirchoff integral with g complex conjugated. Note that if the Kirchoff integral is applied to the field $\phi(\underline{x})$ on S and evaluated at any point $\underline{x}$ inside D, it is identically zero: The Kirchoff integral is nonzero only for points outside D. Conversely, $\phi_H(\underline{x})$ is non-zero only for points inside D. Points inside D are of interest for the inverse scattering problem.

It should be noted that ϕ_H is the mathematical expression for the reconstruction obtained from a hologram (ϕ in Eqn 3) recorded on S. ϕ_H is, in general, known for inverse problems, since ϕ is known over S. ϕ is measured over S for the inverse source and medium problems.

Applying Gauss' theorem to eqn 3 converts the surface integral into a volume integral:

$$\phi_H = \int dV \; (g^* \nabla^2 \phi - \phi \nabla^2 g^*) \tag{4}$$

From eqn 1,

$$\nabla^2 \phi = -K^2 \phi - \rho \tag{5}$$

and by complex conjugation of eqn 1 for g,

$$\nabla^2 g^* = -k^2 g^* - \delta \tag{6}$$

Substitution of eqns 5 and 6 into eqn 4 gives

$$\phi_H = \int dV \left[g^* (-k^2 \phi - \rho) - \phi (-k^2 g^* - \delta) \right]$$
$$= \int dV \; (\phi \delta - g^* \rho) \tag{7}$$

and carrying out the integration over the delta fn,

$$\phi_H = \phi - \int dV \; g^* \rho \tag{8}$$

Direct scattering theory gives the result that

$$\phi = \int dVg\rho + \oint ds(g \nabla \phi - \phi \nabla g)$$
$$= \int dVg\rho + \phi_i \tag{9}$$

In eqn 8, the first integral is just the superpostion integral over the sources. The second term is the Kirchoff integral and is associated with the incident field, ϕ_i. For the inverse scattering problems, ϕ_i can be assumed to be known without loss of generality (e.g. it is the known probing field for the inverse medium case).

Eqns 8 and 9 are two independent simultaneous equations in two unknowns, ϕ and ρ. Substitution of eqn 9 into eqn 8 yields

$$\phi_H = \int dV\, g\, \rho - \int dV\, g^*\rho + \phi_i$$

$$= \int dv\, (g - g^*)\rho + \phi_i \tag{10}$$

$$\text{or} \quad \phi_H(\underline{x}) = 2i \int dV'\, \text{Im}\, g(\underline{x} - \underline{x}')\rho(\underline{x}') + \phi_i(\underline{x}) \tag{11}$$

where Im denotes the imaginary part. Eqn 11 is the basic equation of the Exact Inverse Scattering Theory. It is an integral, convolution equation for the single unknown $\rho(\underline{x})$. It can be solved by standard deconvolution techniques.

To solve an inverse source problem, such as acoustical holography, the following steps have to be taken:

A. Compute $\phi_H(\underline{x})$, using the measured field values in eqn 3 (note that the surface of integration, S, is the measurement surface).

B. Solve eqn 11 for $\rho(\underline{x})$, using $\phi_H(\underline{x})$ from A and the known incident field, $\phi_i(\underline{x})$.

RECORDING OF GENERALIZED HOLOGRAM

A generalized hologram is constructed by recording the field and its normal derivative over a closed surface surrounding the source as shown in Fig 1. For acoustic cases, this means that both the pressure and its normal derivative (normal component of the fluid acceleration) would need to be recorded. However, by judicious selection of the shape of the recording surface the requirement for the normal derivative (which would be difficult to measure in practice) can be relaxed. For example, by taking the surface to consist of two parallel planes on either side of the source such as shown in Fig 1(b) only the pressure field need be recorded. In this case the procedure reduces to making conventional holograms over these two planes.

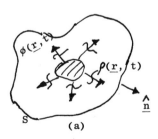
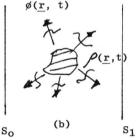

Fig 1 (a) Generalized hologram constructed by recording the pressure field and its normal derivative everywhere on arbitrary closed surface S surrounding source. (b) Only the pressure field need be recorded for case where S consists of two parallel infinite planes S_0 and S_1.

The image is formed in a second step by allowing the recorded field and normal derivative to backpropagate into the space region containing the source.

LIST OF THE ADVANTAGES AND EXTRA INFORMATIONS GIVEN BY GENHOL OVER CONVENT-
IONAL ACOUSTICAL HOLOGRAPHY:

Conventional acoustical holography suffers from the following significant restrictions and limitations:

(1)   The hologram is recorded with single frequency radiation. No broadband
      or noise sources are used.

(2)   The hologram is recorded with a reference wave and primarily phase
      information only is retained with a "square-law" detector.

(3)   The wavelength of the radiation limits the spatial resolution of the
      reconstruction. This means, for example, that two point sources
      cannot be resolved if they are separated by less than a wavelength.

(4)   A hologram which records a specific scalar field can only be used to
      reconstruct that same field. Thus, in conventional acoustical
      holography, a measurement of the sound pressure field cannot be used
      to reconstruct an independent particle velocity field or the vector
      intensity field, and one is unable to map the source or flow of
      acoustic intensity.

(5)   A conventional hologram must be recorded many wavelengths from the
      source (i.e. in the Fresnel or Fraunhofer zone). Thus, due to the
      practical limitation in hologram size, the hologram may subtend a
      small solid angle from the source. A directional source may not be
      properly recorded because of this, and important information might
      be missing.

GENHOL does not have the above restrictions. For example, the
recording of the sound pressure field on a two-dimensional surface can be
used to determine not only the three-dimensional sound pressure field but
also the particle velocity field, the acoustic vector intensity field, the
surface velocity and intensity of a vibrating source, etc. Furthermore,
each data point in the hologram need not be simple phase information from
single frequency radiation, but may be a complete time sequence recording
from incoherent noise radiation; in this case one may not only reconstruct
a three-dimensional field, but may also observe its evolution in time. An
interesting application would be the visualization of energy flow from a
transient source. GENHOL also removes the generally assumed limitations
of conventional holography such as the limited field of view resulting
from conventional recording requirements.

NEARFIELD ACCOUSTICAL HOLOGRAPHY [2] (NAH)

Nearfield acoustical holography (NAH) is the practical application
of GENHOL in an actual experimental measurement system. It is called
nearfield because the distance of the hologram from the object has to be
less than λ = wavelength for evanescent waves to be recorded. NAH works
well for audio frequency sound waves but not for ultrasonic frequencies
which is difficult to perform experimentally. This is because for audio-
frequencies, say f = 500 Hz, λ = 2.3 ft and for ultrasonic frequencies,

say f = 5 MHz, λ = 2.3 x 10^{-4} ft

In medical imaging the distance of the hologram from the object is
usually of the order of few hundred times of the wavelength. This is why
NAH can never be used for ultrasonic frequencies. NAH is even more suitable
for infrasonic frequencies such as in geophysical applications.

APPLICATIONS OF GENHOL (NAH)

Note that all these applications are of audio frequency range where
NAH/GENHOL is experimentally feasible.

Mapping of Acoustic Reactive Intensity

We choose the Green's function to be

$$g\ (x,y,z) = \ -\frac{1}{2\pi}\ \frac{\partial}{\partial \alpha}\ \left.\frac{\exp\left[\ i(2\pi/\lambda)\ (x^2 + y^2 + \alpha^2)^{\frac{1}{2}}\ \right]}{(x^2 + y^2 + \alpha^2)^{\frac{1}{2}}}\right|_{\alpha\ =\ z} \qquad (12)$$

The incident field ϕ_i (x) is given by sound pressure amplitude and
phase in the infinite plane 1. The transform g is found analytically

$$\hat{g}\ (k_x,\ k_y) = \begin{cases} \exp\left\{ id\left[\ (2\pi/\lambda)^2 - k^2\right]^{\frac{1}{2}}\right\}, & k \leqq 2\pi/\lambda \\ \exp\left\{ -d\left[k^2 - (2\pi/\lambda)^2\right]^{\frac{1}{2}}\right\}, & k > 2\pi/\lambda \end{cases}$$

where $\ k^2\ =\ k_x^2 + k_y^2$

It should be noted that $\hat{g}$ for $k < 2\pi/\lambda$ represents the radiation of
sound into the far field and $\hat{g}$ for $k > 2\pi/\lambda$ represents the rapid exponential decay of the nonradiating nearfield of the sources, composed of
evanescent waves.

It should be noted that for NAH, the recording of the sound pressure
field on a two-dimensional surface can be used to determine the three-
dimensional acoustic reactive intensity field.

ϕ (x') has to be measured on S.

This is the surface of integration and measurement surface. This is
also sound pressure field. The ϕ_H(x) can be computed from eqn (3) using
the measured field values. The next step solve eqn (11) for P(x), the
required reactive intensity field using ϕ_H(x) from above and the unknown
incident field ϕ_i(x).

Indentification of Broadband Noise Source

Let the broadband noise source be represented by

$$p\ (x,t) = \sum^{\infty} p_o\ (\omega t - kx)$$
$$t = -\infty \qquad (13)$$

The incident field ϕ (x) will be given by eqn (13) on plane I and
the field ϕ (x) to be measured will be given by eqn (13) on the measurement
surface S.

Following the same procedures as in B. by first mapping the acoustic
intensity, the noise source will be given by location of concentration
of acoustic intensity vector.

Application of NAH to identify broadband noise source has the advantages
over conventional method of plotting acoustic intensity vectors using the
two-microphone technique that more complete information can be obtained
in shorter time, with less risk of including less false dates. Also
NAH enables FFT algorithm to be used.

Active Cancellation of 3-D Broadband Noise (ANA)

We rederive GENHOL from Huygens' principle:

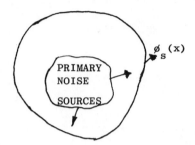

Fig 2. Illustrates GENHOL in terms of Huygens" principle.

Huygens' principle states that the sound field $\phi_p(x)$ due to the unwanted primary noise sources on the surface Sp can be reproduced exactly by suppressing the primary sources and replacing it with an array of secondary noise sources $\phi_s(x)$ on the Huygens' surface S_s.

We first start from Helmholtz equation $(\nabla^2 + k^2)\, \phi = 0$ (14)

with the waveno k and its general solution in terms of a two-dimensional inverse Fourier integral

$$\phi(x,y,z) = \frac{1}{(2\pi)^2} \int_{-\infty}^{\infty} \int_{-\infty}^{\infty} \phi(K_x, K_y, K)\, e^{\pm jz\sqrt{k^2 - K_x^2 - K_y^2}} \cdot e^{j(K_x x + K_y y)}\, dK_x\, dK_y$$

(15)

Here K_x and K_y denote the Fourier variables with respect to x and y.

The mathematical relationship of Huygens' principle is given by the Kirchoff integral as a solution of (15).

$$\phi_s = \oint (\phi_B^n g - \phi_B \frac{\partial g}{\partial n})\, dS$$

(16)

where $\underline{n}$ denotes the outward normal on S_p and the sources ϕ_B and ϕ_B^n are given by the total field

$$\phi(x) = \phi_p(x) + \phi_s(x) \quad \text{on} \quad S_p \quad \text{through}$$

$$\phi_B(x) = \phi|_{S_p}$$

(17)

$$\phi_B^n(x) = \nabla \phi \cdot \underline{n}|_{S_p}$$

(18)

g is the time harmonic free space Green's function accounting for the propagation of elementary wavelets emanating from the surface S_p with amplitudes given by the surface distributions ϕ_B and ϕ_B^n. According to (16) the scattered field is formed as the envelope of all these wavelets.

Generalized holography requires an inversion of eqn (16) using back-propagation argument, in terms of

$$\phi_H = \oint_{S_s} (\phi_p^{M,n} g^* - \phi_p^M \frac{\partial g^*}{\partial n})\, dS$$

(19)

This equation is a formal application of Huygens' principle to the measurement surface S_s where the array of secondary sources are.

516

Hence the secondary or Cancelling noises are given by ϕ_H in eqn (19).

It should be noted that eqn (19) is equivalent to eqn (3) derived from Bojarski's exact scattering theory.

Applying Gauss' theorem eqn (19) can be reduced to the equivalent form of eqn (11).

Here the cancelling secondary noise sources for ANA of 3-D broadband noise sources can be solved once the primary noise sources to be cancelled and the Green's function is fixed, by solving eqn (3) or (19) and eqn (11).

To illustrate this, we choose a spherical sound wave as the primary noise souce:

$$\rho(\omega, t) = \frac{A}{r} e^{j\omega(t - kr)} \tag{20}$$

where r = radial distance, A = wave amplitude.

The Green's function is chosen as

$$g(x,y,z) = -\frac{1}{2\pi} \frac{\partial}{\partial \alpha} \left. \frac{\exp\left[i(2\pi/\lambda)(x^2 + y^2 + \alpha^2)^{\frac{1}{2}} \right]}{(x^2 + y^2 + \alpha^2)^{\frac{1}{2}}} \right|_{\alpha = z} \tag{21}$$

The Fourier transform of g(x,y.z) is found as

$$\hat{g}(K_x, K_y) = \begin{cases} \exp\left\{ id\left[(2\pi/\lambda)^2 - k^2 \right]^{\frac{1}{2}} \right\}, & k \lesssim 2\pi/\lambda \\ \exp\left\{ -d\left[k^2 - (2\pi/\lambda)^2 \right]^{\frac{1}{2}} \right\}, & k > 2\pi/\lambda \end{cases} \tag{22}$$

where $k^2 = K_x^2 + K_y^2$. We restrict the field point to lie in the second plane H defined by $Z = Z_H = Z_I + d$. The first plane is an infinite plane I defined by $Z = Z_I$.

It should be noted that $\hat{g}_d$ for $k < 2\pi/\lambda$ represents the radiation of sound into the far field and $\hat{g}_d$ for $k > 2\pi/\lambda$ represents the rapid exponential decay of the nonradiating near field of the sources, composed of evanescent waves.

The Bojarski integral of eqn (11) can be expressed as

$$\phi_H = 2 j \int \rho g \, dV \tag{23}$$

where ρ represents the primary noise source.

Performing Fourier transform on (23),

$$\hat{\phi}_H = 2 j \hat{\rho} \hat{g} \tag{24}$$

where ρ is given by eqn (20) and g by eqn (22)

The method of solving the above convolution integral is by Fast Fourier transformation technique. To do FFT, we must first convert the convolution integral and approximate it as a discrete convolution. Then evaluation and inversion of this convolution integral can be carried out swiftly by way of Discrete Fourier transformation (DFT) and convolution theorem using FFT algorithm to compute DFT and IDFT.

To evaluate the convolution integral numerically or to make it experimentally useful, we have to reduce the integral over an infinite plane to an integral over a limited region.

The application of NAH to ANA can be treated as an inversion problem.

The theory behind the approximate solution of using the FFT to solve the convolution integral and the necessary conditions are most easily seen if the Fourier transform version of the continuous convolution integral is examined. By the convolution theorem of Fourier transforms, the Bojarski integral can be written as:

$$\phi_H(x,y,z) = F^{-1}\left\{ F[\rho(x,y,z_I)] \cdot F[g(x,y,z-z_I)] \right\} \qquad (25)$$

$$\text{or} \quad \hat{\phi}_H(k_x, k_y, z) = \hat{\rho}(k_x, k_y, z_I) \cdot \hat{g}(k_x, k_y, z - z_I)$$

$$= \hat{\rho}(k_x, k_y, z_I) \cdot e^{jkz(z - z_I)} \qquad (26)$$

where $k_z = (k^2 - k_x^2 - k_y^2)^{\frac{1}{2}}$, $k = \omega/c$

F and F^{-1} represent the Fourier transform and Inverse Fourier transform respectively.

Returning to the numerical problem, the inversion can be written

$$\hat{\rho}(k_x, k_y, z_I) = \hat{\phi}_H(k_x, K_y, z) / \hat{g}(k_x, k_y, z - z_I) \qquad (27)$$

Computationally, the experimental restriction to performing inverse reconstruction only over small distances is fortunate. A large part of the evanescent components will not have decayed to the point where inversion, at least in terms of the continuous transforms, will require the numerically difficult division of extremely small data values by comparably small Green's function values.

Experimentally, it has been observed that if the DFT of the data array is treated as equivalent to the actual Fourier transform of the field, the IDFT treated as equivalent to the actual Inverse Fourier transform and a straightforward inversion attempted,

$$\hat{\rho}(x,y,z_I) \simeq IDFT\left\{ DFT[\phi_H(x,y,z)] / \hat{g}(k_x, k_y, z - z_I) \right\} \qquad (28)$$

the results tend to oscillate about the actual values at near the maximum spatial frequency evaluated by the DFT.

REFERENCES

1. N. N. Bojarski: Exact Inverse Scattering Theory. Radio Science 16 (1981) 1025.
2. J. J. Maynard and E. G. Williams: Nearfield Holography, a New Technique for Noise Radiation Measurement. Proceedings of Noise Con 81, pp. 19 - 23, 1981.

JOINT FOURIER TRANSFORM CROSS-CORRELATION FOR LIVER ECHOTEXTURE

CLASSIFICATION

Paolo Sirotti °, and Giorgio Rizzatto *

° Dipartimento di Elettrotecnica Elettronica Informatica
University of Trieste
Via A. Valerio, 10
34124 Trieste, Italy

* General Hospital of Gorizia
Via Vittorio Veneto, 171
34170 Gorizia, Italy

ABSTRACT

Tissue characterization of liver echographic scans was obtained using
an optical-digital procedure of direct correlation between the unknown
texture and a set of reference textures.
The method, tested on a selected group of static liver B-scans, gave a 90%
accuracy. To date the search is being carried out by collecting and evaluating new cases of diffuse liver diseases: a set of 21 linear dynamic
scans has been processed obtaining a 76.2% sensitivity in the correct recognition of a pathologic state. Considering only the cases with grade 1
fibrosis and/or grade 1 fatty infiltration a 69.2% sensitivity was achieved.

INTRODUCTION

The direct comparison between an unknown texture and a set of reference
textures may be a discriminating criterion to classify echotextures (Sirotti
and Rizzatto, 1984). Cross-correlation functions between unknown and reference textures were obtained using both all-optical and optical-digital
methods (Sirotti and Rizzatto, 1984).

Up to now the optical-digital Joint Fourier Transform (JFT) classification has proved to be the most practicable method. Tissue characterization
of liver echographic scans was obtained using a procedure of direct correlation between the unknown texture and a set of reference textures:

- the JFT of both the reference images and the unknown one is obtained
  in a coherent optical system;

- JFT is on-line entered in a digital image processing system; this retransforms the intensity of the JFT and gives the correlations among input images;

- finally the cross-correlation functions are digitally compared.

This mixed configuration keeps speed and parallel processing of optical methods, adding flexibility and objectivity of digital processing. This technique provided a 90% accuracy in a selected group of static liver B-scans (Sirotti, Rizzatto and Di Stefano, 1985).

CLINICAL CONSIDERATIONS

Due to technological developments ultrasound is increasingly detecting small focal lesions; its sensitivity is very high. Pathological classification of these lesions is easy when fine-needle aspiration methods and citology are performed. Based on these considerations we have defi--nitely decided to deal only with diffuse diseases, mainly liver disorders. Their incidence is significative, mostly induced by alcohol or drugs in the North of Italy, by hepatitis and its chronic outcome in the Center and the South.

Different degrees of fibrosis and fatty infiltrations, often mixed, characterize these pathologies: it has been well demonstrated that they disrupt parenchymal textures (Birnholz, 1979; Fellingham and Graham Sommer, 1984; Rizzatto et al., 1982). Moreover we have already proved that JFT method allows to recognize echotexture alterations when they are still out of the visual perception (Sirotti, Rizzatto and Di Stefano, 1985; Sirotti and Rizzatto, 1985).

ACTUAL RESEARCH - FIRST NEW RESULTS

Basic aims of the actual research are: recognition of texture alterations when conventional B-scans dynamic images are subjectively normal; selection of the scanning format (linear, convex and sector) more fit for texture analysis; grading of fibrosis and/or fatty changes.

The cases are being collected under very strict conditions. Ecographic scans are obtained with an unchanging combination of dynamic scanner, dynamic range, transducer and recording system: white-on-black display mode is used. Interesting area is restricted within the beam focal zone; it must be poor in vessels and limited to the liver segments where biopsy is performed. The images are reviewed to valuate intra-and interobserver variations related to textural differentiations. The scans are finally classified according to the results of liver biopsies performed with the Menghini needle. A definite histological grading of fatty change and fibrosis is obtained using both semi-quantitative and quantitative methods.

Up to date we have evaluated linear scans of 21 patients, that fully responded to the above mentioned conditions.
Although dynamic scans keep less informative contents than the static scans, we have found a 76.2% sensitivity in the correct recognition of a pathologic state. Moreover if we consider only the cases with very limited alterations

on histology, i.e. grade 1 fibrosis (fibrous expansion of the portal
spaces) and grade 1 fatty infiltrations (less than 15% of cells involved),
a 69.2% sensitivity was achieved. This result turns out to be very interesting as all these last cases were considered normally echotextured by
the involved physicians.

The evaluation on possible extensions of JFT correlation for grading
purposes was limited as we could not obtain a sufficient number of cases
with pure fatty infiltration.

REFERENCES

Birnholz, J.C., 1979, Ultrasound evaluation of diffuse liver disease,
in: "Clinics in Diagnostic Ultrasound", Vol. I, 23:33.

Fellingham, L.L. and Graham Sommer, F., 1984, Ultrasonic Characterization of Tissue Structure in the In Vivo Human Liver and
Spleen, IEEE Trans. Sonics Ultrason., Vol. SU-31, No. 4,
418:428

Rizzatto, G., Sirotti, P., Bazzocchi, M., Boltro, E., Busilacchi, P.,
Candiani, F., Ferrari, F., Giuseppetti, G.M., Lo Russo, G.,
Mirk, P., Maresca, G., Rubaltelli, L., Volterrani, L.,
Zappasodi, F., 1982, Standardized Ultrasonic Valuation of
Diffuse Liver Diseases, in: "Ultrasound 1982", ed. R.A.
Lerski, P. Morley, Pergamon Press Ltd., Oxford.

Sirotti, P., Rizzatto, G., 1984, Coherent optical texture recognition
of digital ultrasonic images, IEEE Trans. Sonics Ultrason.,
Vol. SU-31, No. 4, 436:440

Sirotti, P., Rizzatto, G., Di Stefano, E., 1985, Optical-digital Joint
Fourier Transform classification of liver echotexture, in:
"Acoustical Imaging", Vol. 14, 765:768, ed. A.J. Berkhout,
J. Ridder, L.F. van der Wal, Plenum Press, New York and
London.

Sirotti, P., Rizzatto, G., 1985, Coherent Optical Cross-Correlation
for Ultrasonic Texture Classification, in: "Ultrasonic
Tissue Characterization and Echographic Imaging 5. Proceedings of the fifth European Communities Workshop, ed. J.M.
Thijssen and V. Mazzeo, Ferrara.

A TWO-ELEMENT ANNULAR ARRAY OF SHORT FIXED FOCAL LENGTH

FOR DYNAMIC FOCUSING

Nils Sponheim

Center for Industrial Research
P.O. Box 350, Blindern
0314 Oslo 3
Norway

ABSTRACT

A two-element annular array for dynamic focusing has been designed. It is combined with a lens of short, fixed focal length and is to be used in a mechanically scanned transducer for simultaneous 2D cardiographic echo imaging and 2D doppler flow chart mapping. The goal has been to minimize the number of elements, since it is difficult to make annular arrays with many elements having high sensitivity and equal impulse responses. High sensitivity is needed for the Doppler application and equal impulse responses are needed for dynamic focusing in the echo imaging application. A study of the on-axis spatial impulse response has led to a formula for the required number of annular elements. It has also suggested that one should combine the array with a lens of short fixed focal length to obtain best results in dynamic focusing. To test this new design principle experimentally we have made a two-element transducer and measured the impulse response and sensitivity of each element as well as the transient beam pattern. The measurements are in good agreement with calculations based on the transmission line model and the spatial impulse response method. The array produces a narrow beam close to the diffraction limit in the desired depth range.

1. INTRODUCTION

In cardiological applications acoustical imaging has often been combined with Doppler measurements to find the blood velocity and also the velocity of the walls and the valves [1]. Although Doppler measurements do not require as high resolution as the imaging, the weak scattering from the blood cells requires transducers of very high sensitivity. With the imaging systems made so far it has been possible to measure the velocity at only one image point in real time, whereas it would be desirable to make a 2D flow chart map in real time and to superimpose it on the echo image. This requires a transducer with resolution appropriate for imaging and sensitivity appropriate for Doppler measurements. In this paper we present a transducer design to meet these requirements.

In cardiological ultrasound imaging systems two different concepts have been used to perform sector scanning. The phased array is electronically steered and focused, while the annular array is electronically focused, but mechanically scanned. The number of elements in a phased array determines the number of steering directions. In practise the number has ranged from 16 to 128. For annular arrays the number of elements has been less than 10. It is difficult to make an array with many elements since differences in shape and cross-coupling between the elements lead to unequal impulse responses. Also the heavier mechanical support results in reduced sensitivity of each element. Because of the high sensitivity required in the Doppler application we therefore chose an annular array rather than a phased array.

Since an annular array with many elements has reduced sensitivity and is difficult to make it is important to determine the minimum number of elements required. We have developed a theory for determining this number and also shown how the number can be further reduced by using a lens of short focal length. Also, we have designed a two-element transducer combined with a lens and measured its sensitivity, impulse response and beam pattern. The measurements have been compared with calculations based on the spatial impulse response method and the transmission line model.

2. THEORY

To study transient ultrasonic fields from radiating pistons the spatial impulse response method has been widely used [2, 3, 4]. The method is based on factoring the integrand in the Rayleigh integral [5] into a surface velocity $v(t)$ times a spatial impulse response $h(\vec{r},t)$ where $\vec{r}$ is the position of the observation point and t is the time. The velocity potential $\varphi(\vec{r},t)$ is then given by

$$\varphi(\vec{r},t) = v(t) * h(\vec{r},t) \tag{1}$$

where * denotes convolution. Thus the spatial impulse response is the velocity potential when the surface is excited with a δ-pulse. The technique requires that the surface velocity is the same over the radiating surface, but apodization and focusing are included in the spatial impulse response by an amplitude factor $A(\vec{r}_0)$ and a time delay $\tau(\vec{r}_0)$ which both may vary with the position $\vec{r}_0$ on the radiating surface S.

$$h(\vec{r},t) = \int_S \frac{A(\vec{r}_0)}{2\pi R} \delta(t - R/c - \tau(\vec{r}_0)) dS \tag{2}$$

Here δ is the Dirac delta function. $R = |\vec{r} - \vec{r}_0|$ is the distance from the excitation point to the observation point and c is the sound velocity.

As shown in Fig. 1 all points on a plane surface S having the same distance to a point O lie on circles centered at the projection of O on S. If the surface is excited by a δ-pulse, contributions from all points on one circle will arrive simultaneously at O. The first contribution comes from the center, and contributions from circles of increasingly larger diameters arrive successively until finally the contribution arrives from

524

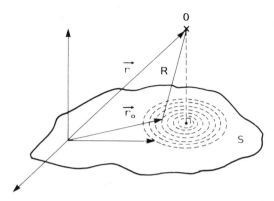

Fig. 1. Geometry showing the observation point 0 at position r and the source point $\vec{r}_0$ on the surface S. R is the distance between the source and observation point.

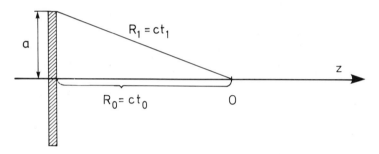

Fig. 2. Geometry showing an on-axis observation point 0 in front of a plane disc of radius a. R_0 and R_1 are the distances from 0 to respectively the center and the edge of the surface.

the edge of the surface. Therefore, if the excitation surface S is a circular disc, it is easy to find the on-axis impulse response. The contribution from the center and from the edge of the disc will arrive at times t_0 and t_1, respectively, where, as shown in Fig. 2.

$$t_0 = R_0/c = z/c \qquad (3)$$

$$t_1 = R_1/c = \frac{1}{c} [z^2 + a^2]^{1/2} \qquad (4)$$

with a being the radius of the disc. For $t_0 < t < t_1$ the on-axis impulse response is independent of time and equal to the sound velocity c, at all other times it vanishes. Thus it is a rectangular function of time as shown in Fig. 3 [6,7]. For a plane aperture the time interval between t_0

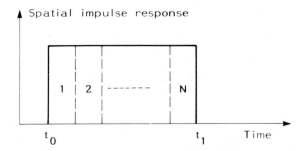

Fig. 3. The on-axis impulse response of a circular plane disc
consisting of N annular elements without any time delay.
t_0 and t_1 are the travel times from the observation point
to respectively the center and the edge of the disc.

and t_1 will decrease as the axial distance increases, and in the far field
the rectangular function approaches a δ-pulse. According to Eqs (3) and
(4) the length of the on-axis spatial impulse response at the distance z
from a plane circular disc of radius a is:

$$t_1 - t_0 = \frac{1}{c} [\ [z^2 + a^2 \ ]^{1/2} - z \ ] \tag{5}$$

Consider a plane array of N concentric annular elements and let the
outer radius of the n'th element be

$$a_n = [\frac{n}{N}]^{1/2} a \qquad\qquad (n = 1,2,\ldots, N) \tag{6}$$

where a_N = a is the outer radius of the outermost element. Then the area
is the same for all the elements. If this array is to be focused at a
distance f_2 the time delay between successive elements must be

$$\Delta t = \frac{1}{c} [(f_2^2 + a_{n+1}^2)^{1/2} - (f_2^2 + a_n^2)^{1/2}] \approx \frac{a^2}{2f_2 Nc} \tag{7}$$

Thus, in the parabolic approximation, which is considered adequate here
[8], Δt is independent of n, so that the time delay between the first and
the n'th element will be

$$\Delta t_n = (n-1) \Delta t \tag{8}$$

We have shown above that the on-axis response of a circular disc is a
rectangular function of time. Therefore, if we have a plane concentric
array of annular elements without time delay, the on-axis response of each

526

element will also be a rectangular function, and the responses of
neighboring elements will be delayed as illustrated in Fig. 3. Here
element no. 1 is the center element and element no. N the peripheral
element. If the elements are focused, i.e., are given time delays as
described in Eqs. (7) and (8), the responses of all elements will coincide
at a distance f_2 from the transducer, and the length of the impulse
response of the focused array will be N times shorter than for the
unfocused array. Ideally we want to make the impulse response as close to
a δ-pulse as possible. A reasonable objective is a response shorter than
half a period λ/2c, where λ is the wavelength, i.e.,

$$\frac{t_1 - t_0}{N} < \frac{\lambda}{2c} \tag{9}$$

To meet this objective the number of elements must satisfy the
requirement

$$N > \frac{[f_2^2 + a^2]^{1/2} - f_2}{\lambda/2} \tag{10}$$

where we have used Eq. (5) with z = f_2. Although this estimate is
oversimplified, since we have not considered the field off-axis, it may
serve as a rule of thumb.

    Calculations of the off-axis impulse response are more complicated.
But for a circular transducer a solution in terms of elementary functions
has been found [7, 9]. This solution can also be used for annular arrays
and has been used in the calculations of this paper. The pressure p is
related to the spatial impulse response by the equation

$$p(\vec{r}, t) = \varrho \frac{\partial}{\partial t} v (t) * h(\vec{r}, t) \tag{11}$$

where v(t) is the velocity of the exciting surface and ϱ is the density of
the medium. The surface velocity pulse used in the calculations is the one
shown in Fig. 10.a. This pulse was obtained from computations based on the
transmission line model [10] for a PZT element with one quarterwave
matching layer.

    The required number of elements in a plane concentric annular array
of focal length f_2, follows from expression (10) from which we see that
the shorter the focal length, the larger the number of elements. Thus if
the desired imaging depth ranges from 20 mm to 150 mm, we must choose N in
accordance with the shortest focal length of f_2 = 20 mm. Consider a plane
transducer of radius a = 6.35 mm, whose center frequency is 3 MHz
corresponding to a wavelength of 0.5 mm in water. For f_2 = 20 mm
expression (10) gives N>3.9 so that 4 elements are required. To check this
result we have calculated the beam diameter as a function of depth for 2,4
and 8 elements, using the surface velocity pulse shown in Fig. 10.a. The
results are shown in Fig. 4. Note that we have used dynamic focusing,
which means that we have adjusted the focal length to be equal to the
depth. This is the optimum choice of focal length if the narrowest
possible beam is desired [6], a result which can also be shown to hold in
general [11, 12]. In Fig. 4 we see that the beams using 4 and 8 elements

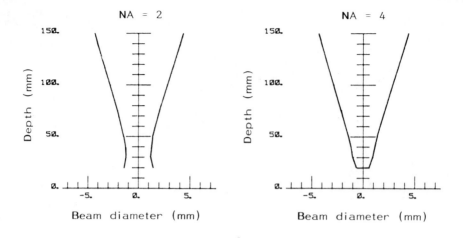

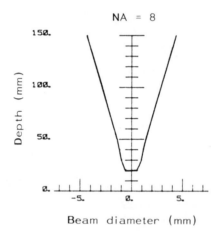

Fig. 4. Beam diameter as a function of depth for a transducer with NA elements. The transducer diameter is 12.7 mm. The excitation pulse is as shown in Fig. 10.a with a center frequency of 3 MHz.

are essentially equal. The beam using 2 elements has a larger diameter in the near field than the other two. At a depth of 20 mm the beam diameter using 2 elements is more than twice the beam diameter using 4 and 8 elements. This shows, as predicted, that for a plane transducer the largest number of elements are needed close to the aperture. Fig. 5 shows the beam profiles at a depth z of 20 mm using 2, 4 and 8 elements. Again, the focal length is equal to the depth. We now clearly see that two elements are not sufficient to give a good focus at a depth of 20 mm. An increase to 4 elements gives a dramatic improvement of the skirts in addition to the reduction in beam diameter mentioned above. A further increase to 8 elements gives an additional improvement, but little compared to the one obtained by going from 2 to 4 elements. Therefore we conclude that 4 elements are needed and that expression (10) can be used to find the number of elements necessary to focus at a depth f_2. The beam profiles in Fig. 5 are obtained from the temporal pulses computed from Eq. (11) by using peak detection, and the beam diameters in Fig. 4 are obtained from the beam profiles by using the half value beam width.

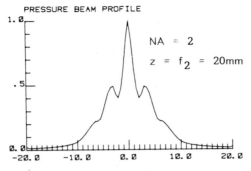

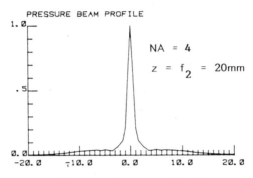

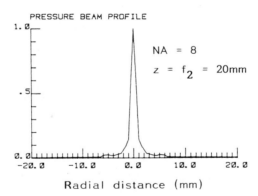

Fig. 5. Pressure beam profiles in the focal plane at a depth of 20 mm of an annular array with NA elements as a function of distance from the axis. The transducer diameter is 12.7 mm. The excitation pulse is as shown in Fig. 10.a with a center frequency of 3 MHz.

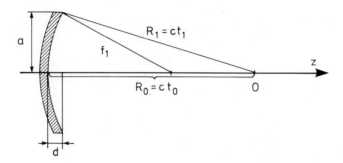

Fig. 6. Geometry showing an on-axis observation point O in front of a
spherical transducer of aperture radius a and focal length f_1.
R_0 and R_1 are the distances from O to respectively the center
and the edge of the surface, and d is the sag of the transducer.

We now proceed by looking at a transducer of fixed focal length
resulting from either a spherical radiating surface or a lens. Let us
consider a spherical surface with an aperture radius a and with radius of
curvature f_1, equal to the focal length as shown in Fig. 6. R_0 and R_1 are
the distances from O to respectively the center and the edge of the
aperture. We also define

$$t_0 = R_0/c = z/c \qquad (12)$$

and

$$t_1 = R_1/c = \frac{1}{c} [a^2 + (z-d)^2]^{1/2} \qquad (13)$$

which are the travel times from O to the center and the edge respectively.
The parameter d given by

$$d = f_1[1-[1-(a/f_1)^2]^{1/2}] \qquad (14)$$

is the sag of the surface as shown in Fig. 6. For focused apertures the
far field resides in the focal plane and the spatial impulse response at
the focal point will be a δ-pulse as a function of time. This is true in
general for all focused apertures. At axial points beyond the focal point
the contribution from the edge will come first, so that t_0 will be greater
that t_1. The on-axis spatial impulse response in the time interval between
t_0 and t_1 will still be independent of time [6], but vary with depth

$$h(0,t) = \begin{cases} c\,\dfrac{f_1}{|f_1-z|} & \text{between } t_0 \text{ and } t_1 \\[2mm] 0 & \text{otherwise} \end{cases} \qquad (15)$$

Thus also for a spherical surface the on-axis impulse response is a rectangular function of time and its length is given by

$$|t_1 - t_0| = \frac{1}{c} \left[\left[(z - d)^2 + a^2 \right]^{1/2} - z \right] \tag{16}$$

Also in this case the length of the impulse response is divided by the number of elements if we have an annular array in which each element is given a proper time delay. For a system having a fixed focal length f_1 and an adjustable focal length f_2 the total focal length f is given by the well-known thin lens formula of paraxial geometrical optics [13].

$$f^{-1} = f_1^{-1} + f_2^{-1} \tag{17}$$

Using Eq. (17) to replace f_2 in Eq. (7) we get the proper time delay between neighboring elements

$$\Delta t = \frac{a^2}{2Nc} (f^{-1} - f_1^{-1}) \tag{18}$$

and the time delay between the first and the n'th element is again given by Eq. (8).

We now investigate the possibilities of this combination, in the same manner as before, i.e., by analysing the on-axis impulse response. Suppose our aim is to focus properly in the range of 20-150 mm, in which we need an on-axis response shorter than half a period. With a fixed focal length f_1 of 75 mm and an aperture radius a of 6.85 mm, the length $|t_1 - t_0|$ of the on-axis response is 0.57 μs at a depth of 20 mm and 0.10 μs at a

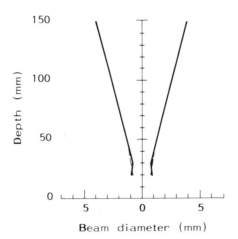

Fig. 7. Calculated (———) and measured (------) beam diameter as a function of depth for a two-element transducer with one matching layer when optimum focal length is used at all depths. The aperture diameter is 13.7 mm, the fixed focal length is 55 mm and the center frequency of the pulse is 3 MHz.

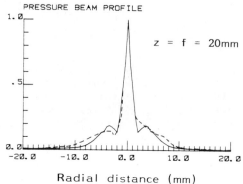

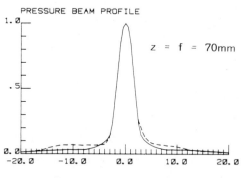

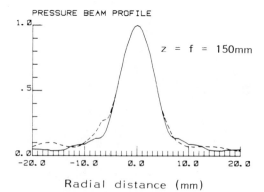

Fig. 8.   Calculated (———) and measured(------) beam profiles as a function
of distance from the axis at depth z for a two-element transducer
with one matching layer when optimum focal length is used at all
depths. The aperture diameter is 13.7 mm, the fixed focal length
is 55 mm and the center frequency of the pulse is 3 MHz.

depth of 150 mm according to Eq. (16). To get an on-axis response shorter than 0.17 µs, which is half a period at 3 MHz it is necessary to use four elements at depth 20 mm. At a depth of 150 mm however, the response is short enough with one element. It might therefore be better to choose a fixed focus that gives a response of the same length at 20 mm and 150 mm. With a fixed focal length of 36 mm we get an on-axis response of length 0.34 µs both at 20 mm and 150 mm according to Eq. (16). Thus it suffices to use two elements to obtain an on-axis response shorter than 0.17 µs both at 20 mm and 150 mm. This solution also has the practical advantage that the timedelay needed at 20 mm and 150 mm is equal with only opposite sign. But calculations show high sidelobes in the far field. A better solution is a fixed focal length of 55 mm. If dynamic focusing is used and the excitation pulse of Fig. 10.a is used, the beam diameter is as shown in Fig. 7 (solid curve). By dynamic focusing we now mean that the total focal length has been adjusted to be equal to the observation depth at all depths. The calculated beam profiles in Fig. 8 at depths 20 mm, 70 mm and 150 mm (solid curves) show a well-behaved beam. Also, on comparing these results with the previous results for the plane two-element transducer in Fig. 4 and Fig. 5 (NA=2), we see that the near field can be considerably improved by using a fixed focus in addition to the electronically steered focus.

3. EXPERIMENTS

On the basis of the preceding calculations we have made a two-element transducer as shown in Fig. 9. The PZT-elements have silver electrodes and a quarter wave thick filled epoxy is molded on the front. The backing is a porous material which gives sufficient mechanical support but a negligible acoustic load. This construction is meant to give short pulses, but at the same time high efficiency.

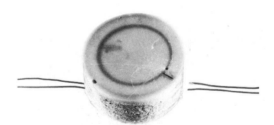

Fig. 9. The two-element transducer used in the measurements.

The efficiency was measured by using an ultrasound power meter [14]. One element at a time was supplied with a continuous 3 MHz voltage and the acoustic power was measured for each element, the efficiency being the ratio between the electric power at the input and the acoustic power at the output. The measured efficiency was 88% for the center element and 57% for the peripheral element. Calculations by the transmission line model gives an efficiency of 92% when the losses in the PZT are accounted for. Thus for the center element the agreement is excellent; for the peripheral element the deviation between theory and measurement may be due to a somewhat heavier backing caused by the gluing at the edge. However, the sensitivity of the transducer is good enough for the Doppler measurements.

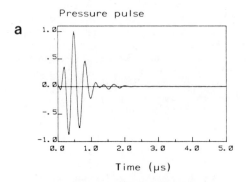

Pressure pulse

a

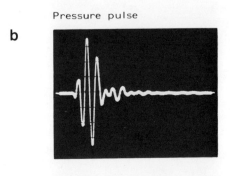

Pressure pulse

b

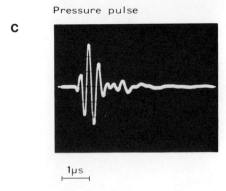

Pressure pulse

c

1μs

Fig. 10. Pressure pulses from the 3MHz PZT-element with one quarter
wave matching layer and porous backing.
a) Calculated
b) Measured center element
c) Measured peripheral element

The measured pulses from each of the two elements are shown in Fig. 10.b and 10.c. Comparing these with the calculated pulse in Fig. 10.a, we find good agreement for the main part of each measured pulse, but small differences between the tails. The measurements were carried out in a water tank using a PVDF-hydrophone with an aperture diameter of 1 mm and a bandwidth larger than 10 MHz. The measurements of the beam diameter and the beam profiles are shown as the dotted lines in Figs. 7 and 8, respectively. The agreement between calculated and measured results is very good both for the beam diameter and the main lobe of each beam profile, but differences can be observed between the skirts of the profiles. But these differences are not vital, and they might be due to differences in the pulses from the two elements and also to the fact that the transducer does not radiate entirely as a piston. The calculations and the measurements show however that the proposed design with two elements and a fixed focal length of 55 mm produces a narrow and well-behaved beam.

4. CONCLUSIONS

In this paper we have presented a design of a transducer for simultaneous 2D echo imaging and 2D flow chart mapping. By studying the on-axis spatial impulse response of a circular aperture we have obtained a formula, which gives the number of elements required to focus at a certain depth, and we have also found a way to reduce this number by using a lens of short focal length. This reduction has made it possible to achieve the desired sensitivity for Doppler measurements without reducing the resolution for echo imaging.

ACKNOWLEDGEMENTS

The author is indebted to Kjell Arne Ingebrigtsen, Vingmed A.S., Horten, Norway and Helge Engan, The Norwegian Institute of Technology, Trondheim, Norway, and also to Jakob Stamnes, Norwave A.S, Oslo, Norway for reviewing this paper. This work was supported by grants from The Norwegian Institute of Technology and from Vingmed A.S.

REFERENCES

1. L. Halte, B.A. Angelsen, "Doppler ultrasound in Cardiology - Physical Principles and Clinical Applications", New York, Lea and Fabiger 1982.

2. P.R. Stepanishen, "The time-dependent force and radiation impedance on a poston in a rigid infinite planar baffle", JASA 49, 841-849, (1971).

3. P.R. Stepanishen, "Transient Radiation from Postons in an Infinite Planar Baffle", JASA 49, 1627-1638, (1971).

4. P.R. Stepanishen, "Wide Bandwidth Acoustic Near and Far Field Transients from Baffled Postons" Proc. 1977 IEEE Ultrason. Symp., 113-118.

5. J.W. Strutt (Lord Rayleigh), "Theory of Sound", Vol. 2, Dover, New York, 1945.

6. N. Sponheim, "Focusing of annular arrays". Submitted to IEEE ultrasonics, Ferroelectrics and Frequency Control.

7. N. Sponheim, "Transient Ultrasonic fields of efficient broadband piezoelectric transducers". Dr.ing.-thesis, The Norwegian Institute of Technology, 1985.

8. D.R. Dietz, S.J. Norton, M. Linzer, "Wideband annular array response", Proc. 1978 IEEE Ultrason. Symp., 206-211.

9. M. Arditi, F.S. Foster, J.W. Hunt, "Transient fields of concave annular arrays", Ultrason. Imag. 3, 37-61, (1981).

10. R. Krimholtz, D. Leedom, G. Matthaei, "New Equivalent Circuits for Elementary Piezoelectric Transducers", Electronics Letters 6, 398-399, (1970).

11. J.H. Erkkilla, "On the maximum intensity in the focal volume", Opt. Commun. 43, 313-314, (1982).

12. J. Stamnes, "Waves in focal regions", Chapter 12.2, Adam Hilger, Bristol, 1986.

13. E. Hecht, A. Zajac, "Optics", Addison-Wesley, USA, 1979. JASA 72, 1121-1123, (1982).

14. H. Engan, "An ultrasound power meter", JASA 72, 1121-1123, (1982).

ACOUSTIC IMAGING OF SOLID OBJECTS IN AIR USING A SMALL SET OF

TRANSDUCERS: III. EXPERIMENTAL DEMONSTRATION

J.M. Richardson, K.A. Marsh, G. Rivera,
M. Lasher and J.F. Martin

Rockwell International Science Center
Thousand Oaks, CA 91360

ABSTRACT

   We describe an algorithm that produces three-dimensional acoustic
images of simple objects in air using an array containing only a small
number of transducers. Each transducer provides a pulse-echo measurement in an appropriate incident direction. Our algorithm uses entire
waveforms (i.e., it is not limited to simple time-of-flight measurement), and is based on the Kirchhoff approximation together with the
assumption that the scatterer is a rigid body. We further assume that
the body is flat-bottomed with its upper surface represented by a
single-valued elevation function. The imaging algorithm employs an
iterative technique involving smoothing and linearization at each stage.
Evaluation of the imaging algorithm by means of synthetic and experimental test data will be discussed.

Introduction

   Our approach to the problem of acoustic imaging of solid objects in
air is a probabilistic one, based on measurement models using the
Kirchhoff approximation for the scattering of acoustic waves. The measured data consist of pulse-echo waveforms taken in a small number of
incident directions. The a priori information is generally in the form
of a statistical ensemble of possible spatial distributions of acoustic
impedance. For the case of of solid objects in air, it is assumed that
the acoustic impedance of the object is infinite (i.e., all acoustic
energy is reflected), and hence everywhere in space the image can be
represented by a three-dimensional characteristic function with only two
possible values at each point, which can be defined as 0 (in air) and 1
(in the object). In the case to be considered here, it is not necessary
to know this function everywhere, but rather it will suffice to know the
elevation function of the visible surface, seen from some viewpoint.

   In this paper we confine our attention to the case of a flat-bottomed object resting on a table where the upper surface of the object

---

* To be more specific, this means that only the top surface contributes
  significantly to the scattering process.

can be represented by a single-valued elevation function. The appropriate formulation of the imaging problem and an iterative method of solution are given detailed discussions in the two earlier papers in this series (Richardson and Marsh, 1984, 1985). In the present paper, we present only a brief review of this method. In the last section, the evaluation of the algorithm with experimental test data is discussed.

Formulation of the Problem

We assume that an unknown solid object rests upon a rigid table within a known three-dimensional localization domain. A set of pulse-echo scattering measurements is made under conditions such that the localization domain and each transducer are in the far field of each other. We will define the incident wave to be the wave that would exist in the absence of the object and the scattered wave as the increment due to the presence of the object.

In formulating the measurement model, we limit our investigation to the case of objects described by single-valued elevation functions. We will use the Kirchhoff approximation for the scattering of acoustical waves under the assumption that the surfaces of the object and the table can be regarded as perfectly rigid. For the sake of simplicity, we will limit our discussion to situations in which acoustical shadows either cannot occur or can be neglected.

The appropriate measurement model is represented by the following expression

$$f(t,\vec{e}) = - \frac{\alpha c}{2\vec{e} \cdot \vec{e}_z} \sum_{\underline{r}} \delta\underline{r}$$
$$[p'(t - 2c^{-1}\vec{e}\cdot\underline{r} - 2c^{-1}\vec{e}\cdot\vec{e}_z \ Z(\underline{r})) \quad\quad (2.1)$$
$$-p'(t - 2c^{-1}\vec{e}\cdot\underline{r})] + \nu(t,\vec{e}) \quad .$$

The symbols in the above expression are defined below:

$f(t,\vec{e})$ = a possible measured scattered waveform at time t coming from a transducer having an incident wave direction $\vec{e}$.

$\nu(t,\vec{e})$ = experimental error associated with $f(t,\vec{e})$.

$p'(t)$ = time derivative of $p(t)$, the measurement system response function. The latter is defined to be the waveform produced by the measurement system if a fictitious scatterer with an impulse response function $R(t) = \delta(t)$ is positioned at the origin.

$\underline{r}$ = two dimensional vector $\vec{e}_x x + \vec{e}_y y$ giving positions in the xy-plane (the plane of the table top). It takes values on a two-dimensional mesh spanning the localization domain D_L. An elementary area of the mesh is denoted by $\delta\underline{r}$.

$Z(\underline{r})$ = elevation function (i.e., the value of the vertical coordinate z on the top surface at a horizontal position $\underline{r}$).

$\vec{e}_z$ = unit vector pointing in the +z direction.

α = constant dependent upon the properties of air.

c = velocity of acoustic waves in air.

The time t is assumed to take a discrete set of values corresponding to an appropriate sampling rate over a specified observation interval. The localization domain D_L (now two-dimensional) is defined by the
inequalities: $-1/2$ L $\leqslant$ x $<$ $1/2$ L and $-1/2$ L $\leqslant$ y $<$ $1/2$ L.

To give a complete description of the measurement model, we must
specify the a priori statistics of $Z(\underline{r})$ and $\nu(t,e)$. Here, we assume
that both entities are Gaussian random vectors with the properties

$$EZ(\underline{r}) = 0 \quad , \tag{2.2a}$$

$$EZ(\underline{r})Z(\underline{r}') = \delta_{\underline{rr}'} \, \sigma_Z^2 \quad , \tag{2.2b}$$

$$E\nu(t,\vec{e}) = 0 \quad , \tag{2.3a}$$

$$E\nu(t,\vec{e})\nu(t',\vec{e}') = \delta_{tt'} \, \delta_{\vec{e}\vec{e}'} \, \sigma_\nu^2 \quad , \tag{2.3b}$$

$$EZ(\underline{r})\nu(t,\vec{e}) = 0 \quad . \tag{2.4}$$

In Eqs. (2.2b) and (2.3b) the Kronecker deltas, $\delta_{\underline{rr}'}$, $\delta_{tt'}$, and $\delta_{\vec{e}\vec{e}'}$,
are generalized in an obvious way to the case of noninteger and, in some
cases, nonscalar subscripts. It is reasonable to assume that $Z(\underline{r})$ has a
positivity constraint. However, in order to focus exclusively on the
problems ensuing from the nonlinear dependence upon $Z(\underline{r})$ in the measurement model (2.1), we will defer this case to a later communication.

Our problem is to determine the most probable elevation function
given the results of scattering measurements. In more specific mathematical terms, our problem is to find the function Z that maximizes the
a posteriori probability denoted by $P(Z|f)$. Here, the symbol Z repre-
sents the values of $Z(\underline{r})$ for all $\underline{r}$ and, similarly, f represents the
values of $f(t,\vec{e})$ for all t and $\vec{e}$. We will now use the relation

$$P(Z|f) = P(f|Z)P(Z)/P(f) \tag{2.5}$$

where in the maximization process P(f) may be regarded as constant. The
factor $P(f|Z)$ is determined entirely by the model (2.1) and the a priori
statistical properties of the measurement error $\nu(t,\vec{e})$. The factor $P(Z)$
is determined by the a priori statistical properties of the elevation
function $Z(\underline{r})$.

Method of Solution

The determination of the most probable elevation function given the
results of scattering measurements, i.e., the determination of $Z(\underline{r})$ that
maximizes $P(Z|f)$, cannot be carried out by purely analytical means be-
cause of the nonlinear dependence upon $Z(\underline{r})$ in the measurement model
(2.1).

Our approach to the solution of this problem involves an iterative
procedure in which $f(t,\vec{e})$ and p'(t) are initially subjected to a common
smoothing operation that has the property that the smoothed version of
p'[$t-2c^{-1}\vec{e} \cdot \underline{r} - 2c^{-1}\vec{e} \cdot \vec{e}_z \, Z(\underline{r})$] can be linearized with respect to $Z(\underline{r})$.
Later stages of the procedure involve successive unsmoothing and linear-
izations with respect to incremental corrections to $Z(\underline{r})$.

Let us first consider the case in which the characteristic wavelength involved in p(t) is large compared with a characteristic eleva-

tion function Z^*, e.g., the a priori r.m.s. value of $Z(\underline{r})$. This means that $p'(t)$ can be regarded as linear to a sufficient level of accuracy in any time interval of length $2c^{-1} \vec{e} \vec{e}_z Z^*$. Thus, we can expand Eq. (2.1) in a power series in $Z(\underline{r})$, omitting second and higher power terms, with the result

$$f(t,\vec{e}) = \alpha \sum_{\underline{r}} \delta\underline{r}p''(t - 2c^{-1}\vec{e}.\underline{r})Z(\underline{r})$$

$$+ \nu(t,\vec{e}) \quad . \tag{3.1}$$

This is a linear model with Gaussian statistics, a case in which the optimal estimate (i.e., the most probable value given the measurement) is well known. It is given by the expression

$$\hat{Z}(\underline{r}) = \sigma_Z^2 \delta\underline{r}\alpha \sum_{t,\vec{e}} \sum_{t',\vec{e}'} p''(t - 2c^{-1}\vec{e}.\underline{r})$$

$$\times C_f(t,\vec{e}; t',\vec{e}')^{-1} f(t',\vec{e}') \quad , \tag{3.2}$$

where $C_f(t,\vec{e}; t',\vec{e}')^{-1}$ is the matrix inverse of

$$C_f(t,\vec{e};t',\vec{e}') = \sigma_Z^2 \delta\underline{r}\alpha^2 \sum_{\underline{r}} [\delta\underline{r}p''(t - 2c^{-1}\vec{e}.\underline{r})$$

$$\times p''(t' - 2c^{-1}\vec{e}'.\underline{r})] \tag{3.3}$$

$$+ \delta_{tt'} \delta_{\vec{e}\vec{e}'} \sigma_\nu^2 \quad .$$

A point worth noting is that in Eq. (3.2) the function $f(t,\vec{e})$ should be replaced by the set of actually measured values when the estimate is based upon measurements.

These results suggest an iterative method for the general case. As we have already indicated, the basic idea is to use a linearization with respect to the incremental correction in $Z(\underline{r})$ combined with a low-pass filtering operation, applied to $f(t,\vec{e})$ and $p(t)$ but not to $\nu(t,\vec{e})$, in order to make the linearization valid. In more explicit mathematical detail, we assume that the filtered versions of $f(t,e)$ and $p(t)$ are given by

$$f_m(t,\vec{e}) = H_m(t)*f(t,\vec{e}) \quad , \tag{3.4a}$$

$$p_m(t) = H_m(t)*p(t) \quad , \tag{3.4b}$$

where * denotes temporal convolution and $H_m(t)$ is the time-domain transfer function representing the low-pass filter associated with the mth stage. The exact model for the filtered measurement process for the mth stage is clearly given by

$$f_m(t,\vec{e}) = - \frac{\alpha c}{2\vec{e}\cdot\vec{e}_z} \sum_{\underline{r}} \delta\underline{r}[p_m'(t - 2c^{-1}\vec{e}\cdot\underline{r}$$

$$- 2c^{-1}\vec{e}\cdot\vec{e}_z \ Z(\underline{r})) - p_m'(t - 2c^{-1}\vec{e}\cdot\underline{r})]$$

$$+ \nu(t,\vec{e}) \quad . \tag{3.5}$$

The remainder of the iterative procedure is conveniently described in terms of abbreviated notation. To this end, we rewrite Eq. (3.5) in the form

$$f_m = g_m(Z) + \nu \tag{3.6}$$

in which the correspondence with Eq. (3.5) is obvious, except perhaps for the fact that in the above expression, Z is a vector whose components are $Z(\underline{r})$. Linearization with respect to the deviation of Z from the previous estimate Z_{m-1} yields the result

$$f_m = g_m \ (\hat{Z}_{m-1}) + A_m \ (Z - \hat{Z}_{m-1}) + \nu \tag{3.7}$$

where A_m is a matrix (in general not square) defined by

$$A_m^T = (\frac{\partial}{\partial Z} g_m \ (Z)^T)_{Z = \hat{Z}_{m-1}} \quad . \tag{3.8}$$

The best estimate $\hat{Z}_m$ for the present stage can be readily obtained by a straightforward application of linear least m.s. estimation theory as was done for Eq. (3.1).

The next step in the recursive procedure is to select a time-domain transfer function $H_{m+1}(t)$ corresponding to a higher frequency roll-off in the low-pass filter (this represents an incremental unsmoothing of the previously smoothed $f(t,\vec{e})$ and $p(t)$). We then use $Z_m(\underline{r})$ as a new point in state space about which the measurement model is to be linearized. We then obtain eventually a new estimate $Z_{m+1}(\underline{r})$.

The total iterative procedure is straightforward, at least in principle. We commence with $Z_0(\underline{r}) = 0$, or some other initial estimate, and a choice of $H_1(t)$ such that the characteristic wavelengths involved in the smoothed version of $f(t,\vec{e})$ and $p(t)$ are sufficiently long. The recursion process is carried on until the difference between successive approximations becomes sufficiently small according to a suitable criterion.

Computational Example

In this section, we present an example of the above iterative approach using synthetic test data. The main purpose of this computation is to provide some insight into what imaging performance is possible with a relatively sparse set of scattering measurements in the absence of scattering theory errors and measurement error. The first type of error is avoided by using the same Kirchhoff approximation in both the preparation of synthetic data and the imaging procedure; however, a major part of the Kirchhoff error is avoided by limiting our treatment to cases in which acoustical shadowing does not exist, and in which the slopes of the elevation function are, in general, not too large. The second type of error, i.e., that due to imperfect measurement, is avoided by setting $\sigma_\nu = 0$ in the preparation of test data. It is to be emphasized that in the imaging algorithm a nonvanishing level of noise is assumed.

In the preparation of such test data, we assume that the solid object of interest is a regular tetrahedron with various degrees of squashing. Specifically, we assume that the tetrahedron rests upon the rigid table with its vertical scale reduced by 0.75, 0.5 and 0.25, respectively. These assumed solid objects are depicted in Fig. 1a. The bottom face is bounded by an equilateral triangle whose sides are assumed to have a common length of 13.75 mm. In this example we have assumed a set of five pulse echo measurements each with an incident direction

$$-\vec{e} = (\vec{e}_x \cos \phi + \vec{e}_y \sin \phi) \sin \theta + \vec{e}_z \cos \theta$$

(4.1)

given by the values of azimuthal and polar angles, ϕ and θ, respectively, tabulated below

| $\theta =$ | 0 | 54.7° | 54.7° | 54.7° | 54.7° | , |
| $\phi =$ | − | 0° | 90° | 135° | 225° | . |

The nonuniform spacing of the azimuthal angles was chosen to avoid (at least partially) certain ambiguities associated with excessive symmetry of the measurement system.

The constant α will be taken equal to 1 since its common value occurs in both the preparation of synthetic test data and the imaging problem and can be regarded as self-cancelling. The velocity of sound

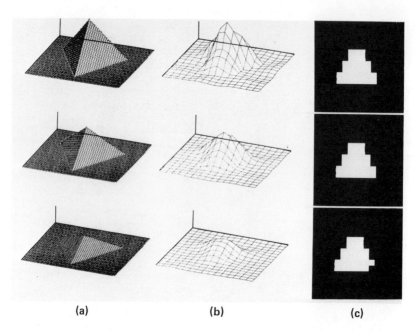

(a)   (b)   (c)

Fig. 1 Imaging of squashed tetrahedra using synthetic data: (a) true image; (b) reconstructed image; (c) x-section, 30% maximum.

in air, c, is assumed to be 345 m s^{-1} = 0.345 mm $(\mu s)^{-1}$. We will use a signal-to-noise ratio η defined by

$$\eta = \tilde{f}(t,\vec{e})_{max}/\sigma_\nu \qquad (4.2)$$

where $\tilde{f}(t,\vec{e})_{max}$ is the maximum (with respect to t and $\vec{e}$) of the waveform corresponding to noiseless synthetic test data and where σ_ν is the standard deviation of $\nu(t,\vec{e})$, as defined by Eq. (2.3b). The function p(t) is given in the frequency domain by a Hanning window between the frequency limits F_{min} and F_{max}.

In Table 1 below, we list the sequence of parameter values used in the present example of the iterative solution. Here, we will assume that each low-pass filtering operation (corresponding to the time-domain convolution of $H_m(t)$ with p(t)) is represented by a Hanning window with upper and lower limits F_{max} and F_{min}. approximately equivalent to changing one Hanning window into another. In the iterations, we will specify the various values of F_{max} assumed, but we will take a fixed value of F_{min} = 1 kHz.

Table 1
Estimation Parameters

Iteration No.	F_{max} (kHz)	$f(t,e)_{max}/\sigma_\nu$
1	10	10
2	10	10
3	10	10
4	20	10
5	30	10
6	30	10
7	40	10
8	40	30

In Fig. 1b, we present the estimated elevation functions Z($\underline{r}$) corresponding to the three assumed squashed tetrahedra shown in Fig. 1a. The comparisons are surprisingly good in view of the sparseness of the measured scattering data. There is clear evidence that the iterative unsmoothing method estimates a number of spatial frequency components of Z($\underline{r}$) that are not directly measured. This is a consequence of the nonlinear dependence of the measurement model on Z($\underline{r}$), as seen in Eq. (2.1). The cross sections of the estimated elevation functions at 30% of maximum level are shown in Fig. 1c. Except for the bottom figure, the cross sections are as close to equilateral triangles as is possible with the rather coarse mesh employed.

Experimental Results

A series of experimental scattering measurements was carried out on a squashed, pentahedron (i.e., a square-based pyramid) with two purposes: 1) to validate the measurement model (2.1); and 2) to demonstrate that the imaging algorithm performs satisfactorily with real data, although under conditions of very low external noise.

The pentahedron was machined out of a block of solid aluminum and its external geometry was four-fold symmetric with a height of 16.6 cm and length of 57.4 cm of each horizontal edge. This object was placed on a turntable to facilitate rotations equivalent to the opposite variations of the azimuthal angle involved in the definition of the incident direction corresponding to each transducer position. Each scattering measurement was made with separate transmitting and receiving transducers placed sufficiently close together to approximate a pulse-echo situation. To achieve satisfactory interfacing with air (in both transmit and receive modes), we made use of hi-fi technology with a tweeter as the transmitter and a microphone as the receiver. The total measurement system response function p(t) (appearing in Eq. (2.1) and defined subsequently) is characterized by a temporal frequency band extending from approximately 3 kHz to 30 kHz (at 20% of maximum amplitude). To reduce external noise to the lowest possible level, the scattering measurements were made in an anechoic chamber. Care was taken to insure that the transducer system (i.e., the transmitter and receiver combination) was in the far field of the object (more correctly, the localization volume) and vice versa.

Since, in the present treatment, the scattered wave is generally defined as the perturbation of the pressure field due to the pressure of object, it is necessary to make two scattering measurements, i.e., (a) with the pentahedron on the turntable, and (b) with the bare turntable, and then to subtract the waveform of measurement (b) from the waveform of measurement (a). Great care was required in the measurement process to obtain a satisfactory subtraction, including even the control of the air temperature.

Two kinds of calibration measurements were performed in advance: a) the difference between the waveforms obtained from the bare turntable and from the interior of the anechoic chamber with the turntable absent; and b) the difference between the waveforms obtained from a hemispherical object centered on the turntable and from the bare turntable. The first measurement was used to determine (with suitable transformations) the measurement system response function p(t). The second measurement was used to determine precisely the round-trip travel time of a pulse from the transducer system to the origin (in this case, the center of the turntable) and back.

The pulse-echo (approximately) scattering measurements corresponded to a set of azimuthal and polar angle, ϕ and θ, respectively, tabulated below.

θ =	0	45°	45°	45°	45°	45°
ϕ =	–	0°	90°	135°	225°	297°.

The relation between ϕ, θ and $\vec{e}$ is given by Eq. (4.1).

The iterative unsmoothing procedure discussed in Section 3 was applied to the experimental waveforms. The sequence of parameter values used in this procedure was approximately the same as that listed in Table 1, except that in the present case the sequence was more gradual, i.e., here the last line of the table corresponds to the 26th iteration. The images formed at the 17th and 26th iterations are presented in Figs. 2 and 3. In Fig. 2, there is a smoothed pentahedron in the center with a breakdown of the flat area smoothly depicted near the edges. In Fig. 3, the pentahedron is more clearly discernable and the breakdown of the flat area is more sharply defined. It is our conviction that this undesirable breakdown is associated with the failure to remove completely the scattering from the rim of the turntable in the subtraction process discussed above.

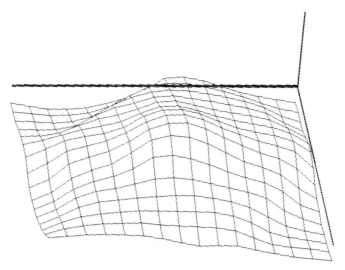

Fig. 2   Imaging of squashed pentahedron using experimental data
(17th iteration).

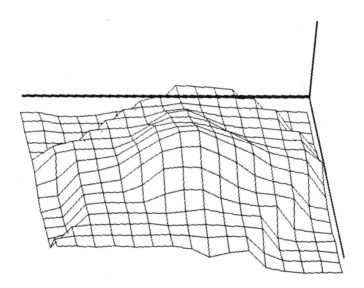

Fig. 3   Imaging of squashed pentahedron using experimental data
(26th iteration).

It is to be noted that in Figs. 2 and 3, the estimated peak heights
of the pentahedron are 19.8 mm and 21.0 mm, respectively, which are to
be compared with the true value of 16.6 mm. Normally, one would expect
the estimated values to be less than the true value with an asymptotic
trend of the estimated values toward the true value as the iterative

unsmoothing process proceeds. We believe that the excessive values of the estimated heights are due to small systematic errors in the determination of the roundtrip travel time from the transducer system to the origin.

Although more work clearly needs to be done, the imaging results based on experimental data suggest strongly the feasibility of the acoustical imaging of simple solid objects using a broadband transducer in a limited set of positions. There is clear evidence of the deduction of spatial frequency components of the elevation function on a well-distributed set of points in two-dimensional k-space outside of the set corresponding to the components directly measured.

References

Richardson, J.M. and Marsh, K.A., 1984, "Acoustic Imaging of Solid Objects in Air Using a Small Set of Transducers," Proc. of 1984 IEEE Ultrasonics Symp., p. 83.

Richardson, J.M. and Marsh, K.A., 1985, "Acoustic Imaging of Solid Objects in Air Using a Small Set of Transducers II. Probabilistic Ambiguities and Selection of Transducer Configurations," presented at 1985 IEEE Ultrasonics Symp.

A BROADBAND-HOLOGRAPHY IMAGING SYSTEM FOR NONDESTRUCTIVE EVALUATION

G. Prokoph, H. Ermert and M. Kröning[*]

Department of Electrical Engineering
University of Erlangen-Nuremberg
Cauerstr. 9, D-8520 Erlangen, FRG

[*]Kraftwerk-Union AG, D-8520 Erlangen, FRG

INTRODUCTION

Acoustical Holography has become a powerful means in computerized non-destructive testing. To obtain a good axial resolution the conventional monofrequent concept /1/ was extended to Multifrequency Holography /2/. Here the data-acquisition has to be repeated several times using a series of different frequencies. A further step is to excite the system with broadband signals, to obtain the object information over a certain range of frequencies within a single measurement procedure. This leads to the principle of "Broadband Holography", a reconstruction scheme, which is similar to the well known LSAFT algorithm /3/.

Broadband Holography is based on the same theoretical principles as the multifrequent concept, but it offers a regardable acceleration in data-acquisition. In the system described here, it is possible to adapt the system properties to the desired application by varying the transmitted signal. Furthermore, an analog preprocessing unit (down mixing) is included which reduces the requirements to A/D-converter in use. This paper shows the theoretical foundations of the imaging concept, describes the experimental setup and presents reconstructions of artificial and natural defects in steel.

THE THEORETICAL FOUNDATIONS OF THE IMAGING CONCEPT

Most of the theoretical foundations of the algorithm have already been discussed in /2/. Therefore, in this case a brief review should be sufficient. The geometrical relations are shown in Fig. 1. A transducer is moved across a linear aperture, from which the object area is to be viewed. It is excited by broadband pulses $F_{TR}(\omega)$ and receives the echo-signals $F_R(\omega, x_A)$ at the various aperture positions x_A. Both signals can be represented in the frequency domain ω. It is now possible to form an image-function as follows:

$$B(x,z) = \left| \int_{x_A} \int_{\omega} F_R(\omega, x_A) \cdot F_F^*(\omega, x_A, x, z) \, d\omega \, dx_A \right| \qquad (1)$$

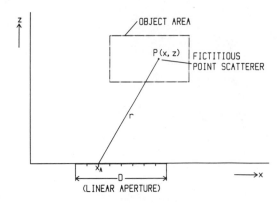

FIGURE 1: Geometrical relations of reconstruction

Equation (1) describes a spatial matched filter. The received signals F_R are compared with fictitious calculated signals, which would appear at position x_A, if there were an isolated scattering point at location $P(x,z)$. $B(x,z)$ represents the image intensity of the corresponding pixel.

The fictitious received signal can be seen as a filtered and time-delayed version of the transmitted waveform:

$$F_F(\omega,x_A,x,z) = F_{TR}(\omega) \cdot H(\omega) \cdot e^{-j\omega\tau_\ell(x_A,x,z)} \tag{2}$$

Here $H(\omega)$ is the superposition of all linear distortions in the system caused by transducer and electronic circuitry. τ_ℓ is the time of flight an ultrasonic pulse needs to propagate from the transducer at position x_A to the location of the fictitious point scatterer and back to the probe. τ_ℓ is dependent on the geometrical relations and can be expressed as follows:

$$\tau_\ell = 2/c \cdot \sqrt{(x - x_A)^2 + z^2} \tag{3}$$

The propagation factor $1/r^2$ is neglected in Equ. (2). This can be done in the case of a small object area, which is far enough away from the aperture. Inserting (2) in (1) we obtain:

$$B(x,z) = \left| \int_{x_A} \int_\omega F_R(\omega,x_A) \cdot F_{TR}^*(\omega) \cdot H(\omega)^* \cdot e^{j\omega\tau_\ell(x_A,x,z)} \, d\omega \, dx_A \right| \tag{4}$$

We now introduce a modified received signal which is defined as

$$F_R'(\omega, x_A) = F_R(\omega, x_A) \cdot F_{TR}^{*}(\omega) \cdot H(\omega)^{*} \tag{5}$$

F_R' is the received signal filtered by the product of the complex conjugate of the transmitted signal and the complex conjugate system transfer-function. Equation (4) can now be reduced to

$$B(x,z) = \left| \int_{x_A} \int_{\omega} F_R'(\omega, x_A) \cdot e^{j\omega \tau_{\ell}(x_A, x, z)} \, d\omega \, dx_A \right| \tag{6}$$

The inner integral represents a Fourier transform from the frequency into the time domain. Taking this into account Equation (6) can be re-written as follows:

$$B(x,z) = \left| \int_{x_A} f_R'(\tau_{\ell}, x_A) \cdot dx_A \right| \tag{7}$$

where $f_R'(\tau_{\ell}, x_A)$ is the complex valued inverse Fourier transform of $F_R'(\omega, x_A)$. Since the aperture is sampled at discrete points, the integral becomes a summation:

$$B(x,z) = \left| \sum_{\ell=1}^{NXA} f_R'(\tau_{\ell}, x_A) \right| \tag{8}$$

The index ℓ denotes the discrete aperture position.

Verbally, the reconstruction procedure can be seen as the summation of the complex valued and filtered A-scans according to their time of flight. To obtain the complex valued received signal an imaginary part must be formed and added to the real part, directly measured with a tran-sient recorder. The imaginary part $f_{RI}(t)$ may be evaluated from the real part $f_{RR}(t)$ by means of a Hilbert transform. This can be done with the help of a Fourier transform or - directly in the time domain - using an appropriate Finite Impulse Response digital filter. So we obtain Equation (9):

$$f_R(t) = f_{RR}(t) + j \cdot f_{RI}(t) = f_{RR}(t) + j \cdot HI(f_{RR}(t)) \tag{9}$$

where HI denotes the Hilbert transform operation.

THE CONCEPT OF OPTIMIZED TRANSMITTED SIGNALS

In the last paragraph we mentioned that it is necessary for the re-construction to form modified received signals by a linear filter-ope-ration and by adding the imaginary part. This leads to the system diagram in Figure 2a. Because of the linearity, it is possible to perform the filter-operation at any position in the system. Especially the transmitted signal can be filtered (Fig. 2b). It is also allowed to include the filtering process in the generation of the transmitted waveform. This can be done by using a function-synthesizer, which is able to generate arbitrary waveforms. So we achieve a further reduction of the computerized reconstruction-process, because the filtering needs no longer to be performed numerically.

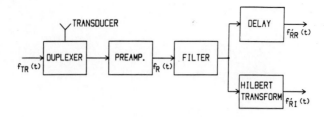

a) Filtering the received signals

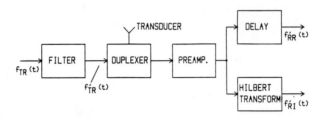

b) Filtering the transmitted waveform

FIGURE 2: Two possibilities to perform the necessary filter operation

Furthermore, the use of an arbitrary waveform-synthesizer allows us to adapt the system properties to different applications by choosing appropriate transmitted waveforms.

Inverse Filtering

If an optimum axial resolution is desirable, the transmitted signal should be chosen for the shortest possible echoes. This leads to the concept of inverse filtering. To calculate the related transmitted waveform it is necessary to know about the system transfer-function $H(\omega)$. The measurement of $H(\omega)$ can be performed by exciting the system with a pulse of short duration. The echo of a test reflector has to be recorded and to be Fourier transformed. The transmitted waveform is then defined as:

$$F_{TR}(\omega) = G(\omega)/H(\omega) \qquad (10)$$

where $G(\omega)$ is a window-function which has to be introduced due to the limited bandwidth. Appropriate windowing can be performed by different well known windows. In our experiments we used a truncated cosine (Tukey-

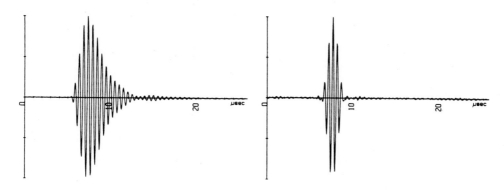

a) Measured impulse response

b) Measured response to an
   optimized excitation
   (inverse filtering)

FIGURE 3: Effects of using optimized transmitted waveforms

window). Figure 3 demonstrates the results obtained by inverse filtering.
Using a transmitted waveform calculated according to equation (10) leads
to a considerable reduction of echo-signal-duration.

Matched Filtering

A high attenuation in the media or a long distance from the aperture
to the object area often lead to a poor signal-to-noise-ratio. Under
those circumstances it is desirable to optimize the echoes for maximum
energy. $F_{TR}(\omega)$ has to be chosen as the complex conjugate of the system
transfer-function.

$$F_{TR}(\omega) = H(\omega)^{*} \qquad (11)$$

In time domain this means that the transducer has to be excited with the
time-inverse impulse-response.

Angle-Dependent Filtering

To take full use of a large aperture it is desirable to apply transducers with a wide beam. Unfortunately their transfer-characteristic is
angle-dependent even in the farfield region. These difficulties can be
overcome by using different transmitted signals related to special angle
ranges. In the case of a large object area it might be necessary to use
several transmitted waveforms at a single aperture point. A similar
range-dependent optimization can be done by defining several depth zones.

SYSTEM RESOLUTION

The axial resolution depends on the envelope of the received echoes.
It becomes optimal when using a transmitted waveform according to equation (10). When $G(\omega)$ is a truncated cosine with a total bandwidth of
$\Delta\omega = 2\pi B$ the axial resolution can be evaluated in a closed form:

$$\delta_{a} = 2c/B \qquad (12)$$

where c denotes the velocity of sound.

It is rather difficult to find a closed form expression of the lateral resolution. The analysis leads to integrals, which can only be evaluated numerically. The lateral resolution improves with the aperture size and the center-frequency and gets worse with the distance from the aperture. In the special case that the object area is located in a central position in front of the aperture it is possible to obtain an approximation:

$$\delta_\ell = 0.82 \; (z \cdot \lambda)/D \tag{13}$$

where D = aperture size
    z = distance of the object area
    λ = wavelength of the center frequency.

ANALOG PREPROCESSING UNIT AND SIGNAL-RESTORATION

Time domain measurement implies considerable requirements of the data-acquisition unit. Due to the poor resolution of available A/D-converters and transient recorders at high sampling rates, the system dynamic range might suffer and becomes too small for certain applications. To overcome this problem, we included an analog preprocessing unit, which makes use of the band-pass properties of the received signals. A well-known principle in communications is to describe band-limited signals f(t), which occupy a spectral range of $\omega_0 \mp \omega_1$, as follows:

$$f(t) = n(t) \cdot \cos \omega_0 t \; + \; q(t) \cdot \sin \omega_0 t \tag{14}$$

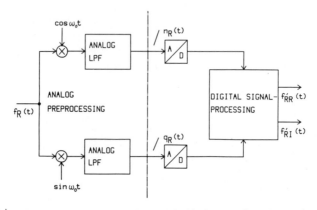

FIGURE 4: Analog preprocessing and digital signal restoration

where $n(t)$ is the in-phase component and $q(t)$ is the quadrature component referring to the band center frequency ω_0. The components have a spectral range from DC to ω_1. They can be obtained by multiplying $f(t)$ with two orthogonal carriers of ω_0 and a succeeding low-pass filtering (Fig. 4). Applying the above analog preprocessing principle leads to a remarkable reduction of the necessary sampling rate. For example, when using a band from 4 MHz to 6 MHz in the imaging system, the Nyquist theorem tells us to perform the digitization at a sampling rate of at least 12 Megasamples per second. The related components occupy only a spectral range from DC to 1 MHz. The corresponding minimum sampling rate is only 2 Megasamples per second. Thus A/D-converters with a high amplitude resolution (12 to 14 bits) become applicable.

The preprocessing unit can easily be adapted to different measurement frequencies by varying the carrier ω_0. To retain the high dynamic capability of the A/D-converter, great care must be taken on the analog component design. In our system we used double-balanced high-level Schottky-mixers which guarantee a sufficient dynamic range and low distortions due to intermodulation.

The image reconstruction requires the complex extension of the received signals. Therefore, the remaining task is to form $f_{RR}(t)$ and $f_{RI}(t)$ from $n_R(t)$ and $q_R(t)$ (Equation 9). It is obvious that for the evaluation of $f_{RR}(t)$ Equation (14) can directly be applied. In a similar way we obtain $f_{RI}(t)$:

$$f_{RR}(t) = n_R(t) \cdot \cos \omega_0 t \; + \; q_R(t) \cdot \sin \omega_0 t \qquad (15\text{ a})$$

$$f_{RI}(t) = n_R(t) \cdot \sin \omega_0 t \; - \; q_R(t) \cdot \cos \omega_0 t \qquad (15\text{ b})$$

Both operations can easily be performed in a digital signal-processing unit. Before multiplying with the orthogonal carriers, it is necessary to evaluate the components at a higher sampling rate. This can be done by resampling the digitized components with an appropriate rate. Thus, zero-elements are inserted between the original values. To obtain a correct interpolation a digital low-pass filter has to be applied to the series of samples. A hardware realization of the signal-processing described above is possible, but presently we perform the signal-restoration tion in the computer using a modified algorithm.

First we form the complex valued signal

$$c(t) = n_R(t) - j \cdot q_R(t) \qquad (16)$$

and calculate the corresponding spectrum:

$$C(\omega) = N_R(\omega) - j \cdot Q_R(\omega) \qquad (17)$$

An operation, equivalent to the above interpolation process in time domain is to add an appropriate number of zero-elements to the FFT-vector in frequency domain (trigonometric interpolation /4/). The multiplication with a carrier becomes a frequency shift:

$$C'(\omega) = C(\omega - \omega_0) = N_R(\omega - \omega_0) - j \cdot Q_R(\omega - \omega_0) \qquad (18)$$

An inverse Fourier transform leads to the corresponding time representation:

$$
\begin{aligned}
c'(t) &= n_R(t) \cdot e^{j\omega_0 t} - q_R(t) \cdot e^{j\omega_0 t} \\
&= n_R(t) \cdot \cos\omega_0 t + q_R(t) \cdot \sin\omega_0 t + j \cdot (n_R(t) \sin\omega_0 t - q_R(t) \cos\omega_0 t) \\
&= f_{RR}(t) + j \cdot f_{RI}(t)
\end{aligned}
\tag{19}
$$

It can be seen from Equation (19) that this method delivers directly the complex valued input-signal for the reconstruction process.

A TOMOGRAPHIC APPROACH

The lateral resolution of the imaging system increases with the aperture size. On the other hand, when using very large apertures, errors in time of flight calculation become more and more significant, so that the quality of reconstruction might suffer. This leads to the concept of partial synthetic apertures. Thus, the aperture is divided in several overlapping subregions. The reconstruction-process is performed for all parts independently. The resulting images are superimposed by adding them according to their spatial relations. This principle leads to a loss of lateral resolution but helps to reduce reconstruction errors due to improper phase cancellation.

Additionally there are some advantages. The object area is viewed from the partial apertures by different angles. This means a better reconstruction of reflecting plane and vaulted mirrors. The algorithm becomes similar to the limited angle reflection CT concept, applied in medicine /5/. Further filtering of the obtained images can improve the results.

Another possibility is to superimpose reconstructions, received by making use of different wave-types (shear and pressure waves) of the same transducer which leads to more object information concentrated in one image.

EXPERIMENTAL SETUP

Central system controller was a HP 9825 A desktop computer (see Fig. 5), which served to load the arbitrary waveform generator, to read the data from the transient recorder (Gould TR 4500) and to move the transducer with the help of a position controller. All analog parts except the power amplifier (ENI A 150), as well as the clock generator and the image memory are self-designed non commercial units.

Reconstructions were performed in a signal processor MSP 78 /6/, a special bit-slice minicomputer optimized for digital signal-processing or on a Control Data Cyber 845 general purpose computer. The resulting images were displayed either on a 256 grey scale or on a 3 x 256 RGB video monitor.

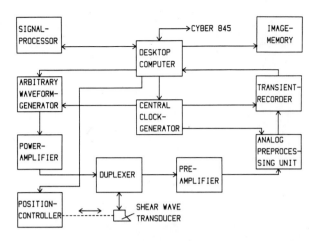

FIGURE 5: Experimental setup

The transducers used were special holography types supplied by the Kraftwerk Union AG, Erlangen and optimized for wide-angle beams. They work in a frequency range from 1.5 MHz to 3.5 MHz.

RESULTS

Finally, we present images of artificial and natural defects in steel. To give a better impression, photographs of the test objects are included. The artificial defects (Fig. 6) were five 2 mm holes drilled into a steel block. The natural crack (Fig. 7) has a size of about 50 mm. In both cases the aperture (length 40 mm) was located on the top left side of the object area. The apertures were sampled in steps of 0.5 mm. This leads to 81 aperture points. The frequency range was from 1.5 MHz to 3.5 MHz. A transmitting waveform according to Equation 10 (inverse filtering) was used.

CONCLUSION

The foundations of Broadband Holography were described as an extension of the multifrequent concept. The imaging properties can be altered by changing the waveform of the transmitted pulse. An analog preprocessing unit (down-mixing) helps to reduce the requirements to the data-acquisition unit. In practical experiments images of artificial and natural defects were generated.

This work was supported by the Kraftwerk Union AG, Erlangen.

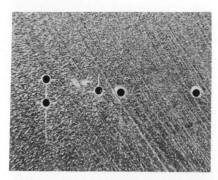

Figure 6: Photograph (a) and reconstruction (b) of an artificial
detect in a steel block

a)

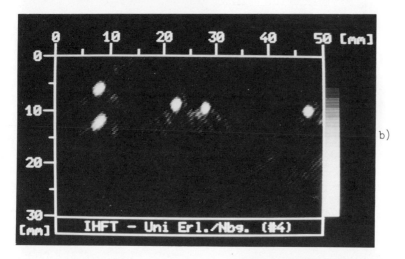

b)

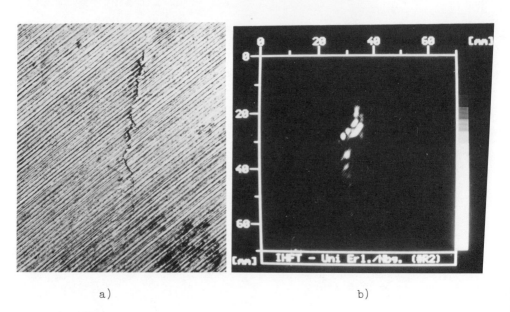

a)   b)

Figure 7: Photograph (a) and reconstruction (b) of a natural crack in
a steel block

REFERENCES

/1/ Ahmed, M., Wang, K., Metherell, A., Holography and its Applications
to Acoustic Imaging. Proceedings of IEEE, 67:4, pp. 466 - 483 (April
1979).

/2/ Ermert, H., Karg, R., Multifrequency Acoustical Holography, IEEE
Transactions on Sonics and Ultrasonics, SU - 26:4, pp 279 - 286 (July
1979).

/3/ Langenberg, K. J., Berger, M., Kreutter, Th., Mayer, K., Schmitz, V.,
SAFT Signal Processing, Preprint of a paper to be published in NDT
International,(1986).

/4/ Papoulis, A., Signal Analysis, McGraw Hill, New York (1977).

/5/ Röhrlein, G., Ermert, H., Limited Angle Reflection Mode Computerized
Tomography, 14th Symposium on Acoustical Imaging, pp 413 - 424,
(1985).

/6/ Kolb, H. J., Schloß, J., Ein Mikrosignalprozessor in Bit-Slice-Tech-
nik, Ausgewählte Arbeiten über Nachrichtentechnik Nr. 38, edited by
W. Schüßler, Erlangen (1979).

/7/ Nagai, K., Multifrequency Acoustical Holography Using a Narrow Pulse,
IEEE Transactions on Sonics and Ultrasonics, SU-31:3, pp 151 - 156,
(May 1984).

EFFICIENT ACOUSTICAL HOLOGRAPHY

AND PHASE IMAGING WITH HIGH RESOLUTION AT 3.6 MHz

USING A LIQUID CRYSTAL CONVERTOR

Jean-Luc Dion

Laboratoire d'Électronique industrielle, Département d'Ingénierie
Université du Québec à Trois-Rivières
Trois-Rivières, Québec, G9A 5H7

INTRODUCTION

For some time, the field of acoustical holography at megahertz frequencies has suffered a decline due to various causes such as complexity of implementation, excessive computation times, artifacts due to coherence, etc. Overall, the lack of fast and relatively simple means of conversion of the acoustical hologram into a visible image has been a decisive factor. As we know, three main field detection and recording techniques have evolved in the last twenty years or so:

a) One- or two-dimensional scanning with a transducer or a transducer array. [1-3]
b) Levitation of a liquid surface. [4-6]
c) Nematic liquid crystal convertor. [7-12]

The first technique, because of the finite size of transducers, is generally limited to frequencies below 1 MHz. It is also rather slow, due to long computing times. For these reasons it has suffered some loss of interest in the last years in favor of the non-holographic systems. Liquid surface acoustical holography has seemed promising since it is a real-time process, but the technique has some serious drawbacks related to its operating principles that limit the applications.

The technique that we have conceived and developed in the last years has evolved from our discovery of a direct coupling of the ultrasonic field with the direction of nematic liquid crystal molecules in an oriented thick layer between specially designed windows; a structural distortion is produced since the molecules tend to orient themselves perpendicular to the acoustic displacement. When an acoustical hologram is formed on the cell or convertor, a distortion is produced according to the amplitude and phase of the ultrasonic field. With an appropriate optical system using a simple incoherent light source, this hologram is directly visible as a fringed image. As such, it can hardly be interpreted. We use a relatively simple analog or digital processing technique to "unfringe" the hologram, to produce either intensity or phase images. The present system operates at about 3.5 MHz and produces a high resolution image in about 10 to 60 seconds depending on the type of image required and the processing technique used. Resolution power is nearly one wavelength, that is less than 1 mm at the actual frequency. We will present the operating principles of the system, with images of various materials. The first phase images and interferometric acoustic holograms ever made with this technique will be shown, illustrating its possibilities in the field of non-destructive testing of materials.

OPERATING PRINCIPLES

Nematic liquid crystal convertor

A cross-section of the LCC is shown in fig. 1. The stratified walls are made of two glass sheets separated by a polymeric layer having a total thickness of about 350 micrometers. This structure is highly transparent to ultrasonic waves at 3.6 MHz for widely varying angles of incidence. This is an essential condition for this particular acoustic interaction to take place and be exploited [13]. The liquid crystal (LC) has the homotropic structure (molecules perpendicular to the walls) and its thickness is about 250 μm. Under the action of the acoustic field, the molecules tend to orient their long axis perpendicular to the acoustic displacement. The torque has been demonstrated [13,14] to be given by:

$$C = \frac{2aI\Delta\alpha}{v} \sin 2\phi \;\; Nm/m \; , \tag{1}$$

where a is the thickness of the layer, I the acoustic intensity, $\Delta\alpha$ the anisotropy of acoustic attenuation, v the propagation velocity in the LC, and ϕ the angle between the acoustic displacement and the long molecular axis. This produces a distortion of the LC structure which is made visible when the cell is placed between crossed polarizers whose axes make an angle of 45° with the plane of acoustic displacement. When two coherent acoustic waves are made to interfere in the plane of the LC layer, the induced distortion produces visible fringes. [10] The nematic compound has positive dielectric anisotropy, allowing rapid reorientation of the molecules in an AC electric field produced between a semi-transparent electrode on one wall and the opposite water surface across the LC. This provides fast erasure of the hologram.

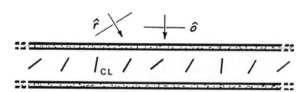

Fig. 1   Cross-section of a nematic liquid crystal convertor showing the reorienting action of the ultrasonic field.

Ultrasonic imaging system

The ultrasonic LC holographic camera is shown schematically in fig. 2. The heart of the system is the liquid crystal cell or convertor (LCC) C described above. The object to be examined is irradiated in a separate tank by transducer T_0, and the energy transmitted to the second tank is focussed on C by an hydro-acoustic lens (Fig. 3), after reflection on the acoustic mirror M_a (glass plate). The LCC is highly transparent to ultrasonic waves at the operating frequency of 3.6 MHz which are finally absorbed after reflection by M_a'. A plane reference wave coming from transducer T_r passes through M_a and interferes with the object wave in the liquid crystal layer C. The ultrasonic control system generates appropriate pulsed sinusoidal signals with variable delay between the reference and object channels to produce overlapping of wave trains on C. The two beams being coherent, a stable interference pattern or hologram is produced in the layer where they interact with the molecular orientation.

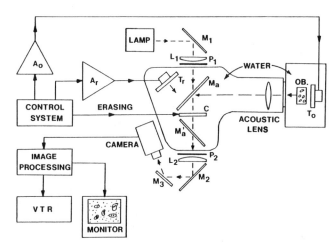

Fig. 2   Schematic of the nematic liquid crystal holographic camera.

This pattern is an image hologram (fringed image) which is made directly visible by means of a cylindrical (parallel) polarized light beam produced by an assemby of incandescent light source, lenses, polarizers and mirrors. The fringe contrast is a function of the object wave intensity for a given reference wave intensity. Their position is a function of the phase of the object wave. A video camera provides corresponding signals for the image processing system. One video line is essentially formed of a quasi-sinusoidal carrier signal, amplitude modulated by the fringe contrast, and phase modulated by the fringe position or object wave phase. A typical hologram, as seen on the convertor is shown in fig. 4

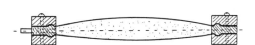

Fig. 3 Liquid-filled acoustic
lens. Polyester membranes
(Mylar), 50 micron-thick,
between brass rings, clear
diameter 120 mm.
Liquid: fluorinated compound
FC-75- (3-M, Inc.).
Focal length 15 cm.

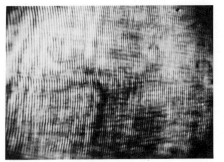

Fig. 4 Typical image-hologram
as photographed on the
liquid crystal cell
(LCC).

Image processing

The "unfringing" of the hologram to obtain an intensity image is readily done by analog techniques that give instant conversion [10,12]. Phase images and interferometric holograms require video frame recording and processing which are now achieved by digital techniques in a few seconds. We use a MATROX 8086 image processing system with 512 X 512, 8-bit color pixels capacity.

Intensity imaging As described in principle in previous publications, a visible image corresponding to acoustic intensities may be obtained essentially by amplitude demodulation of the video signal. Along one line, this signal may be approximated by [10,12]

$$S(t) = C(t) + A(t) \cos\{\omega_1 t + \psi(t)\}, \qquad (2)$$

where $C(t)$ is a low frequency component corresponding to background brightness, and $A(t) \cos(...)$ is a carrier signal whose amplitude $A(t)$ is modulated by the acoustic intensity. Its phase $\psi(t)$ is modulated by the fringes position according to the phase of the object wave.

Digital processing for intensity imaging is simulated in fig. 5. In 5-a, we see the digital sampling of 15 fringes whose contrast in the second part is twice that in the first, at 5 samples per period. Fig. 5-b shows the running average over 5 samples (low-pass filtering). Then, the absolute difference between the previous samples is taken, achieving full-wave rectification of the difference: the result is shown at double scale in 5-c. Finally, the running average on 5 samples, done twice, is shown in fig. 5-d, this last signal representing the modulation amplitude of the carrier signal. Fig. 6 shows the results obtained with a striped pattern (6-a) simulating a hologram as taken by a video camera. Fig. 6-b is given in about 20 seconds by the digital processing described above. It shows the rendition of various shades of gray corresponding to fringe contrast. Our experience shows that analog processing is more efficient for this purpose though: an unfringed image is obtained in real-time. The following images were unfringed analogically. In practice, the carrier signal corresponding to the fringes have an average frequency of about 1.5 MHz.

Holographic phase imaging and interferometry [15,16] To obtain a phase image corresponding to the fringe shift which is a function of the phase of the ultrasonic wave, a reference signal is required. This can be done by recording a hologram of the background. One related video line may be approximated by

$$S_o(t) = C_o(t) + A_o(t) \cos\{\omega_1 t + \psi_o(t)\}, \qquad (3)$$

while the corresponding line of the object hologram is given by Eq. 2. The difference between Eq. 2 and 3 gives the interferometric hologram signal $S'(t)$. It is easily shown that:

$$S'(t) = C'(t) + A'(t) \cos\{\omega_1 t + \psi'(t)\}, \qquad (4)$$

where, if we simplify to $\psi_o(t) = 0$:

$$A'(t) = \{A^2 - 2A_o A \cos\psi(t) + A_o^2\}^{1/2} \qquad (5)$$

Therefore, the carrier amplitude $A'(t)$ will follow the phase of the object wave which is related to $\psi(t)$. In practice, with the processor, we take the difference of (4) and (5), after subtracting a constant from (4) so that no negative values are obtained. What results is the difference

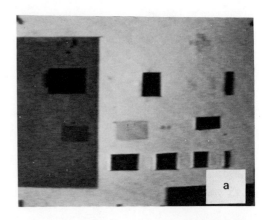

a

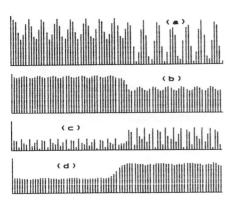

(a)

(b)

(c)

(d)

Fig. 5 Simulation of the digital
processing for intensity
imaging.

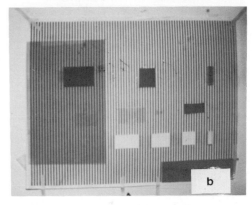

b

Fig. 6 Simulation of a hologram
using a striped pattern
with various contrast values
(a), and the resulting image
with digital unfringing (b).

hologram: fringes appear where there is a difference between the two
holograms. Then, this digitized differential hologram is "unfringed" by
the digital or the analog technique, giving the phase or difference image.
As we will see later, this operation eliminates many artifacts due to some
LCC imperfections, since whatever is present in both holograms is
eliminated by subtraction. A simulation of the technique is shown in Fig.
7. Fig. 7-a is the same striped pattern as in Fig. 6-a, simulating
fringes of various contrasts with different mean levels, while 7-b differs
by an added rectangle with fringes shifted relative to the background.
The difference of the two leaves only the rectangle with contrasted
fringes, as shown in Fig. 7-c. When the corresponding video signal is fed
to the analog or the digital unfringing systems, we obtain the white
rectangle shown in Fig. 7-d. We notice that the small area with lower
fringe contrast visible in 7-a and c is rendered as a dark spot in 7-d.

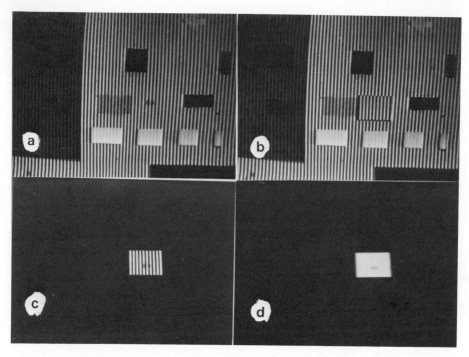

Fig. 7   Simulation of phase imaging and interferential holography.

EXPERIMENTAL RESULTS

Various results using digital and/or analog processing applied to ultrasonic holography with a liquid crystal convertor are shown in the following figures representing intensity or phase images. We used an operating frequency of 3.6 MHz, at which the wavelength of ultrasound in water at 25° C is about 0.42 mm. In most cases, we used the full lens opening of 120 mm, and the Rayleigh criterion gives a resolution of about 1 mm in the object plane, at 200 mm from the lens. The sharpness of the various images indicates that this is attained and even surpassed, since the response of the LCC with the whole system is non-linear. All images were photographed on a TV monitor.

Intensity imaging

Fig. 8-a shows an embossed plastic flag of Québec, with an irregular thickness of about 2 mm. The stripes are about 3 mm wide. The image-hologram of this object is shown in Fig. 4. Fig. 8-b is the processed intensity image of the specimen placed between acrylic plates, 2 mm thick, where the empty space was filled with parafin oil; left and right inverted. This demonstrates resolution better than the optical Rayleigh criterion. Fig. 9-a represents the processed image of a graphite-epoxy composite plate, about 2 mm thick, with induced circular delaminations . The smallest has a diameter of about 3 mm. The specimen was provided by CANADAIR Ltd, of Montréal. Fig. 9-b is the same as the preceeding one, where small air bubbles retained between the specimen and the transducer produced the additional spots. The sharpness of the edges is to be noticed, as is the mottled appearance related to this particular structure. These show that abnormalities are quite easily visualized in this type of material, with theoretical image resolution achieved. Such images are typically obtained in less than 8 seconds, using simply analog processing of the video signal.

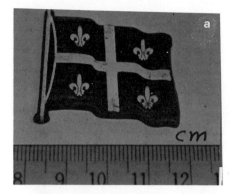 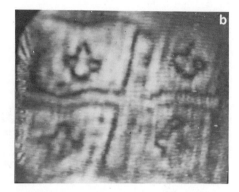

Fig. 8 (a) Embossed plastic specimen, about 2 mm thick.
(b) Intensity image of the specimen.

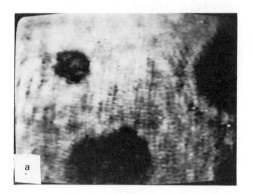 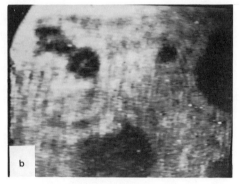

Fig. 9 (a) Intensity image of a graphite-epoxy composite plate with induced circular delaminations: the smallest has a diameter of 3 mm.
(b) Same as the preceding one with air bubbles on the surface.

On the other hand, digital processing allows some improvements of image quality which we have begun to study. Particularly, artifacts which are present when only the reference transducer T_r is energized are radically eliminated when the background image (with T_r alone) is partially subtracted from the hologram of the object before unfringing. Other artifacts are either dark or white spots due to imperfections of the LCC, or random fringes due to multiple reflections or lack of uniformity of the reference field. Fig. 10-a shows a specimen in the form of a small water-filled plexiglas box which can be deformed slightly by increasing the pressure with a syringe. It contains a few small metal washers and pieces of 100 micron-thick mylar. In 10-b, we see the straightforward image of a part of the specimen obtained with analog unfringing: several white spots can be seen due to imperfections of the LCC, along with various parasitic fringes produced by multiple reflections of the reference beam in particular. Fig. 10-c shows the enhanced hologram obtained after subtracting part of the background image from the original hologram and level multiplication. Fig. 10-d illustrates the improvement in the final image; the various artifacts are radically eliminated. We notice in 10-b and 10-d that the characteristic features of the star washer at the bottom are visible: points of the internal star pattern are less than 1 mm apart, imbedded in epoxy cement.

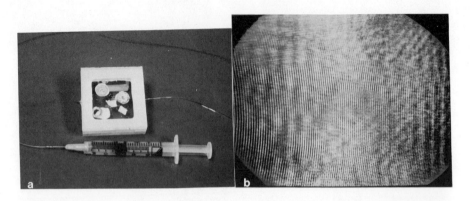

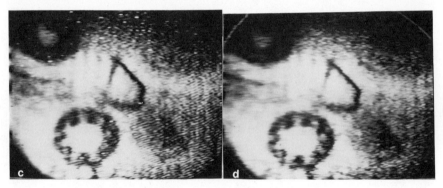

Fig. 10 (a) Inflatable plexiglas specimen with cemented metal and plastic parts inside.
        (b) Direct intensity image of the specimen.
        (c) Processed hologram of the specimen.
        (d) Processed image to be compared with (b).

Phase imaging We demonstrate here the possibility of making visible, by means of phase imaging, objects that are hardly visible with the preceding technique since they produce negligible attenuation of ultrasonic energy, and therefore produce negligible variation of white level in the processed image. Fig. 11-a is the intensity image of a polyester stripe (Mylar), 8 mm wide and 250 μm thick. Only the edges are visible because of diffraction effects. As such, it would be impossible to conclude as to the nature of the object. A hologram of the background, without the object is then taken and subtracted from the object hologram. This leaves the difference hologram shown in Fig. 11-b; fringes exists only where there is a difference between the two holograms. A phase shift of 180° between ultrasonic waves in the two cases gives the maximum fringe contrast in the interferometric hologram. When this last hologram is unfringed, it gives the white stripe of Fig. 11-c, the phase image of the object. In Fig. 11-d, we see the phase image of a four-step specimen made by cementing four stripes of Mylar, 25 μm thick and 5 mm wide. The phase-shift produced by the 25 μm part which is about 2 mm wide, is only about 15° as given by calculations. We may distinguish the four parallel zones representing the increasing thickness from the top to the bottom of the picture.

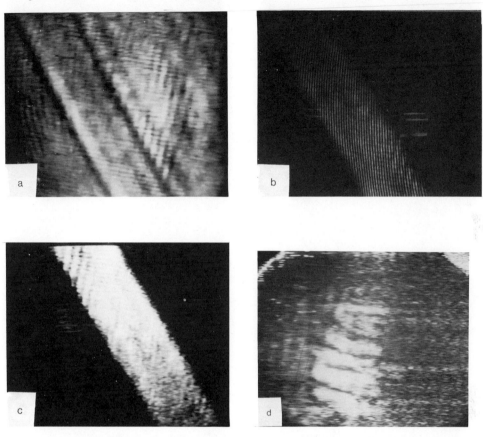

Fig. 11 (a) Intensity image of 250 μm thick, 8 mm wide, mylar strip.
(b) Difference between background and object holograms.
(c) Phase image of mylar strip.
(d) Phase image of four step mylar specimen, 25 to 100 μm thick.

Interferometric holography   Finally, with the deformable specimen of Fig. 10-a, we show the possibilities of the system in making visible structural variations which take place in an object between two successive instants. The first image in Fig. 12-a was taken with no pressure applied on the syringe. Its image-hologram was then recorded. Another hologram was taken after applying a pressure on the syringe that produced an increase of thickness in the center of about 50 microns. A constant was subtracted from every pixel of the first one which was then subtracted from the second one. The processed (unfringed) image resulting from this operation is shown in Fig. 12-b. The difference between these two images represents the change produced in thickness of the specimen. Irregular stresses due to the square shape of the specimen, and the presence of cemented objects inside, produce this particular pattern difference.

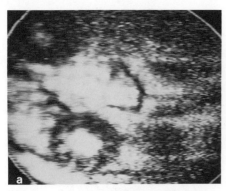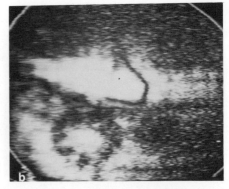

Fig. 12 (a) Intensity image of specimen of Fig. 10-a; no pressure
        applied.
      (b) Image resulting from the unfringing of the interferen-
        tial hologram, after applying pressure.

CONCLUSION

   We have shown that ultrasonic holography at about 3.5 MHz can, in a
few seconds, yield practical amplitude (or intensity) images at high
resolving power using a special nematic liquid crystal convertor (LCC).
The system incorporating digital image processing can also easily achieve
phase imaging and interferometric ultrasonic holography. The LCC is
essentially a quadratic two-dimensional detector which can directly
convert an ultrasonic hologram into a visible hologram and provide a high
resolution image of the ultrasonic field in its plane, after a rather
simple image processing. It is more or less the equivalent for ultrasonic
energy of the photographic film for light, with the additional advantage
of near real-time processing. Several improvements are still possible,
mainly in the LCC which is a fairly delicate device to assemble. It is
believed that its operating frequency could eventually be raised over 10
MHz where the resolving power could be better than 300 micrometers. The
system should normally find several applications in the field of
non-destructive testing of materials, as an intermediate system between
the ultrasonic microscope and the various scanning devices at lower
frequencies.

REFERENCES

1. B. HOSTEN and J. ROUX, " Visualisation numérique d'un champ ultrasonore aérien", Acustica, v. 40, pp. 240-245, 1978.
2. M. AHMED, K.Y. WANG and A.F. METHERELL, "Holography and its
   applications to acoustic imaging", Proc. IEEE, v.67, No 4, pp.
   466-483, 1979.
3. Y. AOKI, "Image reconstruction by computer" in Acoustical
   holography, Acoustical Holography,, v. 5, P.S. GREEN, ed., (Plenum
   Press, N.Y., 1974), pp. 551-572.
4. B.B. BRENDEN, "History and present status of liquid surface
   acoustical holography", J. Acoust. Soc. Amer., v. 58, pp. 951-955,
   1975.
5. A.V. CLARK, Jr., "On obtaining maximum performance from liquid
   surface levitation holography", Acoustical Imaging, v. 8, A.F.
   METHEREL, ed., (Plenum Press, 1980), pp. 417-454.

6. "ARTHIR: Acoustical real-time holographic image reproduction", HTIAC Newsletter, v. 7, No 11, 1980, U.S. Dept. of Def. Inf. Analysis Center.

7. P. GREGUSS, "A new liquid crystal acoustical-to-optical display", Acustica, V. 29, pp. 52-58, 1973.

8. J.N. PERBET, M. HARENG, S. LE BERRE and B. MOUREY, "Visualisation d'images acoustiques à l'aide d'un cristal liquide nématique", Revue Tech. Thomson-CSF, 11, No 4, pp. 837-870, 1979.

9. O.A. KAPUSTINA and V.N. LUPANOV, "Acousto-optical properties of a nematic crystal layer with homogeneous orientation", Sov. Phys. JETP, v. 44, No 6, pp. 1225-1228, 1976.

10. J.L. DION, A. LEBLANC and A.D. JACOB, "Pseudo-holographic acoustical imaging with a liquid crystal convertor", Acoustical Imaging, v. 10, A.F. METHERELL, ed., (Plenum Press, 1982), pp. 151-166.

11. J.L. DION, Canadian Patent No. 1, 112, 750; U.S. Patent No. 4, 338, 821; European Patent No. 0,010,492.

12. J.L. DION, A. MALUTTA and J. BUSSIÈRE, "Caméra ultrasonore à cristal liquide", Advanced NDE Technology / Développements Récents en Evaluation non-destructive, Symposium, 1982, Institut de Génie des Matériaux, C.N.R.C., Boucherville, (Québec).

13. JEAN-LUC DION, "Un nouvel effet des ultrasons sur l'orientation d'un cristal liquide, C.R. Acad. Sc. Paris, 284, série B, pp. 219-222, 1977.

14. J.L. DION and A.D. JACOB, "A new hypothesis on ultrasonic interaction with a nematic liquid crystal", Appl. Phys. Lett., v.31, No 8 (1977), pp. 490-493.

15. B.P. HILDEBRAND and K. SUZUKI, "Acoustical holographic interferometry", Jap. J. Appl. Phys., v. 14, No 6, pp. 805-813, 1975.

16. J. PASTEUR and Y. SEYZERIAT, "Holographie acoustique; application au traitement optique de l'information acoustique", Optica Acta, v. 24, No 8, pp. 859-875, 1977.

NDE IN MULTILAYERS: THEORY, COMPUTER

SIMULATION AND EXPERIMENTS

J.-P. Zhang and Y. Wei

Department of Biomedical Engineering
Nanjing Institute of Technology
People's Republic of China

ABSTRACT

Two recurrence formulae have been deduced to make time-efficient predictions of normal and off-normal responses respectively by computer. The discussion of obvious influences of significant factors on the responses makes it true to direct the practical flaw detection. Finally, after being processed the experimental data obtained prove that the theory and computer simulation are satisfactory to some extent.

INTRODUCTION

Wave motion in layered media has been studied for several decades. The theory of the solution to the wave motion equation, referred to as the direct problem, has been perfectly described, 1,2,3,4,5 and the algorithms for the inverse problem of the wave equation have more been developed over recent years, 6,7,8,9,10 as the non-destructive imaging of the interior properties of objects always results in finding out the algorithms for inverse problems. But most of the algorithms are available only to one wave mode longitudinal or transverse wave) and non-attenuative media, furthermore, they generally appear to be unstable and non-unique. Therefore, as for NDE in attenuative multilayers, such as composite structures consisting of metal layers bonded with non-mental layers by adhesives, other methods have to be developed, one of which will be discussed later in this paper.

The conventional methods used for NDE in multilayers are mainly acoustic resonance and impedance methods 11,12,13. These methods have poor longtudinal resolution when they are used to detect flaws in adhesive layers and cannot be applied to determine the elastic properties of adhesive layers quantitatively, which makes the analysis of bond strength impossible. So a method which uses compact ultrasonic pulse to excite multilayers and signal processing techniques 14,15,16,17,18 may solve the above problems. This method was presented in published papers, 19,20 and has been further described for its theory, computer simulation, and experiments in this paper.

The paper's outline is as follows. First, we use the theory of elasticity to deduce two recurrence formulae for quickly predicting the responses of normal and off-normal incident pulses respectively, and suggest the concept of propagator-tree in off-normal incidence. Next comes a section on computer simulation and the discussion of the influences of two factors – bandwidth and flaws on predicted responses. In the following section, experimental data are obtained and compared with simulated results. The last section is summary and conclusions.

THEORY OF ELASTIC PULSE WAVE PROPAGATING IN MULTILAYERS

The action of an incident pulse wave on media is a transient process. The propagation of an ultrasonic pulse (regarded as an elastic wave) in frequency dependently attenuative layers turns out to be rather complicated. In this paper, wave motion in two dimensional isotopic multilayers is discussed by fourier expansion.

Let a planar elastic wave with displacement vector $\vec{U}_e(\vec{r},t)$ be incident on a multilayer, and the amplitude of a planar sinuidial wave $\vec{U}_e(\vec{r},w)$ can be expressed as follows:

$$\vec{U}_e(\vec{r},\omega) = \int \vec{U}_e(\vec{r},t)\, e^{-i\omega t}\, dt \tag{1}$$

where $\vec{r}$ is position vector; t time variable and w angular frequency.

If nonlinear effects are neglected, the response $\vec{U}_o(\vec{r},t)$ of the multilayer can be written as

$$\vec{U}_o(\vec{r},t) = \int \vec{H}(\vec{r},\omega) \times \vec{U}_e(\vec{r},\omega)\, e^{i\omega t}\, dt \tag{2}$$

here, $\vec{H}(\vec{r},w)$ is called transfer function of the multilayer, which characterizes the multilayer. Later we will only deduce the expression of $\vec{H}(\vec{r},w)$ theoretically.

Complex Potentials

In an isotropic attenuative medium which has complex elastic constants $\lambda(w)$ and $\mu(w)$, the relation between stress $S_{ij}(\vec{r},w)$ and displacement $U(\vec{r},w)$ is simplified to

$$S_{ij}(\vec{r},\omega) = \delta_{ij}\,\lambda(\omega)\, U_{k,k}(\vec{r},\omega) + \mu(\omega)(U_{i,j}(\vec{r},\omega) + U_{j,i}(\vec{r},\omega)) \tag{3}$$

where repeated subscripts denotes sum Σ and comma (,) between two subscripts denotes patial derivative, for example $U_{k,k}(\vec{r},w) = \sum_{k=1}^{3} \partial U_k(\vec{r},w)/\partial r_k$

The motion equation of displacement $\vec{U}(\vec{r},w)$ is

$$U_{k,jj}(\vec{r},\omega) + (\lambda(\omega)+\mu(\omega))\, U_{j,jk}(\vec{r},\omega) = -\rho\omega^2\, U_k(\vec{r},\omega) \tag{4}$$

in equation (4), ρ is the density of the medium.

It is convenient to study the wave motion induced by the passage of an elastic planar wave through two dimensional multilayers by means of complex scalar potential $\Phi(\vec{r},w)$ aand comples vector potential $\vec{\Psi}(\vec{r},t)$. With these two potentials, displacement $\vec{U}(\vec{r},w)$ can be expressed as follows:

$$\vec{U}(\vec{r},\omega) = \text{grad}\ \phi(\vec{r},\omega) + \text{curl}\ \vec{\Psi}(\vec{r},\omega) \tag{5}$$

So merging equation (5) into (4) leads to two separated potential wave equations:

$$\nabla^2\phi(\vec{r},\omega) + K_p^2\ \phi(\vec{r},\omega) = 0 \tag{6}$$

$$\nabla^2 \vec{\Psi}(\vec{r},\omega) + K_s^2\ \vec{\Psi}(\vec{r},\omega) = 0 \tag{7}$$

Recurrence Formula for Responses in Normal Incidence

In fig. 1 the mode is N isotropic homogeneous layers overlapped along the Y axis together with upper infinite halfspace 0 and lower infinite halfspace

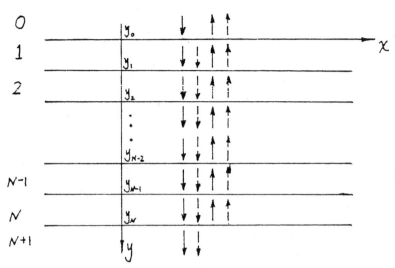

Fig. 1 Multilayered Model

where the comples wave numbers $K_p = \omega \sqrt{\rho/(\lambda(\omega)+2\mu(\omega))}$ and $K_s = \omega \sqrt{\rho/\mu(\omega)}$.

N+1. The thickness of each layer is $d(y_k)$ (k=1,2...,N) and elastic parameters are $\lambda(y_k,w) \mu(y_k,w)$ (k=0,1,..,N,N+1). When a longitudinal wave normally impinges on the first interface, the transverse vector protential $\vec{\psi}(\vec{r},w)$ disappears. As for the incidence of transverse waves, scalar potential $\Phi(\vec{r},w)$ disappears, and the deduction of recurrence formula is similar with the following one.

The solution of equation (6) in kth layer is

$$\Phi(y,\omega) = A'(y_k,\omega) e^{i(y+y_k)K(y_k,\omega)} + B'(y_k,\omega) e^{-i(y+y_k)K(y_k,\omega)} \qquad (8)$$

where $y_k = \sum_{j=1}^{k} d_j$, $K(y_k,\omega) = K_p(y_k,\omega)$.

With the continuity of the displacement and normal stress, we obtain following recurrence formula for transfer function of the multilayer.

$$\frac{B(y_{k-1},\omega)}{A(y_{k-1},\omega)} = \frac{R(y_{k-1},y_k) + e^{-i\phi_k} B(y_k,\omega)/A(y_k,\omega)}{1 + R(y_{k-1},y_k) e^{-i\phi_k} B(y_k,\omega)/A(y_k,\omega)} \qquad (9)$$

where $A(y_k,\omega) = \rho(y_k) A'(y_k,\omega)$; $B(y_k,\omega) = \rho(y_k) B'(y_k,\omega)$; $R(y_{k-1},y_k) = (K(y_k,\omega)\rho(y_{k-1}) - K(y_{k-1},\omega)\rho(y_k))/(K(y_k,\omega)\rho(y_{k-1}) + K(y_{k-1},\omega)\rho(y_k))$; $\phi_k = K(y_k,\omega) d_k$.

After the interative computation of equation (9) we have the transfer function $Hy(o,w) = B(o,w)/A(o,w)$. Furthermore normal responses result for different incident pulse $u_y(o,t)$.

573

Recurrence Formula for Response in Off-Normal Incidence

When a longitudinal wave or transverse wave impinges on the first interface in Fig. 1, reflection, transmission and mode conversion on the boundries appear simultaneously with the wave's propagating through the multilayer. But in every isotropic homogeneous layer, the propagation of the longitudinal wave is thought to be independent of that of the transverse wave, and vice versa. Supposing the polarization of displacement is on the X-Y plane, we have $\Psi_x(x,y,w)=\Psi_x(x,y,w)=0$, so the transverse vector potential $\vec{\Psi}(\vec{r},w)=\Psi(x,y,w)\ \vec{a}_z$.

With above conditions, the solution of equation (6) and (7) may have the following expressions:

$$\phi(x,y,\omega)=A'(y_k,\omega)e^{i(L(y_k,\omega)x+M(y_k,\omega)(y+\bar{y}_k))}+B'(y_k,\omega)\cdot$$
$$\cdot e^{i(L(y_k,\omega)x-M(y_k,\omega)(y+\bar{y}_k))} \tag{10}$$

$$\psi(x,y,\omega)=C'(y_k,\omega)e^{i(l(y_k,\omega)x+m(y_k,\omega)(y+\bar{y}_k))}+D'(y_k,\omega)$$
$$e^{i(l(y_k,\omega)x-m(y_k,\omega)(y+\bar{y}_k))} \tag{11}$$

where $L^2(y_k,\omega)+M^2(y_k,\omega)=K_p^2(y_k,\omega)\ ;\ l^2(y_k,\omega)+m^2(y_k,\omega)=K_s^2(y_k,\omega)\ ;$
$\bar{y}_k=\sum_{j=1}^{k}d_j.$

On the boundaries from (k-1)th to kth and kth to (k+1)th layer, considering the continuity of normal stress and displacement, we deduce two equations:

$$L(y_0,\omega)=l(y_0,\omega)=\cdots=L(y_k,\omega)=l(y_k,\omega)=\cdots=L(y_{N+1},\omega)=l(y_{N+1},\omega)=L \tag{12}$$

$$[Q(y_{k-1})][X^l(y_{k-1})]=[Q(y_k)][X^u(y_k)]$$
$$=([Q(y_k)][D(y_k)][Q(y_k)]^{-1})[Q(y_{k+1})][X^u(y_{k+1})] \tag{13}$$

Matrix equation (13) is a recurrence formula, in which $[x^l(y_k)]$ and $[x^u(y_k)]$ are column vectors of the amplitude of displacement on the upper and lower boundary of kth layer respectively; inverse matrix $[Q(y_k)]^{-1}$ is supposed to exist, which is true if the incident angle with normal is not equal to the critical angle. Square matrix $[Q(y_k)]$ and $[Q(y_k)]^{-1}$, diagonal matrix $[D(y_k)]$ can be expressed concisely; the interested readers may refer to reference 21.

Let propagator matrix $[P(y_k)]=[Q(y_k)]\ [D(y_k)]\ [Q(y_k)]^{-1}$. Its detailed expression is quite complicated and can be found in reference[21], but it has an important characteristic that its determinant is equal to unity.

From the interative computation of the matrix equation (13), we obtain transfer function $\bar{H}(\vec{r},w)$ $H_x(0,0,w)/A(0,0,w)$ and $H_y(0,0,w)=B(0,0,w)/A(0,0,w)$ for the incidence of a longitudinal wave, or $H_x(0,0,w)=D(0,0,w)/C(0,0,w)$, and $H_y(0,0,w)=B(0,0,w)/C(0,0,w)$ for the incidence of transverse wave.

Propagator-Tree

In order to trace the propagation of an incident beam and approximate its transverse deviation by an ideal planar wave and make the complicated propagation more clear, we have proposed the concept of propagator-tree as shown in Fig. 2.

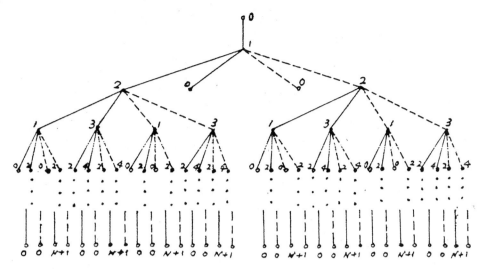

Fig. 2. Propagator-Tree

In Fig. 2. we see the following rules:

(1)   Dashed and solid lines represent the propagation of transverse
waves and that of longitudinal waves respectively.

(2)   A node corresponds to a layer, 0 to upper infinite halfspace and
N+1 to lower infinite halfspace.

(3)   From every node, except 0 and N+1 nodes, four branches always
come out to the next nodes, the numbers of which are always decreased or
increased by 1; meanwhile the coefficients of decomposition are those of
reflection, transmission and mode conversion.

(4)   Every branch has a propagator which makes phase shifts and
attenuation.

(5)   The decomposition comes to an end only if the number of the
branched node turns to be 0 of N+1, and any connection from 0 to 0 or 0 to
N+1 is a path of reflection or transmission.

With the above rules, it is easy to trace the path of propagation
which is to be sorted out and predict the transfer function of this path.

COMPUTER SIMULATION

Based on the recurrence formulae (9) and (13), responses of the multilayer are able to be quickly predicted on computers if the incident pulse
$U_e(t)$ is known. However, from these two formulae it is difficult to deduce
any analytical expression which shows the variance of the responses with
bandwidth or the existence of flaws in adhesive layers.   The available
approach is that we discuss the influence of the bandwidth or the existing
of flaws on the responses directly from the simulated results.

First of all, the incident pulse transmitted by the transducer can be simulated by the following expression:

$$u_e(t) = \begin{cases} 0 & t < 0 \\ u(t_0)e^{-a_1(t_0-t)}\cos(\omega_0(t_0-t)) & 0 \leqslant t \leqslant t_0 \\ u(t_0)e^{-a_2(t-t_0)}\cos(\omega_0(t-t_0)) & t_0 < t \leqslant t_N \\ 0 & t > t_N \end{cases} \qquad (14)$$

where t_N is the length of the sample window; time t_0 at which the membrane of the transducer vibrates to the maximum and the centre frequency w both depend on the properties of the transducer. So the bandwidth could be supposed to be only relevant to two variables a_1 and a_2. Later we discuss the influence of these two variables instead if the direct bandwidth in frequency domain.

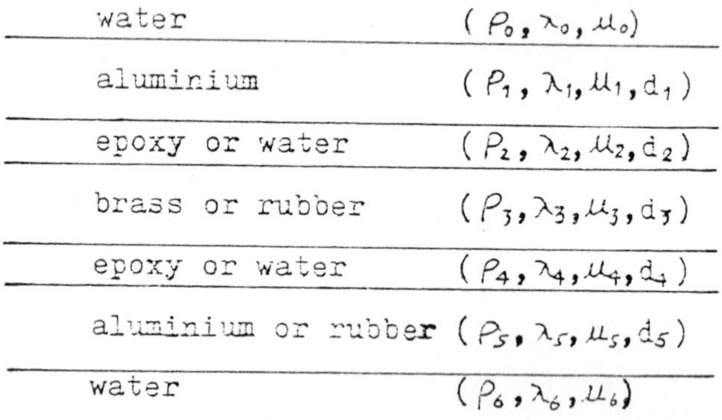

water	$(\rho_0, \lambda_0, \mu_0)$
aluminium	$(\rho_1, \lambda_1, \mu_1, d_1)$
epoxy or water	$(\rho_2, \lambda_2, \mu_2, d_2)$
brass or rubber	$(\rho_3, \lambda_3, \mu_3, d_3)$
epoxy or water	$(\rho_4, \lambda_4, \mu_4, d_4)$
aluminium or rubber	$(\rho_5, \lambda_5, \mu_5, d_5)$
water	$(\rho_6, \lambda_6, \mu_6)$

Fig. 3   Layered model. Halfspace 0 and 6 are water; layers 2 and 4 are epoxy; others are metal (aluminium or brass) or non-metal (rubber). Their elastic properties are listed in Table 1.

In Fig. 3, we display the model of the multilayer, which consists of five layers and their parameters are listed in Table 1.

It must be pointed out that the following two subsections are on normal incidence, and we don't take up off-normal incidence until next phase.

The Influences of Bandwidth

When two sequential reflected pulses from the multilayer arrive at the transducer, they generally overlap due to limited bandwidth and attenuation effects caused by the nonelasticity of the multilayer. If we want to part these two sequential reflected pulses from each other, we must increase the bandwidth to meet our requirement. By deducing, the following expression obtained may be used to approximate one of the two variables a_1

Table 1. Elastic Parameters of the Layered Model

layer	parameter	ρ (kg/m^3)	λ (newton/m^2)	μ (newton/m^2)	d m
o	water	1000	$2.25 \times 10^9 + i0$	$0 + i0$	/
1	aluminium	2700	$6.59 \times 10^{10} + i0$	$2.27 \times 10^{10} + i0$	5×10^{-3}
2	epoxy	2420	$8.84 \times 10^9 + i0$	$2.67 \times 10^9 + i0$	2×10^{-4}
2	water	1000	$2.25 \times 10^9 + i0$	$0 + i0$	
3	brass	8420	$1.11 \times 10^{11} + i0$	$3.47 \times 10^{10} + i0$	4.5×10^{-3}
3	rubber	2900	$(14+i5) \times 10^8$	$(4+i10) \times 10^8$	
4	epoxy	2420	$8.84 \times 10^9 + i0$	$2.67 \times 10^9 + i0$	2×10^{-4}
4	water	1000	$2.25 \times 10^9 + i0$	$0 + i0$	
5	aluminium	2700	$6.59 \times 10^{10} + i0$	$2.27 \times 10^{10} + i0$	5×10^{-3}
5	rubber	2900	$(14+i5) \times 10^8$	$(4+i10) \times 10^8$	
6	water	1000	$2.25 \times 10^9 + i0$	$0 + i0$	/

and a_2, and with these, the bandwidth can be prescribed previously:

$$a_2 \geqslant \frac{2a_1 \ln 10}{(\Delta t - \Delta t_1)a_1 - 2\ln 10} \tag{15}$$

where Δt is relevant to the time resolution and Δt_1 which depends on the attenuation of the multilayer; as shown in Fig. 4, can be calculated from simulated results.

Now we illustrate the influences of the bandwidth on responses of the multilayer by several simulated results.

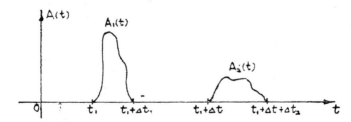

Fig. 4. Two sequential responses of an impulse, which orderly broadened by Δt_1 and Δt_2 due to attenuation

First, if the reflected pulse from the frontface of aluminium layer 1 is separated from the successively reflected pulse from the back of the same layer, then $\Delta t = 1.5576 \times 10^{-6}$; $\Delta t_1 = 0$; $f_0 = 5\text{MHz}$; $a_1 = 2 \times 10$ s , from inequality (15) obtained $a_2 > 3.47 \times 10$ s^{-1}, furthermore the equivalent bandwidth $\Delta f > 1\text{MHz}$. Fig. 5 shows the corresponding response, from which it is clear that the result is in accord with the requirement.

Second, for the adhesive layer 2, if we ask for the same requirement as above case, then we have $a_1 = 6 \times 10^7$ s ; $\Delta t = 1.6529 \times 10^7$ s; $\Delta t_1 = 0$, $f_o = 5$MHz, and after computing inequality (15) $a_2 \geq 5.2 \times 10^7$ s and the equivalent bandwidth $\Delta f \geq 6$MHz. In Fig. 6, the corresponding simulated response with this

Max= .32 , Min=-.52

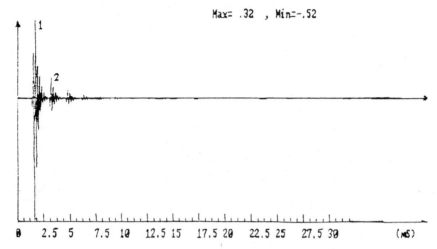

Fig. 5   Simulated response, in which two pulses 1 and 2. reflected from the front and back face of aluminium layer 1 are parted from each other in time domain.

case has been displayed, so it is seen the agreement is reached.

Finally, we take the attenuation effects into consideration. The attenuation effects of the non-metal layer are supposed to be the linear function of frequency and so dominant that the dispersion effects could be neglected, that is, the complex wave number $k = w/c - i\alpha w$, where α is the attenuation coefficient.

Max= .317 , Min=-.524

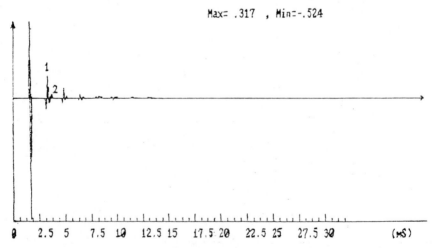

Fig.6. Pulse 1 is front reflected and pulse 2 is back reflected from adhesive layer 2; they are separated from each other

With regard to the front and back reflected pulses of rubber layer 3, we obtain the following expression which shows the relationship between the attenuation coefficient α_3 and the thickness d_3 of the non-metal layer:

$$0 \leqslant \alpha_3 \leqslant (\frac{1}{C_3} - \frac{\ln 10}{2a_1 d_3}) / \sqrt{\frac{1}{x}} - 1 \qquad (16)$$

In this inequality, C_3 is the velocity of planar wave in the non-metal and x is the overlap percent of these back and front reflected pulses.

When the parameters of the non-metal layer don't satisfy the inequality expression (16), the front reflected pulse can't be completely separated from the successively reflected back pulse in time domain.

Influences of the Existence of Flaws in Adhesive Layers

At present, we only deal with the flaws which are equivalent to disbonds and taken into account the the air layer's replacing the adhesive layer where flaws exist. For NDE in multilayers, at first step we want to solve the following problem: which layer do the disbonds exist in?

Consider the following four models of multilayers: (a). water-aluminium-epoxy-rubber-epoxy-aluminium-water, (b). water-aluminium-air-rubber-epoxy-aluminium-water, (c). water-aluminium-epoxy-rubber-air-aluminium-water. By computer simulation, the resulted spectra shown in Fig. 7 to Fig. 10 correspond the above four cases sequentially.

From these four spectra we note the following points:

1. Owing to the attenuation of the rubber layer, in higher frequency region there is no information about the disbonds below the rubber layer, as shown in Fig. 7. and Fig. 9. So it is necessary to low down the centre frequency of the incident pulse so that the deeper flaws can be detected, such as $f < 2MHz$ in this example.

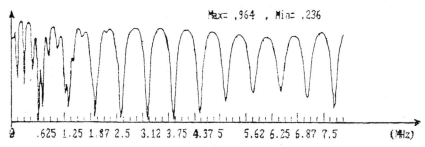

Fig. 7. The spectrum corresponding to no flaws; the more frequent oscillation in lower frequency region contain information about deeper layers than the rubber layer.

2. When there are disbonds in the upmost adhesive layer, the disbonds in the lower adhesive layers are generally masked, as shown in

Fig. 8, and Fig. 10. with their similarity. Detecting by an incident pulse in the higher frequency region can make it certain whether the above phenomenon does happen, and the above failure is avoided by off-normal incidence.

3. The feature extraction method can be used to detect the disbonds in adhesive layers, such as maxima, minima, their numbers and the energy in subregions of frequency.

The above three main points may direct the practical NDE in multilayers. In the next research phase we will study the influences of the distribution and size of flaws.

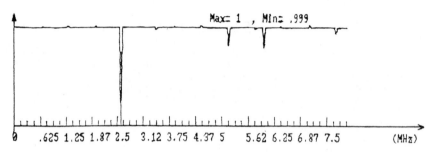

Fig. 8 The spectrum corresponding to flaws only in first adhesive layer.

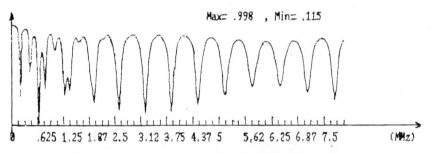

Fig. 9. The spectrum corresponding to flaws only in second adhesive layer; in higher frequency region there is no information about the flaws.

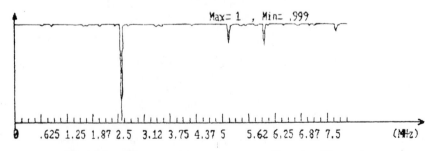

Fig. 10. The spectrum corresponding to flaws in both adhesive layer.

580

EXPERIMENTS

Our experimental results are only preliminary. The digital signal processing techniques, such as spectrum analysis, inverse filtering and cepstrum analysis, have been used to process the obtained data so as to improve the feasibility and reliability of flaw detection in multilayers, but these aren't described here.

During setting up the experimental devices, we pay more attention to the bandwidth and sensitivity requirements, which are critical to flaw detection in deeper adhesive layers. The layered structure of the specimen is made up of five layers immersed in water: aluminium-epoxy-brass-epoxy-aluminium, whose parameters are the same as listed in Table 1.

The experimental results obtained are shown in Fig. 11. to Fig. 13. which sequentially represents each typical spectrum of amplitude in three cases; no disbonds, disbonds only in first epoxy layer, disbonds only in second epoxy layer. In these figures, the corresponding simulated spectrum is also displayed as a dashed curve for comparison.

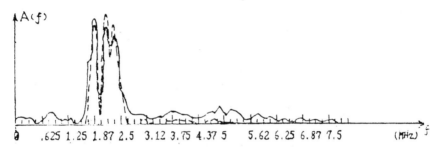

Fig. 11. Solid curve represents experimental spectrum belonging to no flaws; dashed curve is simulalted spectrum in corresponding case.

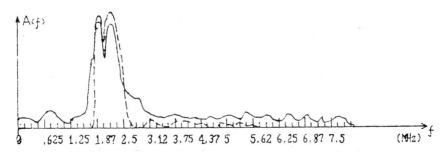

Fig. 12. Experimental spectrum (solid curve) and simulated spectrum (dashed line) when there are disbonds only in first adhesive layer.

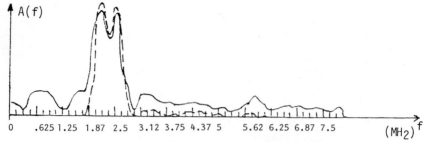

Fig. 13.   Experimental spectrum (solid curve) and
simulated spectrum (dashed line) when there
are disbonds only in second adhesive layer.

First, what can be observed from the shown spectra are the most
significant features: in the effective band (about 1.7–2.5MHz in our
experiments), the frequency points of maxima and minima of experimental
spectra are the same as those of corresponding simulated ones. But we also
see there is a little discrepancy between the amplitudes of them.
Therefore, the above significant features can be easily applied to examine
which adhesive layer is disbonded.

Beyond the effective bond, in experimental cases, due to noises
spectrum, ripples result.

SUMMARY

It is possible to quickly predict the complicated responses of
multilayers, and various influences on practical flaw detection may be
first discussed thoroughly by simulation, which is much more economical.
The experimental results are mostly in accord with the simulated   ones.
The disbonds in different achesive layers can be positively detected with
digital signal processing techniques.   But further improvement on both
theory and experiment must be made to eliminate the discrepancy and image
the distribution of flaws (not only disbonds) in different depths of
adhesive layers.

REFERENCES

1. L.M. Brekhovskikh, Waves in Layered Media, Academic Press, 1980

2. B.A.Auld, Acoustic Fields and Waves in Solids, A Wiley-
    Interscience Publication, 1973

3. B.L.N. Kennett, Seismic Wave Propagation in Stratified Media,
    Cambridge University Press, 1980

4. J.A. Hudson, The Execitation and Propagation of Elastic Waves,
    Cambridge University Press, 1980

5. R.M. Christensen, Theory of, Viscoelasticity; An Introduction Second
    Edition, Academic Press, 1979

6. A.N. Tikhonov and V.Y. Arsenin, Solutions of III-Posed Problems, A
    Wiley-Interscience Publication, 1979.

7. Inverse Source Problems in Optics Edited by H.P. Baltes. Springer-Verlag Berlin Heidelberg, 1978

8. Linear Inverse Theory, by Doug Oldenburg, University of British Columbia,   Aug., 1984

9. K.J. Langenberg, D. Bruck and M. Fischer, "Inverse Scattering Algorithms,"New Procedures in Nondestructive Testing, edited by P. Holler, Springer-Verlag Berlin Heidelberg, 1983

10. R.G. Newton, "Inversion of Reflection Data for Layered Media: A Review of Exact Methods", Geophys, J.R. Astr. Soc., Vol. 65, 1981

11. Y.V. Lange, "Low-Frequency Acoustic Methods and Means of Nondestructive Testing for Multilayer Structures and Products of Plastics," 10th World Conference on Non-Distructive Testing, 1980

12. J. Szilzrd, Ultrasonic Testing: Non-Conventional Techniques, A Wiley Interscience Publication, pp. 263-296, 1982

13. C. Wong, et al., "Sound Resonance Testing for Curve Structures," Symposium on the Third Conference of NDT Institutiuon of CMES,Sept., 1984

14. E.A. Robinson and S. Treitel, Geophysical Signal Analysis.Prentice-Hall, Englewood Cliffs, N.J., 1980

15. A.V. Kak and K.A. Dines, "Signal Processing of Broad-Band Pulsed Ultrasound," IEEE Trans. on Biol. Eng., July, 1978

16. Programs for Digital Signal Processing, edited by the Digital Signal Processing Committee, IEEE Press, 1979

17. A.V. Oppenheim and R.W. Schafer, Digital Signal Processing,Prentice-Hall, Inc., Englewood Cliffs, New Jersey, 1975

18. D.G. Childers, D.P. Skinner and R.C. Kemerait, "The Cepstrum: A Guide to Processing", Proc. the IEEE, Vol. 65, No. 10, Oct., 1977

19. R. Shanker, et.al., Acoustic NDE of Multilayered Composites, Phase 1: Acoustic Model Development and Inspection of Bronze Rubber Structure,Rept. No. TETRAT-A-6139, Jul., 1982

20. R. Shanker, et al., PSAcoustic NDE of Multilayered Composits, Phase 2: Angle Beam Model Validation and Inspection of Bronze-Rubber Structures, Final Technical Report, AD A127253, Mar., 1983

21. J.-P. Zhang, The Computation and Examination of Elastic Pulses Reflected from Layered Media, post-Graduate's Paper, 1985

SYNTHETIC APERTURE SONAR FOR SUB-BOTTOM IMAGING

M.K. Dutkiewicz and P.N. Denbigh

Central Acoustics Laboratory
Department of Electrical and Electronic Engineering
University of Cape Town, Rondebosch 7700, R.S.A.

ABSTRACT

Many of the difficulties which arise in a medium range synthetic aperture sidescan sonar are avoided when the synthetic aperture method is applied to sub-bottom imaging. Preliminary results have been obtained and show the technique to be viable.

INTRODUCTION

Outstanding success has been achieved in radar terrain mapping by using synthetic apertures to achieve fine along-track resolution[1]. A wealth of literature exists on the implementation of the technique, which was primarily developed in the 1960's.

Attempts to extend the technique to sonar applications have, however, not met with the same degree of success. Since Cutrona's benchmark paper[2] a number of attempts have been made to build synthetic aperture sonar systems[3,4]. These attempts have met with success under controlled conditions using 'good' targets. Attempts to extend the technique to use in sidescan sea bed mapping applications are believed to have been largely unsuccessful and this is because of two major problems which do not occur in radar

1) In spite of the lesser operating ranges the low propagation velocity of sound causes the two-way propagation times to be much larger for a sideways looking sonar than for an equivalent radar. This is liable to cause a severe undersampling of the synthetic aperture at typical towing speeds.

2) The inertia of a boat or towed body is much less than that of an aircraft or satellite. This together with the influence of swell and waves can result in deviations of the sampling positions from a straight line path. The deviations may constitute an unacceptably large fraction of a wavelength.

It appears from the foregoing, that a large number of difficulties associated with implementing synthetic apertures in sonar would be overcome if work were carried out at low frequencies and short ranges. Such an application is sub-bottom imaging. It has been shown[5] that it is possible to achieve coherence over long linear arrays in the ocean at low frequencies.

REVIEW OF SUB-BOTTOM IMAGING

Acoustic methods are used to image objects and layers beneath the sea bed and may fall into one of two broad categories, namely seismic profiling and sub-bottom profiling. Seismic profiling usually uses a single explosive or explosive type source and multiple omnidirectional receive hydrophones mounted in a long streamer behind the survey ship. Penetration depths are considerable and the signal processing is aimed particularly at emphasizing strata using reflection or refraction methods[6]. On the other hand sub-bottom profiling usually combines a boomer, air gun, or tone burst source with a single directional hydrophone receiver, both commonly mounted on a "fish" towed close to the sea bed. The maximum penetration is modest compared with seismic systems and, depending upon the type of sediment and the frequency range in which most of the transmit energy is contained, might be between 1m and 100m.

A large amount of research has been carried out into the characteristics of various sediments and a good summary can be found in Hamilton[7]. One of the important features is the largely empirical observation that the attenuation of sound in sediments is proportional to frequency. For sand we have $\alpha = 0.5f(kHz)$ dB/m; for clays we have $\alpha = 0.1f(kHz)$ dB/m. Penetration is clearly increased by a decrease in frequency but the penalty for a given size of receiver is a broadening of the beam. As an example, a typical operating frequency of 4kHz corresponds to a wavelength of 0.375m so that a receiver 0.5m in diameter has very little directionality. For reflecting strata this is not particularly disadvantageous. The first return shows up clearly as a sharp transition between white and black on the chart recording and the only effect of a wide beam is to cause a broadening of the black bands corresponding to strata. For the imaging of buried objects, however, a broad beam is very disadvantageous as the resolution of closely spaced objects is then very poor. At a range of 15m, for example, the lateral resolution corresponding to the 0.5m diameter receiver discussed would be 11.25m.

Clearly there is a need for high lateral resolution sub-bottom imaging. Examples of application are mine detection, treasure hunting, and the checking of buried pipelines. A technique that appears to be suitable for this type of use is that of parametric arrays. These produce narrow, low frequency beams, but a big problem is the conversion efficiency. The source level tends to be insufficient for any great penetration depth although improvements are achievable using pulse compression[8]. Another technique that suggests itself is that of synthetic apertures. This technique has a number of advantages over existing techniques.

(i)   Providing a long array can be synthesized, fine resolution can be achieved.

(ii)   A large amount of information is stored at the time of measurement, giving a great deal of versatility in the use of the information. The beam can be steered and focused in order to look for details of interest. For example the optimal detection process for a point target may be different from that for a faceted target. For a faceted target it may depend on the angle of the facet. As another example amplitude shading can be applied to reduce sidelobe levels.

(iii) Source level (and thus penetration) is high since a conventional
      transducer is used.

Problems with synthetic apertures include the degradation of performance due
to towing path irregularities, and beam distortion due to refraction at the
sediment-water interface. Early work on the project has shown little
degradation due to the latter effect and that, if required, corrections may
be incorporated into the processing algorithm. The problem of towing path
irregularities is alleviated by working at fairly long wavelengths (e.g.
30cm).

THEORY OF SYNTHETIC APERTURES

      A synthetic aperture is generated in a similar fashion to a
conventional array except that, instead of having a long line array of
elements, a single element is traversed across the space and the return
echoes at each position are stored (typically in digital or optical form).
After the full aperture has been traversed, the array is synthesized. At
this stage a variety of different beams can be realized. What follows is a
brief development of the theory. For a more detailed treatment see
Cutrona[1].

For a conventional physical array the beam pattern is given by

$$D(\theta) = \frac{\sin \left(\frac{\pi N d_e}{\lambda} \sin \theta \right)}{\sin \left(\frac{\pi d_e}{\lambda} \sin \theta \right)}$$

where N = number of points in array, d_e = element spacing.

In the synthetic case the transmitter and receiver both move and are indeed
usually the same transducer. The path length to a target changes twice as much
with the position of this transducer as it would with the position of an
element across the receive physical array for the case of a stationary
transmitter.

$$\text{Hence} \qquad D(\theta) = \frac{\sin \left(\frac{2\pi N d_e}{\lambda} \sin \theta \right)}{\sin \left(\frac{2\pi d_e}{\lambda} \sin \theta \right)} \qquad (1)$$

This will be termed a two-way pattern. For apertures which are large in
wavelengths this gives an angular resolution of $\lambda/2Nd_e$ for synthetic case, as
compared to λ/Nd_e for a real array. The sidelobes for the two-way pattern
are 13.2dB down on the main beam. This is appreciable but may be reduced by an
amplitude shading of the aperture.

Further, by analogy to a real array, grating sidelobes will occur when the
denominator in Eq.1 is zero.

i.e. when $\quad \frac{2\pi d_e}{\lambda} \sin \theta = \frac{\pi}{2} \qquad$ or $\qquad \sin \theta = \frac{\lambda}{2d_e}$

These will disappear providing the aperture samples are spaced closer than
$\lambda/2$.

We have $L_e = (N-1)d_e = Nd_e$ for large N. It follows from the angular
resolution of $\lambda/2Nd_e$ that the along-track resolution is given by

$$\delta = \frac{R\lambda}{2L_e} \qquad (2)$$

where R is the range of the target and L_e is the length of the synthetic aperture. Depending on whether the aperture is focused or unfocused a variety of different values of L_e can be achieved.

(i) unfocused. In this case the aperture length is limited by requiring the target to be in the far field of the aperture.

i.e. $\quad R \geq \dfrac{L_e^2}{\lambda} \quad$ giving $\quad L_e \leq (R\lambda)^{0.5}$

Therefore resolution $\quad \delta \geq \dfrac{(R\lambda)^{0.5}}{2}$

(ii) focused: If the aperture is focused, the aperture may be as long as the distance for which the target is insonified by the physical transducer.

Hence $L_e = \dfrac{R\lambda}{D} \quad$, where D is the transducer diameter.

Combining this with eq.(2) gives $\delta = D/2$. It will be noted that this is independent of range and wavelength. At times, it may prove advantageous to focus the array but not to use the full aperture. Under these circumstances $\delta = D/2\gamma$ where γ equals the fraction of the maximum possible aperture.

Further degradation of resolution occurs due to phase errors. These are primarily caused by tow path irregularities. A theoretical treatment of this is available[9]. Experimental results illustrating this effect as well as other features mentioned earlier will be shown later.

EXPERIMENTAL WORK

The system built to realise synthetic apertures used a single transducer for both transmission and reception. Data capture was performed in the field on a HP-86 microcomputer, using a single A/D converter with quadrature sampling. This was later transferred to a UNIVAC mainframe computer where the amplitude and phase of the receive signal was calculated for every range bin of each transmission. Each transmission corresponded to a different sampling point along the synthetic aperture. Processing was carried out for each image point in turn and began with a calculation of the two way propagation distances to each of the sampling points on the synthetic aperture. On the basis of this the phase correction needed to make all receive signals co-phasal was calculated. This was then applied to the contents of the range bin which corresponded most closely to the two way propagation distance. The corrected signals for all the aperture positions were then summed vectorially to yield the target strength for that image point. This is equivalent to realising a curved array centred about the image point. The procedure was carried out for each point in the image space in turn and the displays generated used a SACLANT graphics package. These displays show along-track distance versus range with the vertical axis being an indicator of the target strength. The experimental work began with laboratory tests under carefully controlled conditions, and progressed to reservoir tests, and finally to tests at sea. As a point of interest it has not always been found advantageous to apply amplitude shading to the data. This is because targets move in and out of the skirts of the physical beam as the transducer is scanned across the aperture, and this imposes a very effective natural amplitude shading.

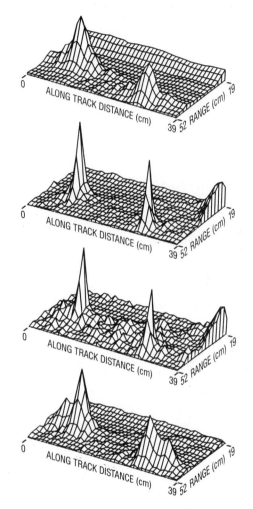

Figure 1. Images of two mid-water targets: (a) 10cm. unfocused aperture;
(b) 39cm. focused aperture; (c) focused aperture with random
phase errors; (d) focused aperture with 10% velocity error.

200kHz tank tests

Two ping pong balls were used as mid water targets and were imaged using a 200kHz transducer. The size of the transducer used was 8mm square. Transmission and reception were performed with the transducer stationary at each position along the aperture. A total of 78 aperture points spaced 5mm apart were used. The results shown in Fig. 1 are gratifying, showing the expected improvement in resolution as the aperture length is increased. It should be noted, in this and subsequent images, that the vertical displacement represents intensity and not target height.

When making synthetic aperture measurements under less controlled conditions, at sea for example, it is to be expected that the data will contain phase errors due to sideways perturbations of the transducer position; also because an incorrect velocity might be assumed in the processing. Work has been done in which the tank data has been perturbed by random phase errors and by a systematic 10% velocity error. The effect is shown in Fig. 1 and has been to degrade resolution and to increase sidelobes.

Reservoir Tests

Experiments were carried out from a floating laboratory on a fresh water reservoir. The reservoir was known to contain scattered rocks lying in a bed of silt. The laboratory had a 4.5m long rectangular hole cut in the floor. The transducer was suspended in the water from a trolley which ran on rails along the length of the hole. Apertures 4.5m long were created by pulling this trolley by hand at constant velocity along the length of the laboratory.

The transducer used was taken from a conventional sub-bottom profiling array. It operated at a resonant frequency of 4.5kHz and gave a beamwidth of 100 degrees. The transducer bandwidth allowed a pulse of 1ms length to be transmitted, corresponding to a range resolution of 0.75m. At the frequency used, the attenuation in the sediment was approximately 3dB/m which, because of the two-way travel time, gave an attenuation of 6dB per metre of penetration.

The initial experiments were conducted with the transducer looking directly downwards, as is usual in sub-bottom profiling. However, a problem arises that would not, for example, occur with a parametric array. Although the processing of the synthetic aperture leads to a good along-track resolution, the lateral resolution remains unchanged and is poor. A perspective view of the geometry is shown in Fig. 2.

Fig. 3(a) represents a vertical cross-section of the beam corresponding to Fig. 2 and shows the resolution cell. Directly beneath the transducer, in the centre of the physical beam, the sensitivity is maximum. However the attenuation of the sediment reduces the return echo. To the side of the transducer, in the skirts of the physical beam, the sensitivity is lower but the penetration into the sediment is less, so that the return echo is less attenuated. Although sub-bottom strata may still be imaged satisfactorily due to their specularity, small objects are likely to appear stronger when they are located to the side of the transducer than when they are beneath it. Bearing in mind that the intention of a high resolution sub-bottom profiler is to image small targets, it is apparent that the image will be very difficult to interpret.

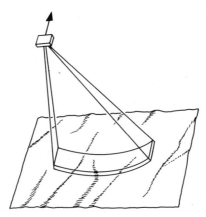

Fig. 2.   Intersection of synthesized fan beam with sea bed.

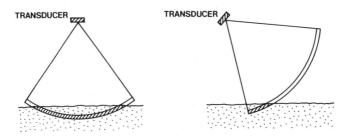

Fig. 3. Intersection of synthesized fan beam with sea bed
a) echo sounding mode   b) sidescan mode

       Because of the foregoing problems, the preferred mode of operation now
is to use the system as a short-range sidescan sonar in which the use of low
frequencies enables bottom penetration. After synthetic aperture
processing, the resolution cell is as shown in Fig. 3(b). Essentially, the
geometry is the same as in Fig. 3(a) except that, because the transducer is
now tilted sideways, the sensitivity to targets directly beneath the
transducer is greatly diminished. The dominant echoes may be expected to
come in from the side and, because of the sediment attenuation, they may be
expected to arise in the top metre or so of the sediment. The volume making
a significant contribution to the return signal at any instant now becomes
relatively small and, because of this, the reconstructed image becomes much
more amenable to interpretation. However, in spite of the reduced
sensitivity and high sediment attenuation in the vertical direction, the
large reflections from strata can still dominate the return signal. In
order to diminish still further the returns from beneath the transducer, a
pressure release reflecting baffle was used beneath the transducer. This was
in order to shadow from the transducer that part of the bed of the reservoir
directly beneath it.

       As an example of the performance of the system Fig. 4(a) shows the
unprocessed amplitude data collected using the low frequency transducer.

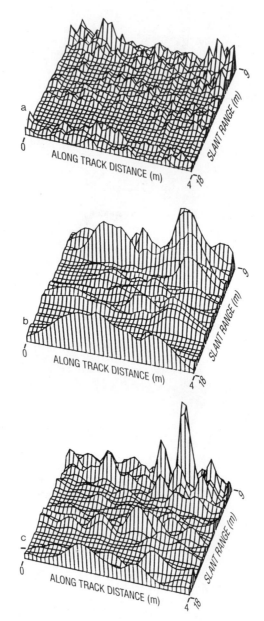

Figure 4. Images at reservoir site: (a) unprocessed data; (b) 2m. synthetic aperture; (c) 4m. synthetic aperture.

Figs. 4(b) and 4(c) show the reconstructed images obtained over a 4m along-track distance using aperture lengths of 2m and 4m respectively. For the 4m case, the complete aperture data is used for all the points in the image, i.e. the beam is focused and steered to each point in the image plane. For the case of a 2m aperture where 4m of data is available, the section of the data used is moved (Fig. 5). The central 2m of the image is obtained by selecting the appropriate section of the data and using focusing but no beam deflection. The outer 1m parts of the image are obtained by deflecting the beam. A comparison of Figs. 4(b) and 4(c) clearly shows that the detail of the images is improved as the aperture size is increased.

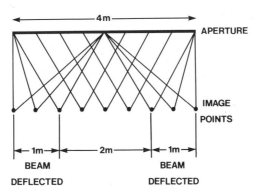

Fig. 5. Use of data for image reconstruction.

It is important to know whether bottom penetration has been achieved and, although not entirely conclusive, it has proved useful to compare the images with those obtained using a conventional 300kHz sidescan system where only surface structure can be expected. Such an image is shown in Fig. 6(a). The transducer was pointing slightly foreward of the broadside direction and hence there is a slight displacement of the image compared with that of the 4m synthetic aperture image which is repeated in Fig. 6(b). Comparison aided by the marking of six targets A to F which are common to both images. The differences in the relative strengths of these targets between these two images may be due to the difference in sensitivities at the two frequencies to the submerged parts of these targets. The areas marked G and H in Fig. 6(b) are not apparent in Fig. 6(a) thus suggesting that these targets are completely submerged. Unfortunately it has not been possible yet to back up this conclusion by visual observations of the bed of the reservoir.

Sea Tests

In order to image a larger area and to test the system under realistic operational conditions, tests were carried out at sea. The same transducer as used previously in the reservoir tests was mounted rigidly between the hulls of a twin engined catamaran. The sideways looking configuration was again adopted but, because of water resistance, the baffle beneath the transducer was discarded. The speed measured by a taffrail log was 1.1 m/s but images produced using this value were found to be totally unsatisfactory. For example images obtained from beams at different squint angles, but directed at the same area of the sea bed by using different blocks of synthetic aperture data, did not give coincident feature. By trial and error the true velocity relative to the sea bed was found to be 1.6 m/s. Based upon this value and the known interpulse period it followed that

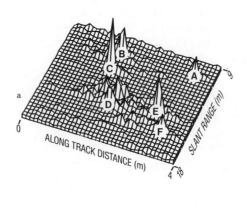

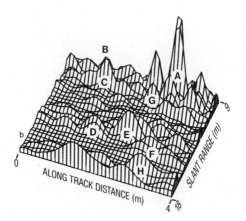

Figure 6. Images at reservoir site: (a) 300kHz sidescan; (b) 4.5kHz
synthetic aperture.

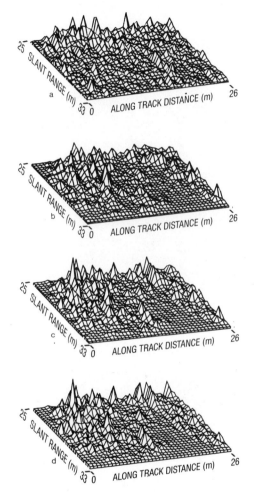

Figure 7. Images of sea bed at 10° squint angle: (a) unprocessed;
(b) 4m. synthetic aperture; (c) 8m. synthetic aperture;
(d) 12m. synthetic aperture.

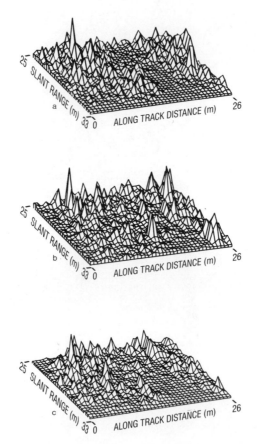

Figure 8. Images of sea bed using 8m. synthetic aperture: (a) -10° squint angle; (b) broadside; (c) +10° squint angle.

receive signals were recorded every 0.19m over total track lengths of 85m. The 0.19m corresponded to a theoretical prediction of grating sidelobes at 60°. The sensitivity of the physical transducer was well down at this angle.

One of the practical problems encountered in the sea trials was a very strong acoustic interference signal, attributed to the transmit signal undergoing multiple reflections between the hulls of the catamaran and returning to the transducer to overlap the wanted sea bed echoes. This acoustic interference was therefore confined to the broadside direction. The problem was overcome by forming a squint beam in the reconstruction processing which was insensitive to the broadside interference.

Unprocessed data corresponding to an area near some semi-submerged pillars is shown in Fig.7(a). No meaningful feature can be seen. The remaining images of Fig.7 are reconstructions of the same area using different lengths of apertures and a beam which is steered 10° ahead of broadside. Considerable feature is now apparent, with the resolution being improved by increasing the aperture length from 4m to 8m but not significantly when going from 8m to 12m. The processing incorporated a Hamming amplitude shading function as given by $w(z) = 0.54 + 0.46 \cos (2\pi z/L)$. This was done because the natural shading of targets discussed earlier, where targets move in and out of the physical beam, was no longer effective at the increased ranges.

Considerable confidence in the images is gained if similar feature is generated when using different blocks of data. This can be tested by imaging the same area with the beam at different squint angles. Fig. 8 shows images for squint angles of -10°, 0°, and +10°. It is seen that there is a strong similarity between them. The broadside image is of degraded quality because of the acoustic interference problem mentioned earlier. The difference between the fore and aft beam images is attributed to the faceted nature of typical targets such as rocks and, in this case, pillars.

DISCUSSION

The tank tests and the reservoir tests have confirmed that, under controlled conditions, the principle of synthetic aperture imaging is viable. There is good evidence, though not yet entirely conclusive, that targets beneath the bed of the reservoir are being imaged. Useful images have been produced applying the synthetic aperture technique at sea, but only after trial and error adjustments have been made to the supposed boat velocity as measured by a taffrail log. The useful aperture length was limited by coherence problems to about 8m. The explanation for this can only be speculative but is probably related to unwanted boat movement. It seems likely that the problem would be reduced if the transducer were mounted in a fish and towed with a cable configuration that provided little coupling to the movements of the mother boat. Based upon the reservoir tests it seems likely that bottom penetration has been achieved but further work needs to be done to establish its extent.

CONCLUSIONS

The feasibility of synthetic aperture techniques for short range low frequency imaging has been demonstrated. In contrast to the parametric array the use of synthetic aperture techniques for sub-bottom imaging does not suffer from a low source level. However the beam resulting from a synthetic aperture is narrow in one direction only and is not a pencil beam.

The disadvantage of a fan beam is greatly reduced by using the system in sideways looking mode. Indeed the fan beam may even be regarded as advantageous as the sidescan mode of operation gives a very much faster rate of survey than the echo-sounder mode of the conventional sub-bottom profiler. Another point in favour of the synthetic aperture may well prove to be the ease with which the surveyed area may be examined from different angles, thus easing the interpretation.

REFERENCES

1. L.J. Cutrona, Synthetic Aperture Radar, Chap. 23 of "Radar Handbook", M.I. Skolnik (ed.) McGraw-Hill, New York, 1970.
2. L.J. Cutrona, "Comparison of sonar system performance achievable using synthetic-aperture techniques with the performance achievable by more conventional means", J.Acoust. Soc. Am.,58(2),336-348(1975)
3. T.Sato, O.Ikeda, "Sequential synthetic aperture sonar system-a prototype of a synthetic aperture sonar system", IEEE Trans. on Sonics and Ultrasonics, Vol. SU-24, No.4, July 1977.
4. Loggins et al., "Results from rail synthetic aperture experiments", J. Acoust. Soc. Am., 71(S1), S85(1982).
5. R. Williams, "Creating an acoustic synthetic aperture in the ocean", J. Acoust. Soc. Am., 60(1), 60-73(1976).
6. M. Dobrin, Introduction to Geophysical Prospecting, McGraw-Hill, New York, 1976.
7. E.L. Hamilton, "Compressional wave attenuation in marine sediments", Geophysics, 37, 620-646(1972).
8. H.O. Berktay, et al., "Sub-bottom profiling using parametric sources", Proceedings of the Institute of Acoustics Conference on Underwater Applications of Non-Linear Acoustics, Bath, Sept. 1979.
9. W. Brown, "Synthetic Aperture Radar" , IEEE Trans. on Aerospace and Electronic Systems, Vol. AES-3, No.2, March 1967.

VERTICAL SEISMIC PROFILING DEPTH

MIGRATION OF A SALT DOME FLANK - A SUMMARY

N. D. Whitmore and Larry R. Lines

Amoco Production Co.
P.O. Box 3385
Tulsa, OK   74102

INTRODUCTION

Vertical Seismic Profiles (VSPs) supply information about both
velocity and subsurface interface locations. Properly designed VSPs can
be used to map steeply dipping interfaces such as salt dome flanks. Mapping subsurface interfaces with VSP data requires careful survey design,
appropriate data processing, interval velocity estimation, and reflector
mapping. The first of these four ingredients is satisfied in most cases
by preacquisition modeling. The second is accomplished by careful data
processing. The initial velocity estimates are provided by seismic tomography. Velocity model refinement is accomplished by a combination of
iterative modeling and iterative least squares inversion. Finally, the
resultant interval velocities are used in depth migration of the processed
VSP. These four ingredients have been combined to map a salt dome flank.

(from Geophysics, 51, 1087-1109)

Method

Vertical Seismic Profiles (VSPs) have been employed for many years to
help determine the lithology and velocity in the vicinity of the borehole.
In recent years, VSPs have been used more and more frequently in an
attempt to map structure. This short note discusses a VSP survey which
was designed, recorded, and processed to map a salt dome flank. The
details of the study are discussed by Whitmore and Lines, 1986, in a
detailed paper in Geophysics.

The paper provides a case history of the preacquisition planning and
post-acquisition processing of a VSP specifically obtained for mapping
structure. The four areas discussed are: preacquisition modeling and
migration, data processing, velocity model determination, and depth migration of the VSPs. The modeling and migration section demonstrates feasibility that a VSP survey can indeed locate a salt dome flank. A cursory
description of the migration principle as given in Figure 1, uses the
imaging principle due to Claerbout (1971) and the backwards time propagation described by Whitmore (1983). The section on data processing discusses the basic preconditioning of the VSP data applied to make the processed VSP suitable for input to depth migration. Velocity determination
involves straight ray tomography as described by McMechan, 1983, and the

modeling of rays that obey Snell's law. Seismic tomography is used to provide an initial estimate of the velocity structure by using direct arrivals. The direct arrivals and reflections are then modeled by applying ray tracing, wherein the combination of iterative modeling of least squares inversion is used to produce a set of dipping layers. The velocity structure estimated from the VSPs provides reasonable agreement with the model obtained independently by surface seismic measurements. Details of the velocity estimation steps are given by Lines and Whitmore (1986). The procedure of combining tomography and migration have also been applied to seismic data by Stork and Clayton (1985) and by Bording, Lines, Scales and Treitel (1986). The results of depth migration of the processed VSPs agree with the results of travel time inversion and ray tracing.

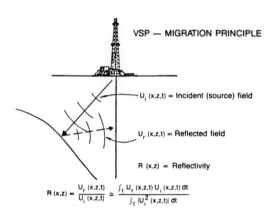

Fig. 1   Illustration of VSP Depth Migration Principles
(from Geophysics, 51, 1087-1109)

Conclusions

The combination of many techniques involving modeling, traveltime inversion, and depth migration, can be used to successfully image reflected arrivals on vertical seismic profiles. In this case, the procedure was used to successfully map a Salt Dome Flank.

References

Bording, R. P., Lines, L. R., Scales, J. A., and Treitel, S. 1986, Principles of Seismic Travel Time Tomography, Submitted to Geophys. Jour. R. Astr. Soc.

Claerbout, J. F., 1971, "Toward a Unified Theory of Reflector Mapping," Geophysics, v. 36, p. 467-481.

McMechan, G. A., 1983, "Seismic Tomography in Boreholes: Geophys. J. Roy Astr. Soc., 74, 601-612.

Lines, L. R., and Whitmore, N. D., 1986, Travel Time Inversion of Offset Vertical Seismic Profiles -- a Real Data Case," manuscript submitted for publication in BSSA.

Stork, C. and Clayton, R. W., 1985, "Iterative Tomographic and Migration Reconstruction of Seismic Images," Presented at the 55th Annual SEG Meeting in Washington, D.C.

Whitmore, N. D., 1983, Iterative depth migration by backward time propagation: paper presented at the 1983 SEG meeting in Las Vegas, Nevada.

Whitmore, N. D. and Lines, L. R., 1986, "VSP Depth Migration of A Salt
    Dome Flank," Geophysics 51, p. 1087-1109.

A SENSOR-EFFICIENT ALGORITHM FOR ARRAY PROCESSING

T. E. Cichocki† and M. Kaveh*

†Raytheon Company
Hartwell Road
Bedford, MA 01730

*Department of Electrical Engineering
University of Minnesota
Minneapolis, MN 55455

ABSTRACT

This paper presents the derivation and some statistical properties of a new use of Prony's algorithm for the estimation of the angles of arrival of plane waves received in noise. The technique, called the Sensor Efficient Method (SEM), has applications for signal returns that are wide band or multi-frequency.

INTRODUCTION

The problem of locating a target or targets by use of an array of sensors has been the focus of research efforts for some time, having applications involving radar, sonar, ultrasonic biomedicine, etc. The case at hand involves the solution to the angular resolution problem (it is assumed that the range determination problem is solved by appropriate selection of the waveform).

If the signals transmitted/ reflected by the targets are represented by plane waves then the 1-th received signal sampled at the k-th sensor, after complex demodulation, is

$$x_k(\ell) = \sum_{i=1}^{NT} A_{i\ell}(e^{j\Phi_{i\ell}}) \, e^{j2\pi(k-1)e_i D/\lambda} + n_k(\ell), \tag{1}$$

where $A_{i\ell}$ and $\Phi_{i\ell}$ refer to the ℓ-th sample (ℓ-th snapshot) amplitude and phase of the i-th plane wave, NT is the number of targets, D is the array element spacing, λ is the wavelength and $e_i = \sin\theta_i$ with θ_i the (AOA) of the i-th wave referenced to the array broadside.

It is this signal which is processed by any of a number of algorithms to obtain information concerning the number of targets, their directions relative to antenna boresight, etc. Many of these algorithms are based on the approach of spatial spectral estimation. They include conventional Fourier techniques (periodogram, Blackman-Tukey), rational transfer function methods; autoregressive and autorepressive-moving-average, Pisarenko and Prony. These algorithms are reviewed in [1]. An extension to the wideband model is given in [2]. A common requirement for all these methods is that the number of sensors be greater than the number of targets. In this paper we extend Prony's method, in the wideband signal case, so that this requirement is no longer necessary.

DEVELOPMENT OF THE ALGORITHM

The extended Prony's method generates an approximation to a finite-length data record in the form of sum of complex exponentials [3]. That data is fit with the model

$$\xi(n) = \sum_{i=1}^{NT} b_i e^{j\omega_i n} \quad 1 \leqslant n \leqslant N , \ NT < N, \tag{2}$$

where b_i is the complex amplitude and ω_i is the frequency of the i-th component. Define the system rooting polynomial,

$$\psi(Z) = \prod_{i=1}^{NT} (Z-Z_i) = \sum_{i=0}^{NT} a_i Z^{NT-i} , \quad a_0 = 1 \tag{3}$$

Letting $Z_k = e^{j\omega_k}$, we have

$$\xi(n-i) = \sum_{k=1}^{NT} b_k Z_k^{n-i} . \tag{4}$$

So,

$$\sum_{i=0}^{NT} a_i \xi(n-i) = \sum_{k=1}^{NT} b_k Z_k^{n-NT} \sum_{i=1}^{NT} a_i Z_k^{NT-i} = \sum_{k=1}^{NT} b_k Z_k^{n-NT} \psi(Z)\big|_{Z=Z_k} = 0. \tag{5}$$

We now note that $\{\xi(n)\}$ is a noise-less model for the data $x(n)$. Using (6), we can therefore estimate a_i by minimizing Q_1 with respect to a_i given by

$$Q_1 = \sum_{n=NT+1}^{N} |x(n) + \sum_{i=1}^{NT} a_i x(n-i)|^2. \tag{7}$$

Thus, a_i estimation can be viewed as estimation of the parameters of an autoregressive process, for which many algorithms exist (see e.g., [1]). In particular, it is well-known that the autocorrelation function (ACF) of $x(n)$ in (1), for the case of white measurement noise is given by

$$R_x(n) = \sum_{i=1}^{NT} \alpha_i e^{j2\pi e_i nD/\lambda} + \sigma^2 \delta(n), \tag{8}$$

where $\delta(n)$ is the Kronecker delta, σ^2 is the noise variance and α_i is the i-th target return power. This ACF satisfies the extended Yule-Walker equations. That is, given an estimate, $\hat{R}(n)$, of the ACF, a_i may be estimated by minimizing Q_a given by

$$Q_a = \sum_{n=1}^{NL} |\hat{R}_x(n) + \sum_{i=1}^{NT} a_i \hat{R}_x(n-i)|^2 . \tag{9}$$

Once a_i are estimated from (7) or (9), they can be substituted in (3) and the roots of $\Psi(Z)$ found. These roots are of the form

$$z_i = e^{j\hat{\omega}_i} ,$$

with $\hat{\omega}_i = \dfrac{2\pi \hat{e}_i D}{\lambda}$, giving an estimate of the i-th spatial frequency,

resulting in an estimate of the i-th AOA. After the determination of $\hat{\omega}_i$, the component powers can be determined by linear-least squares fit of sum of complex exponentials to the estimated ACF.

Note the system constraints that are implied when using an algorithm with the "reduced data set" in the form of the ACF estimates:

1 - From the set of recursive linear equations

$$\hat{R}_x(n) = \sum_{i=1}^{NT} a_i R_x(n-1). \qquad\qquad NT + 1 \leqslant n \leqslant NL$$

For a unique (least-squares) solution we must have

$$NL \geqslant 2NT \qquad or \qquad N \geqslant 2NT + 1$$

where NL is the number of ACF lags needed and N is the number of sensors.

2 - To obtain an unambiguous estimate of target direction.

$$-\pi \leqslant 2\pi e_i D/\lambda \leqslant \pi \qquad or \qquad \lambda/D \geqslant 2|e_i|_{max} = 2$$

THE SENSOR EFFICIENT METHOD (SEM)

A key point to realize is that the first constraint at the end of the previous section applies to any NL consecutive lags of the ACF estimates (rather than just the first NL lags), so long as $NL \geqslant 2NT$. It is this point which led to the development of the technique called the "Sensor-Efficient Method" (SEM). We begin by defining $\lambda_1 \triangleq \lambda/n$, $\lambda_2 \triangleq \lambda/(n+1)$, $\lambda_3 \triangleq \lambda/(n+2)$, etc. for any set of consecutive integers, n, n + 1, n + 2,... The model ACF for consecutive lags, assuming equal component powers, can be expressed as

$$R_x(n) = \sum_{i=1}^{NT} |A|^2 e^{j2\pi e_i nD/\lambda} = \sum_{i=1}^{NT} |A|^2 e^{j2\pi e_i D/\lambda_1} = R_1(1)$$

$$R_x(n+1) = \sum_{i=1}^{NT} |A|^2 e^{j2\pi e_i (n+1)D/\lambda} = \sum_{i=1}^{NT} |A|^2 e^{j2\pi e_i D/\lambda_2} = R_2(1)$$

$$R_x(n+2) = \sum_{i=1}^{NT} |A|^2 e^{j2\pi e_i (n+2)D/\lambda} = \sum_{i=1}^{NT} |A|^2 e^{j2\pi e_i D/\lambda_3} = R_3(1)$$

$$R_x(n+k) = \sum_{i=1}^{NT} |A|^2 e^{j2\pi e_i(n+k)D/\lambda} = \sum_{i=1}^{NT} |A|^2 e^{j2\pi e_i D/\lambda_{k-1}} = R_{k+1}(1)$$

Therefore successive lags of the ACF at frequency λ are equal to the first lags of the ACF at wavelengths $[\lambda_i]$, if these wavelengths are chosen to match the specific structure shown [and if the amplitudes of the individual target returns are the same (or known ratios) at each of the λ_i]. This leads the SEM variations of the extended Prony's algorithm described earlier.

The most noteworthy result of using such a "multifrequency reduced data set" is seen in examining the analogy to the previously shown constraint on the number of sensors. Given a return signal composed of NUM frequencies:

$$R_n(1) = -\sum_{i=1}^{NT} a_i R_{n-i}(1) \qquad NT + 1 \leqslant n \leqslant NUM.$$

Since only two sensors, i.e. $N = 2$, are needed to estimate $R_n(1)$,

$$NUM \geqslant 2NT.$$

i.e. - at the expense of increased signal complexity, it is possible to operate with only two sensors.

ALGORITHM PERFORMANCE

In examining the performance of the algorithm, attention will be centered on the accuracy of estimated AOA's and resolution of closely spaced targets. Lacking specific closed-form expressions for the statistics of the algorithm outputs, the measure of accuracy will be its performance relative to the Cramer-Rao bound, which states:

For any unbiased estimate of the nonrandom parameters given by the elements of a vector $\underline{\theta}$, the variance of the estimates is bounded by [4]

$$\sigma_i^2 = E\lfloor[\theta_i(\underline{x}) - \theta_i]^2\rfloor \geqslant j^{ii}$$

where J^{ii} is the ii^{th} element in the square matrix J^{-1} and $\underline{x}$ is the date used in estimation. The elements of $\underline{J}$, the Fisher information Matrix, are given by:

$$J_{ij} = E\{\frac{\partial \ln[p(\underline{x};\theta)]}{\partial\theta_i} \frac{\partial \ln[p(\underline{x};\theta)]}{\partial\theta_j}\} ,$$

where p is the probability density function of the statistic $\underline{x}$.

The bound is examined for four specific multifrequency cases:

1 - One target, multiple random snapshots.
2 - One target, multiple fixed snapshots.
3 - One target, multiple snapshots, reduced data set in the form of ACF estimates .
4 - Two targets, multiple snapshots, reduced data set, in the form of the ACF estimates.

The appropriate statistic for each of these four cases is substituted

606

into $p(\underline{x}; \underline{\theta})$, which is assumed to be multivariate complex Gaussian, to obtain the specific probability density function which is then used to compute the terms in the information matrix. The results of this computation are briefly summarized.

For cases 1 and 2 (single target, measured data) with NS snapshots, the bound on the variance of the directional estimate is given by [5]

$$\sigma_e^2 \geqslant \frac{1}{SNR(NS)} \sum_{i=1}^{NUM} (2\pi/\lambda_i)^2 , \qquad (10)$$

where SNR is the signal-to-noise power ratio: $SNR = \frac{|A|^2}{\sigma_n^2}$. For case 3

(single target, reduced data set), the bound is given by:

$$\sigma_e^2 \geqslant \frac{4(2SNR + 1)\sigma^4}{NUM} 2|A|^4 \sum_{i=1}^{NUM} (2\pi/\lambda_i)^2 (NS)$$

which means, at high SNR,

$$\sigma_e^2 \geqslant \frac{\sum_{i=1}^{NUM} (2\pi/\lambda_i)^2}{SNR(NS)}$$

A comparison of the results for cases 1, 2, and 3 highlights a very important feature -- at reasonable SNR, no accuracy is lost by using the reduced data set rather than the entire set of measured sensor outputs. This is particularly important in the case of Prony's method. To use multiple snapshots with the entire measured data set would require doing the algorithm computation for each individual snapshot and then averaging the results. However, to use multiple snapshots with the reduced data set requires computation of only the ACF estimates for each snapshot, averaging them, and then performing algorithm computation only once. This savings in computation is the rational for using the set of ACF estimates as the data to be processed.

For case 4, while no simple closed-form expression has yet been obtained, the analysis has shown [5] that the bounds on the variance of the directional estimate for a 2-target return are:

1 - dependent upon $1/NS$,
2 - $e_i - e_2 \rightarrow 0 \Rightarrow \sigma_e^2 \rightarrow \infty$, as expected
3 - are not strongly dependent on the SNR.

To compute the expected resolution for the SEM algorithm an analogy to the multisensor case is required. As discussed in the previous section, the mathematical structure of the multifrequency ACF is that of a true (non-timelimited) ACF multiplied by an "equivalent SEM window". In such a case, conventional Fourier techniques will distinguish peaks in

the frequency domain only if $e_i - e_2 \geqslant \frac{\lambda}{D(NUM)}$. This result furnishes a

rationale for selecting the frequency parameters NUM, λ; i.e. - given a specific resolution requirement, the number and spacing of the frequencies can be selected to meet it. This resolution value is that obtainable using Fourier techniques on the given data, and lacking other information, will be used as a first estimate of the SEM performance in distinguishing multiple targets.

SIMULATION RESULTS

The results of interest consisted primarily of SEM accuracy and resolving power (using ACF estimates) as a function of various system parameters (SNR, NS, etc). The experimentally observed behavior of the variance of the directional estimates is depicted in Figs. 1-3.

    1 - In the one target case, the dependence upon SNR and 1/NS, as well as the non-dependence upon location are evident.
    2 - In the two target case, the dependence upon 1/NS and the non-dependence upon SNR are clear.

While this behavior follows the theoretically expected performance in a relative sense, the numerical values of variances obtained are considerably higher than the C/R bound. Therefore, a final variation of SEM is proposed which requires the solution of a nonlinear least-squares problem:

$$\min_{e_i} Q_1 = \min_{e_i} \sum_{n=1}^{NUM} |R_n(1) + \sum_{i=1}^{NT} |A|^2 e^{j2\pi e_i \lambda_n}|^2. \tag{11}$$

To perform the indicated minimization, an iterative computer solution of the resulting nonlinear equations was accomplished. Using the outputs of the previously detailed SEM Extended Prony's Method as the initial parameter values estimate was found to be sufficiently accurate to assure convergence to the correct solution after a quite modest number of iterations.

The final version, consisting of using the Extended Prony's Method on the reduced data set, and then using its output as the initial guess in an iterative nonlinear least-squares (NNLSQ) estimator, is referred to as the Complete Sensor Efficient Method (CSEM). As can be seen in Figs. 4-6, the inclusion of this additional NLLSQ processing results in a directional estimate with variance approaching the C/R bound.

The difficulty in evaluating algorithm performance with respect to distinguishing multiple targets is due to the subjectivity in the definition of resolution: what criteria must be met by a spectral estimate to consider two targets distinguishable? For this initial investigation, it was decided to consider targets having estimates with variances less than $(e_1 - e_2)/3$ to be resolved. Based upon this criterion, Figs. 7 shows that the resolution of the CSEM algorithm is approximately 0.6 - 0.7 equivalent beam widths (EBW).

To determine whether it is the processing by Prony's Method or the particular selection of the $[\lambda_i]$ which is responsible for the improvement in resolution over a typical two-sensor/single frequency array (see Fig. 10), the conventional method (FFT) was also applied to ACF estimates from properly chosen frequency bands. The results are shown in Figs. 8 and 9.

Based on the experimental observations concerning resolution, it seems reasonable to conclude that:

    1 - The SEM algorithm is a 2-sensor technique which has the capability of resolving targets well inside the beamwidth of a standard 2-sensor array.

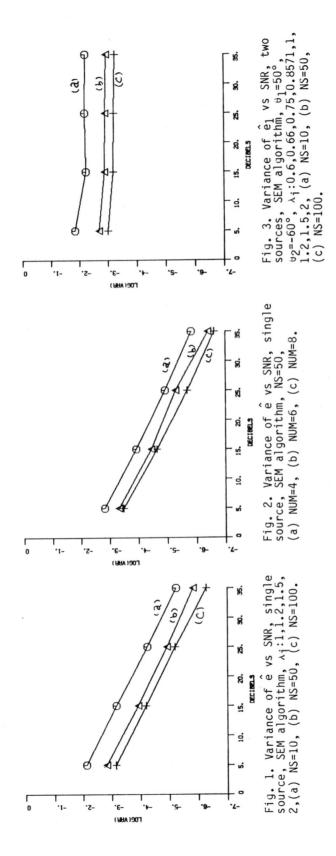

Fig. 3. Variance of $\hat{e}_1$ vs SNR, two sources, SEM algorithm, $\theta_1=50°$, $\theta_2=-60°$, λ_i:0.6,0.66,0.75,0.8571,1, 1.2,1.5,2, (a) NS=10, (b) NS=50, (c) NS=100.

Fig. 2. Variance of $\hat{e}$ vs SNR, single source, SEM algorithm, NS=50, (a) NUM=4, (b) NUM=6, (c) NUM=8.

Fig. 1. Variance of $\hat{e}$ vs SNR, single source, SEM algorithm, λ_i:1,1.2,1.5, 2,(a) NS=10, (b) NS=50, (c) NS=100.

609

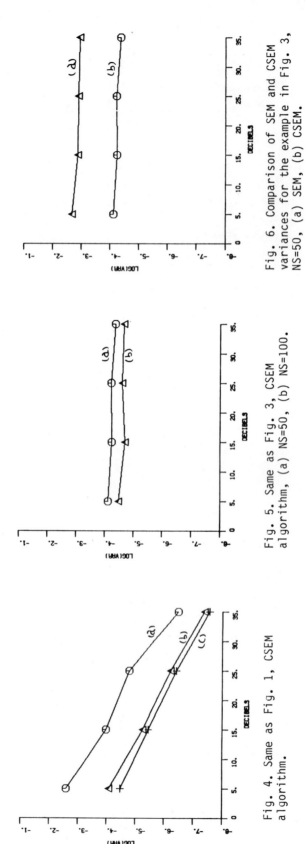

Fig. 6. Comparison of SEM and CSEM variances for the example in Fig. 3, NS=50, (a) SEM, (b) CSEM.

Fig. 5. Same as Fig. 3, CSEM algorithm, (a) NS=50, (b) NS=100.

Fig. 4. Same as Fig. 1, CSEM algorithm.

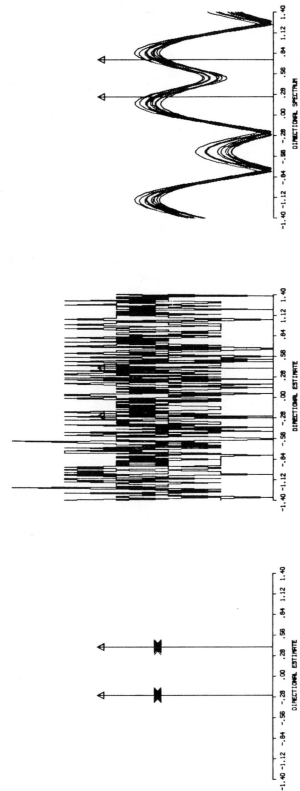

Fig. 7. Samples of estimates of e_1 and e_2 using the SEM algorithm, $e_1-e_2=1$ effective beamwidth, NS=100, SNR=20 dB, λ_i:0.5, 0.666,1,2.

Fig. 8. Samples of the single frequency 2-sensor DFT spectrum of two sources, $e_1-e_2=0.5$, $\lambda=2$, SNR=20 dB.

Fig. 9. Samples of the 4-frequency DFT spectrum, $e_1-e_2=0.75$ effective beamwidths, NS=100, SNR=20 dB, $\lambda_i=0.5$, 0.66,1,2,.

611

2 - The actual resolution can be related to the "effective beamwidth" (EBW) of the array, which is determined by the particular choice of $[\lambda_i]$. The achievable resolution appears to be about 0.6 - 0.7 EBW.

3 - The resolution is a function of SNR and NS only to a secondary degree (i.e. - as ACF estimates improve, the performance will approach the actual resolution limit determined by the $[\lambda_i]$.

CONCLUSIONS

In conclusion, it can be said that the feasibility of using a 2-sensor array to detect multiple targets has been clearly demonstrated by the SEM/CSEM algorithm detailed in this paper. The algorithm opens the door to several intriguing avenues of research.

For the sake of mathematical ease, the class of return signals considered here was made rather specific (wideband approximating pure sinusoids in noise, known amplitude ratios, etc.). The next logical step would appear to be to generalize the class of returns to models approximating sums of true narrowband signals, and finally to a true wideband signal.

Also, while considering the increased complexity involved in analysing these systems, a key point to remember is that one of the highlights of the SEM algorithm is its use as an initializer. Therefore, the efficacy of such an approach may ultimately be to obtain a sufficiently accurate first guess for use in other more traditional processing methods.

The relationships affecting SEM/CSEM performance in the multiple target case, particularly with respect to $[\lambda_i]$ and e_1 -e_2 and their interactions require more intensive investigation. In addition to mathematical analysis, computer simulation detailing the response would prove valuable.

In closing, it can be said that the SEM/CSEM algorithm demonstrates an extremely effective approach in processing directional estimates in the array problem, when the data is in a somewhat restricted class of signals. It is a 2-sensor technique producing amplitude and directional estimates, with accuracy approaching the C/R bound, and resolution capability far exceeding that of regular 2-sensor array techniques. It also appears to be quite promising as a technique in itself or an aid used in conjunction with other methods to process and obtain estimates from an even wider class of signals encountered in the array processing problem.

ACKNOWLEDGEMENT

This work was supported in part by the National Science Foundation under Grant ECS-8414316 and in part by the Office of Naval Research under Grant #N00014-86-K-0410.

REFERENCES

1. S. M. Kay and S. L. Marple, Spectrum Analysis - a Modern Perspective, Proc. IEEE, 69: 1380 (1981).

2. H. Wang and M. Kaveh, Coherent Signal-Subspace Processing for the Detection and Estimation of Angles of Arrival of Multiple Wideband Sources, IEEE Trans. on ASSP, 33: 823 (1985).

3. M. E. Van Blaricum, Problems and Solutions Associated with Proney's Method for Processing Transient Data, IEEE Trans. on Antennas and Prop., 26: 174 (1978).

4. H. Van Trees, "Detection, Estimation and Modulation Theory," Wiley, New York (1968).

5. T. E. Cichocki, "A Sensor-Efficient Method for Wideband Array Processing," Ph.D. Thesis, University of Minnesota, 1986.

ACOUSTICAL IMAGING AND POINT PROCESSES

J.M. Richardson and K.A. Marsh

Rockwell International Science Center
Thousand Oaks, CA 91360

ABSTRACT

There are many situations in acoustical imaging (active or passive)
where the possible sources or scatterers to be detected or discriminated
against are points, or, more generally, are represented by models in
which some kind of point process is embedded. A point process is a random set of points (random both in number and positions) in some kind of
state space. Examples of imaging problems involving point processes may
be found in nondestructive evaluation (including acoustic emission),
underwater surveillance (e.g., bearing estimation), medical imaging
(e.g., in the case where the detection of echogenic nodules in breast
tissue is desired), etc. In this paper, we will address the problem of
estimating the average local density of points in some appropriate state
space, given a set of measured signals. This density function or a
suitable slice or projection of it constitutes the image. Most earlier
treatments of this problem involve either 1) an approach that is exact
for a single-point model, but which involves an inaccurate ad hoc extension to the many-point case, or 2) an approximate approach involving
linear estimators with or without the use of an underlying many-point
model. Neither of these approaches can yield algorithms that can resolve two point sources that are too close to be resolvable according to
conventional optical criteria. We present here a third approach, based
on a many-point model, where the estimation procedure is sufficiently
accurate to preserve the essential "pointyness" of the model. Our estimation procedure involves the solution of a hierarchy of integro-differential equations, appropriately truncated, in which the independent variable is a parameter defining the a priori density bias. Computational
examples will be presented and discussed.

INTRODUCTION

An important aspect of the decision-theoretic approach to acoustical imaging (in fact, to imaging in general) is the use of a priori
information in the development of the imaging algorithm. There is, for
a given measurement process, a direct relationship between the performance of an optimal algorithm and the restrictiveness of the a priori
information. Perhaps the most restrictive kind of a priori information
within the scope of legitimate imaging problems (as contrasted with rec-

ognition problems) is that represented by a point process, or, more
generally, by some kind of statistical ensemble in which a point process
is embedded. A point process can be simply defined as a random act of
points in some kind of state space where the random set involves random
numbers of points as well as random positions.

Next to Gaussian random processes, point processes are possibly the
most frequently occurring type of random process in information science.
Examples of acoustical imaging problems involving point processes may be
found in nondestructive evaluation (including acoustic emission), underwater surveillance (e.g., bearing estimation), medical imaging (e.g., in
the case where the detection of echogenic nodules in breast tissue is
desired), etc.

In this paper, we will discuss a general formulation of estimation
problems involving point processes and a particular method of solution
involving a hierarchy of integro-differential equations, in which the
independent progress variable is a certain kind of a priori density
parameter to be defined later. An application to the problem of bearing
estimation in underwater surveillance will be worked out and computational tests with synthetic data will be presented and discussed.

MATHEMATICAL PRELIMINARIES

It is appropriate to define the state of a many-object system by a
set of representative points in a single-object state space. In the
general discussion presented here and in the two following sections, the
word "object" will be used to denote an entity whose state is represented by a point in an appropriate state space. In the case of spherical voids, for example, a point in the single-object state space, or z-
space as we will call it, is given by the radius and center position of
the void. In the case of noncoherent sources, such as might occur in
the problem of bearing estimation, a point in single-object state space
is given by the bearing and power of the source. To avoid the somewhat
awkward problems associated with the nonunique labeling of the representative points, it is convenient to adopt an occupation number formalism.
To this end, we partition z-space into a large number of small domains
D_i, i = 1, ..., p, and denote the volume of D_i by δz and its nominal
center position by z_i. The state of the many-object system is given by
the set of occupation numbers n_i, ..., n_p, implying that there are n_i
objects with representative points in D_i. More explicitly, the many-
object state x is defined by

$$x^T = (n_i, ..., n_p) \quad .$$ (2.1)

Since we intend to take the limit* $\delta z_i \to 0$, i = 1, ..., p (with a compensating increase in the dimensionality of p) at a later state in the
analysis, it is reasonable to assume that the probability of multiple
occupancy (i.e., $n_i > 1$ for any i) is negligible, and thus we will limit
the possible values of each n_i to 0 and 1. For example, if only one
object were present with a single-object state z_i, the many-object state
x would take the form

---

* It is, of course, necessary to assume that each domain D_i must shrink

   down in all directions.

$$x^T = (0, \ldots, n_i = 1, \ldots, 0) \quad .$$ (2.2)

The generalization to larger numbers of objects is obvious.

3. THE MEASUREMENT MODEL AND STATEMENT OF THE GENERAL ESTIMATION PROBLEM

It is possible to express the measurement model in the simple form

$$y = Fx + \nu$$ (3.1)

where $y =$ an M-dimensional vector representing the possible results of measurement

$\nu =$ an M-dimensional vector representing experimental error and any other perturbing random effects (e.g., scattering from random inhomogeneities not represented by x)

$x =$ a p-dimensional vector representing the state of the many-object system as discussed in the last section

$F =$ an Mxp-dimensional matrix representing the deterministic response of the measurement system.

We assume for the moment that y, ν and F are all real (the state vector x is real by definition).

The term Fx requires further discussion. In more explicit terms, it can be written in the form

$$Fx = \sum_i f(z_i) \, n_i \quad ,$$ (3.2)

where $f(z_i)$ is the noiseless measurement vector that would be obtained if the total many-object system contained only one object and this was located at $z = z_i$ in single-object state space. It is to be stressed that, while the general model given by Eq. (3.1) is linear in x, the dependence on z for the case of one object is, in general, nonlinear. Obvious generalizations of this statement apply to cases in which larger numbers of objects are present. The fact that Eq. (3.1) is linear in x arises from the assumption that in the measurement process different objects contribute independently.

The description of the measurement model must include a discussion of the a priori statistical properties of x and ν. We assume that x and ν are statistically independent. The measurement error ν is assumed to be a Gaussian random vector with the properties

$$E\nu = 0$$ (3.3a)

$$E\nu\nu^T = C_\nu \quad ,$$ (3.3b)

where C_ν is the covariance matrix of ν. The statistical properties of x are given by the expression

$$P(x) = \exp(\lambda + \alpha N) \, P^o(x) \quad ,$$ (3.4)

where N is the total number of objects given by

$$N = \sum_i n_i \quad , \tag{3.5}$$

α is a real constant and λ is a normalization constant defined by the expression

$$\exp(-\lambda) = \sum_x \exp(\alpha N) \, P^o(x) \quad . \tag{3.6}$$

The summation on x involves all possible values of the occupation numbers n_i. The quantity $P^o(x)$ is the so-called standard probability given by the expression

$$P^o(x) = \prod_i P^o(n_i) \quad , \tag{3.7}$$

where

$$P^o(n_i = 0) = 1 - \rho^o(z_i) \, \delta z_i \tag{3.8a}$$

$$P^o(n_i = 1) = \rho^o(z_i) \, \delta z_i \quad . \tag{3.8b}$$

In the above expressions, $\rho^o(z_i)$ is the standard density in single-object state space, i.e., z-space, evaluated at $z = z_i$.

In the above formulation, all of the involved quantities were assumed to be real. In many cases, it is more convenient for y, ν and F to be complex (e.g., in the temporal frequency representation of the scattering process). To convert the above equations to a complex form, it is necessary only to apply an appropriate unitary transformation U to Eq. (3.1), thereby obtaining

$$y' = F'x + \nu' \quad , \tag{3.9}$$

where

$$y' = Uy \tag{3.10}$$

$$F' = UF \tag{3.11}$$

$$\nu' = U\nu \quad . \tag{3.12}$$

Equation (3.3b) must be replaced by

$$E(\nu')(\nu')^\dagger = UC_\nu U^\dagger \overset{\Delta}{=} C'_\nu \quad , \tag{3.13}$$

where $(\ )^\dagger$ is the Hermitian conjugate of $(\ )$. Equations (3.4) to (3.8b) relating to the state vector x are unchanged.

In the subsequent analysis, we will, for the sake of generality, assume the complex case. With the dropping of the primes, this assumption simply means in the writing of formulas that the transpose $(\ )^T$

618

must be replaced by the Hermitian conjugate ( )†. The situation in which quantities are real may now, of course, be regarded as a special case.

We turn now to the consideration of the a posteriori average local density of representative points in single-object state space. In explicit mathematical terms, this quantity is given by the expression

$$\rho(z_i|y)\delta z_i = E(n_i|y)$$

$$= \sum_x n_i \ P(x|y) \quad , \tag{3.14}$$

where $P(x|y)$ is a posteriori probability of x conditioned on the measurement vector y. This quantity is given by

$$P(x|y) = P(y|x) \ P(x)/P(y)$$

$$= P(y|x) \ P(x)/\sum_x P(y|x) \ P(x) \quad , \tag{3.15}$$

where $P(y|x)$ is, in turn, given by

$$P(y|x) = A \ \exp(- \frac{1}{2} \ (y-Fx)^\dagger \ C_\nu^{-1} \ (y-Fx)) \quad , \tag{3.16}$$

in which A is a normalization constant. Substituting Eqs. (3.4) and (3.16) into Eq. (3.15), we obtain

$$P(x|y) = \exp(\mu - \frac{1}{2} \ (y-Fx)^\dagger \ C_\nu^{-1} \ (y-Fx) + \alpha N) \ P^o(x) \quad , \tag{3.17}$$

in which μ is a new normalization constant given by

$$\exp(-\mu) = \sum_x \exp(- \frac{1}{2} \ (y-Fx)^\dagger \ C_\nu^{-1} \ (y-Fx) + \alpha N) \ P^o(x) \quad . \tag{3.18}$$

It will be necessary at a later stage in our analysis to compare the a posteriori average local density $\rho(z_i|y)$ with the a priori average local density $\rho(z_i)$ given by

$$\rho(z_i) \ \delta z_i = E \ n_i = \sum_x n_i \ P(x) \quad , \tag{3.19}$$

where $P(x)$ is given by Eqs. (3.4) and (3.6).

One can also consider higher order average local densities, both a priori and a posteriori, defined by the relations

$$\rho(z_i,z_j) \ \delta z_i \delta z_j = \sum_x n_i n_j \ P(x) \quad , \tag{3.20}$$

619

$$\rho(z_i, z_j | y) \, \delta z_i \delta z_j = \sum_x n_i n_j \, P(x|y) \quad , \tag{3.21}$$

where it is, of course, understood that $i \neq j$. The definitions of still higher order average local densities are obvious. For the sake of convenience, we will henceforth refer to the average local densities simply as densities.

The a priori densities $\rho(z_i)$, $\rho(z_i, z_j)$, etc., are easy to compute since we have assumed no a priori correlations between the occupation numbers for different domains. Using Eqs. (3.4) – (3.8b) and Eq. (3.19), we obtain

$$\rho(z_i) \, \delta z_i = \frac{\exp(\alpha) \, \rho^\circ(z_i) \, \delta z_i}{1 + (\exp(\alpha) - 1) \, \rho^\circ(z_i) \delta z_i} \quad , \tag{3.22}$$

which, in the limit $\delta z_i \to 0$ becomes

$$\rho(z) = \exp(\alpha) \, \rho^\circ(z) \quad . \tag{3.23}$$

It can be readily shown that the second-order density is given by

$$\rho(z, z') = \exp(2\alpha) \, \rho^\circ(z) \, \rho^\circ(z')$$
$$= \rho(z) \, \rho(z') \quad . \tag{3.24}$$

However, in the a posteriori case, no such simple relations can be derived for $\rho(z|y)$, $\rho(z'|y)$, etc., and furthermore it is not in general true that the second-order density can be factored into a product of first-order densities. Thus, the latter observation implies that the conditioning on measurements induces a correlation between the occupation numbers of different domains, a phenomenon that can be inferred from an examination of the quadratic expression in x in the exponent of Eq. (3.17).

At this point, it is appropriate to emphasize that several different forms of optimal estimates can be considered depending on the type of optimality criterion selected. For example, if we choose a mean square error criterion, then the optimal estimate is the a posteriori average value, e.g., $n_i = (n_i|y)$ in the case in which n_i is the quantity to be estimated. Clearly, this optimal criterion underlies the treatment discussed here. However, one could choose the best score (the average fraction of correct estimates in the ensemble of test data corresponding to the measurement model), in which case the optimal estimate is the a posteriori most probable value, e.g., the most probable set of occupation numbers n_i (assuming that a suitable definition of "most probable" can be defined). It is possible to use the a posteriori average values of various combinations of occupation numbers as a point of departure for determining the most probable values, or one can consider a more direct approach to this objective. The latter course has been pursued by Hebbert and Barkakati (1986) in their treatment of the bearing estimation problem. The relation between their approach and ours remains to be investigated.

AN APPROXIMATE SOLUTION FOR $\rho(z|y)$ BASED UPON A HIERARCHY OF EQUATIONS

Although the exact solution for $\rho(z|y)$ and $\rho(z,z'|y)$ is given in a formal sense by Eqs. (3.14), (3.16) and (3.21), it is impossible in a practical sense to carry out by any conceivable combination of analytical and computational processes for an arbitrary value of α. The reader is reminded that the components of the state vector x are not continuous variables. If they were and if $\log P(x)$ were quadratic in x, then the problem would be readily solvable. However, this is not the case, and thus an approximate procedure must be devised.

We observe that as $\alpha \to \infty$, i.e., the system of many-objects becomes very dilute <u>a priori</u>, the conditional density $\rho(z_i|y)$ has a limiting behavior given by

$$\exp(-\alpha) \rho(z|y) \to \exp(y^\dagger \, C_\nu^{-1} \, f(z) - \frac{1}{2} f(z)^\dagger \, C_\nu^{-1} \, f(z)) \, \rho^o(z) \quad (4.1)$$

after taking the limit $\delta z_i \to 0$. This relatively simple result suggests that it might be worthwhile to devise a method that is based on the consideration of the behavior of $P(x|y)$ as α increasess from $-\infty$ to some desired value.

Such a method can be obtained by consideration of the differential equation

$$\frac{\partial}{\partial \alpha} P(x|y) = (N - E(N|y)) \, P(x|y)$$

$$= \sum_i (n_i - E(n_i|y)) \, P(x|y) \quad , \quad (4.2)$$

where, as previously stated, $N = \sum_i n_i$ is the total number of objects present.

The above result is simply derived from Eq. (3.17) by direct differentiation with respect to α and by noting from Eq. (3.18) that

$$\frac{\partial \mu}{\partial \alpha} = -E(N|y) \quad . \quad (4.3)$$

A similar equation can be derived from $P(x)$, namely

$$\frac{\partial}{\partial \alpha} P(x) = (N - EN) \, P(x) \quad , \quad (4.4)$$

by differentiating Eq. (3.4) with respect to α and using Eq. (3.6) to deduce that

$$\frac{\partial \lambda}{\partial \alpha} = -EN \quad . \tag{4.5}$$

Due to the lack of a priori correlation between occupation numbers for different domains, the unconditional average densities of various orders can be simply obtained in closed form, and thus there is not need for an approximate procedure in this part of the problem.

Starting with the differential equation, (4.2), we can derive an infinite hierarchy of equations for the various orders of a posteriori densities by multiplying both sides of Eq. (4.2) by n_j, $n_j n_k$, $n_j n_k n_l$, etc., and then summing on x. We obtain the first member of the hierarchy in the form

$$\frac{\partial}{\partial \alpha} E(n_j|y) = E(n_j|y) - E(n_j|y)^2$$

$$+ \sum_i{}' (E(n_i n_j|y - E(n_i|y) E(n_i|y)) \quad , \tag{4.6}$$

where the prime on the summation sign denotes the omission of the term in which $i = j$. Using the definitions (3.14) and (3.21) and taking the limit $\delta z_i \to 0$ for all i, we obtain the result

$$\frac{\partial}{\partial \alpha} \rho(z|y) = \rho(z|y) + \int dz'(\rho(z,z'|y) - \rho(z|y) \rho(z'|y)) \quad . \tag{4.7}$$

The next member of the hierarchy is obtained by a somewhat similar procedure, with the final result

$$\frac{\partial}{\partial \alpha} \rho(z,z'|y) = 2\rho(z,z'|y)$$

$$+ \int dz'' (\rho(z,z',z'')|y) - \rho(z,z'|y) \rho(z''|y)) \quad . \tag{4.8}$$

We will not discuss the higher members here.

It is interesting to note that, outside of the fact that $\log P(x|y)$ contains an isolated additive term αN, the hierarchy is completely independent of the structure of $P(x|y)$. These structural details enter the solution through the "initial" conditions (i.e., the values of the various conditional densities in the limit $\alpha \to -\infty$) to be used in the solution of the hierarchy of integro-differential equations. These conditions are obtained by analyzing the behavior of $P(x|y)$ given by Eq. (3.17) as $\alpha \to -\infty$. We will postpone further investigation of these questions until the hierarchy is transformed into a more convenient form.

The above hierarchy of equations may be reminiscent (at least to some readers) of certain hierarchies of equations used in classical statistical mechanics. For a review of such developments, the reader is referred to the monograph by Ruelle (1969).

Following the common practice in classical statistical mechanics, we will introduce correlation factors $g(z,z'|y)$, $g(z,z',z''|y)$, etc., defined by the relations

$$\rho(z,z'|y) = \rho(z|y)\, \rho(z'|y)\, g(z,z'|y) \tag{4.9}$$

$$\rho(z,z',z''|y) = \rho(z|y)\, \rho(z'|y)\, \rho(z''|y)\, g(z,z'|y)$$
$$g(z',z''|y)\, g(z'',z|y)\, g(z,z',z''|y) \tag{4.10}$$

etc. It is understood that all of the g functions are unchanged by permuting the order of the various z arguments, i.e., $g(z,z'|y) = g(z',z|y)$, etc. We will introduce a new variable, γ, replacing α in accordance with the relation

$$\gamma = \exp(\alpha) \quad . \tag{4.11}$$

It can be shown that γ is proportional to $\rho(z|y)$ when γ is very small. We accordingly introduce a reduced density $\sigma(z|y)$, defined by the relation

$$\rho(z|y) = \gamma\sigma(z|y) \quad . \tag{4.12}$$

The reduced density approaches a function independent of γ as $\gamma \to 0$.

With the above modifications, the first member of the hierarchy, i.e., Eq. (4.6), reduces to

$$\frac{\partial}{\partial\gamma} \log \sigma(z|y) = \int dz'\, \sigma(z'|y)\, (g(z,z'|y)-1) \tag{4.13}$$

and the second number, Eq. (4.8), reduces to

$$\frac{\partial}{\partial\gamma} \log g(z,z'|y) = \int dz''\, \sigma(z''|y)[(g(z,z''|y)-1)(g(z',z''|)-1)$$

$$+ g(z,z''|y)g(z',z''|y)(g(z,z',z''|y)-1)] \quad .\tag{4.14}$$

By analyzing the behavior of $E(n_i|y)$ and $E(n_i n_j|y)$ as $\gamma \to 0$ (or $\alpha \to -\infty$), we obtain the initial conditions

$$\sigma(z|y)\big|_{\gamma=0} = \exp(y^\dagger\, c_\nu^{-1}\, f(z) - \tfrac{1}{2} f(z)^\dagger\, c_\nu^{-1}\, f(z))\, \rho^o(z) \tag{4.15}$$

$$g(z,z'|y)\big|_{\gamma=0} = \exp(-f(z)^\dagger\, c_\nu^{-1}\, f(z')) \quad . \tag{4.16}$$

It is easy to show that all of the higher order g functions have an initial value of 1.

We will henceforth call the above hierarchy of integro-differential equations the densification hierarchy because of the fact that it transforms a set of densities of various orders (more appropriately, a set of reduced densities and correlation factors) from a situation with a low a priori density bias to one with a high a priori density bias. As shown in Fig. 1, one can regard this procedure as involving the consideration of a continuous sequence of measurement models, each containing a different a priori density bias represented by the parameter γ.

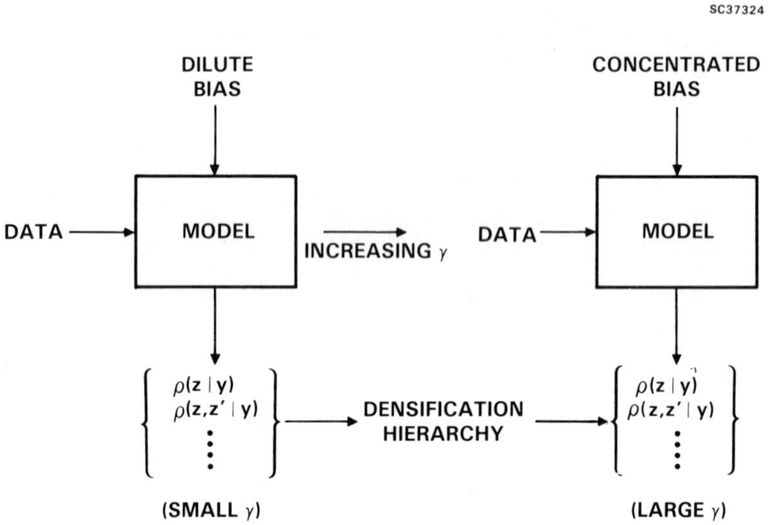

SC37324

DILUTE
BIAS

CONCENTRATED
BIAS

DATA → MODEL

INCREASING γ

DATA → MODEL

$$\left\{ \begin{array}{c} \rho(z \mid y) \\ \rho(z,z' \mid y) \\ \vdots \end{array} \right\}$$ DENSIFICATION HIERARCHY $$\left\{ \begin{array}{c} \rho(z \mid y) \\ \rho(z,z' \mid y) \\ \vdots \end{array} \right\}$$

(SMALL γ)

(LARGE γ)

Fig. 1   Continuum of measurement models and the densification hierarchy.

There remains the problem of selecting the terminal value of γ in the integration of the above hierarchy. We could decide in advance what the terminal value should be, i.e., the desired a priori probability P(x) is completely specified. Another possibility is that value of the parameter γ is unknown a priori, but which can be determined from the measured data represented by the vector y. Regarding γ as a random variable to be estimated by the maximum likelihood procedure, we obtain the an estimate given by the condition

$$E(N \mid y) = EN \quad , \tag{4.17}$$

i.e., the best estimate of γ, the desired (i.e., terminal) value, is consistent with the equality of the a priori and a posteriori average values of the total number of objects. In terms of $\sigma(z \mid y)$ and $\rho^0(z)$, this condition can be expressed in the form

$$\int dz(\sigma(z \mid y) - \rho^0(z)) = 0 \quad . \tag{4.18}$$

In the present treatment, this equation will be used as the stopping rule for the integration of the hierarchy of integro-differential equations.

To obtain a practical computational scheme for the infinite hierarchy, whose first two members are Eqs. (4.13) and (4.14), we must introduce a truncation approximation that yields a finite hierarchy of tractable complexity. Here, we will employ a particular truncation approximation in which terms in Eq.(4.14) proportional to $g(z,z',z''|y)-1$ are neglected. This reduces the hierarchy to two members given by Eqs. (4.13) and (4.14), but with the last line of Eq. (4.14) omitted. In the specific applications discussed below, we will introduce additional approximations with the objective of reducing computational effort still further.

APPLICATION TO BEARING ESTIMATION

In this section, we will show how the point-process formalism developed in the last section can be applied to the problem of bearing estimation in underwater surveillance. We assume a physical setup exemplified schematically by Fig. 2, in which noncoherent localized sources of sound of various powers radiate more or less isotropically in the horizontal plane. We assume here that the stratified nature of the ocean affects only the vertical structure of the transmitted waves to an appreciable extent. The waves from all sources impinge on a linear array of hydrophones. As shown, the estimation process occurs in two steps: 1) the formation of a "conventional" image; and 2) the improvement of this image by an algorithm based on a suitable point-process model. The whole estimation process could be performed in one step, if desired.

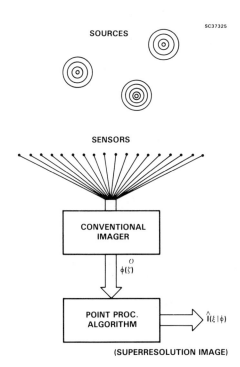

Fig. 2 Schematic setup for
        the bearing estima-
        tion problem.

The reason for the choice of two steps is that the first step, i.e., the "conventional" imaging process to be described below, reduces the remaining problem to one that is described by a standard measurement model of the form (3.1) or (3.2).

The first step involving the so-called "conventional" imaging process for noncoherent sources starts with the determination of the cross power spectral densities for the outputs of various pairs of transducers. These complex quantities, one of which is denoted by $V(m,m')$ for the case of hydrophones m and m', are called visibility functions. It is well known (Devaney, 1979) that the visibility function $V(m,m')$ is given by

$$V(m,m') = (4\pi)^{-2}|q|^2 \sum_i \alpha_i \exp(i\omega e^{-1}\xi_i(x_m-x_{m'}))n_i$$
$$+ v(m,m') \tag{5.1a}$$

where $q = q(\omega)$ is the response of a transducer in the frequency domain

α_i = power of a source represented by a point in cell i

ε = velocity of sound

ξ_i = $\sin\theta_i$, where θ_i is the bearing of a source represented by a point in cell i

x_m = position of nth transducer on the x-axis

n_i = occupation number of cell i

$v(m,m')$ = random experimental error associated with $V(m,m')$

We assume that the variable ξ_i (or ξ in general) is confined to the localization domain $[-\frac{1}{2}\xi_o, \frac{1}{2}\xi_o]$.

It is easily seen that the deterministic part of the visibility function $V(m,m')$ is a Fourier component of the true image defined by

$$\psi(\xi) = \sum_i \alpha_i \delta(\xi-\xi_i)n_i \tag{5.2}$$

corresponding to the "spatial" frequency

$$-\omega c^{-1}(x_m-x_{m'}) \qquad . \tag{5.3}$$

Here, ξ is a dimensionless variable related to a possible bearing, and the above "spatial" frequency is correspondingly dimensionless. Thus, we see that the set of visibility functions, aside from measurement error provides a bandwidth-limited representation of $\psi(\xi)$, which we can express in the form

$$\overline{\psi}(\zeta) = \sum_i \alpha_i f(\zeta-\xi_i)n_i \qquad , \tag{5.4}$$

where $f(\zeta)$ is a point-spread function embodying the bandwidth limitations. In the computational example, we will assume the

$$f(\zeta) = a \text{ sine } b \zeta \qquad (5.5)$$

corresponding to a continuous band of "spatial frequencies (see Eq. (5.3)) in the interval $[-b,b]$. The amplitude scale factor a will not be discussed.

Re-introducing experimental error, we obtain the equivalent measurement model

$$\phi(\zeta) = \overline{\phi}(\zeta) + \nu(\zeta)$$

$$= \sum_i \alpha_i \ f(\zeta - \xi_i) n_i + \nu(\zeta) \qquad , \qquad (5.1b)$$

in which the new measurement noise $\nu(\zeta)$ is an appropriate Fourier transform of $\nu(m,m')$. It is clear that the bearing (more correctly, the sine of the bearing) and power (ξ and α, respectively) correspond to the single-object state z in the general formulation.

To complete the specification of the measurement model, we must define the a priori statistical properties of $\nu(\zeta)$ and the n_i. Because of the nature of $\nu(m,m')$, the random process $\nu(\zeta)$ will have a positive mean. We will subtract this term from both sides of Eq. (5.5) and accordingly redefine a new $\nu(\zeta)$ with zero mean. We assume, as usual, that $\nu(\zeta)$ is a Gaussian random process with the properties

$$E \ \nu(\zeta) = 0 \qquad (5.6a)$$

$$E \ \nu(\zeta) \ \nu(\zeta') = S_\nu \delta(\zeta - \zeta') \qquad . \qquad (5.6b)$$

The statistical properties of the n_i are assumed to be statistically independent of $\nu(\zeta)$. At this stage, we introduce another assumption: namely, that α is a discrete-valued variable, while ξ is still continuous-valued. Without going into the detailed modifications in the general theory of point processes required by the presence of a discrete-valued, single-object state variable, we will discuss the end results. As in the general discussion, the a priori statistical properties of the n_i are defined by the parameter γ and the standard density $\rho^0(\xi,\alpha)$, which is now interpreted as the standard density in ξ-space for a given value of α. Thus, $\sum_\alpha \rho^0(\xi,\alpha)$ is the standard density in ξ-space of sources of all powers.

The truncated densification hierarchy now takes the form

$$\frac{\partial}{\partial y} \log \sigma(\xi,\alpha|\phi) = \int d\xi' \sum_{\alpha'} \sigma(\xi',\alpha'|\phi) \qquad (5.7)$$

627

$$\frac{\partial}{\partial \gamma} \log \left(1 + h(\xi, \alpha; \xi', \alpha' | \phi)\right)$$

$$\frac{\partial}{\partial \gamma} \log \left(1 + h(\xi, \alpha; \xi', \alpha' | \phi)\right)$$

$$= \int d\xi'' \sum_{\alpha''} \sigma(\xi'', \alpha'' | \phi) \, h(\xi, \alpha; \xi'', \alpha'' | \phi) \, h(\xi', \alpha'; \xi'', \alpha'' | \phi) \qquad (5.8)$$

where $\sigma(\xi, \alpha | \phi)$ is the a posteriori reduced density and $1 + h(\xi, \alpha; \xi', \alpha' | \phi)$ is the a posteriori correlation factor (corresponding to $g(z, z' | y)$ in Section 4). The quantity $\gamma\sigma(\xi, \alpha | \phi)$ is the a posteriori density of sources in ξ-space for a given intensity α. The truncation approximation, reducing the infinite hierarchy to the above two-member hierarchy, involves neglecting the deviation of the third-order correlation factor (corresponding to $g(z, z', z'' | y)$ in the general theory) from unity.

The initial (i.e., $\gamma = 0$) conditions for the above integro-differential equations are

$$\sigma(\xi, \alpha | \phi) \big|_{\gamma=0} = \exp(S_\nu^{-1} \alpha \int d\zeta \, \phi(\zeta) f(\zeta - \xi)$$

$$- \frac{1}{2} \alpha^2 \int d\zeta \, f^2(\zeta)) \rho^o(\xi, \alpha) \qquad (5.9)$$

$$1 + h(\xi, \alpha; \xi', \alpha' | \phi) \big|_{\gamma=0}$$

$$= \exp(-S_\nu^{-1} \alpha \alpha' \int d\zeta \, f(\zeta - \xi) f(\zeta - \xi')) \qquad . \qquad (5.10)$$

The terminal value of γ is given by the stopping rule

$$\int d\xi \sum_{\alpha} \left(\sigma(\xi, \alpha | \phi) - \rho^o(\xi, \alpha)\right) = 0 \qquad . \qquad (5.11)$$

All of the integrations in ξ and ζ in the above equations span the localization domain $[-\frac{1}{2}\xi_0, \frac{1}{2}\xi_0]$.

Our ultimate objectives include the calculation of the a posteriori intensity (power per unit interval in ξ-space) given by

$$I(\xi | \phi) = E(\psi(\xi) | \phi)$$

$$= \sum_{\alpha} \alpha \, \rho(\xi, \alpha | \phi) \qquad , \qquad (5.12)$$

where $\psi(\xi)$ is the true image defined by Eq. (5.2).

For the sake of reducing computational labor, we introduce an additional approximation that implies that $h(\xi, \alpha; \xi', \alpha' | \phi)$ is a function only of the difference $\xi - \xi'$. Specifically, we assume that $f(\zeta)$ is periodic with a period ξ_0 (corresponding to the localization domain $[-\frac{1}{2}\xi_0, \frac{1}{2}\xi_0]$) and we replace $\sigma(\xi, \alpha | \phi)$ by its average on ξ, i.e.

$$\sigma(\xi,\alpha|\phi) \rightarrow \overline{\sigma}(\alpha|\phi) \qquad , \tag{5.13a}$$

$$\overline{\sigma}(\alpha|\phi) = \xi_o^{-1} \int d\xi \ \sigma(\xi,\alpha|\phi) \qquad . \tag{5.13b}$$

This approximation reduces the number of bits required for storing the correlation factor.

To investigate the nature of the estimation process based on the densification hierarchy, we have considered several computational examples using synthetic test data. In the generation of the synthetic test data, we assume a true image given by

$$\widetilde{\psi}(\xi) = \alpha_1\delta(\xi-\xi_1) + \alpha_2\delta(\xi-\xi_2) \tag{5.14}$$

corresponding to two single-source states with bearings and powers given by (ξ_1,α_1) and (ξ_2,α_2), respectively. The conventional image is then given by

$$\widetilde{\phi}(\zeta) = \int d\xi \ f(\zeta-\xi) \ \widetilde{\psi}(\xi) + \widetilde{\nu}(\zeta)$$

$$= \alpha_1 f(\zeta-\xi_1) + \alpha_2 f(\psi-\xi_2) + \widetilde{\nu}(\zeta) \qquad , \tag{5.15}$$

where $f(\zeta)$ is given by Eq. (5.5) and $\widetilde{\nu}(\zeta)$ is a sample of Gaussian white noise. The generation of synthetic test data is illustrated with and without noise in Fig. 3.

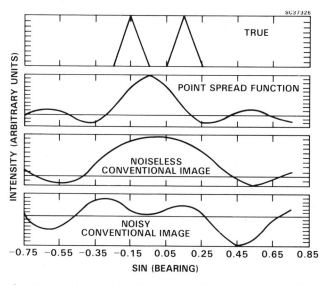

Fig. 3 Generation of noiseless and noisy synthetic data.

In the computable forms of both the test data generation and the densification hierarchy, the variables ξ and ζ will be defined on a discrete mesh extending over the localization domain $[-\frac{1}{2}\xi_o, \frac{1}{2}\xi_o]$, i.e., we set

$$\xi = -\frac{1}{2}\xi_o + s\delta\xi \quad , \tag{5.16}$$

where $s = 0,1,\ldots,15$ and $\delta\xi = \xi_o/15$. The integral $\delta d\xi h(\xi)$ is replaced by the discrete summation $\frac{1}{16}\sum_{s=0}^{15} h(-\frac{1}{2}\xi_o + s\delta\xi)$ with an analogous expression for an integration on ζ.

The measurement model (5.16) stays as written for the case of discrete-valued ξ_i, ξ and ζ. The a priori statistical description of $\nu(\xi)$ must be changed by replacing S_ν by σ_ν^2 (where σ_ν is the standard deviation) and replacing $\delta(\zeta-\zeta')$ by a Kronecker delta in Eq. (5.6b). The a priori statistical properties of the n_i stand as written. Here, we make the special assumption that $\rho^o(\xi,\alpha) = 5$ and that α takes the values 0.8, 1.0 and 1.2.

The next step is the integration of the truncated densification hierarchy (5.7) and (5.8) with the additional approximation (5.13a) and (5.13b) incorporated. The initial conditions (5.9) and (5.10) are modified by the substitution of S_ν by σ^2 and the integration by the discrete summation discussed above. The integration is terminated by the stopping rule (5.11) appropriately reformulated in discrete form. It is to be emphasized that the truncated densification hierarchy is now a large system of ordinary differential equations that can be integrated by elementary methods. In this integration, we use an increment $\delta\gamma = 0.001$.

Numerical values assumed for other parameters are: $\delta\xi = 0.1$ (corresponds to $\xi_o = 1.5$ or $|\theta|_{max} \approx 45°$), $a = 1$ and $b = 13.8$. Our measure of signal-to-noise (S/N) ratio is

$$S/N = \tilde{\phi}(\zeta)_{max}/\sigma_\nu \quad , \tag{5.17}$$

thereby giving a relation between S/N and σ_ν for each set of synthetic data. In all cases, the synthetic data involved the bearings $\xi_1 = -0.5$ and $\xi_2 = 0.15$, with various values of α_1 and α_2 to be specified in individual cases.

We first consider two cases of noiseless data, but with S/N = 1 in the imaging algorithm. In the first case, we assume sources of equal power ($\alpha_1 = \alpha_2 = 1$) in the synthetic data. The results of integrating the truncated densification hierarchy is depicted in Fig. 4. Specifically, we show the evolution of the spatial distribution of estimated intensity $I(\xi|\phi)$ (given by Eq. (5.12)) as a function of γ, from the initial value $\gamma = 0$ to the terminal value ($\gamma \approx 0.1$), determined by the stopping rule (Eq. (5.11)). It is interesting to note that in the initial phase of the evolution of $I(\xi|\phi)$ it is difficult to perceive the presence of two sources, while in the terminal phase there is rapid improvement in the resolution of the sources. The final estimated in-

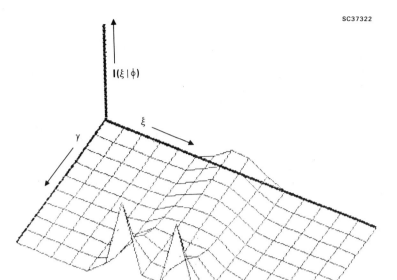

SC37322

$I(\xi|\phi)$

ξ

γ

Fig. 4 Evolution of estimated intensity distribution $I(\xi|\phi)$ with
increasing γ. Noiseless synthetic data; two assumed sources
with equal powers ($\alpha_1 = \alpha_2 = 1$).

tensity distribution agrees perfectly with the assumed intensity distribution within the resolution limits imposed by the mesh spacing ($\delta\xi$ =
0.1).

In the second case with noiseless data, we assume two unequal
powers corresponding to $\alpha_1 = 0.8$ and $\alpha_2 = 1.2$. As shown in Fig. 5, the
estimated intensity distribution evolves into a final form with clearly
perceptible separate sources. It is interesting to note that their peak
positions are correct (within the resolution limits imposed by the mesh
spacing). The relative values of the peak intensities are qualitatively
correct. It is also of interest to note that the stopping rule did not
become operative until a significantly higher value of γ was reached.

In the third case, we reconsider the case of equal sources corresponding to $\alpha_1 = \alpha_2 = 1$, but now with noise in the test data (with S/N =
1). We chose a random sample of such noise. The evolution of the estimated intensity distribution is shown in Fig. 6. In the initial phase,
the contribution of the second source at $\xi = \xi_2 = 0.15$ is barely perceptible. This is because the present noise sample reduced the contribution of second source to $\widetilde{\phi}(\zeta)$ and because the exponential dependence
on $\widetilde{\phi}(\zeta)$ in the initial condition (5.9) exaggerated the reduction. This
accidental occurrence makes the present case look very much like the
second case. In the terminal phase, two clearly perceptible peaks have
formed with the correct separation (again, within the resolution limits
imposed by the mesh) and with approximately the correct ratio of peak
intensities. However, the peak positions have shifted to the left by
0.1 in the ξ-axis. It is to be noted that the terminal value of γ is
much larger than that in the first case.

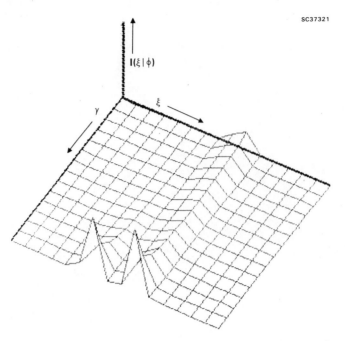

SC37321

Fig. 5 Evolution of estimated intensity distribution $I(\xi|\phi)$ with increasing γ. Noiseless synthetic data; two assumed sources with unequal powers ($\alpha 1 = 0.8$, $\alpha 2 = 1.2$).

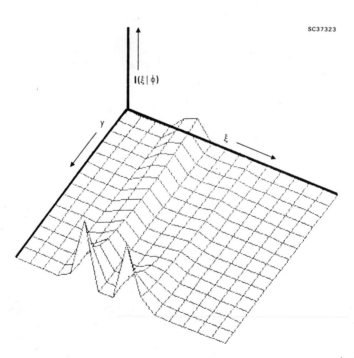

SC37323

Fig. 6 Evolution of estimated intensity distribution $I(\xi|\phi)$ with increasing γ. Noisy synthetic data (S/N = 1); two assumed sources with equal powers ($\alpha 1 = \alpha 2 = 1$).

A second computation of the last case was made with another random sample of noise in the synthetic data. Here, the integration on γ proceeded to very large values of γ without satisfying the stopping rule. Clearly, a more systematic investigation of the effect of noise needs to be made.

COMMENTS

It clear from the above application of point process theory to bearing estimation that the integration of the truncated densification hierarchy yields a terminal image (i.e., the estimated intensity distribution) showing a significant degree of super resolution in the presence of substantial noise. It is to be noted that this formalism involves an adaptive feature in the stopping rule that determines the terminal value of the a priori density parameter γ in a manner dependent upon the measured data. This example also suggests that truncation of the hierarchy at the second member preserves the underlying "pointyness" of the model. Some earlier investigations have suggested that truncation at the first member does not preserve this property to a sufficient degree.

It is also to be stressed that the above formalism can be applied to any imaging problem involving point processes as long as this problem fits into the general framework.

ACKNOWLEDGEMENT

This investigation was supported by Independent Research and Development funds of Rockwell International.

REFERENCES

Devaney, A.J., 1979, "The Inverse Problem for Random Sources," J. Math. Phys. 20 (8), pp. 1687-1691.

Hebbert, R.S. and Barkakati, L.T., 1986, "High-Resolution Transforming by Fitting a Plane-Wave Model to Acoustic Data," J. Acoust. Soc. Am. 79 (6), pp. 1844-1849.

Ruelle, D., 1969, Statistical Mechanics-Rigorous Results, Chap. 4, Benjamin, NY.

HIGH-RESOLUTION ACOUSTICAL IMAGE RECONSTRUCTION

ALGORITHM FOR FINITE-SIZE OBJECTS: THE CASCADE FORM

Hua Lee

Department of Electrical and Computer Engineering
University of Illinois at Urbana-Champaign
Urbana, Illinois 61801

Abstract- Backward propagation has been one of the most widely used algorithms for acoustical image reconstruction and it is known that the resolution of the resultant images is governed by Rayleigh-criterion. The quality of the image reconstruction can be significantly improved by utilizing additional constraints such as the finite spatial-frequency bandwidth of the resultant wavefield and the finite size of the source region.

It has been shown that we can utilize the finite frequency bandwidth information to improve resolution by wavefield extrapolation. Recently, a more advanced reconstruction algorithm is formulated by using both the finite bandwidth and source size information for super-resolution imaging. However, the construction of the linear matrix operator of this algorithm is not computationally efficient because the elements of the matrix can not be formulated in closed form.

This paper introduces the formulation of the optimal image reconstruction algorithm in a cascade form. Both the finite frequency bandwidth and source size are utilized for resolution enhancement. The enhancement matrix operation consists of three independent matrix operators: one for wavefield extrapolation, one for backward propagation, and one for spatial frequency bandwidth extension. All these operators are formulated independently in closed form to be computationally efficient. The formulation can also be used to evaluate the performance and limitation of discrete acoustical imaging systems in terms of the computation and resolution with respect to data acquisition, aperture size, source size, and noise level.

Introduction

For holographic acoustical image reconstruction, the backward propagation method represents the earliest development of image reconstruction algorithms [1,2]. It is popularly used in various inverse scattering problems because of the simplicity in terms of algorithm structure and stability in the presence of noise. The resolution of the images reconstructed by backward propagation is half wavelength for systems with infinite apertures. This is due to the loss of the evanescent wave components during propagation. For systems with finite size receiving apertures, the resolution limit is governed by Raleigh criterion. Since then, because of the emphasis of high-resolution reconstruction, many algorithms have been developed by utilizing a priori knowledge of the source distribution, spatial frequency bandwidth, or finite size of the source region [3-8]. With the

635

assumption of discrete source distribution, discrete mode algorithms are developed in iterative and non–iterative forms [3,4,6]. Using the finite frequency bandwidth, we also formulated algorithms for image enhancement by wave–field extrapolation[5]. To maximize the information content of data acquisition, optimal sampling is then formulated [8]. Recently, the optimal image reconstruction algorithm has been developed for the partial-discrete mode by considering all available constraints including finite source size, sample spacing, and spatial-frequency bandwidth [9].

The basic structure of the optimal algorithm consists of a linear matrix operation and followed by backward propagation. The significance of the development of the optimal algorithm is that it provides a clear description of the enhancement of image resolution, system performance and sensitivity corresponding to the available constraints. However, the formation of the matrix operation is not computationally efficient because of the complex structure of the elements. Therefore, in this paper, we provide an alternative formulation of the optimal algorithm such that the enhancement matrix operator is partitioned into three independent operations. These operators are independently associated with the constraints and are in closed form. This format will not only enable us to improve the computation of the image reconstruction, but also to identify the contribution of the constraints independently to resolution enhancement.

Background

For coherent acoustical imaging systems, the linear and space–invariant relationship between the source distribution $p(x)$ and the complex amplitude of the resultant wave–field $q(x)$ can be represented by a linear convolution integral

$$q(x) = \int_{-d}^{d} p(x') h(x-x') dx' \qquad (1)$$

The space-limited source distribution is bounded within the interval $(-d, d)$. The impulse response of the systems which widely known as the Green's function is given by

$$h(x) = \frac{1}{j\lambda r} \exp(j2\pi r/\lambda) \qquad (2)$$

where λ is the wavelength and $r = |x|$.

In practice, for most systems with discrete data acquisition devices, only a finite number of wave–field data samples are detected at a finite-size aperture and available for image reconstruction. Assume that the sample spacing of the received wave–field is uniform, then Eq. (1) becomes

$$q(n) \overset{\Delta}{=} q(x)|_{x=n\Delta x} \qquad (3)$$

$$= \int_{-d}^{d} p(x') h(n\Delta x - x') dx'$$

where Δx is the sample spacing and $q(n)$ denotes the detected wave–field sequence.

636

Then we can describe the image reconstruction as an optimization procedure that the objective is to solve for the continuous space-limited source distribution p(x) based on N uniformly-spaced wave-field data samples q(n). This is to estimate an infinite-dimensional unknown function with only a finite number of measurements.

Consider a vector space with the associated inner product defined as

$$<a(x), b(x)> = \int_{-d}^{d} a(x)b^{*}(x) \, dx \qquad (4)$$

Hence we can rewrite Eq. (3) as

$$q(n) = \int_{-d}^{d} p(x') \, h(n\Delta x - x') \, dx' \qquad (5)$$

$$= <p(x), h^{*}(n\Delta x - x)>$$

The optimal (minimum-norm) solution exists in an N-dimensional subspace can be written in the form of

$$\hat{p}(x) = \sum_{n=1}^{N} s(n) \, h^{*}(n\Delta x - x) \qquad (6)$$

where s(n) denotes the optimal coefficient sequence of the combination in the subspace.

The optimal solution must satisfy the measurement constraints given by Eq. (3)

$$q(n) = <\hat{p}(x), h^{*}(n\Delta x - x)> \qquad (7)$$

$$= \int_{-d}^{d} \left[\sum_{k=1}^{N} s(k) \, h^{*}(k\Delta x - x) \right] h(n\Delta x - x) \, dx$$

$$= \sum_{k=1}^{N} s(k) \int_{-d}^{d} h(n\Delta x - x) h^{*}(k\Delta x - x) \, dx$$

We define

$$H(n,k) \overset{\Delta}{=} < h(n\Delta x - x), h(k\Delta x - x)> \qquad (8)$$

$$= \int_{-d}^{d} h(n\Delta x - x)\, h^{*}(k\Delta x - x)\, dx$$

Then Eq. (7) can be written as

$$q(n) = \sum_{k=1}^{N} s(k)\, H(n,k) \tag{9-a}$$

and alternatively we can write it in matrix form

$$[q] = [H][S] \tag{9-b}$$

where [s] and [q] are the vector representations of the sequences $s(n)$ and $q(n)$ respectively, and [H] is a square matrix with its elements $H(n,k)$.

According to this formulation, the optimal image reconstruction algorithm can be described as follows:

Step 1: Formulate [H] matrix according to Eq. (8).

Step 2: Obtain optimal coefficients $s(n)$.

Step 3: Perform image reconstruction according to Eq. (6).

The sequence $s(n)$ is found by applying the inverse of [H] to the received data sequence. This matrix operation is an enhancement process which fully utilizes the information of the finite source size and the finite transfer function bandwidth. It should be also pointed out that the optimal image is formed by backward propagating the enhanced wave-field samples to the source region (-d, d). Fig. (1) shows the diagram of the procedure of the optimal image reconstruction algorithm.

Discrete Band-Limited Spectral Estimation and Signal Extrapolation

It can be seen from the algorithm structure that the enhancement matrix operation is the only basic difference between the optimal algorithm and the conventional backward propagation method. Because there is no closed form available to generate the matrix elements $H(n,k)$, the formation of the enhancement operator becomes computationally complicated and often inaccurate during practical implementation and execution of the algorithm. Therefore, we need to partition the optimal algorithm into three cascade components.

First we need to review the band-limited spectral estimation technique by discrete signal extrapolation [10,11]. The band-limited spectral estimation problem is to obtain the continuous spectrum based on a finite number of space domain data samples. When the estimation objective is the band-limited space-domain signal which is equivalent to the spectrum, this technique is known as the discrete band-limited signal extrapolation. Consider a band-limited space function $w(x)$ with cutoff frequency f_c. We are given a finite number of uniformly-spaced data samples to estimate the band-limited spectrum $W(f)$. The relationship between the space-domain data samples and the unknown spectrum can be written as

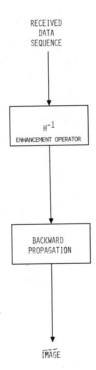

Fig. 2   Diagram of the Optimal Imaging Algorithm
in Cascade Form.

$$w(n) = w(x)|_{x=n\Delta x} = F^{-1}\{W(f)\}|_{x=n\Delta x} \qquad (10)$$

$$= \int\limits_{-f_c}^{f_c} W(f)\exp(j2\pi f n\Delta x)\,df$$

Define a finite-size control-point sequence $c(n)$ and the sample spacing of the control points is $\Delta x'$. The control-point sequence gives the same spectral distribution $W(f)$ within the lowpass frequency band.

$$W(f) = F\{\sum_{k=1}^{N} c(k)\,\delta(x-k\Delta x')\} \qquad (11)$$

$$= \sum_{k=1}^{N} c(k)\exp(-j2\pi f k\Delta x')$$

Combining Eqs. (10) and (11), we have the linear relation between the received waveform and control-point sequences.

$$w(n) = \int\limits_{-f_c}^{f_c} \left[\sum_{k=1}^{N} c(k)\exp(-j2\pi f k\Delta x') \right] \exp(j2\pi f n\Delta x)\,df \qquad (12)$$

$$= \sum_{k=1}^{N} c(k) \int\limits_{-f_c}^{f_c} \exp[j2\pi f(n\Delta x - k\Delta x')]\,df$$

$$= \sum_{k=1}^{N} c(k)\, \frac{\sin[2\pi f_c(n\Delta x - k\Delta')]}{\pi(n\Delta x - k\Delta x')}$$

Let

$$A(n,k) \overset{\Delta}{=} \frac{\sin[2\pi f_c(n\Delta x - k\Delta x')]}{\pi(n\Delta x - k\Delta x')} \qquad (13)$$

Then we can rewrite the linear relationship in matrix form

$$[W] = [A]\,[C] \qquad (14\text{-}a)$$

where [w] and [c] are the column-vector representations of the received data and control-point sequences respectively. Subsequently, the control-point sequence can be obtained by a similar matrix operation

$$[C] = [A]^{-1} [W] \tag{14-b}$$

Once the control-point sequence is computed, the band-limited spectral distribution can be evaluated according to Eq. (11).

This spectral estimation technique and the optimal algorithm described in the previous section have striking similarities. Both of them consist of a matrix operation and followed by a matched filter and the enhancement is achieved by the matrix operation. The significant advantage of the spectral estimation technique is that the elements of the [A] matrix is in closed form and can be easily computed given the cutoff frequency, signal sample and control-point spacings.

The Cascade Form

The linear space-invariant relationship given by Eq. (1) can be also written as a multiplication operation in the spatial-frequency domain

$$Q(f) = F\{q(x)\} \tag{15}$$

$$= H(f) P(f)$$

$$= F\{h(x)\} F\{p(x)\}$$

It is known that the transfer function associated with wave propagation is lowpass with the cutoff frequency $1/\lambda$ when the propagating distance z is large

$$H(f) = F\{h(x)\} \tag{16}$$

$$\cong \begin{cases} \exp\left[j2\pi z_0 \left[\dfrac{1}{\lambda^2} - f^2\right]^{1/2}\right] & |f| < \dfrac{1}{\lambda} \\ \\ 0 & \text{otherwise} \end{cases}$$

This effect is due to the attenuation of the evanescent wave components during the propagation. This implies that the resultant wave-field is a band-limited signal with a known cutoff frequency. To improve the matrix inversion as well as the formation of the spectral distribution, we choose half-wavelength as the control-point spacing which is corresponding to the Nyquist rate. Then the elements of the associated [A] matrix are

$$A(n,k) = 2f_c \, \text{sinc}[2\pi f_c(n\Delta x - k\Delta x')] \tag{17}$$

$$= \frac{2}{\lambda} \, \text{sinc}[\frac{2\pi}{\lambda}(n\Delta x - k\frac{\lambda}{2})]$$

$$= \frac{2}{\lambda} \, \text{sinc}[\pi(n\beta - k)]$$

641

where $0 < \beta = \Delta x / \Delta x' < 1$.

Subsequently, we compute for the control-point sequence according to Eq. (14-b). From the control-point sequence, we take M spatial-frequency data samples within the frequency band $(-1/\lambda, 1/\lambda)$. The number of frequency samples must be larger than the total number of wave-field samples in order to retain the information content. If the frequency samples are uniformly-spaced, the frequency spacing is

$$\Delta f = \frac{2}{\lambda M} \tag{18}$$

These frequency samples can be obtained by first padding zeros to the control-point sequence and then taking an M-point discrete Fourier transform (DFT).

$$Q(k) \stackrel{\Delta}{=} Q(f)|_{f=k\Delta f} \tag{19}$$

$$= \sum_{n} c(n) \exp[-j2\pi(k\Delta f)n\Delta x']$$

$$= \sum_{n} c(n) \exp[-j2\pi nk/M]$$

The spectrum of the source distribution and the wave-field spectrum is related by the transfer function corresponding to the propagation which is only a phase term within the cutoff. Therefore, we can obtain M frequency samples of the source distribution by performing phase correction on $Q(k)$

$$P(k) = P(f)|_{f=k\Delta f} = Q(k) H(f)|_{f=k\Delta f} \tag{20}$$

Now we have an estimation problem with the dual structure that M uniformly-spaced frequency samples are available and the estimation objective is the unknown space-limited source distribution bounded within the region $(-d, d)$. Corresponding to the source size, we choose the Nyquist rate as the frequency-domain control-point spacing

$$\Delta f' = \frac{1}{2d} \tag{21}$$

Similar to the spectral estimation process we described, we form another matrix [A'] using the frequency sample spacing, control-point spacing, and the source size.

$$A'(n,k) = 2d \; \text{sinc}[2\pi d(k\frac{2}{M\lambda} - n\frac{1}{2d})] \tag{22}$$

$$= 2d \; \text{sinc}[\pi(k\alpha - n)]$$

where

$$0 < \alpha = 2d\, \Delta f = \frac{4d}{M\lambda} \leqslant 1 \tag{23}$$

Then the frequency-domain control-point sequence $C(k)$ can be computed by a matrix operation.

$$[C] = [A']^{-1}[Q] \tag{24}$$

Finally, the optimal solution of the space-limited source distribution can be formulated as

$$\hat{p}(x) = F^{-1}\{\sum_k C(k)\,\delta(f - \frac{k}{2d})\} \tag{25}$$

$$= \sum_k C(k)\exp[j\pi kx/d]$$

If we wish to observe the source distribution by evaluating L uniform samples over the source region, we can similarly pad zeros to the frequency control-points $C(k)$ and take an L-point DFT.

$$\hat{p}(n) = \hat{p}(x)\Big|_{x=n\frac{2d}{L}} \tag{26}$$

$$= \sum_k C(k)\exp[j2\pi nk/L]$$

Algorithm Structure

From the analysis given in the previous section, we can represent the structure of the algorithm using a cascade form in terms of matrix operators

$$[\hat{p}] = [IDFT]\,[A']^{-1}[\Phi]\,[DFT]\,[A]^{-1}\,[q] \tag{27}$$

where $[q]$ and $[\hat{p}]$ are the vector forms of the received data and resultant image sequences respectively. The square matrix $[\Phi]$ is a diagonal phase-correction matrix which is responsible for backward propagation operation in the spatial-frequency domain. The matrix $[A]^{-1}$ is the space-domain enhancement operator constructed by using the knowledge of finite spatial-frequency bandwidth. Similarly, the matrix $[A']^{-1}$ is the spatial-frequency domain enhancement operator constructed based on the finite size of the source. One of the most significant advantage of the cascade structure is that the algorithm is now partitioned into three independent operations responsible for space-domain enhancement, backward propagation, and frequency-domain enhancement. Fig. (2) shows the diagram of the optimal algorithm in cascade form.

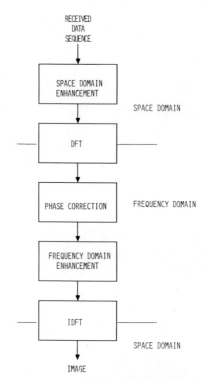

RECEIVED
DATA
SEQUENCE

SPACE DOMAIN
ENHANCEMENT

SPACE DOMAIN

DFT

PHASE CORRECTION

FREQUENCY DOMAIN

FREQUENCY DOMAIN
ENHANCEMENT

IDFT

SPACE DOMAIN

IMAGE

Fig. 1   Diagram of the Optimal Imaging Algorithm
in Direct Form.

It can be seen that the Nyquist rate is the upper limit of the data sample spacing. Enhancement can be achieved only when the spacing is smaller than the Nyquist spacing. If we sample the space or frequency domain signals with Nyquist rate, the matrices [A] and [A′] becomes diagonal. As a result, the matrix operation in the algorithm gives no enhancement to the image reconstruction which is often called the degenerated case. This means that the space-domain enhancement operator will be degenerated when the sample spacing is half-wavelength

$$\Delta x = \frac{\lambda}{2} \qquad\qquad (28\text{-a})$$

Similarly, the frequency-domain enhancement becomes ineffective if the frequency sample spacing is

$$\Delta f = \frac{1}{2d} \qquad\qquad (28\text{-b})$$

If both [A] and [A′] are degenerated, Eq. (27) becomes direct backward propagation which implies that the optimal algorithm does not have resolution improvement over the conventional methods.

$$[\hat{p}] = [\text{IDFT}]\,[\Phi]\,[\text{DFT}]\,[q] \qquad\qquad (29)$$

$$= \text{Backward Propagate } [q]$$

Conclusion

The limitation of image quality is largely due to the uncertainty due to the incomplete information detection of the data acquisition systems. To improve image resolution, one approach is to utilize additional constraints to reduce the ambiguity caused by the uncertainty. The most common constraints available for resolution improvement are the finite size of the source distribution and the finite spatial-frequency bandwidth of the resultant wave-field. The optimal image reconstruction algorithm developed recently successfully incorporate these constraints into an enhancement matrix operator. However, the formation of the enhancement operator remains a very complicated step of the computation process because the formulation is not in closed form. The main objective of this paper is to restructure the optimal algorithm into a format such that is can be implemented efficiently.

In this paper, we first present the general structure of the optimal algorithm with a vector space method. Subsequently, we formulate the signal extrapolation algorithm using the similar technique. Then we can decompose the optimal algorithm into three independent steps. These steps include two signal extrapolation algorithms and one spatial-frequency domain backward propagation. The first extrapolation process is for aperture expansion by using the knowledge of the cutoff frequency of the band-limited resultant wave-field. The second extrapolation steps is to extend the frequency bandwidth by using the constraint of finite source region. This approach will significant improve the computation since all operations are in closed form. In addition, the cascade structure separates the contribution of the constraints and we will be able to identify their effectiveness to image resolution improvement independently.

Acknowledgment

This research is supported by the National Science Foundation under Grants IST-8409633 and ENG-8451484, Motorola Inc., and Hughes Aircraft Co.

References

1. A. J. Devaney, "A Filtered Backpropagation Algorithm for Diffraction Tomography," *Ultrasonic Imaging*, vol. 4, pp. 336-350, 1982.

2. A. J. Devaney, "Inverse Source and Scattering Problem in Ultrasonics," *IEEE Transactions on Sonics and Ultrasonics*, vol. SU-30, no. 6, pp. 355-364, November 1983.

3. Hua Lee and Glen Wade, "High-Resolution Imaging for Systems with Small Apertures," *Journals of Acoustical Society of America*, 72(6), pp. 2033-2035, December 1982. IEEE Computer Society Press, pp. 240-246, 1982.

4. Hua Lee and Glen Wade, "Constructing an Imaging Operator to Enhance Resolution," *Journals of Acoustical Society of America*, 75(2), pp. 499-504, February 1984.

5. Hua Lee, "Resolution Enhancement by Wavefield Extrapolation," *IEEE Transactions on Sonics and Ultrasonics*, vol. SU-31, no. 6, pp. 642-645, November 1984.

6. Hua Lee, "Resolution Enhancement of Backward Propagated Images by Wavefield Orthogonalization," *Journals of Acoustical Society of America*, 77(5), pp. 1845-1848, May 1985.

7. Hua Lee, "Inverse Filter Design for Holographic Imaging Systems with Small Apertures," *Acoustical Imaging*, vol. 14, A. J. Berkhout, J. Ridder, L. F. van der Wal Eds., Plenum Press, New York, pp. 715-718, 1985.

8. Hua Lee and Glen Wade, "Sampling in Digital Holographic Reconstruction," *Journals of Acoustical Society of America*, 75(4), pp. 1291-1293, April 1984.

9. Hua Lee, "Optimal Reconstruction Algorithm for Holographic Imaging of Finite Size Objects," *Journals of Acoustical Society of America*, 80(1), pp. 195-198, July 1986.

10. Hua Lee and Thomas S. Huang, "On Discrete Band-Limited Signal Extrapolation," *Proceedings of the 1985 IEEE International Conference on Acoustics, Speech, and Signal Processing*, pp. 465-468, 1985.

11. Hua Lee, Zse-Cherng Lin, and Thomas S. Huang, "Performance and Limitation of Discrete Band-Limited Extrapolation Algorithms," *1986 International Conference on Acoustics, Speech, and Signal Processing*, pp. 1645-1648, 1986.

UNDERWATER ACOUSTICAL HOLOGRAPHIC IMAGING BY A SQUARE ARRAY SYSTEM

Dejun Zhang[*]

Wuhan Institute of Physics
Academia Sinica
Wuhan,Hubei
The People's Republic of China

ABSTRACT

All the previous theoretical analyses for acoustical holographic imaging are based on the diffraction integral, but most of the underwater man-made objects show mirror reflection character to acoustical waves. Owing to this character, the angular field of view of the imaging system cannot be fully used and the probability of finding an object will be decreased. A new method "multiple sources projection – holograms overlapping – images piecing together method" is presented in this paper. The mathematical expressions also given. A series of experiments were conducted to test the method and study the ability of acoustical holographic imaging for man-made objects using a 64 X 64 square array system. Cylinders of different sizes were used as underwater targets. Results were accorded with theoretical anticipation. The prospect of the system in underwater viewing is also discussed.

INTRODUCTION

In the mid-sixties of this century acoustical holography, as a new imaging method and signal processing technology appeared. After that some forerunners pointed out immediately that acoustical holography whould have good prospect in the application to underwater imaging, and they proposed various models and schemes.[1],[2],[3],[4]

In the mid-seventies some typical underwater imaging systems using acoustical holographic square arrays were built.[5],[6] Since then many specialists made valuable works on the acoustical image reconstruction and signal processing using a computer.[7],[8] However acoustical holographic underwater imaging has made no breakthrough in practical applications up to now. It is held that besides the other reasons the low probability of finding on object and the incomplete nature of acoustical images are also the important reasons. It means put in a nutshell, that the acoustic reflex characteristics of underwater objects need to be studied in a more deep-going way. The recent work dealing with the computer simulation of the cylinder imaging drew a conclusion promptly—mirror effect would be a great problem.[9]

---

[*]Major participants in experiments: Z.Q.Sun, W.G.Du, X.Su, L.Mi, J.M.Gao et al.

A 64 X 64 square array acoustical holographic imaging system was built in 1980 in our institute.[1][2]Using it we have conducted a series of imaging experiments for man-made objects, especially for cylinders. Two different methods have been used in the experiments: conventional holographic method with a single sound source and multiple sources projection method. The experimental results and theoretical analyses show that the system design and imaging quality depend upon the acoustical reflex characteristics of the object. In fact, it is difficult entirely avoiding mirror reflection and using only the diffraction for imaging because of the harsh demands on the gain and the noise immunity of the system. So we must consider how to improve the image quality using more mirror reflection. Correspondingly, when the diffraction integral is used to analyze the imaging procedure, its mathematical form needs to be revised slightly.

ACOUSTIC REFLECTING CHARACTER OF OBJECTS

The acoustical reflecting character of an object has relation to the dimension L of the object and the size t of its surface coarseness. In underwater imaging, for common man-made targets usually $L \gg \lambda$ and $\lambda \gg t$. So they show the mirror reflecting characters to the acoustical wave basically. However, even if for the same target and the same wavelength, the target will show different reflection characters to the different illuminant forms.

For example, when a cylinder which is frequently met with in the underwater imaging is illuminated by a point source in a short distance, the reflection of the cylinder will obey the mirror reflection law, i.e. Snell's law. According to geometrical acoustics we can draw a schematic diagram shown in Fig. (1). Obviously, in this case, what the receiving array can only receive is the reflected wave from one part of the cylinder along the axis direction,the length of that part is the half of the receiving array dimension. Therefore the image reconstructed is also corresponding to this section of the cylinder.

With the increase of the imaging distance, the illuminant wave of the point source would be quite similar to a plane wave. So the reflected field of the cylinder has directional characteristic.

It is known from the theory[11] that if $kL \gg 1$, $z > L^2/\lambda$; $ka \gg 1$, $z > a^2/\lambda$, the target strength in the plane including the axis of cylinder is given by

$$TS \doteq 10 \log \left[\frac{kaL^2}{4\pi} \left[\frac{Sin(kLSin(\phi))}{kLSin(\phi)} \right]^2 Cos^2\phi + \right.$$

$$\left. (\frac{ka^2}{2})^2 \left[\frac{J_1[2kaSin(\pi/2-\phi)]}{kaSin(\pi/2-\phi)} \right]^2 Cos^2(\pi/2-\phi) \right] \quad (1)$$

and in the plane including the radius of the cylinder.[12]

$$TS \doteq 10 \log \{(a/2/z) Sin(\phi'/2) +$$

$$(Cot^2(\phi'/2))(Sin^2(kaSin(\phi')))/2/\pi/k/z$$

$$+ (fast\ undulate\ term\ )\} \quad (2)$$

where $k=2\pi/\lambda$ is the wave number, L the cylinder length, a the cylinder radius, Z the distance from the cylinder center,angle ϕ and ϕ' see Fig.(2).

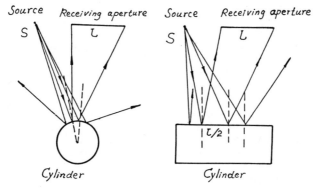

a. In radius plane   b. In axis plane
Fig.1 Geometric representation for mirror reflecting object

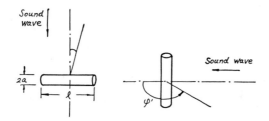

a. In axis plane   b. In radius plane
Fig.2 Reflecting angles of a cylinder to sound wave

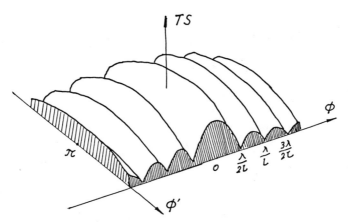

Fig.3 Scheme of the three dimensional reflecting intensity

On these grounds,we can get a scheme of the three dimensional reflecting intensity of the cylinder. It is showed in Fig.(3). From Fig. (3) we can see that the reflected sound field of the cylinder looks like "wave-form". It presages that the hologram of of cylinder in far distance will become "ribbon-form".

MATHEMATICAL DESCRIPTION OF TWO KINDS OF IMAGING METHODS

Firstly, according to above mentioned analysis if using a finite aperture to record the object wave field taking mirror reflection as dominant factor, only some parts of the reflected wave from the object could be received, and the contribution from the other part of the object is very small. It seems the object is affected by an effective aperture function $\sigma_s(x_s,y_s)$. From this point we can still continue to use the diffraction integral formula to the following mathematical description.

Single source imaging method

Under the Fresnel approximation, the process from the object function $U_s(x_s,y_s,\emptyset)$ to the holographic function $U(x,y,z)$ can be written as

$$U(x,y,z)=C_1\int\!\!\!\int_{-\infty}^{\infty} U_s(x_s,y_s,\emptyset)\sigma_s(x_s,y_s)\ \exp\{-jk[(x-x_s)^2+(y-y_s)^2]/2/z\}dx_s dy_s$$

$$=C_1 U''_s(x,y)*h(x,y) \tag{3}$$

where $h(x,y)=\exp\{-jk[(x-x_s)^2+(y-y_s)^2]/2/z\}$

$U''_s(x,y)=U_s(x,y,\emptyset)\sigma_s(x,y)$

are the spatial transmission function and the effective object function respectively; symbol "*" denotes the convolution

The reconstruction process of the object function is an inverse Fresnel transform

$$U''(x_s,y_s)=C_2\int\!\!\!\int_{-\infty}^{\infty} U(x,y,z)\ \exp\{jk[(x-x_s)^2+(y-y_s)^2]/2/z\}dxdy \tag{4}$$

Where C_1, C_2 are constants

If the receiving aperture is a finite one such as a square receiving array with the dimension D,the reconstructed image $U_1(x_1,y_1,\emptyset)$ is an approximation of the function $U_s''(x_s,y_s)$:

$$U_1(x_1,y_1,\emptyset)=C_3\int\!\!\!\int_{-\infty}^{\infty} \mathrm{rect}(x/D)\mathrm{rect}(y/D)U(x,y,z)$$

$$\exp\{jk[(x-x_1)^2+(y-y_1)^2]/2/z\}dxdy \tag{5}$$

where x_1, y_1 are the coordinates on the image plane.

Naturally, it is necessary for Eq.(3),(4),(5) to be discretized when the hologram was discretely sampled and reconstructed numerically.

Multi-source Imaging Method

Assume that the sparse emitting array consists of n sources placed in the receiving plane. When one of them emits a sound pulse, the receiving array would receive a "Single-element hologram" generated by the reflection wave from the relevant part of the object. Letting n sources emit in turn and overlapping these "single-element hologram" we get the "multi-fold hologram". If the latter were used for reconstruction, the images from each "single-element hologram" would be pieced to a more complete image. we call this method "multiple sources projection-holograms overlapping-images piecing together method".

Assume that $U_p(x,y,z)$ is the single-element hologram from the pth source, the multi-fold hologram is

$$U'(x,y,z) = \sum_{p=1}^{n} U_p(x,y,z)$$

$$= B_1 \sum_{p=1}^{n} \int\int_{-\infty}^{\infty} U(x_s, y_s, \emptyset) \sigma_p(x_s, y_s)$$

$$\exp\{-jk[(x_s-x_{tp})^2+(y_s-y_{tp})^2+$$

$$(x-x_s)^2+(y-y_s)^2]/z/2\}dx_s dy_s \qquad (6)$$

where x_{tp}, y_{tp} is the coordinate of the pth source in the receiving plane. $\sigma_p(x_s, y_s)$ the effective aperture function corresponding to the pth source. The reconstruction process of the multi-fold hologram is the same as that of the single-element hologram, i.e.

$$U'_i(x_i, y_i, \emptyset) = B_2 \int\int_{-\infty}^{\infty} rect(x/D)rect(y/D) \, U'(x,y,z)$$

$$\exp\{jk[(x-x_i)^2+(y-y_i)^2]/z/2\}dxdy \qquad (7)$$

It must be pointed out that if the images are reconstructed optically there exist two kinds of ways to overlap the holograms: sequential transmitting and concurrent of the sources. But the former is better than the latter because the latter has additional inter-cohering terms from the different parts of the object. The additional terms lead to extra noise in the image plane.

As a simple illustration let's consider the case of two sources imaging.

Assume that the source 1 generates a object wave $U_1 = A_1 \exp\{j\phi_1\}$ in the receiving plane; and for the source 2, $U_2 = A_2 \exp\{j\phi_2\}$; The reference wave $U_r = A_r \exp\{j\phi_r\}$. In the sequential transmitting model, U_1 and U_2 first make coherence with U_r separately to form two single-element holograms H_1 and H_2, then H_1 plus H_2 to form a two-fold hologram H.

$$H_1 = |U_1 + U_r|^2$$

$$= A_1^2 + A_r^2 + 2A_1 A_r Cos(\phi_1 - \phi_r) \qquad (8)$$

$$H_2 = |U_2 + U_r|^2$$

$$= A_2^2 + A_r^2 + 2A_2 A_r Cos(\phi_2 - \phi_r) \qquad (9)$$

$$H = H_1 + H_2$$

$$= K' + A_r \exp\{j\phi_r\}[A_1 \exp\{-j\phi_1\} + A_2 \exp\{-j\phi_2\}]$$

$$+ A_r \exp\{-j\phi_r\}[A_1 \exp\{j\phi_1\} + A_2 \exp\{j\phi_2\}] \qquad (10)$$

where $\qquad K' = A_1^2 + A_2^2 + 2A_r^2$

In Eq.(10), the second term denotes the real image and the third the conjugate image.

For the concurrent transmitting way, two complex amplitutes U_1 and U_2 are added first, then they make coherence with U_r

$$H = |(U_1 + U_2) + U_r|^2 = A_1{}^2 + A_2{}^2 + A_r{}^2$$

$$+ A_r \exp\{j\phi_r\}[A_1 \exp\{-j\phi_1\} + A_2 \exp\{-j\phi_2\}]$$

$$+ A_r \exp\{-j\phi_r\}[A_1 \exp\{j\phi_1\} + A_2 \exp\{j\phi_2\}]$$

$$+ 2A_1 A_2 \cos(\phi_1 - \phi_2) \tag{11}$$

In Eq.(11), the last term is the additional term.

The simulation of the two overlying ways using one dimensional holography was made by a microcomputer. The parameters of the simulant system were the same as our square array system.[1*] Fig.(4) shows the passive holographic imaging of two point sources located in the object plane, the distance between the two point sources is 16 resolution elements, and the distance to the receiving plane is 10m. Fig.(4a) shows the intensity distribution of the reconstructed image for the concur emitting of the sources, Fig.(4b), for the sequential transmitting. Fig.(5) is the imaging result of two point scatterers in the object plane. Two illuminating sources are located at the both ends of the receiving array. Fig.(5a) corresponds to the concur transmitting and Fig.(5b) the sequential transmitting. From Fig.4-5, we can see that the concur transmitting causes not only the background noise increasing but also the intensity change of the major image sometimes.

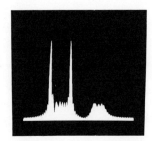

a. Concur transmitting   b. Sequential transmitting
Fig.4 Simulation for passive holographic imaging of two point sources

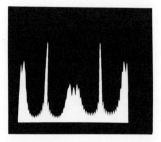 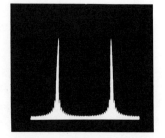

a. Concur transmitting   b. Sequential transmitting
Fig.5 Simulation for holographic imaging of two point scatterers

The reconstruction of a linear object (128 points were arranged at a distance one-fourth of the resolution element dimension) is shown in Fig.(6). In order to simulate the effect of the effective aperture function in the object plane, we assume that the source only illuminates half of the linear object. Fig.(6a) corresponds to the concur transmitting way and Fig.(6b), the sequential transmitting way.

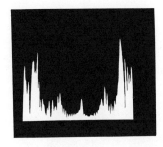
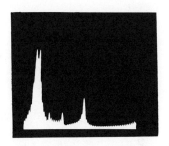

a. Concur transmitting   b. Sequential transmitting
Fig.6 Simulation for holographic imaging of a linear object

EXPERIMENTAL METHOD AND RESULTS

In our square system, the number of receiving array elements is 64X64, the aperture dimension L=760.5mm, the angular field of view $2\beta=23°4'$, the angular resolution $\alpha=21'$ and the frequency f=312.5 KHz. The underwater part of the system includes the receiving array, convex transducers, pre-amplifiers, signal processing channels and a reference signal generator etc. The boat part includes the ultrasonic pulse transmitter, the multi-switcher, the control panel, and the display etc. Two parts are linked up by a long cable. As far as the recording and reconstructing of the holo-gram was concerned, in early experiments the optical system was used; in boat experiments, especially for searching test the "video recording – laser film projection system" was used; now, the microcomputer reconstruc-tion system has been built.

Near Distance Imaging in the Anechoic Water Tank

The schematic diagram of the experiment is shown in Fig.(7). The size of the tank is 6X5X4m³. The face of the square array was towards the bottom of the tank.

Single source illumination imaging. Fig.(8) gives the reconstructed image of ⊟ -shaped target which is made by metal tube with diameter 30mm and the photo of the target.

Fig.(9) gives the reconstructed image of a metal cylinder with diameter 100mm on the pebbles background at a distance of 3m from the array. From Fig.(9) we see that the system can differentiate the cylinder from the background, but only a section of the cylinder was imaged because of the mirror reflection.

Passive imaging of point sources. The targets were composed of three convex transducers installed on a support. The curvature radius of radiating surface of the transducer was 30mm, the effective aperture was 29mm, the interval between them was 250mm. The distance from the target to

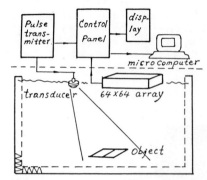

Fig.7 Scheme of experiments in the water tank

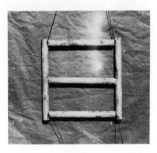 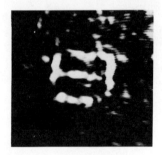

a. object   b. image

Fig.8 Imaging of B--shaped target

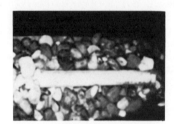 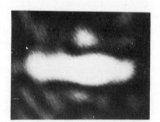

a. object   b. image

Fig.9 Imaging of a cylinder on the pebbles background

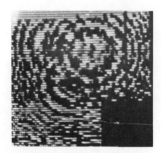 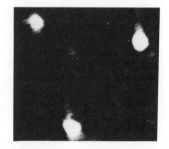

a. hologram   b. image

Fig.10 Passive imaging of three sources concur transmitting

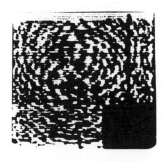 

a. hologram　　　　　　　　b. image

Fig.11 Passive imaging of three sources sequential transmitting

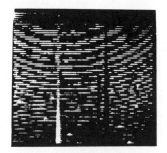 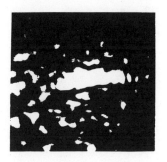

a. hologram　　　　　　　　b. image

Fig.12 Imaging of a cylinder using single source emitting

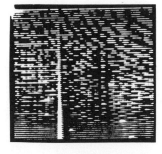 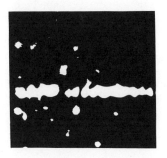

a. hologram　　　　　　　　b. image

Fig.13 Imaging of a cylinder using two sources concur emitting

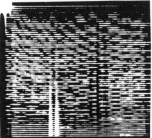

a. hologram　　　　　　　　b. image

Fig.14 Imaging of a cylinder using two sources sequential emitting

the array was 3m. Fig.(10a) is the hologram for the concur transmitting of the sources and Fig.(10b) the reconstructed image. Fig.(11a) is the hologram for the sequence transmitting and Fig.(11b) the reconstructed image. From comparison we see that the sequence transmitting-holograms overlapping way causes less noise.

Imaging of a cylinder using two sources. Two sources were installed on the two opposite sides of the square array, and the distance between the two sources was 550mm. A metal cylinder with 1.5m long and a diameter of 50mm was put under the array and in parallel with the square array. The distance from the cylinder to the array was 2.5m. Fig.(12a) gives the hologram corresponding to single source emitting and Fig.(12b) the reconstructed image. Fig.(13a) the hologram for concur transmitting and Fig.(13b) the reconstructed image. Fig.(14a) the hologram for sequence transmitting and Fig.(14b) the reconstructed image. These results show that using two sources we can see more parts of the cylinder, and the image quality for the sequence transmitting is better than the concur transmitting.

Cylinder Imaging in a Lake

In order to test the effects of Multi-source imaging and the ability of acoustical holographic imaging system for seeking and distinguishing targets, we conducted a series of experiments in a natural lake. The square array was installed in the gapped place of U-shaped boat, and 12 convex transducers were arranged at the four corners of the array and the sides of the boat. The curvature radius of the transducers was 100mm, effective aperture was 70mm. The major size of the cylinder was 3.5m long and its diameter was 0.5m. The schematic diagram of the boat experiments is shown in Fig.(15).

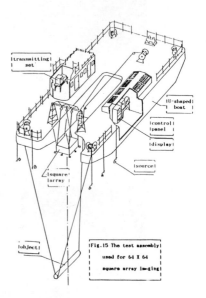

Fig.15 The test assembly used for 64 X 64 square array imaging

Conventional holographic imaging by single source. The cylinder was hanged in different depths under the boat, so we got the holograms and the images of the cylinder in the depths range from 3m to 60m. In the above experiments we found that when the depth exceeded 40m, the hologram became "tape-form" pattern clearly. Fig.(16) gives the reconstructed image of the cylinder in depth of 60m.

Imaging of Cylinder by Multiple Sources. Fig.(17) is the reconstructed image using sequence transmitting of 4 sources located as shown in Fig.(18). The distance from the cylinder to the array was 12m. The continuity of the image doesn't look good because the interval (1.5-3m) between sources is longer than the aperture L of the array.

Fig.(19) shows the reconstructed image using concur transmitting of 7 sources located as shown in Fig.(20). The distance from the cylinder to the array was 12m. Since the interval (about 0.5m) between sources was shorter than L, the major image had some coherent effect, but the image looked as if it was more complete.

The imaging of the cylinder in farther distance (more than 40m) using multiple sources was also made, but the improvement of image quality is not obvious owing to the appearance of "tape-form hologram".

Preliminary Experiments to Search a Target. We threw down the cylinder which arbitrarily sank on the bottom of the lake. The depth of sinking place was 21m. The U-shaped boat loading the system sailed slowly through the water area above the target. One of the reconstructed images obtained by single source is shown in Fig.(21).

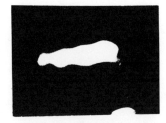

Fig.16   Imaging of a cylinder in depth of 60m

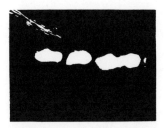

Fig.17 Image of a cylinder by 4 sources sequential emitting

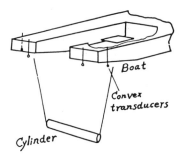

Fig.18   Scheme of experiment for Fig.17

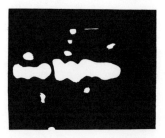

Fig.19 Image of a cylinder by 7 sources concur emitting

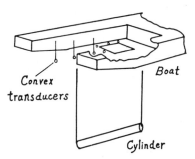

Fig.20   Scheme of experiment for Fig.19

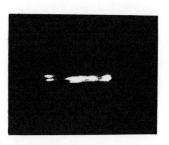

Fig.21 Image of a cylinder sunk on the bottom of the lake

CONCLUSIONS AND ACKNOWLEDGMENTS

In underwater acoustical holographic imaging, the reflected sound field characters of the targets should be studied emphatically. In view of the mirror reflection of man-made targets, the "Multiple sources projection-holograms overlapping-images pieced together method" proposed in the paper has the following advantages: In the near-distance imaging, the obtained images have some completeness, and the angular field of view can be used fully; In farther distance imaging, the probability of finding targets can be increased. From above experiments we can also see that the acoustical holographic square array system has better ability to discern man-made targets including sunken targets and to adapt to boat environment. It could be estimated that the prospect of acoustical holographic underwater imaging is inspiring.

The author wishes to thank Prof. J.P.N. Wei for his direction and to X.H. Xia for the aid in computer simulation.

REFERENCE

[1] P.Greguss,Ultraschall-hologramme,Research Film,5:330(1965)

[2] F.L.Thurstone,Ultrasound holography and visual reconstruction, Proc. Symp. Biomed. Eng.,1:12 (1966)

[3] R.K.Mueller and N.K.Sheridon, Sound holograms and optical reconstruction, App. Phys. L.,9:328 (1966)

[4] G.Wade, et al, An acoustic holographic system for underwater search, PIEEE, 57:2051 (1969)

[5] J.L.Sutton, et al, Description of a Navy Holographic Underwater Acoustic Imaging System (AIS), Acoustical Imaging,Vol.8 (1978)

[6] Kazuhiko Nitadori, et al, An Experimental Underwater Acoustic Imaging System Using Multibeam Scanning, Acoustical Imaging,Vol.8 (1978)

[7] Y.Aoki, Consideration on Super Resolution in a Fresnel Transform Holography, Trans. IECE,62-B No.8 :767 (1979)

[8] P.N.Keating, et al, Holographic Aperture Synthesis Via a Transmitting Array, Acoustical Holography, 6:485 (1975)

[9] Kjell Dalland, et al, Simulation of Imaging Systems for Underwater Viewing, Acoustical Imaging, Vol.13

[10] J.P.N.Wei, et al, Array Systems for Underwater Viewing by Acoustical Holography, Acoustical Imaging, Vol.12

[11] R.J.Urick, Chapter 9, in: "Principles of Underwater Sound for Engineers," McGraw-Hill, New York (1967)

[12] P.Morse and U.Ingard, Chapter 8, in: "Theoretical Acoustics," McGraw-Hill, New York (1968)

IMAGING THE NEARFIELD OF A SUBMERGED-PLATE

USING ACOUSTICAL HOLOGRAPHY

K. E. Eschenberg and S. I. Hayek

Applied Research Laboratory
The Pennsylvania State University
University Park, PA 16802

Abstract

The image of the acoustic field near a driven, submerged plate has been obtained experimentally using underwater nearfield holography. In addition to a discussion of the results, this paper develops theoretical explanation for mechanical and acoustical processes, and describes aspects of the work which may be of interest to others attempting similiar experiments.

1.0 Introduction

Underwater nearfield holography is a process by which the measurement of the pressure at a set of points on a surface in the nearfield of an acoustically radiating object is analyzed to yield the velocity vector field and the acoustic pressure in three dimensional space. If the measurement points are recorded on a surface which is located at a distance of at least one acoustic wavelength from the actively vibrating surface, then processing these data results in an acoustic image that can only resolve sources that are separated spatially by a distance of at least one acoustic wavelength. However, if the measurement points are taken in the nearfield of the source region, then the spatial resolution can be reduced to a fraction of a wavelength.

The imaging process starts by recording the acoustic pressure amplitude and phase with appropriate filtering, amplification and averaging at a set of points lying in a plane. Next, the data is digitized and then digitally calibrated and processed to compute the velocity vector, the pressure and the vector intensity fields on the surface of the radiator or anywhere else in three dimensional space.

2.0 Imaging Formulas

The nearfield imaging process we have used is derived from an ultrasonic imaging method developed by Van Rooy[1] who was one of the first to use the FFT to efficiently implement an "exact" reconstruction (except that the evanescent waves were discarded as being 'unmeasureable'); much of this paper has also been published in a more assesible form[2] At Penn State, Cohen[3] further developed the digital algorithms used in acoustical holography; these simulations demonstrated the value of a nearfield hologram and the importance of using what was called the 'backward tracer' in correctly reconstructing the evanescent waves. More recent work (see, for example, Williams[4]) has investigated the usefulness of nearfield holography in the analysis of plate vibration and the acoustic nearfield of the plate.

2.1 Integral Imaging Formulas

Defining the Fourier transform integrals as

$$\tilde{u}(k_x, k_y) = \frac{1}{2\pi} \int\limits_{-\infty}^{\infty} \int\limits_{-\infty}^{\infty} u(x,y)\, e^{-i(k_x\, x + k_y\, y)}\, dx\, dy, \tag{1}$$

$$u(x,y) = \frac{1}{2\pi} \int\limits_{-\infty}^{\infty} \int\limits_{-\infty}^{\infty} \tilde{u}(k_x, k_y)\, e^{i(k_x\, x + k_y\, y)}\, dk_x\, dk_y, \tag{2}$$

then the transform of the wave equation on the acoustic pressure

$$\nabla^2 p + k^2 p = 0 \tag{3}$$

becomes

$$\frac{d^2 \tilde{p}}{dz^2} + k_z^2\, \tilde{p} = 0, \quad k_z^2 = k^2 - k_x^2 - k_y^2, \tag{4}$$

where the $e^{-i\omega t}$ factor has been omitted. For outgoing waves in z,

$$\tilde{p} = A\, e^{i k_z\, z}, \tag{5}$$

where

$$\begin{aligned} k_z &= \sqrt{k^2 - k_x^2 - k_y^2} \quad \text{if} \quad k^2 > k_x^2 + k_y^2, \\ &= i\sqrt{k_x^2 + k_y^2 - k^2} \quad \text{if} \quad k^2 < k_x^2 + k_y^2, \end{aligned} \tag{6}$$

and A is an arbitrary complex function of k_x and k_y. Note that the evanescent waves (imaginary k_z) are exponentially attenuated. We choose the measurement plane (the hologram) to be located at $z = z_H$, the source plane to be located at z_S, z to be any plane, and require that $z_H > z_S > 0$ and $z > z_S$. Then, the transform of the hologram pressure field $p_H(x, y, z_H)$ is given by

$$\tilde{p}_H(k_x, k_y) = \frac{1}{2\pi} \int\limits_{-\infty}^{\infty} \int\limits_{-\infty}^{\infty} p_H(x, y, z_H)\, e^{-i(k_x\, x + k_y\, y)}\, dx\, dy \tag{7}$$

$$= A\, e^{i k_z\, z_H}, \tag{8}$$

or

$$A = \tilde{p}_H\, e^{-i k_z\, z_H}, \tag{9}$$

so that the transform of the pressure at any field point is

$$\tilde{p} = \tilde{p}_H\, e^{i k_z (z - z_H)}. \tag{10}$$

The inverse transform of the pressure at any field point z can then be written as

$$p = \frac{1}{2\pi} \int\limits_{-\infty}^{\infty} \int\limits_{-\infty}^{\infty} \tilde{p}_H\, e^{i k_z (z - z_H)}\, e^{i(k_x\, x + k_y\, y)}\, dk_x\, dk_y. \tag{11}$$

The velocity vector field at z is given by

$$\vec{v} = \frac{1}{i\omega\rho} \vec{\nabla} p = \frac{1}{2\pi i f \rho} \vec{\nabla} p, \tag{12}$$

$$v_x = \frac{1}{(2\pi)^2} \frac{1}{f\rho} \int\limits_{-\infty}^{\infty} \int\limits_{-\infty}^{\infty} k_x\, \tilde{p}_H\, e^{i k_z (z - z_H)}\, e^{i(k_x\, x + k_y\, y)}\, dk_x\, dk_y, \tag{13}$$

$$v_y = \frac{1}{(2\pi)^2} \frac{1}{f\rho} \int\limits_{-\infty}^{\infty} \int\limits_{-\infty}^{\infty} k_y\, \tilde{p}_H\, e^{i k_z (z - z_H)}\, e^{i(k_x\, x + k_y\, y)}\, dk_x\, dk_y, \tag{14}$$

$$v_z = -\frac{1}{(2\pi)^2} \frac{1}{f\rho} \int\limits_{-\infty}^{\infty} \int\limits_{-\infty}^{\infty} k_z\, \tilde{p}_H\, e^{i k_z (z - z_H)}\, e^{i(k_x\, x + k_y\, y)}\, dk_x\, dk_y, \tag{15}$$

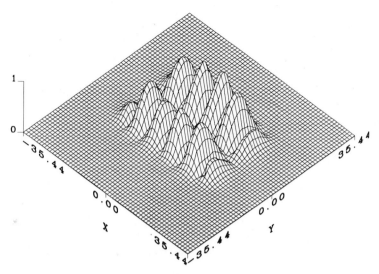

Figure 3.   Amplitude of a hologram versus X and Y in inches for the ribbed plate driven at 171 Hz.

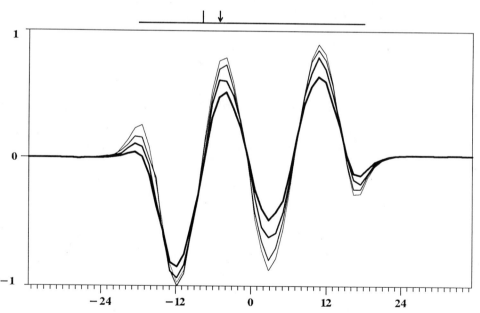

Figure 4.   Real part of a hologram versus X in inches for the ribbed plate driven at 171 Hz. The thin-to-thick curves are for Y=-6.19, -5.06, -3.94 and -2.81 inches, respectively.

where f is the frequency in Hz and ρ is the density. The intensity field at z is given by

$$\vec{I} = \tfrac{1}{2}\Re(p\,\vec{v}^*),\tag{16}$$

$$I_x = \tfrac{1}{2}\Re(p\,v_x^*),\tag{17}$$

$$I_y = \tfrac{1}{2}\Re(p\,v_y^*),\tag{18}$$

$$I_z = \tfrac{1}{2}\Re(p\,v_z^*),\tag{19}$$

where v^* is the complex conjugate of v and $\Re$ is the real part of a complex number.

2.2   Discrete Imaging Formulas

To generate a discrete form of the Fourier transforms used in the previous equations, the spatial improper integrals are converted to definite integrals over the aperture of the measurement plane or surface. Let $2L_x$ and $2L_y$ be the dimensions of the aperature, i.e., $-L_x \le x \le L_x$ and $-L_y \le y \le L_y$. Thus, the spatial increments dx and dy are

$$dx \to \Delta x = \frac{L_x}{M} \quad \text{and} \quad dy \to \Delta y = \frac{L_y}{N},\tag{20}$$

where the integers M and N represent the discrete number of measurement points in L_x and L_y, respectively, so that

$$x = q\Delta x = \frac{qL_x}{M} \quad \text{with} \quad -M \le q \le M,\tag{21}$$

$$y = r\Delta y = \frac{rL_y}{M} \quad \text{with} \quad -N \le r \le N.\tag{22}$$

Since we will also need discrete points in wavenumber-space we let

$$dk_x \to \Delta k_x = \frac{\pi}{L_x} \quad \text{and} \quad dk_y \to \Delta k_y = \frac{\pi}{L_y},\tag{23}$$

so that

$$k_x = m\,\Delta k_x = \frac{m\pi}{L_x} \quad \text{with} \quad -M \le m \le M,\tag{24}$$

$$k_y = n\,\Delta k_y = \frac{n\pi}{L_y} \quad \text{with} \quad -N \le n \le N.\tag{25}$$

The integral Fourier transforms, Eqs. (1) and (2), are now written in their discrete form for u a two-dimensional array of 2M by 2N elements:

$$\tilde{u}(m,n) = \frac{L_x L_y}{2\pi N M} \sum_{q=-M}^{M} \sum_{r=-N}^{N} u(q,r)\, e^{-2i\pi\left(\frac{mq}{2M} + \frac{nr}{2N}\right)},\tag{26}$$

$$= \frac{2L_x L_y}{\pi}\, \text{FFT}[u],\tag{27}$$

$$u(q,r) = \frac{\pi}{2L_x L_y} \sum_{m=-M}^{M} \sum_{n=-N}^{N} \tilde{u}(m,n)\, e^{-2i\pi\left(\frac{mq}{2M} + \frac{nr}{2N}\right)},\tag{28}$$

$$= \frac{\pi}{2L_x L_y}\, \text{IFFT}[\tilde{u}].\tag{29}$$

The symbols **FFT** and **IFFT** represent the typical implementation of the forward and inverse discrete Fourier transform (DFT) using the Fast Fourier Transform algorithm. The factor of $(1/4NM)$ in Eq. (26) could also be absorbed into the definition of the inverse transform algorithm if done so consistently. The integral calculation of the pressure at any field point, Eq. (11), can now be written in its discrete form as

$$p(q,r,z) = \text{IFFT}[\ \text{FFT}[p_H(q,r,z_H)]\ G(m,n)\ ]\tag{30}$$

with the terms which act like a Green's function collected into G,

$$G(m,n) = e^{2i\pi K_z(z-z_H)}, \tag{31}$$

where

$$\begin{aligned} K_z &= \sqrt{K^2 - K_x^2 - K_y^2} \quad \text{if} \quad K^2 > K_x^2 + K_y^2, \\ &= i\sqrt{K_x^2 + K_y^2 - K^2} \quad \text{if} \quad K^2 < K_x^2 + K_y^2, \end{aligned} \tag{32}$$

and

$$K = \frac{1}{\lambda} = \frac{f}{c}, \quad K_x = \frac{m}{2L_x}, \quad K_y = \frac{n}{2L_y}, \tag{33}$$

with λ being the acoustic wavelength. The discrete form of the calculation of the velocity becomes

$$v_x = \frac{1}{\rho f} \, \text{IFFT}[\ K_x \, \text{FFT}[p_H] \ G(m,n) \ ], \tag{34}$$

$$v_y = \frac{1}{\rho f} \, \text{IFFT}[\ K_y \, \text{FFT}[p_H] \ G(m,n) \ ], \tag{35}$$

$$v_z = -\frac{1}{\rho f} \, \text{IFFT}[\ K_z \, \text{FFT}[p_H] \ G(m,n) \ ]. \tag{36}$$

The discrete form of the calculation of the intensity can be obtained by a straight-forward substitution of Eq. (30) and Eqs. (34)-(36) into Eqs. (17)-(19).

2.3 Processing Evanescent Wave Information

In wavenumber-space, the evanescent regions will always contain some 'noise' due to acoustical noise in the test facility, electronic noise in the data acquisition hardware, quantization errors and the computer's limited numerical accuracy. Thus, to help insure that the experimental evanescent data was above this evanescent noise, we recorded the hologram only 3 inches away from the source — this was less than a fifth of a wavelength at even the highest frequency (3635 Hz) we used.

When reconstructing evanescent waves at the source $(z = z_s)$, the Green's function, Eq. (31), becomes an exponential amplifier that grows, for the most extreme case we encountered (171 Hz), to about 1.6×10^{14} or 284 dB. As described in Section 4.0, we feel that the recording system used cannot detect evanescent waves which have attenuated by more than about 12 dB. Thus, those regions in wavenumber-space which call for a reconstruction amplification of more than about 12 dB represent regions which are probably noise and which should be attenuated rather than amplified.

The Green's function, Eq. (31), is replaced with a windowed version such that

$$\begin{aligned} G_W(m,n) &= (1 - \tfrac{1}{2} e^{-6.666(1-K_r/K_C)}) \, G(m,n), \quad &K_r < K_C, \\ &= \tfrac{1}{2} \, G(m,n), \quad &K_r = K_C, \\ &= \tfrac{1}{2} e^{-6.666(K_r/K_C - 1)} \, G(m,n), \quad &K_r > K_C. \end{aligned} \tag{37}$$

where the cylindrical coordinate in wavenumber-space is

$$K_r = \sqrt{K_x^2 + K_y^2}. \tag{38}$$

The factor of 6.666 was selected to yield a relatively sharp slope. The cutoff point of the filter, K_C, was chosen so that at this wavenumber the value of G_W represents an amplification of 12 dB or 3.98. For our experimental system, K_C ranges from 0.11 to 0.13 for frequencies from 171 Hz to 3635 Hz.

It should be noted that this evanescent filter deletes a significant percentage of wavenumber-space. The largest circular region which lies within our square wavenumber-space data has a

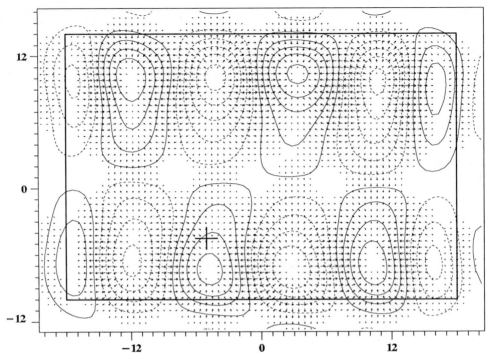

Figure 5. Vector velocity versus X and Y in inches at the surface of the unribbed plate driven at 171 Hz.

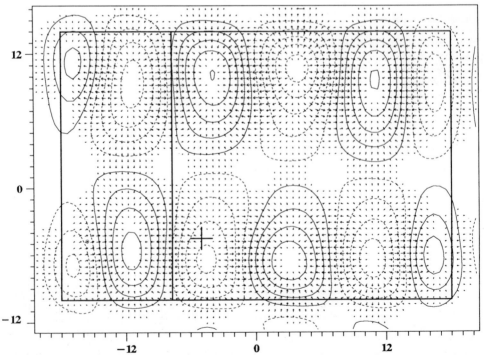

Figure 6. Vector velocity versus X and Y in inches at the surface of the ribbed plate driven at 171 Hz.

radius K_r of 0.44 while the circular propagating region varies from 0.003 to 0.062 for frequencies from 171 Hz to 3635 Hz.

3.0   The Acoustic Experiment

The ARL anechoic-tank test facility used for these experiments is a 26ft by 17.5ft by 18ft deep tank which is structurally isolated from the rest of the building and lined with acoustic absorbing material. Experience with this facility indicated that we would be able to ignore the reflections at the boundaries if the test object was no larger than a few feet across and was centered in the tank.

Point-driven flat plates were chosen for the experiment because of their simplicity. As shown in Figure 1, each of the unfinished steel plates tested were hung in a vertical plane by two thin wires tied to the plate along its top edge at small holes drilled into the plate. A second plate was also tested which had a rib welded to its back side (that is, the side away from the hydrophone array). The size of the plates was chosen so that the dimensions of the hologram were at least twice the dimensions of the plate.

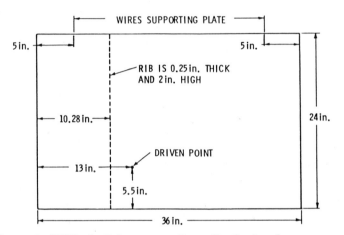

Figure 1. Ribbed plate as seen from the hydrophone array.

The plate was driven by a Wilcoxen electromagnetic shaker equipped with an impedance head and prepared for underwater usage; it was attached via a stud welded to the back side of the plate. Because of the weight of the shaker, it was also supported with a fixture which helped keep the plate in a vertical plane but which may also have introduced some other unknown effects.

In order to choose the frequencies at which holograms would be recorded, an in-water test was made where the impedance head output was recorded as a function of frequency. A total of eight frequencies were chosen so that both low and high mode number resonances would be examined.

When a uniform plate is excited to vibration at one of its resonances, one expects the velocity of the plate to correspond to the specific mode shape for that resonance. For a rectangular plate, these shapes have nodal lines that are parallel to the plate edges. However, the actual radiation of acoustic energy into the farfield may not correspond to that mode order. This is due to the short-circuit of sloshing fluids when the acoustic wavelength is much longer than the structural wavelength — in other words, only helical wavenumbers which are real $(K_z^2 > 0)$ contribute to the farfield acoustic pressure. All the measurements were made well below the coincidence frequency of 51.2 kHz. For such low frequencies, most of the acoustic radiation into the farfield from a uniform plate comes from the neighborhood of the forced excitation.

When a rib-reinforced plate is excited to vibration, the mode shapes and the corresponding resonances shift from those of a uniform plate of the same size and thickness. However, if the rib is not very massive, this shift is not extensive, especially in the lower frequency range. In the mid-frequency range, the mode shape may resemble a plate of a smaller dimension, i.e., corresponding to the plating area between the rib and the three free edges. Furthermore, mode overlap could also cause skew-shaped nodal lines, instead of the expected nodal lines that are parallel to the edges of the rectangular plate. Most of these modes do not radiate because they are short-circuited. However, since the reaction of the rib reinforcement acts like a line force on the plate, one would expect to see some energy radiation from the neighborhood of the rib, especially in the mid to high frequency ranges. Of course, one also expects radiation from the neighborhood of the point force itself.

Analytical predictions of the mode shapes of the plate in air and when submerged in water were made to help in the identification of the imaged velocity distribution as generated by the processing of the acoustic data described in Eqs. (34)-(36).

4.0   The SUNI Data Recording System

The development of the prototype System for Underwater Nearfield Imaging (SUNI) was begun in late 1982 with support from the Office of Naval Research (ONR) in order to apply the methods of nearfield imaging to submerged acoustic sources. This automated system (Figure 2) directs the operation of the underwater scanner and record the results onto magnetic tape; the tape is then carried to the laboratory's VAX 11/782 for processing.

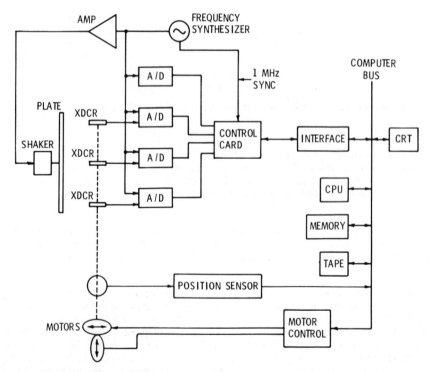

Figure 2.   Diagram of the experimental system. Note that the phase reference is recorded on the first channel. The actual system used 16 transducers.

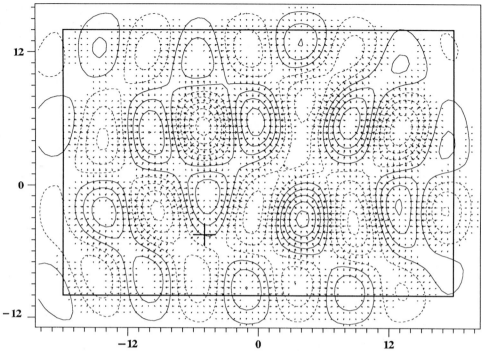

Figure 7.   Vector velocity versus X and Y in inches at the surface of the unribbed
plate driven at 680 Hz.

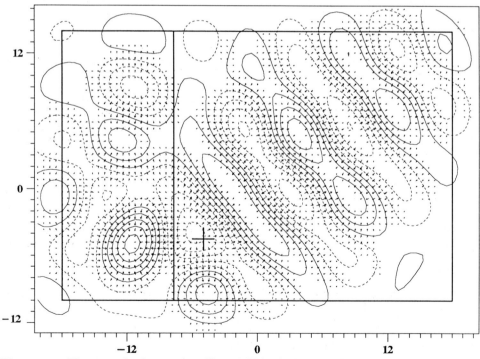

Figure 8.   Vector velocity versus X and Y in inches at the surface of the ribbed
plate driven at 680 Hz.

667

One of the central tenets of the SUNI design was that all devices be under the programable control of a microprocessor and console terminal. This significantly reduces the chance that the operator will forget to set some gain or filter; and, it allows the system to record all settings onto the magnetic tape, along with the data, for a permanent record of the experiment.

The underwater scanner includes a vertical line of 16 Celesco LC-10 hydrophones, spaced 4.5 in apart, which is moved in both the horizontal and vertical directions by stepping motors; it can cover an area as large as 6 ft high and 8 ft wide with a positioning accuracy of about 0.04 in. For these experiments, the scanner was operated over a 6 ft square to obtain an evenly-spaced grid of 64 by 64 sample locations in a plane approximately 3 in away from the surface of the plate. Mechanical speed limitations caused a single hologram recording to take up to 3 hours; a better mechanical design could probably bring this time down to about 30 minutes.

A unique component of SUNI is the data acquisition subsystem which was built in-house; it consists of 25 essentially independent recording channels, each containing its own programmable-gain amplifier (0 dB to 60 dB); a filter (flat, full-octave, or 1/3-octave); a 12-bit A/D converter; and 1,024 words of 12-bit memory. The filter center frequency and the A/D sampling rate, which are the same for all channels, can be set anywhere up to 10 kHz and 40 kHz, respectively. The system also has the capability to acquire data from multi-frequency and pulsed sources with a maximum burst recording rate, using all 25 channels, of a million samples per second.

Since the plates were driven continuously, the 1/3-octave filter was used for all experiments. The sample rate was always 4 times the experimental frequency; thus, we were able to have the microprocessor average the 1,024 samples recorded at each location and then translate the data into a single amplitude and phase before storage on tape. Tests indicated that the amplitude and phase measurements with this filtering and averaging were repeatable to within 0.1 dB and 0.1 degrees, respectively.

In order to calibrate the SUNI system, a USRD Type J9 piston source was precisely located directly in front of each hydrophone, one at a time. A short sequence of sine waves at the test frequency was then transmitted and recorded by the data acquisition system using the same electronics and filters which would later be used to record the hologram. After processing, we were then able to generate amplitude and phase calibrations for each hydrophone channel relative to the entire array. No attempt was made to acquire an absolute calibration.

The microprocessor attempted to optimize the amplifier gain on each channel so that the data had from 7 to 11 bits of precision (the 12th bit always represented the sign). A rough estimate indicates that about 7 bits are needed to represent a sine wave with no more than a few degrees of phase error. Therefore, if the gain was such that a propagating wave component was all but saturating the A/D converters (i.e., all 11 bits were used), then an evanescent wave which was 12 dB lower could be detected but evanescent waves that were more than 18 dB lower would fall below the 7-bit minimum for accurate phase representation. In the worst case, where only 7 bits were used, it would be unlikely that an evanescent wave superimposed upon a propagating wave could be sampled with the desired accuracy. Of course, it is impossible to know in general what mix of evanescent and propagating wave components would be encountered at a given sample location.

5.0   Data Processing

Each set of hologram data was calibrated then doubled in size to 128 by 128 points by adding zeroes in order to avoid FFT wrap-around. In wavenumber-space, the hologram size was again doubled to 256 by 256 points by adding zeroes in order to obtain a doubling of the resolution of the final image.

A FORTRAN program running in batch mode created the reconstructed pressure, velocity and intensity fields for up to 10 selected planes. The program's arrays need a little over 2Mb of main memory while another several megabytes of temporary disk storage is needed, depending upon the number of planes being processed. A 10-plane reconstruction required about 25 minutes of CPU time and yielded about 4.4Mb of data.

6.0 Plotting the Nearfield Image

These experiments generate vast amounts of data. Sucessful understanding of the data depends heavily upon having a plotting system that can provide convenient and rapid study of the acoustical phenomena while handling, invisible to the user, the very complex, three-dimensional scalar and vector data structures.

The system needed to be built using those facilities typically found in a University environment: a good but general-purpose commercial graphics package, and low-resolution graphics CRT terminals for interaction with the user. Hardcopy output was available through shared pen plotters and a small laser printer.

The approach taken was to create a *display pipeline* which was traversed, whenever the user entered the 'refresh' command, by the following subroutine:

```
subroutine display_pipeline
...
if( .not. view_is_ready ) call prepare_view
if( .not. data_is_ready ) call prepare_data
if( .not. work_is_ready ) call prepare_work
if( .not. plot_is_ready ) call prepare_plot
return
end
```

The `prepare_view` module prepares the viewing environment at the CRT terminal including selection of the viewport. The `prepare_data` module compares the 'current' file name to the requested one and, if not the same, obtains the requested data and associated information from a disk file. The `prepare_work` module creates a one-plane, normalized working subset of the data. The final module, `prepare_plot`, creates a windowed subset of the working subset and passes this onto one of five plotting modules: line, contour, hidden-surface, vector or vector plus contour. All plotting is also saved internally in a *segment* so that the user can enter the 'copy' command at any time to have the current segment written to a metafile; this metafile can later be sent to any of the batch plotting devices.

For each of these modules there is a menu which allows the user to inspect and change all parameters which control the operation of that module. A simple main menu allows selection of any of these sub-menus. Whenever a parameter is changed, one of the 'ready' flags is set false so that the appropriate module or modules are re-executed the next time the display pipeline is traversed.

All plots shown in this paper are for data in the X-Y plane of the plate where X runs horizontally and Y runs vertically. The origin of this coordinate system is 2 inches higher than the center of the plate. Thus, the plate runs from -18 to +18 inches in X and from -10 to +14 inches in Y. A small sketch, next to the plot or superimposed upon it, will indicate the plate location, the driven point, and, if appropriate, the rib.

Most plots discussed in the next section use the vector plus contour plot style that depicts the two in-plane vector components as arrows and the out-of-plane component as contour lines with solid or dashed lines for positive or negative components, respectively. In all cases the amplitude of the data has been normalized to the largest value.

7.0 Survey of Experimental Data

A plot of the amplitude ($= \sqrt{\Re^2 + \Im^2}$) of a typical hologram is shown in Figure 3. Although not visible at this scale, there is a slight 'bump', whose magnitude is typically 60 dB below the peak, between regions recorded by different hydrophones indicating that the calibration was not exact. Four horizontal slices through this same hologram in the vicinity of the driven point (at Y=-4.5 inches) are shown in Figure 4.

The calculated vector velocity at the surface of the plates driven at 171 Hz are shown in Figures

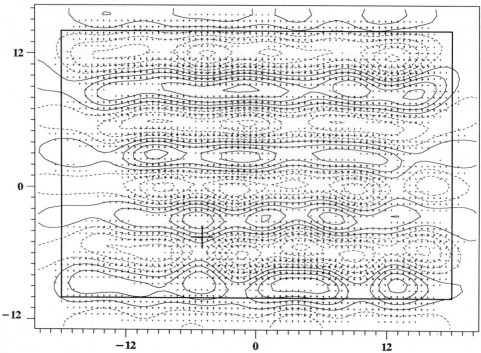

Figure 9.   Vector velocity versus X and Y in inches at the surface of the unribbed plate driven at 1530 Hz.

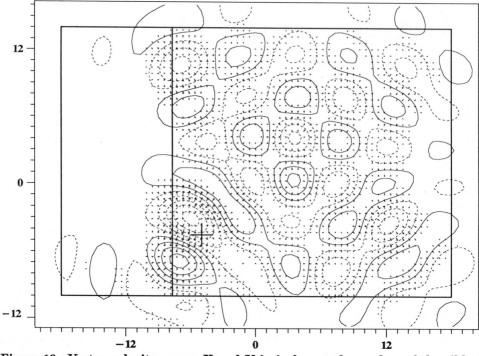

Figure 10. Vector velocity versus X and Y in inches at the surface of the ribbed plate driven at 1530 Hz.

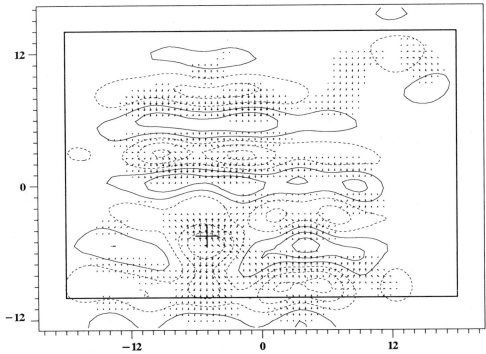

Figure 11. Vector intensity versus X and Y in inches at the surface of the unribbed plate driven at 1530 Hz.

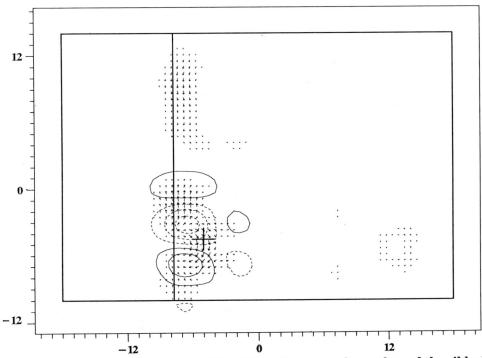

Figure 12. Vector intensity versus X and Y in inches at the surface of the ribbed plate driven at 1530 Hz.

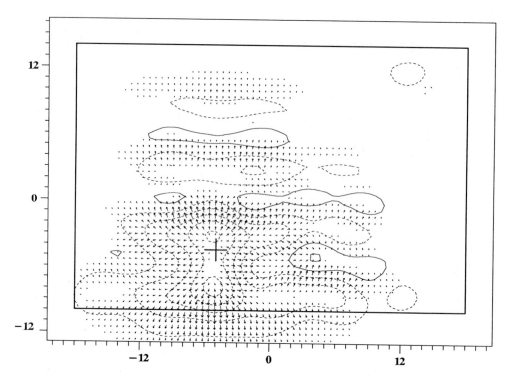

Figure 13. Vector intensity versus X and Y in inches at a distance of 4.25 inches in front of the unribbed plate driven at 1530 Hz.

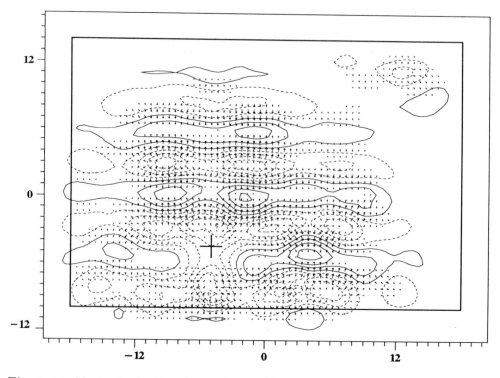

Figure 14. Vector intensity versus X and Y in inches at a distance of 2.25 inches in front of the unribbed plate driven at 1530 Hz.

5 and 6 for the unribbed and ribbed plates, respectively. This frequency corresponds to the (4,1) mode where there are four nodal lines in one dimension and one nodal line in the other (edges aren't counted). In is interesting to note that, except for an arbitrary 180° phase shift between them, the two mode shapes seem to be identical. This can be explained by the fact that for such low mode numbers, the rib is not massive enough to drastically change the mode shape.

The surface velocities are shown in Figures 7 and 8 for the plates driven at the resonance at 680 Hz. The addition of the rib has, at this frequency, separated the plate into two regions. To the right of the rib, a mode superpositon occurs such that the velocity at the surface has a diagonal pattern while to the left of the rib a rectangular pattern is observed.

The surface velocities and intensities for a driving frequency of 1530 Hz are shown in Figures 9-12. The shielding effect of the rib is more pronounced, while the intensity plots seem to show some circular energy flow along the surface of the plates. It should be noted that at these frequencies the radiation from the vicinity of the driver (and rib) has become strong enough to be seen superimposed upon the radiation from the specific mode shape.

The intensity for the unribbed plate driven at 1530 Hz is shown again in Figures 13 and 14 except that the intensity is calculated for planes parallel to the surface of the plate and in front of it. Note that the two circular flows near the driven point merge as the energy propagates away from the plate; this is not suprising since at this frequency the acoustic wavelength is 38 in or slightly longer than the plate.

8.0 Conclusions

These experiments have taught us that the mechanics of an underwater scanner are far more challenging than we expected; a very large amount of time was spent insuring that the array was accurately positioned and that no anomalous signals were present. On-line data processing and plotting would have been very useful in insuring that valid data was being obtained.

We also learned that the creation of this type of plotting software is very difficult and time-consuming — it resulted in more code (about 4200 lines) than the nearfield imaging algorithm (about 930 lines). Nevertheless, the ease and speed with which we could examine the data has, we believe, played an important part in understanding the acoustic phenomena.

Nearfield acoustical holography seems to be a more expedient method for determining the mode shape of objects like plates than alternatives such as accelerometers. The acoustic fields near the surface of the plate match the expected motion of the surface of the plate in a reasonable manner, making nearfield acoustical holography a very useful tool in redesigning underwater systems so as to radiate less energy, or at least less energy into the farfield.

References

1. D. L. Van Rooy, "Digital Ultrasonic Wavefront Reconstruction in the Near Field", IBM Publication No. 320.2402 (19 May 1971)

2. A. L. Boyer, et al., "Reconstruction of Ultrasonic Images by Backward Propogation", Acoustical Holography, 3, page 333 (1971)

3. R. L. Cohen, "Digital Wavefront Reconstruction for Acoustical Applications", Doctoral Dissertation, The Pennsylvania State University (1979)

4. E. G. Williams, H. D. Dardy, and R. G. Fink, "A technique for measurement of structure-borne intensity in plates", J. Acoust. Soc. Am., 78(6), page 2061 (1985)

PARTICIPANTS

Prof. V. Akulichev
Pacific Oceanological
Institute
USSR Academy of Sciences,
7 Radio St.
Vladivostok - 32, USSR
690032

P. Alais
Universtiy of Paris, Lab
Mechanique
2 pl de la Gare de Ceinture
Saint Cyr, France   78210

Yoshinao Aoki
Hokkaido University
N13 W8
Sapporo, Japan

A. Atalar
Middle East Technical
University
Ankara, Turkey

Prof. Dean Ayers
Dept. of Physics and
Astronomy
CSU 1250 Bellflower Blvd.
Longbeach CA.   USA   90840

M. J. Berggren
University of Utah
Dept. of Bioeng.
2059 MEB
Salt Lake City UT   USA
84112

J. Berry
Dept. of Engineering Physics
TUNS
PO Box 1000
Halifax, NS Canada B3J 2X4

Yves H. Berthelot
School of Mechanical
Engineering
Georgia Institute of
Technology
Atlanta Georgia USA 30332

Didier Billon
Thomson Sintra Activites
Sous-Marines
Route de Conquet
Brest CEDEX France 29601

Heinz Brautigam
Bundesamt fur Wehrtechnik
und Beschaffung
12 Fernblick
Eckernforde FRG 2330

Acad. L. M. Brekhovskikh
P.P. Shirshov Institute of
Oceanology
Krasikowa 23
Moscow 117218 USSR

Dr. Richard J. Brind
Admiralty Research
Establishment
DF Division
Portland Dorset UK DT5 2JS

Richard Brown
Arctec Canada Ltd.
311 Legget Drive
Kanata, Ont. Canada K2K 1Z8

V. A. Bulanov
Pacific Oceanological
Institute
7 Radio Street
Vladivostok USSR   690032

Dr. J. A. Burt
York University
4700 Keele Street
Downsview, Ont. Canada
M3J 1P3

A. H. Carter
AT&T Bell Laboratories
Whippany Road
Whippany USA 07981

Paul Everett Chandler
Electrical Engineering
Univ. of Calif., Irvine
Irvine, CA USA 92717

K. Chandrasekaran
Mayo Clinic
Biodynamics Research Unit
200 First Street SW
Rochester MN USA 55905

P. C. H. Chen
UCSB
Dept. of ECE., Univ. of
California
Santa Barbara, CA USA 93106

Thomas L. Clarke
Ocean Acoustics
Division/AOML/NOAA
4301 Rickenbacker Causeway
Miami, FL USA 33149

Dr. R. Cobbold
University of Toronto
Inst. of Biomedical
Engineering
Toronto, Ont. Canada
M5S 1A4

Eugene Colbourne
Dept. of Physics and NICOS
Memorial University of
Newfoundland
St. John's, Nfld. Canada
A1B 3X7

Dr. H. D. Collins
Battelle Northwest
P.O. Box 999, Richland
Washington USA 99352

John Dalen
EIAB-SINTEF GROUP
O. S. Bragstad Pl 6
Trondheim-NTH
Norway N-7034

Marcel R. de la Fonteijne
OLdelft
van Miereveltlaan 9
2612 XE Delft Netherlands

P. N. Denbigh
University of Cape Town
Dept. of Electrical
Engineering
Rondebosch 7700 S. Africa

G. Deniau
ECAN
83990 Saint-Tropez
France

Dr. Larry Deuser
Tracor, Inc.
6500 Tracor Lane
Austin, TX USA 78725

Terry Deveau
Oceanroutes Canada Inc.
Suite 330
1496 Bedford Highway
Bedford, NS Canada
B4A 1E5

Jean-Luc Dion
University du Quebec
C.P. 500 Trois-Rivieres
Quebec Canada G9A 5H7

Dr. B. Granz
SIEMENS AG
Paul-Gossen-Str. 100
Erlangen FRG D-8520

J. F. Greenleaf
Mayo Clinic
Biodynamics Research Unit
200 First St. SW
Rochester MN USA 55905

R. P. Gribble
Battelle Northwest
PSL Bldg. 3000 Area
P.O. Box 999
Richland, WA USA 99352

Prof. D. Guan
The Institute of Acoustics
Academia Sinica
P.O. Box 2712
Beijing China

Thomas E. Hall
Battelle NW
P.O. Box 999
Richland WA USA 99352

D. J. W. Hardie
ARE HM Naval Base
Portland, Dorset
UK DT5 2JS

Logan E. Hargrove
Office of Naval Research
Code 1112
Physics Division
800 N Quincy Street
Arlington, VA USA 22217

Daniel Hauden
LPNO-CNRS
32 Ave. de l'observatoire
Besancon France 25000

A. E. Hay
Dept. of Physics
Memorial University of
Newfoundland
St. John's, Nfld. Canada
A1B 3X7

Robert Hebel
Siemens AG Bereich Med.
Techn. Dept. STUE 2
Henkestrasse 127
Erlangen FRG   8520

Olivind Heier
SIMRAD Subsea A/S
Strandpromenaden 50,
Box 111
Horten   Norway N-3191

Bong Ho
Department of Electrical
Engineering
Michigan State University
East Lansing, Michigan
USA   48864

Dr. F. Horneck
Bundesamt fur Wehrtechnik
und Beschaffung
Postfach 7360
Koblenz FDR 5400

D. A. Hutchins
Department of Physics
Queen's University
Kingston, ONT Canada
K7L 3N6

M. Ikegami
Hokkaido University
N-13 s-8 Kitaku
Sapporo 060   Japan

Junichi Ishii
Hitachi Research Laboratory
4026 Kuji-cho, Hitachi-shi
Ibaraki-ken   Japan 319-12

Samuel Itzikowitz
IDF c\o Naval Attache
Embassy of Israel
3514 International Dr. NW
Washington, DC   USA 20008

Jules S. Jaffe
Woods Hole Oceanographic
Institution
Woods Hole, Bigelow Lab.
Massechussetts USA 02543

S. A. Johnson
Dept. of Bioeng.
University of Utah
Salt Lake City, Utah
USA   84112

Prof. Hugh Jones
Dept. of Engineering
Physics
TUNS, P.O. Box 1000
Halifax, NS Canada
B3J 2X4

A. W. D. Jongens
University of Cape Town
Central Acoustics Lab.
7700 Rondesbosch, S. Africa

Mos Kaveh
University of Minnesota
Elect. Eng. Department
123 Church Street SE
Minneapolis, MN USA 55455

Eino Keranen
Hollming Ltd. Electronics
Naulakatu 3
SF-33100 TRE Finland

S. I. Kim
Drexel University
Philadelphia, PA USA
19104

John R. Klepper
Institute of Applied
Physiology and Medicine
701 16th Avenue
Seattle, WA. USA 98122

John Klepsvik
Seatex A/S
P.O. Box 1961 Moholtan
Trondheim, Norway N-7001

A. Kovacs
Techno Scientific Inc.
205 Champagne
Downsview, ONT Canada

H. Koymen
Middle East Technical
University
Ankara, Turkey 06531

Kurt-Even Kristensen
ELAB/SINTEF Group
OS Bragstad Pl. 6
Trondheim-NTH
Norway N-7034

Boris Kukyanov
Inst. of Oceanology
Krasikova 23
Moscow Krasikova USSR
117218

Dr. Jun-ichi Kushibiki
Tohoku University
Dept. of Electrical
Engineering
Sendai 980   Japan

H. W. Kwan
Department of Engineering
Physics
TUNS P.O. Box 1000
Halifax, NS Canada B3J 2X4

Hua Lee
University of Illinois
Dept. of Electrical Eng.
1406 West Green Street
Urbana, Illinois USA 81801

Dr. Sidney Leeman
Department of Medical
Engineering and Physics
Dulwich Hospital
East Dulwich Grove
London UK   SE228PT

Jorma Lilleberg
Hollming Ltd. Electronics
Box 14
26101 Rauma, Finland

Z. C. Lin
UCSB
1704 Andrews Road
Arcadia, CA   USA 91006

Larry Lines
Amoco Production Co.
P.O. Box 3385
Tulsa, Oklahoma USA 74102

James F. Lynch
Woods Hole Oceanographic
Institution
Woods Hole, Mass. USA 02543

Andrew J. Madry
University of Sydney
Department of Architectural
Science
Sydney N.S.W.
Australia 2006

Andrew Maidment
Ontario Cancer Institute
500 Sherbourne Street
Toronto, ONT Canada

D. K. Mak
PMRL/EMR
568 Booth Street
Ottawa, ONT   Canada
K1A 0G1

Dr. -Ing Juval Mantel
Dr. Mantel & Partners
Inninger Strasse 7a
Muenchen 70
Germany D-8000

Jean-P Mattei
Conseille Scientifique
24 rue Jeanne d'Arc
F-94160
St. Mande   France

Bill McCroskey
Imagtech
5475 Parkside Trail
Solon, Ohio USA 44139

Bruce McDermott
Duke University
Biomedical Engineering
Department
Durham, NC USA 27705

James I. Mehi
University of Toronto
Inst. of Biomedical Eng.
Toronto, Ontario Canada
M5S 1A4

Jinsheng Meng
The Institute of Acoustics
Academia Sinica
Beijing, China

Michael Moles
Ontario Hydro Research
800 Kipling Avenue
Toronto, Ontario Canada

R. K. Mueller
Department of Electrical
Engineering
University of Minnesota
Minneapolis, MN USA 55455

Ole E. Naess
Forus
Postboks 300
Stavenger, Norway N-4001

Peter Nauth
Ges. Z. Ford,
d. Forschung a.d. DKD
Aukammallee 33, Wiesbaden
Germany D-6200

Andre Johann Nepgen
NIMR CSIR
P.O. Box 395
Pretoria 001 S. Africa

Ed Nyland
University of Alberta
Dept. of Physics
Edmonton, Alta. Canada

Shigeo Ohtsuki
Tokyo Institute of Tech.
Midori-ku Nagasuta 4259
Yokohama 227 Japan

M. G. Oravecz
Sonoscan, Inc.
530 East Green Street
Bensenville, IL USA
60106

Bruce H. Pasewark
Naval Research Lab.
Code 5161
Washington DC USA 20375

John Powers
US Naval Postgraduate
School
ECE Dept., Code 62
Monterey CA USA 93943

David D. Prentiss
Nova Scotia Research
Foundation
100 Fenwick Street
Dartmouth, NS Canada

G. Prokoph
Univ. of Erlangen-Nuremberg
Cauershc 9
Erlangen Germany D-8520

Dr. Bernard Querleux
L'Oreal
Boite Postale No. 22
Aulnay-sous-boix
France 93601

B. Richard
Lab de Biophysique
Faculte Cochin
26 rue de Faubourg
Saint-Jacques
Paris cedex 16
France F-75674

John M. Richardson
Rockwell International
Science Centre
1049 Camino Dos Rios
P.O. Box 1085
Thousand Oaks CA
USA 91360

Claude Royer
University of Toronto
4 Taddle Creek
Toronto, Ontario
Canada M5S 1A4

Thomas D. Sachs
University of Vermont
Physics Department
Burlington, VT
USA 05405

Toshio Sannomiya
Tohoku University
Aramaki Aza Aoba
Sendai, Japan 980

Volker Sattler
Bundesamt fur Wehrtechnik
und Beschaffung
Postfach 7360
Koblenz FDR 5400

A. S. Schaafsma
Delft Hydraulics Lab.
P.O. Box 177
2600 MH Delft Netherlands

Mark Schafer
Drexel University
Biomedical Engineering
Philadelphia, PA
USA 19104

Prof. E. C. Shang
Institute of Acoustics
Academia Sinica
P.O. Box 2712
Beijing, China

Jinyu Sheng
Department of Physics
Memorial University of
Newfoundland
St. John's, NFLD
Canada A1B 3X7

Hiroshi Shimizu
Faculty of Engineering
Tohoku University
Aramaki-Aza-Aoba
Sendai 980, Japan

S. Singh
CBME, I.I.T.
Delhi Centre for
Biomedical Engineering
Indian Inst. of Tech.
Delhi, India 110016

Paolo Sirotti
University of Trieste
Via A Valerio 10
Trieste, Italy 34127

Richard Soldner
Siemens AG
Henkesir 127
852 Erlangen, Germany

Nils Sponheim
Centre for Industrial Res.
P.O. Box 350, Blindern
Oslo 3, Norway 0314

Dr. Anrzej Stepnowski
Technical University
of Gdansk
Institute of
Telecommunications
Gdansk, Poland 80-952

Veijo Suorsa
University of Oulu
Department of Electrical
Engineering
Oulo SF-90570, Finland

Thomas Szabo
Hewlett Packard
3000 Minuteman Road
Andover, MA USA 01810

M. Talmant
GPS University Paris 7-
Tour 23
GPS Tour 23, 2 Place
Jussieu
Paris, cedex 05, France
75251

Tat-Jin Teo
Drexel University
Biomedical Engineering
Philadelphia, PA
USA 19104

Robert Ting
US Naval Research Lab.
Underwater Acoustics
P.O. Box 8337
Orlando, FL USA 32856

Jean Claude Tricot
I.D.N.
BP 48 Villeneuve
d'Ascq CEDEX
France 59651

W. H. van den Berg
Shell Research B.V.
Badhuisweg 3, 1031 CM
Amsterdam, Netherlands

C. J. M. Van Ruiten
Institute of Applied
Physics INO
P.O. Box 144
2600 AD Delft, Netherlands

A. G. Voronovich
P.O. Shirsov Institute of
Oceanology
Krasikowa 23
Moscow, USSR 117218

D. Vray
INSA de Lyon
20 Avenue A Einstein
Villeurbanne, France
69621

Robert Waag
Rm. 340, Hopeman Hall
University of Rochester
Rochester, NY USA 14627

Prof. G. Wade
Electrical Engineering
Department
University of California
Santa Barbara, CA USA
93106

J. M. Wagner
E.C.A.N.
St. Tropez, France 83990

Jill A. Wollins
Mayo Clinic Biodynamics
Res. Unit
200 First Street SW
Rochester, MN USA 55905

T. Yamamoto
Hokkaido University
N-13, W-8, Kitaku
Sapporo 060, Japan

Mykola Yaremko
Riverside Research Inst.
330 West 42nd Street
New York, NY USA 10036

Eric Yeatman
Department of Engineering
Physics
TUNS
P.O. Box 1000
Halifax, NS B3J 2X4

Wei Yu
Nanjing Institute of Tech.
Dept. of Biomedical Eng.
Jiangsu Province, China

Manell Zakharia
ICPI Lab de Traitement
du Signal
25 rue de Plat
Lyon CEDEX 02, France
69288

De-Jun Zhang
Wuhan Institute of Physics
Academia Sinica
P.O. Box 241
Wuhan, Hubei, China

Renhe Zhang
Institute of Acoustics
5 Zhongguancun Street
Beijing, China

Prof. Yu Yu Zhitkovsky
P.P. Shirsov Institute
of Oceanology
Krasikowa 23
Moscow, USSR 117218

AUTHOR INDEX

Pan, S.X., 330
Papallardo, M., 225
Papoulis, A., 78, 357, 557
Parker, D.L., 486
Parmon, W., 288
Pasteur, J., 569
Paulraj, A., 54
Penttinen, A., 108
Peragallo, J., 479
Perbert, J.N., 569
Pernod, P., 471
Perrin, Jean, 227
Peyrin, F., 371, 381
Pfannensteil, P., 91
Piwakowski, B., 471
Plummer, J.D., 225
Pohlman, R., 27
Pons, F., 239
Power, John, 67, 459
Powers, John, 117, 145, 191
Powis, P.L., 307
Powis, R., 509
Prassad, S.K., 422
Prokoph, G., 547

Quate, C.F., 288, 401, 441, 452

Rader, C.M., 501
Ramm, O.T.V., 486
Readhead, A.C.S., 54
Reid, John M., 135, 183, 307
Reid, L.D., 253
Richard, Bruno, 227, 238
Richardson, J.M., 47, 537, 546,
      615
Ritman, E.L., 318
Rivera, G., 537
Rizzato, G., 519, 521
Robb, R.A., 318
Robbins, W.P., 383
Robinson, B.S., 201, 422
Robinson, D.E., 238
Robinson, E.A., 583
Roehrlein, Gehard, 341, 357, 557
Rosencwaig, A., 428, 429
Rosenfeld, A., 469
Roucayrol, J.C., 227
Royer, C., 299
Royer, D., 428
Rudd, E.P., 383, 392
Ruelle, D., 633
Rugar, D., 410
Rylander, R.L., 422

Sankar, P.V., 109
Sannomiya, Toshio, 393
Sasaki, Souji, 169
Sato, J., 167
Sato, T., 181, 598
Sawada, H., 318
Schafer, Mark E., 135, 145

Schmitz, V., 251, 509
Schomberg, H., 381
Schomberg, M., 381
Schueler, C.F., 340, 459
Seelen, M.V., 91
Seggie, D.A., 501
Selfridge, A.R., 167
Sanker, P.M., 486
Shanker, R., 583
Shattuck, D.P., 486
Simmons, James A., 27
Singh, Satpal, 481
Sirotti, P., 519, 521
Skilling, H.H., 266
Skorton, D.J., 318
Slaney, M., 369
Smith, I.R., 288, 401
Smith, J.M., 251
Smith, S.W., 486
Sokolov, S.J., 27
Sondhi, M.M., 145
Spencer, M.P., 212
Sponheim, Nils, 523, 535, 536
Stamnes, J., 536
Stenger, F., 193, 359
Stephanishen, P.R., 126, 134, 145,
      191, 535
Stickels, K.R., 318
Stork, C., 600
Strutt, J.W., 535
Suorsa, Veijo, 159
Sutton, J.L., 658
Switzer, D.F., 307
Szilard, J., 583

Tanabe, K., 381
Tandon, S.N., 481
Taouriainen, Antti, 159
Theroux, P., 212
Thurstone, F.L., 27, 69, 658
Tikhonov, A.N., 582
Tom, V.T., 469
Tracey, M.L., 201
Trahey, G.E., 78
Tricot, J.C., 471
Tsao, M.C., 340
Tupholme, G.E., 126

Ulrych, T.J., 191
Urick, R.J., 27, 658

van den Berg, W.H., 147
Van Blaricum, M.E., 613
Van Rooy, D.L., 673
Van Trees, H., 613
Venetsanopoulos, A.N., 469

Waag, R.C., 101
Wade, Glen, 1, 67, 89, 319, 443
Wade, G., 27, 28, 658
Wagner, R.F., 357